THE FETUS IN THREE DIMENSIONS

THE FETUS IN THREE DIMENSIONS

Imaging, Embryology, and Fetoscopy

Asim Kurjak MD PhD
Department of Obstetrics and Gynecology
Medical School, University of Zagreb
Zagreb
Croatia

Guillermo Azumendi MD
Gutenberg Clinic, Ultrasound Unit
Málaga
Spain

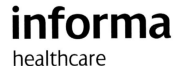

First published in the United Kingdom in 2007 by Informa Healthcare, 4 Park Square, Milton Park, Abingdon, Oxon OX14 4RN. Informa Healthcare is a trading division of Informa UK Ltd. Registered Office: 37/41 Mortimer Street, London W1T 3JH. Registered in England and Wales number 1072954.

Tel: +44 (0)20 7017 6000
Fax: +44 (0)20 7017 6699
Email: info.medicine@tandf.co.uk
Website: www.informahealthcare.com

A CIP record for this book is available from the British Library.
Library of Congress Cataloging-in-Publication Data

Data available on application

ISBN-10: 0 415 37523 1
ISBN-13: 978 0 415 37523 8

Distributed in North and South America by
Taylor and Francis
6000 Broken Sound Parkway, NW, (Suite 300)
Boca Raton, FL 33487, USA

Within Continental USA
Tel: 1 (800) 272 7737; Fax: 1 (800) 374 3401
Outside Continental USA
Tel: (561) 994 0555; Fax: (561) 361 6018
Email: orders@crcpress.com

Distributed in the rest of the world by
Thomson Publishing Services
Cheriton House
North Way
Andover, Hampshire SP10 5BE, UK
Tel: +44 (0)1264 332424
Email: tps.tandfsalesorder@thomson.com

Composition by Scribe Design Ltd, Ashford, Kent, UK
Printed and bound in India by Replika Press Pvt Ltd

Contents

Contributors

Abdallah Adra MD
Department of Obstetrics and Gynecology
American University of Beirut, Medical Center
Beirut
Lebanon

Wiku Andonotopo MD PhD
Department of Health
Ministry of Health
Republic of Indonesia
Jakarta
Indonesia

Guillermo Azumendi MD
Gutenberg Clinic, Ultrasound Unit
Málaga
Spain

María J Barco
Department of Obstetrics and Gynecology
University Clinic Hospital Lozano Bleso
Zaragoza
Spain

Zoran Belics MD PhD
Department of Obstetrics and Gynecology
Semmelweis University
Budapest
Hungary

Fernando Bonilla-Musoles MD PhD
Department of Obstetrics and Gynecology
School of Medicine
Valencia
Spain

Carmina Comas Gabriel PhD
Prenatal Diagnosis Unit
Gutenberg Clinic
Málaga
Spain

Vincenzo D'Addario MD PhD
Fetal Medicine Unit
Department of Obstetrics and Gynecology
University of Bari
Bari
Italy

Luca Di Cagno MD
Fetal Medicine Unit
Department of Obstetrics and Gynecology
University of Bari
Bari
Italy

Tibor Fekete MD
Department of Obstetrics and Gynecology
Semmelweis University
Budapest
Hungary

Mijna Hadders-Algra MD PhD
Developmental Neurology
Groningen
The Netherlands

Radoslav Herman MD PhD
Department of Obstetrics and Gynecology
Medical School, University of Zagreb
Sestre Milosrdnice Hospital
Zagreb
Croatia

Ashok Khurana MD MBBS
The Ultrasound Laboratory
Centre for Advanced Imaging Research Studies
New Delhi
India

Sanja Kupesic MD PhD
Department of Obstetrics and Gynecology
Medical School, University of Zagreb
Zagreb
Croatia

Asim Kurjak MD PhD
Department of Obstetrics and Gynecology
Medical School, University of Zagreb
Zagreb
Croatia

Luiz Eduardo Machado
INTRO
Salvador (Ba)
Brazil

Kazuo Maeda MD PhD
Tottori University
Department of Obstetrics and Gynecology
(Emeritus)
Yonago
Japan

Luis Martinez-Cortes MD PhD
University Hospital of Getafe
Madrid
Spain

Marijana Medic MD
Croatian Institute for Brain Research
Medical School, University of Zagreb
Zagreb
Croatia

Dr Luis T Mercé MD PhD
International Ruber Hospital
Madrid
Spain

Berivoj Miskovic MD MSc
Department of Obstetrics and Gynecology
Medical School, University of Zagreb
Sveti Duh Hospital
Zagreb
Croatia

Vishal Mittal GNIIT
The Ultrasound Laboratory
Centre for Advanced Imaging Research Studies
New Delhi
India

Newton Osborne
Howard University
Washington, DC
USA

Zoltan Papp MD PhD DSc
Department of Obstetrics and Gynecology
Semmelweiss University
Budapest
Hungary

Armando Pintucci MD
Fetal Medicine Unit
Department of Obstetrics and Gynecology
University of Bari
Bari
Italy

Kyong-Hon Pooh
Department of Neurosurgery
National Kagawa Children's Hospital
Kagawa
Japan

Ritsuko K Pooh MD PhD
Division of Fetal Diagnosis
Clinical Research Institute of Fetal Medicine PMC
Pooh Maternity Clinic
Kagawa
Japan

Pilar Prats MD
Department of Obstetrics and Gynecology
Dexeus University Institute
Barcelona
Spain

Aida Salihagic Kadic MD PhD
Department of Obstetrics and Gynecology
Medical School, University of Zagreb
Zagreb
Croatia

Elena Scazzocchio MD
Department of Obstetrics and Gynecology
Dexeus University Institute
Barcelona
Spain

Bernat Serra MD
Department of Obstetrics and Gynecology
Dexeus University Institute
Barcelona
Spain

Milan Stanojević MD PhD
Department of Obstetrics and Gynecology
Medical School, University of Zagreb
Sveti Duh Hospital
Zagreb
Croatia

Juan-Mario Troyano MD PhD
Hospital Universitario de Canarias
Santa Cruz de Tenerife
Canary Islands
Spain

Gino Varga MD
Department of Radiology
Policlinic Nemetova
Zagreb
Croatia

Sanja Zaputovic MD PhD
Department of Obstetrics and Gynecology
Medical School University of Rijeka
Rijeka
Croatia

Foreword

Ian Donald had the epiphany that ultrasound might have application to the visualization of the fetal patient. The past 50 years have been a truly remarkable success story in the translation of Ian Donald's dream to clinical reality due to important technologic breakthroughs and innovative clinical investigation. In the past, grey scale imaging, real time visualization, and Doppler ultrasound have transitioned from novel concept to everyday reality. Today, three and four dimensional ultrasound is the new frontier. The technologic breakthroughs in this area have been tremendous and have been surpassed only by the brilliant insights and arduous efforts of clinical investigators.

The authors of this text: Asim Kurjak and Guillermo Azumendi have been leaders in this effort.

They review in a comprehensive and very readable style the state-of-the-art of three and four dimensional ultrasound in all of its forms. Their list of authors is a who's who of contributors to the field. The spectrum of contributors documents that the development of this technology is truly an international effort. The spectrum of topics is exceptional. Basic anatomy, safety, gynecologic and obstetric utilization, and the evolving area of fetal behavior are elucidated clearly. This book will be of value to all sonologists and sonographers who care for obstetric and gynecologic patients. The only group who will not enjoy this wonderful textbook would be the decreasing number of diehard skeptics of this rapidly evolving and increasingly essential technology.

Frank A Chervenak MD
Given Foundation Professor and Chairman
Department of Obstetrics and Gynecology
New York Weill Cornell Medical Center
New York, NY
USA

Preface

In recent years, there have been dramatic technical advances in diagnostic sonography. The advent of color Doppler, power Doppler, and, more recently, three-dimensional (3D) imaging has led to a revolution in ways of doing and seeing things. These developments now occur at such a rapid pace that unless we keep up with the developing technology, we will inevitably and inexorably fall behind. In order to stay with the leading edge of diagnostic sonography, one has to keep pace with what colleagues are doing around the world.

Sonography has become essential to the modern management of pregnancy, expanding rapidly throughout the last three decades. Starting with the bimodal green dots on the black background of A-mode, we have progressed through the period of black dots on the white background of B-mode static scanning, evolved quickly to mechanical real-time ultrasound with gray-scale displays, then advanced to high-resolution real-time sonography. During a relatively short period of time, we have witnessed this extraordinary progression to the highly mature field of sonography today.

3D sonographic volume imaging has enabled the practitioner to obtain volumes that can be reconstructed in any plane after the patient has left the clinic.

The main advantages of 3D sonography in examining the fetus include scanning in the coronal plane, improved assessment of complex anatomic structures, surface analysis of minor defects, volumetric measuring of organs, 'plastic' transparent imaging of the fetal skeleton, spatial presentation of blood flow arborization, study of fetal behavior, and, finally, storage of scanned volumes and images. Additional progress has been achieved owing to the permanent possibility of repeated analysis of previously saved 3D volumes with additional elimination of redundant structures and artifacts.

Tremendous advances in high-resolution sonography have increased our knowledge of normal fetal development and improved the prenatal diagnosis of a great number of complex fetal anomalies. Close follow-up by serial sonography has expanded our understanding of the natural history of a number of these disorders.

With 4D techniques, sonography will move from the artistic to the standard planes of imaging, which are understandable by many more practitioners.

With the introduction of 3D sonography, a new wave of interest arose, in the hope that the improved spatial awareness and the volumetric and quantitative vascular information could further enhance our ability to assess normal and abnormal early human development.

4D sonography makes it straightforward to comprehend some morphologic dynamics, such as yawning, sucking, smiling, crying, and blinking. This offers a practical means for assessment of neurophysiologic development, as well as for detection of anatomic pathology.

Thus, sonography may become less dependent upon the skill of the operator.

The new technology is both exciting and frustrating. Proper use of 3D equipment has a difficult learning curve, and the international experts contributing to this book offer image quality and technical pearls to assist both the novice sonographer and specialist alike.

A great deal of the material in this book has been written by the two editors, but the other contributors have all been selected for their special expertise in their own chosen fields, their access to outstanding visual material, and their ability to explain its significance in an effective and lucid way. Finally, particular emphasis has been placed on achieving very high-quality reproduction in the printing process in order to do full justice to the wide variety of visual images presented.

Readers of this atlas should find that the emerging advantages of 3D sonography have now become a clinical reality.

AK, GA

1   3D and 4D sonography: How to use it properly – technical advice

Gino Varga, Guillermo Azumendi, and Asim Kurjak

Three-dimensional (3D) sonography should be accepted as a natural development of ultrasound imaging technology. Fast computer processing is essential for 3D and 4D sonography. Due to rapid developments in computer and transducer technology, image quality, number of volume applications, and processing speed have improved significantly. With the machines presently available, volume acquisition and volume display can be achieved in such a way that the fetus can be visualized three-dimensionally in real time providing highly realistic fetal images. Additional 3D/4D techniques with clinical applications have been developed, allowing combinations between different modalities of volume sonography. We will review them in detail in this chapter.

3D DATA ACQUISITION

The first 3D-capable systems were developed in the mid-1990s. 3D acquisition was performed by moving the transducer over the region of interest (ROI) with the operator's hand at a constant speed. There was no proper control of this procedure, and the results of such scanning were of poor quality. This scanning technique was called 'hands-free'. A freehand technique such as this does not require a specially designed transducer.[1] Scans could be performed using a conventional 2D probe.

Volume acquisition systems today use mechanically moved transducers (linear, convex, or transvaginal) (Figure 1.1). The probe itself includes a mechanical movement system for acquiring images and volumes. The information obtained with 3D volume acquisition is superior to a video or cine-loop of 2D information.

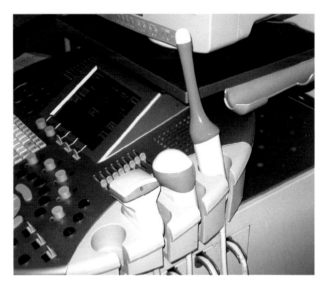

Figure 1.1 Ultrasound probes capable of 2D, 3D, and 4D scanning: linear, convex, and transvaginal probes

On reaching the ROI, the operator must keep the transducer stable while the patient stays still, so that the probe may scan simultaneously. Images are then captured and processed by a computer that will display them three-dimensionally. In the multiplanar volume mode three planes are shown – longitudinal or sagittal (*A*-plane), transverse (*B*-plane), and coronal (*C*-plane) – and an orthogonal reconstruction is obtained, which may be rotated around three axes (x, y, z) (Figure 1.2).

4D IMAGING

Real-time 4D imaging is the continuous, 3D scanning of an object with simultaneous visualization of the *A*-, *B*-, and *C*-planes. Real-time 4D imaging is enabled by

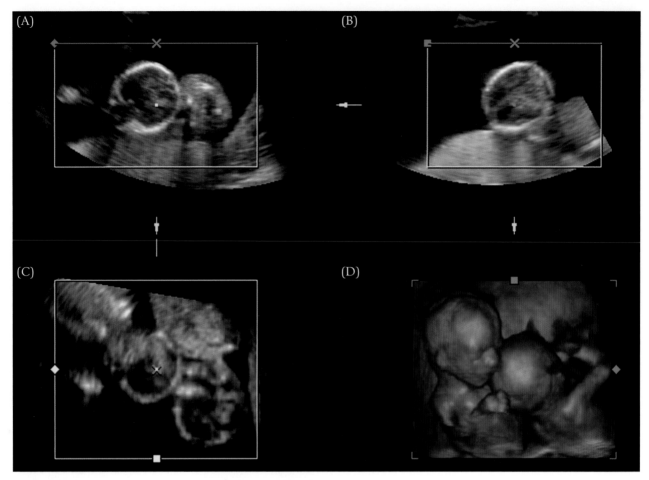

Figure 1.2 Multiplanar image of twins at 16 weeks of gestation. Perpendicular planes: (A) Midsagittal (*A*-plane); (B) transverse (*B*-plane); (C) coronal (*C*-plane); (D) 3D surface reconstruction

specially developed 3D/4D transducer technology that performs sweeping and automatic acquisition of volume data. With a volume acquisition rate of up to 20 volumes/s, the 3D image is continuously updated, providing a live 3D view (Figure 1.3). Movement of the ultrasound beam over the ROI is automatic. Structures that are not selected by the volume box will be cut from the 3D reconstruction. The operator

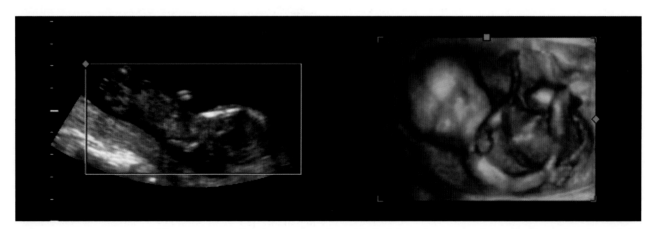

Figure 1.3 Live 4D view of fetus at 14 weeks of gestation. The image of the volume scan from the 2D technique and the real-time 4D image simultaneously present on the screen enable maintenance of good scanning conditions and show a good comparison between the two techniques

determines the speed of the scanning process. A slower speed yields higher resolution, because the number of 2D images/slices within the acquired volume is maximized. Likewise, a larger volume box results in a longer acquisition time and a smaller volume rate (number of volumes/s).

A pixel is the smallest element of a 2D image, while a voxel is the smallest information unit in 3D and 4D imaging. Volume rendering provides visualization of animated voxel-based images on a 2D screen. Fast volume data processing enables calculation of 1–20 volumes/s, depending on the ultrasound system hardware and the size of the rendering box. As 4D imaging is not actually a real-time technique, there is always some delay as a result of the time needed to reconstruct a 3D image from 2D frames. In 4D imaging, it is desirable to achieve as many volumes/s (volume rate) as possible. The number of volumes/s is a trade-off between image quality and volume rate. 3D and 4D image quality depends mostly on 2D image quality.[2] Prior to volume acquisition, it is important to achieve the best possible 2D image quality, adjusting depth, focus position and number of focuses, frequency, and gain. When using color and power Doppler (CDI and PDI) imaging, adjustments of velocity, wall filter, persistence, and Doppler gain are important. Good 4D image acquisition depends on the following important points: ROI, size and volume box size, ROI position and direction of view, and accessibility to the object. The rendering box determines the contents that will be rendered.[3] Structures that are not selected by the volume box will be cut from the 3D reconstruction. The ROI can be altered in size, moved, and rotated in all directions arbitrarily by the operator. Volume data can be acquired from different 2D modes – surface, transparent (maximum, minimum, or X-ray), and light – some of which can be active simultaneously in real time.[4]

RENDERING MODALITIES

Different rendering volume modes are available: minimum mode for tissue structure; maximum-mode visualization of bony structures; surface mode and gradient light for surface anomalies; and X-ray mode showing bones and soft tissue structures on the same image. Vascular structures can be displayed by using 3D volumes based on 2D grayscale images and PDI or CDI modes or by using the B-flow mode. The glass-body mode shows vascular structures with more or less transparent surrounding tissue.

Surface imaging

In the surface rendering mode, only signals from the surface of the ROI are extracted, and are displayed with a plastic-like appearance. Surface rendering examination of fetus focuses the sonographer's attention exclusively on fetal external surface anatomy. This mode is capable of clear visualization of fetal surface anatomy or surface anomalies such as encephalocele, spina bifida, cleft lip/palate, and abdominal wall and limb defects.[5] Furthermore, visualizing the spatial relationship between surface

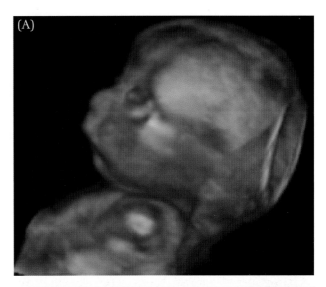

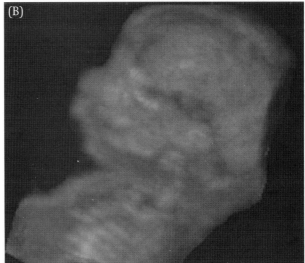

Figure 1.4 3D surface rendering reconstruction of a fetus at 27 weeks of pregnancy. This fetus has a small chin – a possible sign of mandibular micrognathism. (A) Surface rendering mode. (B) Maximum mode: bones, particularly the mandible, are visible in the reconstruction. A significant difference between soft tissue and bones is evident using the maximum-mode rendering algorithm

structures enables accurate diagnosis of subtle malformations and anomalies such as micrognathia, overlapping fingers, hexadactyly, and auricular malposition or malformation.[6] Prenatal diagnosis of facial deformations is very important in prenatal consultation and managment after birth, because these are frequently associated with chromosomal aberrations and genetic syndromes (Figure 1.4). With the advent of 3D/4D sonography, and the improved visualization of the fetal face thus provided, better prenatal diagnosis of cleft palate, micrognathism, etc. is now possible. The most important advantage of 3D sonography is its ability to display a true midsagittal plane of the fetal face. Surface rendering gives the best results when ROI structures are surrounded by fluid or by hypoechoic tissue.[7]

The advantages of 3D sonography are the following:

- The face may be viewed in a standard orientation.
- Defects may be viewed systematically using an interactive display.
- The rendered image provides landmarks for the planar images.

Moreover, in polymalformed fetuses, two or more anomalies can be visualized on a single image. In these situations, 3D imaging offers a realistic reconstruction of fetal external anatomy that enables parents to see and understand fetal conditions (Figures 1.5 and 1.6). This facilitates parental decisions on fetal future and the necessity or otherwise for termination of

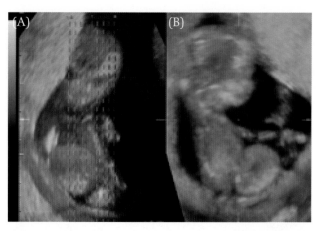

Figure 1.6 Tomographic ultrasound imaging (A) and volume contrast imaging (B) are used for better visualization of malformations: these images show a fetus with omphalocele at 15 weeks of gestation

pregnancy. On the other hand, for parents who have been faced with a polymalformed fetus in a previous pregnancy, confirmation of normal fetal anatomy can allay their fears.[8]

Voxels with grayscale values below a selected threshold value are not shown on the reconstructed image. Selecting the threshold parameter influences the quality of surface rendered images. Surface images can be displayed in the textural mode (Figure 1.7). Grayscale values can be replaced by different colors. The texture mode can also be smoothed, showing smooth structures on volume reconstructions. Texture and smooth surface displays are suitable for use in applications such as imaging of the fetal face, abdominal wall, genitals, umbilical cord, and the surfaces of

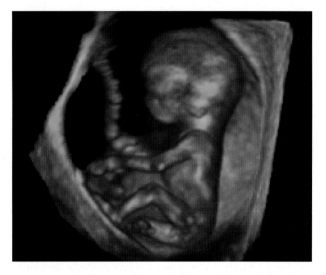

Figure 1.5 Surface rendering of fetus with omphalocele at 15 weeks of gestation

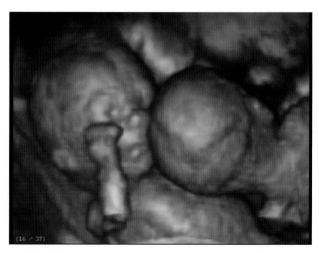

Figure 1.7 Surface texture mode image of twins at 16 weeks of gestation

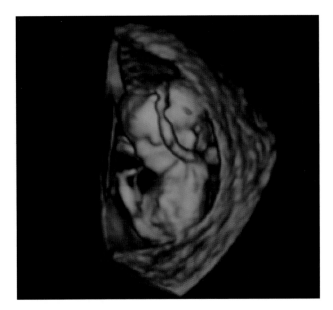

Figure 1.8 Surface view in the gradient light mode: lower limb malformation of a fetus at 13 weeks of gestation

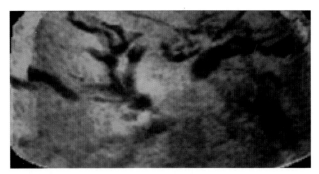

Figure 1.9 Transparent minimum-mode view of dilated intrahepatal bile ducts and hepatic veins as anechoic zones

the urinary bladder. Surfaces can also be displayed in light mode or gradient light mode (Figure 1.8). In the light mode, closer structures appear brighter while more distant structures are displayed darker. A variation of the light mode is the gradient light mode, showing fetus, as there is a virtual illumination from a spot light source.

TRANSPARENT RENDERING MODALITIES

In the transparent mode, in contrast to the surface mode, only the signals from the inner layers of the ROI are extracted, providing spatial reconstruction of the internal structure of the ROI. According to the echogenicity of extracted signals, there are two submodalities: the maximum and minimum modes. In the maximum mode, only the signals of highest echogenicity are extracted from the volume of interest, whereas in the minimum mode, only the signals of lowest echogenicity are extracted. This mode is suitable for visualization of fetal bones, the endometrium, and the breast.

Minimum mode

In this mode, minimum gray values are displayed for visualization of vessels, cystic structures, and parenchyma of different organs. Objects of interest

should be surrounded by hyperechoic structures (Figure 1.9).

Maximum mode

In this mode, maximum gray values of the volume are displayed. The maximum mode is suitable for visualization of fetal bony structures. It is the method of choice for imaging of spatial relationships between bones. Moreover, this modality offers an option of complete visualization of curved bones, such as the ribs, mandible, and clavicle on a single image (Figure 1.10). Evaluation of the whole of the skeleton, particularly the thoracic skeleton, in developing fetuses is often difficult with 2D sonography because of the curvature of the bones. Ribs can be observed

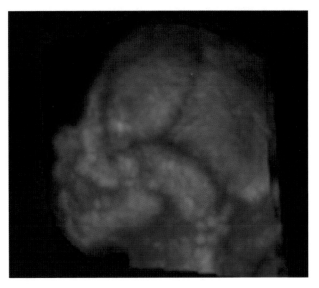

Figure 1.10 Maximum-mode view of the fetal profile at 28 weeks of gestation. The image displays properly developed bones and a normal intermaxillary relationship (compare Figure 1.4B)

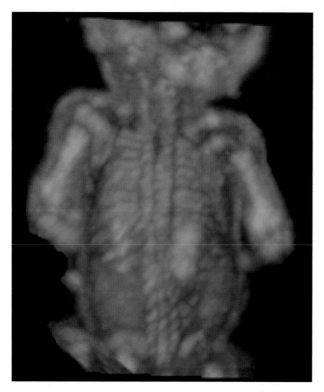

Figure 1.11 Maximum-mode view of the fetal body showing normal spine and thorax

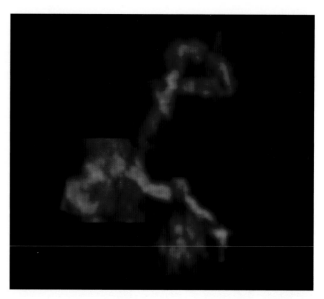

Figure 1.12 3D power Doppler image of the umbilical cord of monochorionic–monoamniotic twins

completely using the 3D transparent mode (Figure 1.11). This modality reduces the echogenicity of soft tissues lying behind echogenic structures, namely the bones. The vertebral column is originally curved anteroposteriorly. If it is pathologically curved laterally, it is impossible to display the whole column in a single sectional image by 2D sonography.[9,10] The advantage of 3D sonography is its ability to visualize both curvatures at the same time. Congenital malformations of the fetal spine can be identified easier using 3D surface and transparent modes together.[11]

X-ray mode

The X-ray mode is a transparent rendering algorithm by which all gray values within the ROI are presented. The reconstructed image looks like an X-ray image. Adjusting the ROI depth as low as possible will improve image contrast.

3D POWER AND COLOR DOPPLER IMAGING

Using PDI and CDI techniques during 3D acquisition, it is possible to view blood vessels and vascular

patterns of the ROI. The technique of 3D PDI has the same limitations as 2D PDI. Flash artifacts and sensitivity to tissue motion are also visible on 3D reconstructions.[12] 3D PDI images generally give a better overall picture of vascular distribution in multiplanar mode and 3D render mode than 2D slices (Figures 1.12 and 1.13).

GLASSBODY RENDERING

Glassbody rendering is a combination of 3D CDI or PDI and grayscale 3D images. This rendering algorithm allows visualization of vascularization in relation to the surrounding anatomy. Grayscale data are presented in some of transparent algorithms such as transparent texture or transparent maximum mode (Figure 1.14).

ELECTRONIC SCALPEL

During 3D and 4D scanning, especially during scanning of the fetus, there are structures that interfere with or are superimposed on the reconstructed image. Overlying and adjacent structures such as the umbilical cord, placenta, and fetal limbs often obscure the structure of interest and must be removed with the electronic scalpel. Electronic scalpel (or MagiCut tool) enables successful removal of overlying structures using 3D imaging. Unwanted structures can be cut off

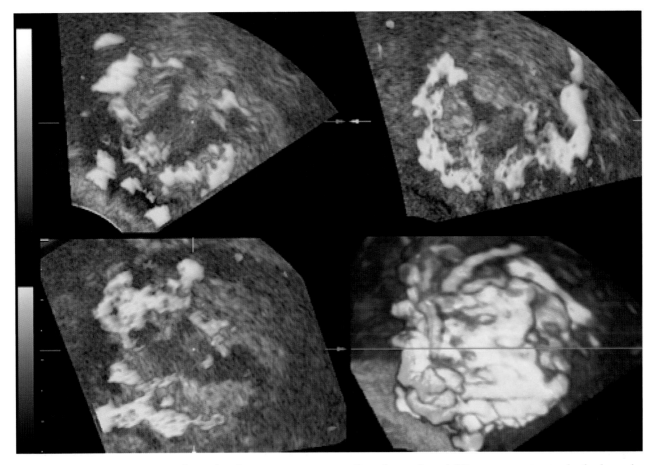

Figure 1.13 Multiplanar image of a total molar pregnancy in power Doppler mode with 3D reconstruction in glassbody mode. Transvaginal power Doppler images show zones of vascularization inside the uterine cavity and proliferation of trophoblastic tissue on grayscale

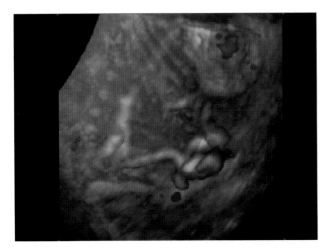

Figure 1.14 Fetal vascularization in glassbody rendering of a fetus at 19 weeks of gestation. The image is a combination of transparent maximum mode and 3D power Doppler

from the image in all three directions along the x-, y-, and z-axes.[13] During real-time scanning, it is possible to change the size, scanning direction, and shape of the

volume box to improve 3D reconstruction, especially during scanning in surface mode rendering algorithms.

ARTIFACTS IN 3D SONOGRAPHY

As with conventional 2D sonography, artifacts are present in 3D or 4D imaging methods. Acoustic shadowing, enhancement, reverberation, refraction, and motion artifacts from vascular pulsation are also present on volumetric reconstructions. There are also artifacts specific to volume acquisition, namely acquisition, rendering, and processing artifacts.

3D AND 4D CINE SEQUENCE

The 4D cine loop allows the examiner to review volumes and choose the best demonstration of the ROI for storage or to make a 3D reconstruction using the postprocessing possibilities of the ultrasound system's software. The volume can be stored on the ultrasound system's database for later processing.[14] The 3D cine mode allows rendering and animation of volume data displayed and rotated on the screen in the desired direction. 3D animation can be stored also as an AVI video file or as an image in standard image data formats (jpg and bitmap).

SPECIAL VOLUME IMAGING MODALITIES

Spatiotemporal image correlation (STIC)

This is a volume ultrasound technique that allows analysis of image data according to their spatial and temporal domain, and processes a dynamic 3D image sequence after an automatic volume sweep. 4D cardiac images are shown on a multiplanar reformatted cross-sectional display and/or a surface-rendered display.[15] STIC is an easy-to-use technique to acquire data on the fetal heart that allows visualization with both 3D static images and 4D sequences (Figure 1.15).

Combination of B-flow (see below) and STIC is also possible with or without use of the inversion mode.

The limitation of B-flow STIC is that it provides no information on blood flow direction. Visualization of the extracardiac great vessels is possible with B-flow STIC; however, intracardiac vascular flow is not clearly detected because of a lack of information on blood flow direction. Combination of both color Doppler STIC with directional information and B-flow STIC with identification of fine vascular flow may be useful for obtaining cardiac vascular information.[16,17]

Inversion mode

The inversion mode is a new rendering algorithm for visualization of fluid-filled anatomic structures. It

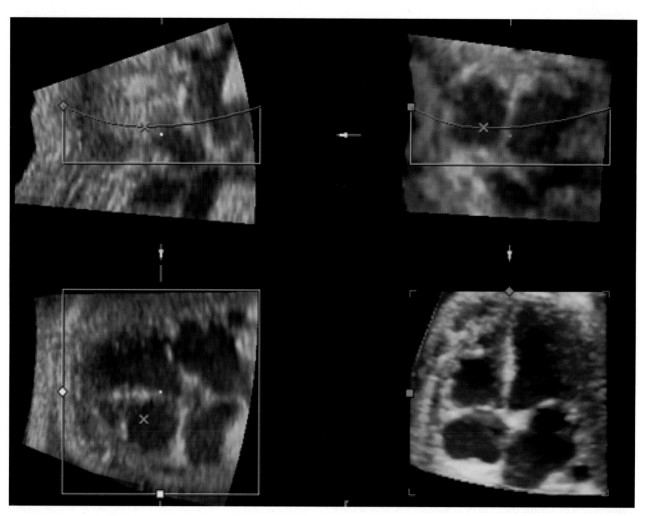

Figure 1.15 Four-chamber view of the fetal heart at 32 weeks of gestation: multiplanar image using the STIC technique

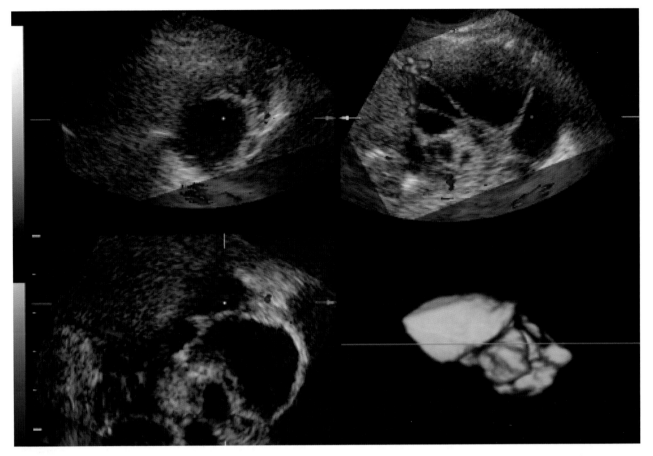

Figure 1.16 Cystic adnexal mass displayed in the multiplanar mode: anechoic cystic zones are displayed using the inversion mode

transforms anechoic structures into solid voxels. Anechoic structures such as the heart chambers, great vessels, and bladder appear on the rendered image, whereas structures that were echogenic prior to grayscale inversion are shown as anechoic. Since this technique does not use color or power Doppler methods as a contrast technique to highlight the blood vessels, it does not have the limitations of Doppler related to the angle of insonation, persistence of color data, and intensity of the Doppler signal. This technique does not differentiate blood vessels from other anechoic structures, but it is a useful new way to examine spatial relationships between fluid-filled structures that can otherwise be difficult to characterize on 2D grayscale images (Figure 1.16).

Volume contrast imaging (VCI)

This volume rendering technique is based on selecting thick slices of tissue data. It is possible to select a slice thickness between 3 and 20 mm. VCI is a volume rendering real-time technique. It simultaneously provides information from 2D conventional imaging and a volume rendered image. The volume rendered image is a combination of surface and transparent maximum mode. VCI provides a marked improvement in tissue contrast resolution, with no speckle pattern (Figure 1.17). There are two ways to use this technique. It is possible to view the VCI image in the A-plane or the C-plane (coronal). VCI-A reveals the same anatomic region as in the 2D ultrasound image, with improved image contrast. VCI-C allows a real-time approach in the coronal plane of the ROI. VCI-C is useful for visualization of planes that are not accessible with conventional grayscale imaging.

Tomographic ultrasound imaging (TUI)

TUI enables simultaneous display of up to nine parallel slices of an ultrasound volume dataset on one display, similar to computed tomography or magnetic resonance imaging (Figures 1.18 and 1.19). It can use

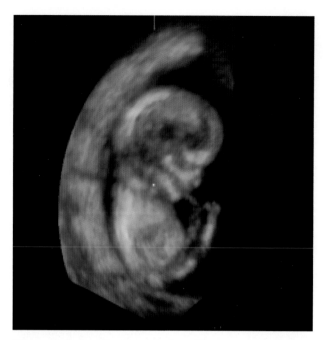

both static 3D and real-time 4D datasets. TUI in combination with STIC provides an easy way to review fetal heart examinations. In combination with transparent volume techniques, PDI, CDI, and VCI, TUI can be very useful in displaying different pathologic changes in abdominal organs and small parts.

B-flow

A recently developed B-flow imaging technology permits grayscale and non-Doppler visualization of fetal blood flow. The most useful characteristic of B-flow is a better resolution with a higher frame rate on the grayscale image. Because of direct visualization of blood reflectors, the peripheral blood vessels can be demonstrated. B-flow is basically a grayscale mode imaging method. Setting of ROI, flow velocity, and pulse repetition frequency (which is usually required in CDI/PDI) is not necessary in B-flow, and an easy rapid switching between conventional 2D imaging and B-flow imaging is possible. Furthermore, as B-flow has

Figure 1.17 Amelia: lower-limb malformation of a fetus at 13 weeks of gestation. Volume contrast imaging provides better contrast than conventional grayscale imaging

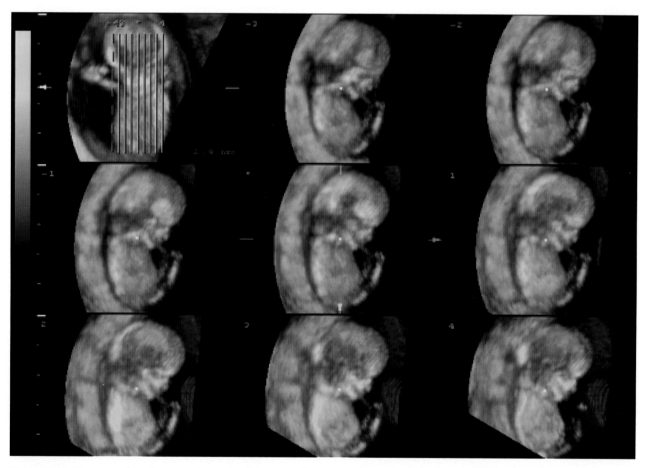

Figure 1.18 Tomographic ultrasound images of the same fetus as in Figure 1.17: eight parallel slices are displayed

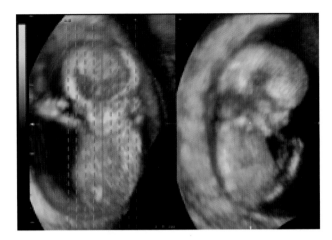

Figure 1.19 Combination of volume contrast imaging and tomographic ultrasound imaging: just one tomographic slice of the region of interest is displayed

no angular dependence, it provides easier acquisition of images than does CDI, regardless of the direction or angle of blood vessels. Vascular flow in blood vessels is more realistically represented and more clearly delineated on B-flow than on CDI/PDI. This is why B-flow may be potentially used as an imaging technique

in fetal cardiac and vascular imaging and may avoid the limitations of CDI/PDI.

Volume calculation (VOCAL)

An important advantage of 3D sonography is the ability to accurately obtain volume measurements even of irregularly shaped structures (Figure 1.20).

IMAGE PROCESSING AND STORAGE OF VOLUMES, IMAGES, OR VIDEO SEQUENCES

Volume data stored on the ultrasound system's database can be processed using integrated system software or sent by network to personal computer or workstation for further processing. It is recommended that volume data be copied to magneto-optic disks or CD/DVD as back-up. In many cases, volume datasets require postprocessing. Specialized software gives numerous possibilities in the postprocessing of saved

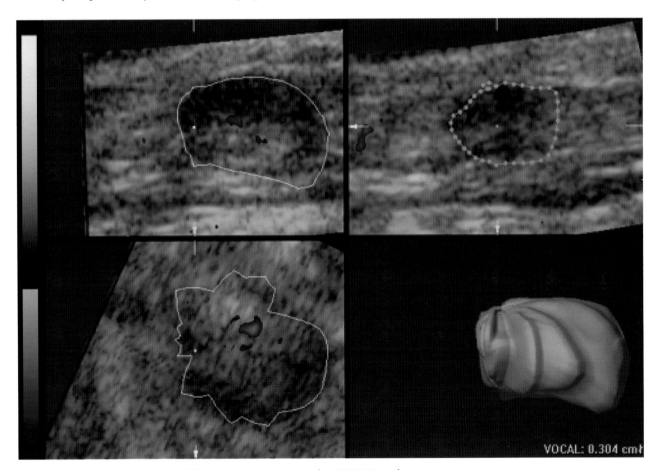

Figure 1.20 Multiplanar image of breast carcinoma using the VOCAL technique

volumes and images. Superimposed and overlapping structures present on screen can be removed using the electronic scalpel. Image brightness and contrast can be set to desired values. Low-level echoes can be filtered out by increasing the threshold values. Angio threshold removes motion artifacts and noise in the CDI and PDI rendering modalities. To improve visualization, different rendering modalities can be applied to saved volume data, such as altering surface rendered data to transparent modalities, or using the inversion mode, static VCI, or TUI. The changes can be simultaneously visible on screen, and processed images can then be stored or 3D-reconstructed.

HOW TO ACHIEVE A GOOD 3D IMAGE

1. Adjusting a 2D image

The basic quality of the 3D image is completely dependent on the 2D information. It is essential to optimize the 2D image before acquiring the volume. This should include setting the correct gain, time gain compensation (TGC), focus settings, and appropriate image size. In addition, different examination objectives have varying requirements. The best 3D and 4D images can only be obtained from an excellent 2D base. Traditional skills remain, as does the need for even greater technical knowledge to optimize the 2D picture before adding 3D, as well as familiarization with an entirely new set of controls.[18,19]

2. Orientation of 2D image

The sonographer must choose a good position in 2D, with an idea of what should appear on the 3D image.

3. Turn on 3D/4D mode

Acquisition of volume datasets is performed using 2D scans with special transducers designed for volume scanning. Volume acquisition starts with a 2D scan and superimposed volume box. The 2D image presented on screen is a central 2D image plane of the volume.

4. Adjust the ROI

The volume box frames the region of interest (ROI). The green line has to be adjusted (position, shape, and

rendering direction): information outside of this green dotted line will be eliminated from the 3D reconstruction. On the 2D screen, two dimensions of the volume box are visible. The volume angle is displayed as a small icon on the screen and represents the third dimension of volume sweep or scanning amplitude. 3D imaging of a fetal surface requires fluid in front of the target organ, while this is of minor importance when imaging the fetal bony spine.

5. Capturing

The volume scan is started by pressing the start key. The sweep time depends on the volume box size and the scan quality that has been set.

6. Multiplanar navigation

After acquisition, the volume data are shown in a multiplanar display on the monitor. The three planes of the multiplanar display (transverse, sagittal, and coronal) are perpendicular to each other. The 3D reconstruction is also visible on screen. The operator can arbitrarily choose a point on the reference image, and rotate the volume and orient the scan planes in order to optimize the rendered image.[20]

7. Rotation and translation

The 3D image can be rotated about the x-, y-, and z-axes. Translation allows displacement of the center of rotation of the 3D reconstructed image, with the orthogonal plates being simultaneously updated. It is important to optimize the threshold value for the best image quality.

8. Electronic scalpel

With this software option, it is possible to remove overlying structures that interfere with the view to the ROI.

9. Choose rendering

Different rendering algorithms can be applied to the ROI. The operator can select between surface, transparent, and light modalities for visualization of the volume.

Training of sonographers must include standard acquisitions of volumes that will be displayed with a minimum of artifact. Sonographers must recognize inadequate volumes that cannot be used due to motion or other artifacts. The training of physicians reviewing the volumes must also include learning how to evaluate anatomy in orientations different from the original acquisition plane. The technique of scanning in 3D has to be learnt, as this is different from that in 2D, and it is necessary to learn how to use an entirely new set of controls.[21] Although interrogation of a 3D volume may enable the operator to visualize the anatomy in planes that are unobtainable with conventional 2D imaging, the basic quality of the 3D image is completely dependent on the 2D information from which it is derived. Thus, it is vital to optimize the 2D image before acquiring the volume.

REFERENCES

1. Guerra FA, Isla AI, Aguilar RC, Fritz EG. Use of freehand three-dimensional ultrasound software in study of the fetal heart. Ultrasound Obstet Gynecol 2000; 16: 329–34.

2. Azumendi G, Kurjak A. Three-dimensional and four-dimensional sonography in the study of the fetal face. Ultrasound Rev Obstet Gynecol 2003; 3: 160–9.

3. Kurjak A, Azumendi G, Vecek N, et al. Fetal hand movements and facial expression in normal pregnancy studied by four-dimensional sonography. J Perinat Med 2003; 31: 496–508.

4. Kurjak A, Vecek N, Hafner T, et al. Prenatal diagnosis: What does four-dimensional ultrasound add? J Perinat Med 2002; 30: 57–62.

5. Mertz E. 3-D ultrasound in prenatal diagnosis. In: Mertz E, ed. Ultrasound in Obstetrics. Stuttgart: Thieme Verlag, 2004.

6. Dyson RL, Pretorius DH, Budorick NE, et al. Three-dimensional ultrasound in the evaluation of fetal anomalies. Ultrasound Obst Gynecol 2000; 30: 40–7.

7. Mangione R, Lacombe D, Carles D, et al. Craniofacial dysmorphology and three-dimensional ultrasound: a prospective study on practicability for prenatal diagnosis. Prenat Diagn 2003; 23: 810–18.

8. Kossoff G. Basic physics and imaging characteristics of ultrasound. World J Surg 2000; 24: 134–42.

9. Benoit B. The value of three-dimensional ultrasonography in the screening of the fetal skeleton. Child Nerv Syst 2003; 19: 403–9.

10. Rotten D, Levaillant JM. Two and three-dimensional sonographic assessment of the fetal face. A systematic analysis of the normal face. Ultrasound Obst Gynecol 2004; 23: 224–31.

11. Yanagihara T, Hata T. Three-dimensional sonographic visualization of fetal skeleton in the second trimester of pregnancy. Gynecol Obstet Invest 2000; 49: 12–16.

12. Chaoui R, Kalache KD, Hartung J. Application of threedimensional power Doppler ultrasound in prenatal diagnosis. Ultrasound Obstet Gynecol 2001; 17: 22–9.

13. Mertz E, Miric-Tesanic D, Welter C. Value of the electronic scalpel (cut mode) in evaluation of the fetal face. Ultrasound Obstet Gynecol 2000; 16: 364–8.

14. Hu W, Wu MT, Liu CP, et al. Left ventricular 4D echocardiogram motion and shape analysis. Ultrasonics 2002; 40: 949–54.

15. Vinals F, Poblete P, Giuliano A. Spatio-temporal image correlation (STIC): a new tool for the prenatal screening of congenital heart defects. Ultrasound Obstet Gynecol 2003; 22: 388–94.

16. Chaoui R, Hoffmann J, Heling KS. Three-dimensional (3D) and 4D color Doppler fetal echocardiography using spatio-temporal image correlation (STIC). Ultrasound Obstet Gynecol 2004; 23: 535–45.

17. De Vore GR, Falkensammer P, Sklansky MS, et al. Spatio-temporal image correlation (STIC): New technology for evaluation of the fetal heart. Ultrasound Obstet Gynecol 2003; 22: 380–7.

18. Timor-Tritsch IE, Platt LD. Three-dimensional ultrasound experience in obstetrics. Curr Opin Obstet Gynecol 2002; 14: 569–75.

19. Lee W. 3D fetal ultrasonography. Clin Ostet Gynecol 2003; 46: 850–67.

20. Arzt W, Tulzer G, Aigner M. Realtime 3D sonography of the normal fetal heart – clinical evaluation. Ultraschall Med 2002; 23: 388–91.

21. Kurjak A, Hafner T, Kos M, et al. Three-dimensional sonography in prenatal diagnosis: a luxury or a necessity? J Perinat Med 2000; 28: 194–209.

2 3D sonoembryology and fetal anatomy

Asim Kurjak, Wiku Andonotopo, and Guillermo Azumendi

INTRODUCTION

The recent development of ultrasound technology has resulted in remarkable progress in visualization of early embryos and fetuses and in the development of sonoembryology. With the use of three- and four-dimensional (3D and 4D) ultrasound, both structural and functional developments in the first 12 weeks of gestation can be assessed more objectively and reliably. New technology has moved embryology from postmortem studies to the in vivo environment. It is the purpose of this chapter to illustrate the potential of 3D/4D sonography in the study of the embryo and early fetus.

PRE-EMBRYONAL PERIOD

Human development as a repeating process from generation to generation starts with fertilization, which usually takes place in the ampulla of the uterine tube. Fertilization is a complex process that involves some preparative steps as well as a set of interactions between sperm and egg. The ejaculated sperm must first undergo a process of maturation, known as capacitation, which is the alteration of its glycoprotein surface under the influence of products secreted from the female reproductive tract. How can we assess this part of early human development by ultrasound?

Transvaginal sonography is considered the most reliable method for monitoring follicular growth (Figure 2.1). It enables accurate prediction of ovulation and detection of any ovulation abnormalities. During in vitro fertilization, the success of the procedure depends on the ability of the ovary to respond to

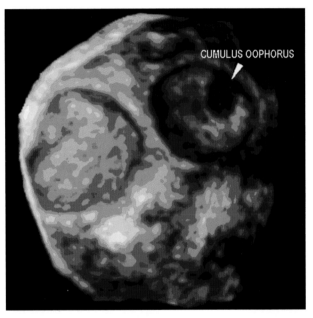

Figure 2.1 3D ultrasound scan of an ovary stimulated by human menopausal gonadotropin. Note the two follicles, in one of which a triangular structure presenting cumulus oophorus is clearly visualized

controlled stimulation by gonadotropins and to develop a reasonable number of mature follicles and oocytes simultaneously. Increased ovarian stromal blood flow velocity has been detected in polycystic ovaries (Figures 2.2 and 2.3), in combination with relatively unchanged impedance to blood flow. This may reflect increased intraovarian perfusion and thus a greater delivery of gonadotropins to the granulosa–thecal cell complex, with a resultant greater number of follicles being produced (Figure 2.4). This mechanism may help to explain why patients with polycystic ovaries tend to respond excessively to the

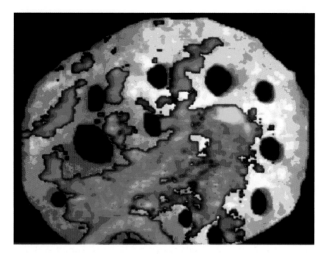

Figure 2.2 3D transvaginal power Doppler scan of a polycystic ovary. Note the peripheral distribution of small follicles and increased vascularity within the ovarian stroma

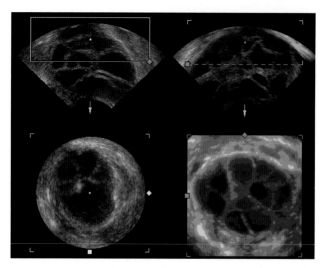

Figure 2.4 Multiplanar view of an ovary in a patient undergoing oocyte retrieval. 3D ultrasound enables better anatomic orientation during penetration of the needle

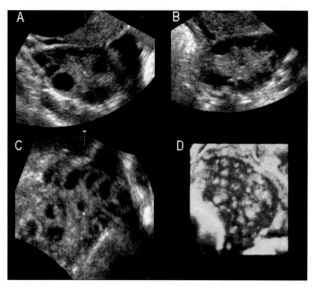

Figure 2.3 Simultaneous 2D (A–C) and 3D (D) images of a polycystic ovary. This method allows direct measurement of the total ovarian volume and estimation of the ovarian stromal volume

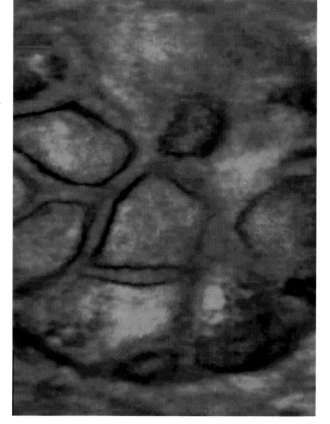

Figure 2.5 3D ultrasound scan of a hyperstimulated ovary

administration of gonadotropins, and may possibly explain their increased risk of ovarian hyperstimulation syndrome (Figure 2.5).[1–4]

The basic structural information provided by conventional scans in the longitudinal and transverse planes can now be augmented by new 3D ultrasound systems that provide an additional view of the coronal or C-plane, which is parallel to the transducer face (Figures 2.3 and 2.4). The computer-generated scan is displayed in three perpendicular planes. Translation or rotation can be carried out in one plane, while maintaining the perpendicular orientation of all three so that serial translation will result in an ultrasound tomogram from which volumetric data can be captured.[1,4]

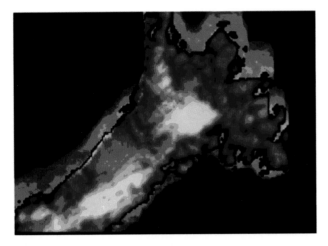

Figure 2.6 Entire length and spillage of contrast medium from the fimbrial end, as demonstrated by echo-enhanced 3D power Doppler hysterosalpingography

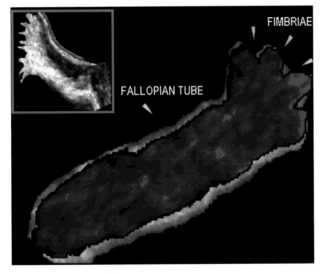

Figure 2.7 3D power Doppler facilitates detection of tubal patency and evaluation of tubal morphology. Inset: 3D hystero-contrast-salpingography using echogenic contrast medium. Note the regular filling of the tube and spillage from the fimbrial end

The normal Fallopian tubes are narrow and usually not seen by transabdominal or transvaginal ultrasound unless they contain fluid within their lumen or are surrounded by fluid (Figure 2.6). Together with developments in ultrasound technique, a totally new concept of diagnostic procedures has been developed. By using 3D volume sections and reconstruction, it is possible to visualize more precisely pathologic processes in Fallopian tubes. Similarly, using 3D power Doppler technology, it is possible to visualize the flow of the contrast through the entire tubal

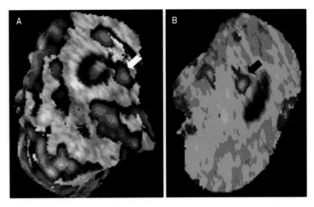

Figure 2.8 At the 4th and 5th weeks of a normal pregnancy, we can observe an endometrium that is more (A) or less (B) vascularized, but it is always possible to distinguish a 3D color signal penetrating to the gestational sac. We call this phenomenon the 'comet sign', and it indicates the implantation site (from: Kurjak A et al. Structural and functional early human development assessed by three-dimensional and four-dimensional sonography. Fertil Steril 2005; 84: 1285–99)

length and its spill in the retrouterine space (Figure 2.7). The 3D power Doppler imaging method appears to have advantages over conventional hysterosalpingography for evaluation of tubal patency.[3,4]

EVENTS FOLLOWING IMPLANTATION

As the embryo and placental structures develop, their vascular network becomes more pronounced.[1–4] Hence, it is possible to observe three separate and yet unified units: the maternal, placental, and fetal portions of the vascular network (Figures 2.8–2.11). The earliest visible sign of pregnancy is a new formed gestational sac that can be seen during the 5th week of pregnancy (Figure 2.12).[1–5] Ultrasonographically, it is presented as a hypoechoic oval structure, surrounded by a hyperechoic ring, situated asymmetrically in the uterine cavity. The gestational sac at this time measures approximately 5 mm and grows 1–2 mm per day. The beginning of the embryochorionic circulation alters the supply of nutrition to intraembryonic tissues, as well as the chorionic mesenchyme. Development of the embryo becomes subject to the circulation of fetal blood. In some cases, avascular degenerated chorionic villi constituting a hydatidiform mole (Figures 2.13–2.15) can coexist with a healthy twin (Figures 2.16 and 2.17): this is a twin pregnancy with one healthy twin and normal placenta, with the other twin being a complete hydatidiform mole. It

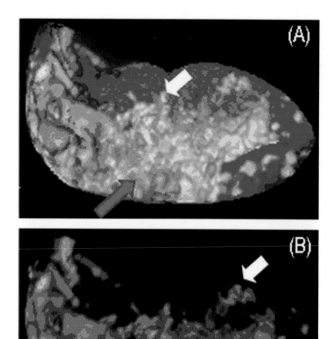

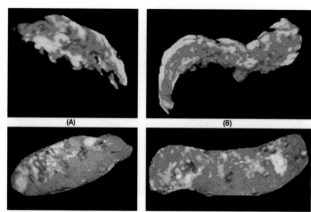

Figure 2.11 Visual analysis demonstrates increased blood flow in both circulations during the 1st trimester of a normal pregnancy. (A) At 10 weeks of gestation. (B) At 12 weeks (from: Kurjak A et al. Structural and functional early human development assessed by three-dimensional and four-dimensional sonography. Fertil Steril 2005; 84: 1285–99)

Figure 2.9 Uterochorionic and intrachorionic circulation at the 12th week of a normal pregnancy. From 6 weeks, we can differentiate between uterochorionic (i.e., spiral and radial vessels: red arrow) and intrachorionic (i.e., intervillous blood flow: white arrow) circulations. (A) Transparent 'glassbody' mode of 3D power Doppler mapping. (B) Color mode of 3D power Doppler angiography (from: Kurjak A et al. Structural and functional early human development assessed by three-dimensional and four-dimensional sonography. Fertil Steril 2005; 84: 1285–99)

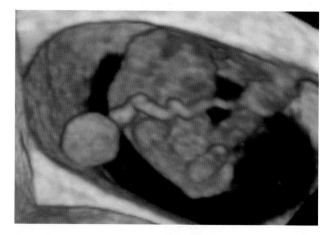

Figure 2.12 3D surface rendering demonstrating embryo and yolk sac structure at 6 weeks of gestation

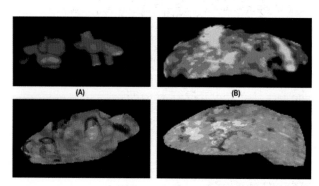

Figure 2.10 Uterochorionic blood flow (color rendering: top) and intervillous blood flow (transparent rendering: below). (A) At 6 weeks of gestation. (B) At 8 weeks (from: Kurjak A et al. Structural and functional early human development assessed by three-dimensional and four-dimensional sonography. Fertil Steril 2005; 84: 1285–99)

originates from fertilization of two eggs – with the mole originating from one and the normal fetus from the other. The complete hydatidiform mole has a paternal origin and diploid karyotype (Figures 2.16 and 2.17).

MATERNAL PORTION

The maternal portion of the placental circulation consists of the main uterine arteries and their branches, which spread throughout the uterus until they reach the decidual plate of the placenta. The main uterine arteries originate from the internal iliac arteries, and they give off branches, which extend

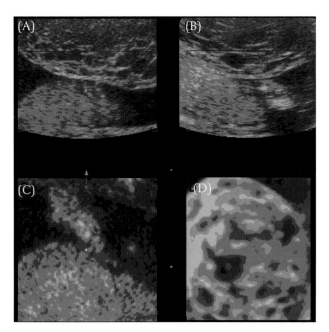

Figure 2.13 Simultaneous 2D ultrasound images (A–C) and 3D image (D) at 22 weeks of gestation showing typical vesicular tissue of a hydatidiform mole

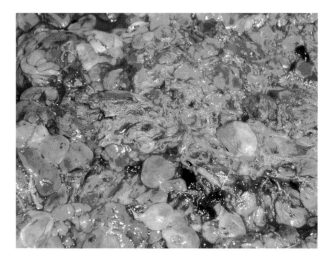

Figure 2.14 Macroscopic classic characteristic of a hydatidiform mole demonstrating vesicular structures

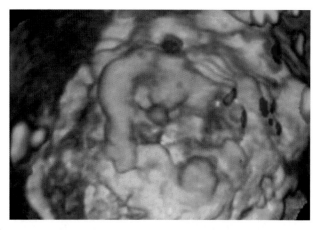

Figure 2.15 3D ultrasound image of a hydatidiform mole showing typical vesicular tissue with high vascularization

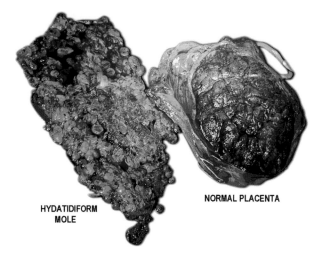

HYDATIDIFORM MOLE

NORMAL PLACENTA

Figure 2.16 Pathologic specimens of pregnancy complicated with hydatidiform mole

inward for about a third of the myometrial thickness without significant branching. At this point, they subdivide into an arcuate wreath encircling the uterus. From this network, there arise smaller branches called the radial arteries, which are directed towards the uterine lumen. The radial arteries branch into basal arteries and endometrial spiral arteries as they pass the myometrial–endometrial border. Basal arteries, which are relatively short, terminate in a capillary bed that serves the stratum basale of the endometrium. The spiral arteries project further into the endometrium

and terminate in a vast capillary network that serves the functional layer of the endometrium. All of them can be clearly identified in the pregnant uterus by their anatomic position and characteristic waveform profile. Intrauterine placental development requires adaptive changes of the uterine vascular environment. The fact that the uterine vascular network elongates and dilates throughout pregnancy is well known from anatomic studies.[2]

Doppler findings

Flow velocity waveforms from small arteries show significantly lower pulsatility and blood velocity compared with the main uterine artery. This phenomenon is a consequence of the branching of the uterine

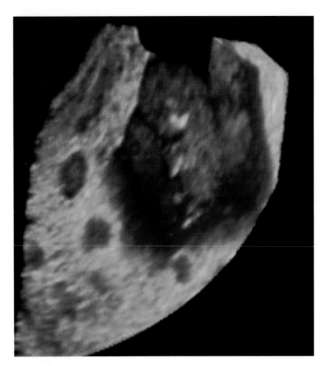

Figure 2.17 Ultrasound image at 9 weeks of gestation showing typical vesicular tissue of a hydatidiform mole (left side), which is clearly delineated from the fetus (right side) and normal placenta

circulation and the increased total vascular cross-sectional area, which results in lower impedance to blood flow. Most authors have demonstrated that the progressive decrement in the impedance to blood flow observed in the main uterine artery during early pregnancy occurs in all the segments of the uteroplacental circulation. Transvaginal color and pulsed Doppler allow identification of the uterine vascular transformation. Furthermore, the invasion of larger maternal blood vessels of higher pressure results in higher velocity and a larger diastolic component of Doppler signal. With advancing gestational age, impedance to blood flow decreases from the main uterine to the spiral arteries. At the same time, an increase in blood flow by means of peak-systolic velocity has a decreasing trend from the uterine, through the arcuate to the radial arteries. The increment in blood flow through the uterine network is probably caused by an urgent need of the placenta and fetus for nourishment.[2]

Uterine arterial blood flow in non-pregnant and pregnant patients

The main uterine artery can be visualized at the level of the internal cervical os, as it approaches the uterus laterally and curves upward alongside the uterine body. Pulsed Doppler waveform profiles of the main uterine artery are characteristic, comprising a high peak-systolic component with a characteristic notch in the protodiastolic part and very low end-diastolic flow. Numerous Doppler studies have demonstrated a gradual decrement in the uterine artery resistance index during the first trimester of pregnancy. The characteristic notch in the protodiastolic part of the sonogram gradually disappears; diastolic flow is characterized by high velocity, and the difference between systolic and diastolic flow velocities decreases. These changes indicate normal development of pregnancy (trophoblast invasion). Obviously, this decrement continues during the 2nd trimester of pregnancy and can be observed in all the segments of the uteroplacental circulation.[2]

Arcuate and radial arterial blood flow in non-pregnant and pregnant patients

Arcuate arteries may be seen within the outer third of the myometrium, while the radial arteries are identified within the two inner thirds. Doppler sonograms of the arcuate and radial arteries are very similar, with moderate peak-systolic and diastolic components of blood flow. However, differences exist in the values of the resistance and pulsatility indices. These are lower in the radial than in the arcuate arteries, corresponding to the lower peripheral impedance to blood flow.[2–4]

Normal finding of spiral arteries in pregnant patients

During early pregnancy, the spiral arteries are progressively converted to non-muscular dilated tortuous channels. The normal musculo-elastic wall is replaced with a mixture of fibrinoid material and fibrous tissue. Easily detected above the chorion (near the placental implantation site), the spiral arteries are characterized by lower resistance index and higher peak systolic velocities followed by turbulent flow. This kind of flow is typical of wide tortuous blood vessels and has the hemodynamic characteristics of an arteriovenous shunt. The active trophoblast induces vascular adaptation, which ensures adequate blood supply to the growing embryo. Pulsed Doppler waveform signals obtained from spiral arteries show low impedance to blood flow and a characteristic spiky outline. The sonogram presents the blood flow from more than one spiral artery. The spiral arteries change their wall structure with gestation and become vessels with completely different hemodynamics in relation to other arteries of the uteroplacental circulation.[2–4]

PLACENTA

Development and ultrasound imaging

Primary chorionic villi develop between the 13th and 15th days after ovulation (during the 4th week of gestation), and mark the beginning of placental development. At the same time, the formation of blood vessels starts in the extraembryonic mesoderm of the yolk sac, the connecting stalk, and the chorion. By 18–21 days (during the 5th week of gestation), the villi have become branched and the mesenchymal cells within the villi have differentiated into blood capillaries and formed an arteriocapillary venous network. Chorionic villi cover the entire surface of the gestational sac until the end of the 8th week. At that time, the villi on the side of the chorion proliferate towards the decidua basalis to form the chorion frondosum, which develops into the definitive placenta. The villi in contact with the decidua capsularis begin to degenerate and form an avascular shell, known as the chorion laeve or smooth chorion. The placenta is mostly derived from fetal tissues, with the maternal component contributing little to the architecture of the definitive placenta. Normal placentation requires a progressive transformation of the spiral arteries and an infiltration of trophoblastic cells into the placental bed. These physiologic changes normally extend into the inner third of the myometrium, and in normal pregnancies, all the spiral arteries are transformed into uteroplacental arteries before 20 weeks of gestation. In some cases of early pregnancy failure and pregnancy-induced hypertension, there is adequate placentation but a defective transformation of spiral arteries.[2–5]

3D power Doppler studies in assessment of early chorionic circulation

New developments on the cutting edge of ultrasound technology have enabled us to expand investigations of early placental vascular supply (Figures 2.8–2.11). 3D power Doppler is able to depict an integral 3D image of the placenta and embryo and their vascular network. Additionally, it is possible to quantify and express numerically data related to vascular signals in the investigated volume.

Development of the process of placentation begins after the first contact between trophoblast and decidua has been established. There are two waves of trophoblastic invasion. The first occurs at 8 weeks of gestation. It is characterized by invasion of interstitial trophoblast into the myometrium and of cytotrophoblast (endothelial trophoblast) into the complete decidua, but not the myometrium. The second wave is characterized just by invasion of endothelial trophoblast into the myometrium, and occurs between 16 and 18 weeks of gestation.

Uteroplacental arteries are not responsive to the autonomic nervous system. In the second lunar month, the intervillous space increases as the result of the extensive branching of the villi. The intervillous space, combined with the villi, is the functional unit of the human placenta, where maternal–fetal metabolic exchange occurs. In this period, many terminal parts of the spiral arteries near the intervillous space contain plugs of cytotrophoblastic cells. At the same time, centrally placed communications between the decidual veins are numerous and large. After 40 days, spiral arteries show direct openings into the intervillous space, and the cytotrophoblastic cells appear within their lumen. The maternal blood reaches the intervillous space through the gaps between the cells of the endovascular trophoblast. These events can be studied by 3D color and power Doppler ultrasound.

During pulsed Doppler analysis, two types of waveform can be visualized: pulsatile arterial-like and continuous venous-like flow. The lumen of the spiral arteries is never completely obstructed by the trophoblastic plugs. These data indicate that establishment of the intervillous circulation is a continuous process rather than an abrupt event at the end of the first trimester.[2–4]

EARLY FETAL DEVELOPMENT (FIGURES 2.18–2.43)

5th week

Characteristic embryologic findings

The deep neural groove and the first somites are present (Figure 2.25). The embryo is almost straight and somites produce conspicuous surface elevation.

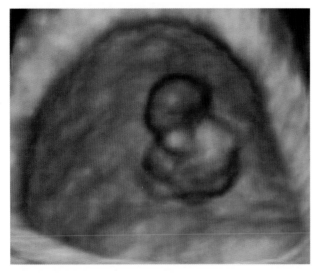

Figure 2.18 3D surface rendering of an embryo at 5 weeks of gestation showing embryonic pole and yolk sac

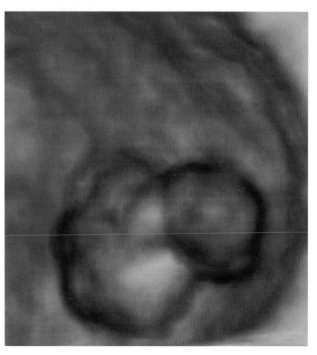

Figure 2.20 3D surface rendering of an embryo at 5 weeks of gestation demonstrating the same structure as seen in Figure 2.19

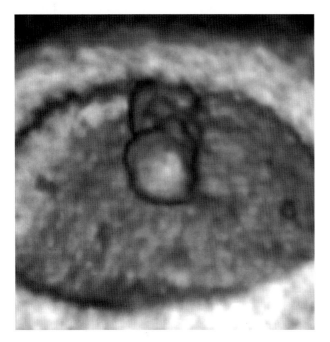

Figure 2.19 3D surface imaging of an embryo at 5 weeks of gestation showing chorionic sac, amniotic sac, and yolk sac

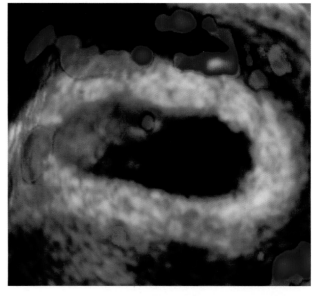

Figure 2.21 3D power Doppler image of gestational sac at 5 weeks of gestation showing the heartbeat of the embryo

The heart prominence is distinct and the optic pits are present. The attenuated tail with its somites is also a characteristic feature.

3D ultrasound findings

The gestational sac can be visualized as a small spherical anechoic structure inside one of the endometrial leafs. 3D sonography enables precise measurement of exponentially expanding gestational sac volume during the 1st trimester (Figures 2.18–2.20). 3D measurement of yolk sac volume and vascularity may be predictive of a pregnancy outcome. Using this non-invasive modality, one can obtain multiplanar and surface images in reduced scanning time. Surface

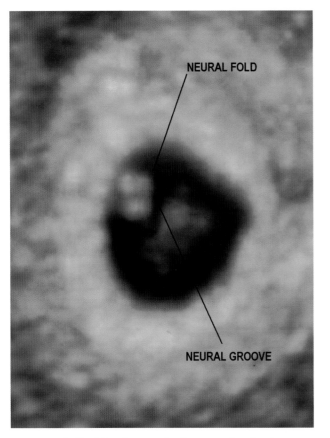

Figure 2.22 By 21st day postfertilization, the development of the notochordal process changes its shape from disk-like to sandal-like. This process, which cannot be visualized with 2D ultrasound, can be seen with 3D imaging

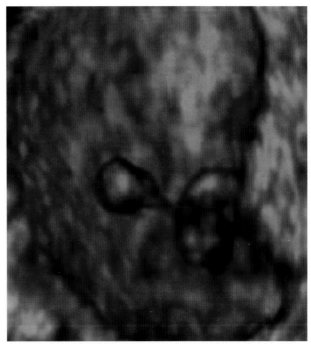

Figure 2.23 An embryo at 6 weeks of gestation depicted by 3D surface rendering

images seem to be beneficial in the evaluation of the yolk sac echogenicity and detection of the hyperechoic yolk sac, which may indicate chromosomal abnormality. Automatic and manual volume calculation allow analysis of the precise relationship between yolk sac and gestational sac volumes, as well as assessment of the correlation between yolk sac volume and crown–rump length (CRL) measurements. Planar mode tomograms are useful for detecting the embryonic pole inside the gestational sac. The embryo itself can be seen 24–48 hours after visualization of the yolk sac, at approximately 33 days after menstruation, at which it is 2–3 mm long. Adjacent to the yolk sac, the embryo can be seen as a small straight line by the end of the 5th week of gestation.

3D power Doppler findings

3D power Doppler reveals intensive vascular activity surrounding the chorionic shell, starting from the first sonographic evidence of the developing pregnancy during the 5th week of gestation (Figure 2.21). The gestational sac can be detected as a tiny ring-shaped structure at the beginning of the 5th week. 3D power Doppler reveals intense vascular activity surrounding it. A hyperechoic chorionic ring is interrupted by color-coded sprouts of early intervillous and spiral artery blood flow. At the end of the 5th week, when the gestational sac exceeds 8 mm, the small secondary yolk sac is visible as the earliest sign of the developing embryo.

6th week

Characteristic embryologic findings

The embryo appears as a C-shaped curve (Figures 2.18–2.20). The growth of the head (caused by the rapid development of the brain) exceeds that of the other regions.

3D ultrasound findings

A rounded bulky head and thinner body characterize 3D image of an embryo during the 6th week of gestation (Figures 2.24–2.26). The head is prominent due to the developing forebrain. Limb buds are rarely visible at this stage of pregnancy. However, the umbil-

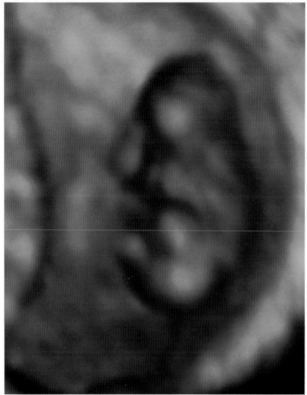

Figure 2.24 3D surface rendering of an embryo at 5–6 weeks of gestation. The head is prominent due to the developing forebrain

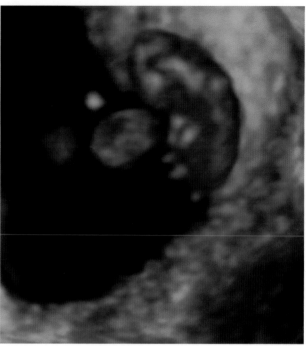

Figure 2.26 A rounded bulky head and a thinner body characterize the 3D image of an embryo during the 6th week of gestation. The head is prominent due to the developing forebrain. Limb buds are rarely visible at this stage of pregnancy

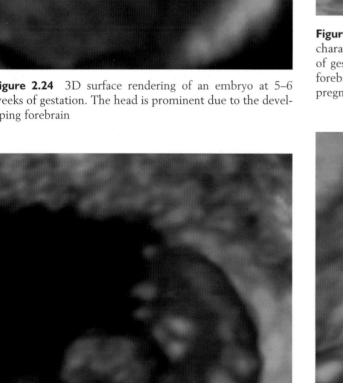

Figure 2.25 3D ultrasound at 6 weeks of gestation. The deep neural groove and the first somites are present. The embryo is almost straight, and the somites produce conspicuous surface elevation

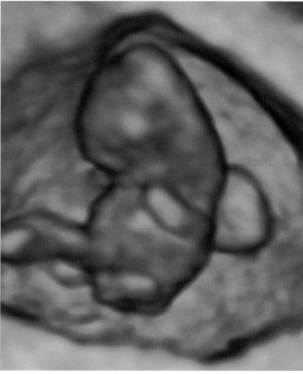

Figure 2.27 An embryo at 7 weeks of gestation demonstrating umbilical veins and the development of anterior and posterior limbs

ical cord and vitelline duct are always clearly seen. At 6 weeks of gestation, the ductus omphalomesentericus can be as much as three to four times the length of the embryo itself. The amniotic membrane is also visible, initially at the dorsal part of the embryo. A few days later, it surrounds the embryo, but not the yolk sac, which remains in the extracelomic cavity.

3D power Doppler findings

Aortic and umbilical blood flow is well depicted. The initial branches of the umbilical vessels are visible at the placental umbilical insertion (Figures 2.28 and 2.29). 3D power Doppler detects embryonic heartbeats as early as 5 weeks and 4 days menstrual age, at an embryo CRL of 3±4 mm. At this very early stage, this finding may help clinicians to diagnose the viability of the pregnancy. Near the end of the 6th week, the first signs of aortic and umbilical blood flow are visible within the trunk of the embryo.

7th week

Characteristic embryologic findings

The head is now much larger in relation to the trunk and is more bent over the cardiac prominence. The trunk and neck have begun to straighten. Hand and foot plates are formed and digital or finger rays have started to appear.

3D ultrasound findings

During the 7th week of gestation, the spine gradually becomes visible, as well as limb buds, lateral to the body. The amnion can be seen as a spherical hyperechoic membrane, still close to the embryo. The chorion frondosum can be distinguished from the chorion laeve. Rapid development of the rhombencephalon (hindbrain) occurs. This process gives even more prominence to the head, which becomes the dominant embryonic structure. Using the multiplanar mode, the developing vesicles of the brain can be depicted as anechoic structures inside the head. The biggest, and usually the only one visible, is the rhombencephalon, situated on the top of the head (vertex). The head is strongly flexed anteriorly, being in contact with the chest (Figures 2.30–2.33). The hypoechogenic brain cavities can be identified, including the separated cerebral hemispheres. The lateral ventricles are shaped like small round vesicles. The

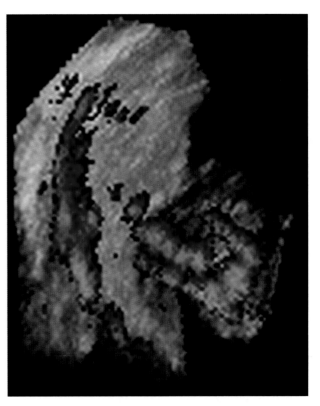

Figure 2.28 3D transvaginal power Doppler can obtain a signal from the uteroplacentar blood flow and from the fetus at the same time during the 6th week of gestation

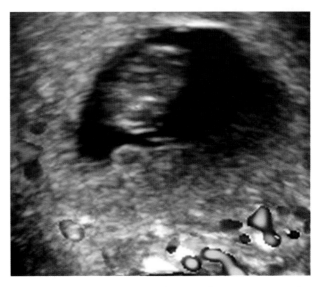

Figure 2.29 3D power Doppler reveals intensive vascular activity surrounding the chorionic shell, starting from the first sonographic evidence of the developing pregnancy during the 6th week of gestation

cavity of the diencephalon (the future third ventricle) runs posterior. In the smallest embryos, the medial telencephalon forms a continuous cavity between the

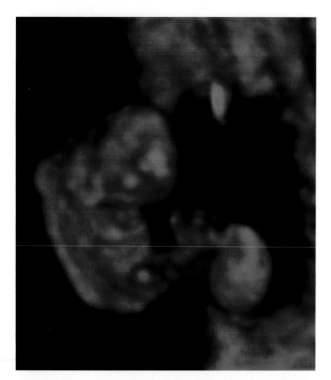

Figure 2.30 3D surface rendering demonstrating the embryo and yolk sac structure at 7 weeks of gestation

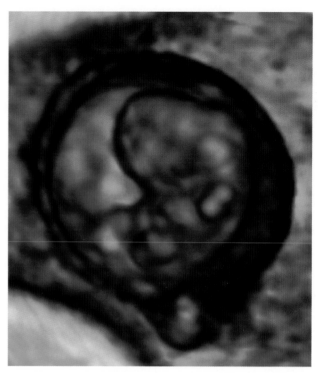

Figure 2.32 3D image: during the 7th week of gestation, the spine gradually becomes visible, as well as limb buds, lateral to the body. The amnion can be seen as a spherical hyperechoic membrane, still close to the embryo

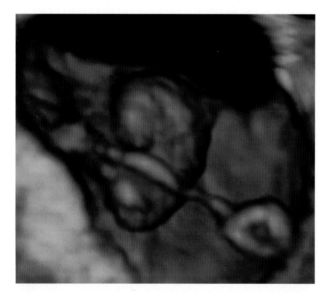

Figure 2.31 3D surface rendering demonstrating the embryo and yolk sac structure at 7 weeks of gestation. Note the whole length of the vitelline duct

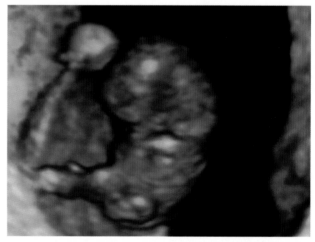

Figure 2.33 3D ultrasound image of an embryo at 7 weeks of gestation. Note the site of implantation in the uterine wall

lateral ventricles. The future foramina of Monroe are wide. In the sagittal plane, the height of the cavity of the diencephalon is slightly greater than that of the mesencephalon. Thus, a wide border between the cavities of the diencephalon and the mesencephalon can be seen. The curved tube-like mesencephalic cavity (the future Sylvian aqueduct) lies anterior, its

rostral part pointing caudally. It straightens considerably during the following weeks.

3D power Doppler findings

Besides the aorta and umbilical blood flow, at the end of the 7th week of gestation, 3D power Doppler

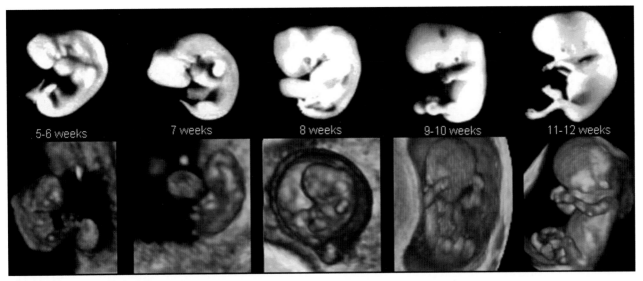

Figure 2.34 Comparison betwen a computer animation model of embryonic development and a series of in vivo images of the human embryo by 3D sonography, emphasizing the development of the embryo in early pregnancy (adapted, with permission, from: Azumendi G, Kurjak A, Andonotopo W, Arenas JB. Three dimensional sonoembryology. In: Kurjak A, Arenas JB, eds. Donald School Textbook of Transvaginal Sonography. London: Taylor and Francis, 2005: 396–407.[4]

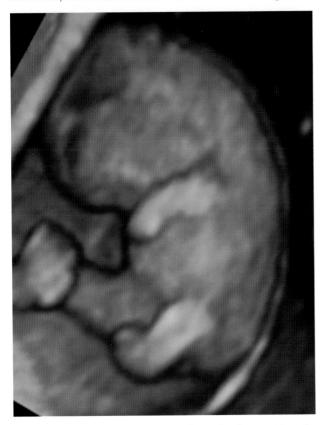

Figure 2.35 3D surface rendering from the fetus at 7 weeks of gestation showing the implantation site and the whole intra- and extra-amniotic structure

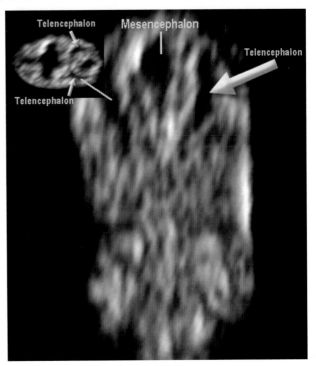

Figure 2.36 Development of the brain at 12 weeks of gestation. Brain structures such as the mesencephalon and telencephalon are visualized, the cerebral hemispheres dominate the brain, but the brain is still immature (from: Benoit B et al. Three-dimensional sonoembryology. J Perinat Med 2002; 30: 63–73)

depicts features of early vascular anatomy on the base of the skull. Vessels are evolving laterally to the mesencephalon and cephalic flexure. As well as the embryonic circulation, 3D power Doppler can obtain blood flow signals from the intervillous space. The gestational sac occupies about one-third of the uterine

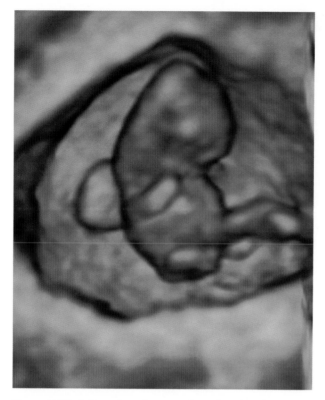

Figure 2.37 A 7-week embryo implanted within the uterus: the chorion (gestational sac) is covered by deciduas, and the embryo, located within the amniotic sac, is attached to the villous chorion by a thick umbilical cord

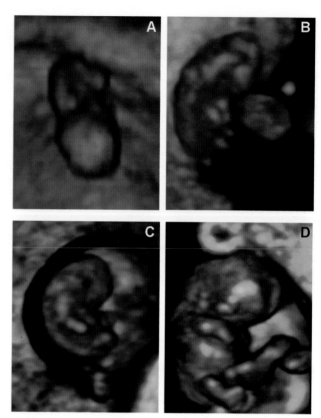

Figure 2.38 Chronological 3D images of embryonic development at (A) 5 weeks of gestation; (B) 6 weeks; (C) 7 weeks; (D) 8 weeks

volume. The main landmark now is an echogenic fetal pole consisting of the embryo adjacent to a cystic yolk sac. The intracranial circulation becomes visible during the 7th week of gestation. At this time, discrete pulsations of the internal carotid arteries are detectable at the base of the skull (Figure 2.39A).

8th week

Characteristic embryologic findings

By the beginning of the 8th week of gestation, the embryo has developed a skeleton, which is mostly cartilaginous and gives form to its body. The communication between the primitive gut and the yolk sac has been reduced to a relatively small duct (the yolk stalk).

3D ultrasound findings

The most characteristic finding is a complete visualization of the limbs, which end in thicker areas that correspond to the future hands and feet. The shape of

the face begins to appear, but is not clearly seen (Figures 2.38D, 2.42, and 2.43). The great majority of embryos show a cranial pole flexion that makes it almost impossible to see the face. Insertion of the umbilical cord is visible on the anterior abdominal wall. During the 8th week of gestation, there is expansion of the ventricular system of the brain (lateral, third, and midbrain ventricles). Due to these processes, the head erects from the anterior flexion. The vertex is now located over the position of the midbrain. The structures of the viscerocranium are not visible, because of their small size. During the 8th and 9th weeks, the developing intestine herniates into the proximal umbilical cord.

3D power Doppler findings

During the 8th week of gestation, the herniation of the intestine into the proximal umbilical cord can be assessed using this technique (see 3D power Doppler findings – 8th week). By the 8th week, the embryo is between 10 and 16 mm long, and the CRL can easily be measured. The rate of visualization of the fetal

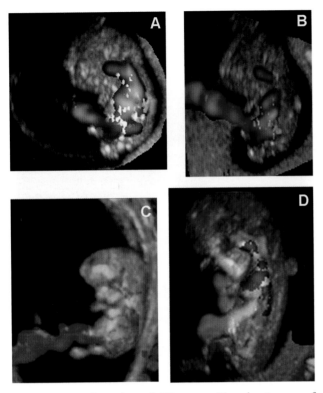

Figure 2.39 Chronological 3D power Doppler images of early development of fetal circulation: (A) 7 weeks of gestation; (B) 8 weeks; (C) 9 weeks; (D) 12 weeks

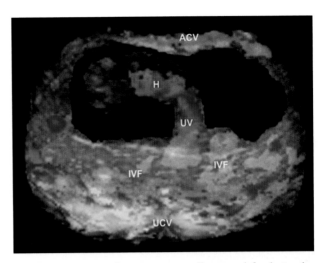

Figure 2.40 Uterochorionic, intervillous, and fetal circulation at 8 weeks of a normal pregnancy. UCV, uterochorionic (spiral and radial) vessels; IVF, intervillous blood flow; UV, umbilical vessels; H, heart; DV, ductus venosus; CV, cerebral vessels (from: Kurjak A et al. Structural and functional early human development assessed by three-dimensional and four-dimensional sonography. Fertil Steril 2005; 84: 1285–99)

aorta and umbilical artery is higher (Figures 2.39B and 2.40). Blood flow in the fetal heart and aorta as well as in the umbilical artery and intracranially is clearly visualized. At this stage of gestation, 3D power Doppler imaging allows visualization of the entire fetal circulation.

9th–10th weeks

Characteristic embryologic findings

The head is more rounded and constitutes almost half of the embryo (Figure 2.44B). The hands and feet approach each other. The upper limbs develop faster than the lower limbs, and toward the end of the 9th week, the fingers are almost entirely formed. The intestines are in the umbilical cord (physiologic midgut herniation).

3D ultrasound findings

Transvaginal 3D ultrasound produces remarkably well-defined facial images as early as 9 weeks of gestation. Sometimes, even the external ear can be depicted using

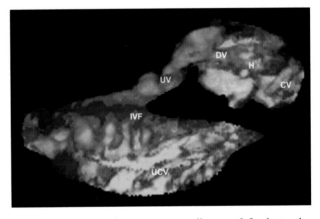

Figure 2.41 Uterochorionic, intervillous and fetal circulation at 10 weeks of a normal pregnancy. UCV, uterochorionic (spiral and radial) vessels; IVF, intervillous blood flow; UV, umbilical vessels; H, heart; DV, ductus venosus; ACV, antichorionic vessels (from: Kurjak A et al. Structural and functional early human development assessed by three-dimensional and four-dimensional sonography. Fertil Steril 2005; 84: 1285–99)

3D surface imaging. Herniation of the midgut is still present, as it is a consequence of the rapid growth of the bowel and liver before closure of the abdominal wall. Although this is a physiologic phenomenon, it does not appear in each fetus. Possibly, it cannot always be visualized, or else its size may vary. At 10 weeks of gestation, the bowel undergoes two turns of 180°,

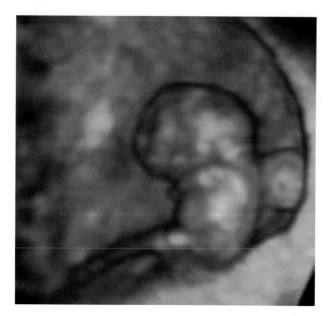

Figure 2.42 3D surface rendering of fetus at 8 weeks of gestation showing early limb bud structure and the whole length of the umbilical cord

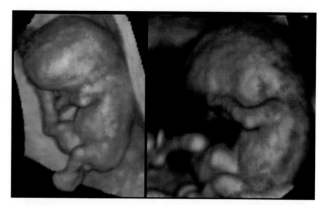

Figure 2.43 The whole body of the fetus at 8 weeks of gestation can be seen on 3D surface rendering

returning to its original position, at the same time that closure and development of the abdominal wall end. The cerebral hemispheres continue to develop during the 9th and 10th weeks of gestation. Lateral ventricles containing hyperechoic choroid plexuses are visible. The head is clearly divided from the body by the neck. The external ear is sometimes depicted in the 3D surface image. Herniation of the midgut is present. The dorsal column – the early spine – can be examined in its entire length. The arms with elbows and the legs with knees are clearly visible. The feet can be seen approaching the midline. The size of the lateral ventricles increases rapidly. While the third ventricle is still relatively wide at the beginning of the 9th week, its anteromedial part narrows due to the growth of the thalami. In the fetuses with CRL of 25 mm and more, there is a clear gap between the rhombencephalic and mesencephalic cavities due to the growing cerebellum. The isthmus rhombencephaly is narrow, and in most cases is not visible in its complete length. The cavity of the diencephalon decreases in larger fetuses (CRL 25 mm), and becomes narrow, especially at its upper anterior part. The spine is still characterized by two echogenic parallel lines.

3D power Doppler findings

Fetal structures are now clearly discernible, being represented by distinct parts of the fetal body – head,

trunk, and limbs. The head measures two-thirds of the entire body and becomes a distinct anatomic structure. The common and internal carotid arteries may be visualized at the end of the 8th week of gestation and the beginning of the 9th. A cerebral circulation (circle of Willis and its major branches) can be documented at 8 weeks in the form of discrete pulsations of the intracerebral part of the internal carotid artery. From the 9th week, arterial pulsations can be detected on transverse section, lateral to the mesencephalon and cephalic flexure (Figures 2.39C and 2.41).

11th week

Characteristic embryologic findings

The midgut herniation disappears. The fetal kidneys produce urine that is excreted into the amniotic fluid.

3D ultrasound findings

During the 11th week of gestation, development of the head and neck continues. Facial details such as nose, orbits, maxilla, and mandibles are often visible (Figures 2.44C, 2.50, and 2.51). The herniated midgut returns into the abdominal cavity. Its persistence after 11 weeks of gestation is suggestive of an omphalocele. Planar mode imaging enables detailed analysis of the embryonic body with visualization of the stomach and urinary bladder. Kidneys are often visible. The arms and legs continue to develop. During the 11th and 14th weeks of pregnancy, 3D ultrasound technique of measuring nuchal translucency has allowed a high rate of detection of chromosomal abnormalities (Figures 2.44–2.47). It has been possible to obtain the

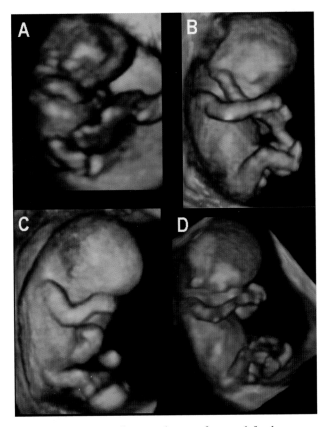

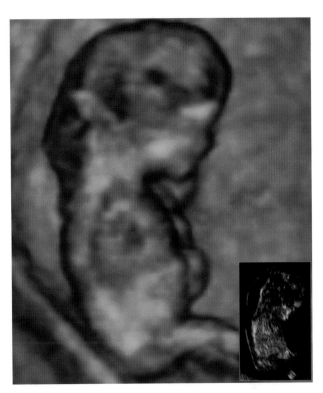

Figure 2.45 Early fetus depicted by 3D surface rendering at 11 weeks of gestation, showing increased nuchal translucency. Inset: 2D imaging of the same fetus

Figure 2.44 3D surface rendering of normal fetal appearance: (A) at 8–9 weeks of gestation; (B) at 10 weeks; (C) at 11 weeks; (D) at 12 weeks demonstrating completed morphologic development. The limbs are completely developed and their segments are discernible

midsagittal section and measure nuchal translucency using 3D transvaginal sonography. The ability of 3D ultrasound to distinguish between the nuchal region and the amnion will aid greatly in this very important screening examination. Transabdominal scanning is often a more reliable method for obtaining measurement of nuchal thickness because of the lack of flexibility of movement of the transvaginal probe in the vaginal vault.[1,3–5]

12th week

Characteristic embryologic findings

Fetal sex is clearly distinguishable by 12 weeks of gestation. The neck is well defined, the face is broad, and the eyes are widely separated. By the end of the 12th week, erythropoiesis decreases in the liver and begins in the spleen. The decidua capsularis adheres to the decidua parietalis.

3D ultrasound findings

Visualization by 3D ultrasound in the 12th week of gestation enables more detailed analysis of fetal anatomy, especially the limbs. It is possible to count fingers and toes. The growing cerebellum is clearly visible (Figure 2.36). The lateral ventricles dominate the brain.

3D power Doppler findings at the 11th and 12th weeks of gestation

With the use of 3D power Doppler, it is possible to depict major branches of the aorta: the common iliac and renal arteries. The circle of Willis and its branches are easily visible. From this week onwards, a more detailed anatomic survey can be obtained, including the cerebral and cardiovascular systems and the digestive and urinary tracts. At this stage, the pulsations of the middle cerebral artery can easily be discerned as a separate vessel. However, until the end of the 10th week of gestation, the ultrasonically detected vascular network should be called the intracranial circulation (Figure 2.39D). Until the end of the 1st trimester, the

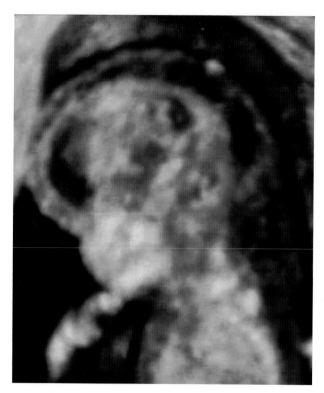

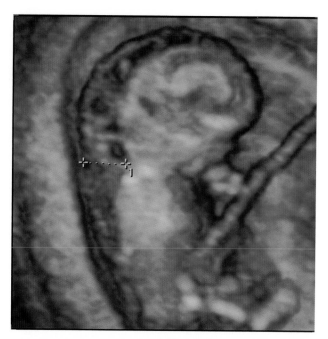

Figure 2.48 Increased nuchal translucency can be seen on 3D surface rendering in a fetus complicated by trisomy 21 at 12 weeks of gestation

Figure 2.46 Cystic hygroma of a fetus at 12 weeks of gestation complicated by Turner syndrome can be seen in the nuchal region by 3D imaging

absence of end-diastolic blood flow in fetal and placental components of the circulation is a normal physiologic finding.

DEVELOPMENT OF LIMBS, HEAD, AND FACE

The ability to visualize fetal hands, fingers, feet, and toes is better with 3D ultrasonography in the late 1st to 2nd trimester (Figures 2.49–2.94). Long bones can be visualized as hyperechoic elongated structures inside the upper and lower extremities. Detailed 3D analysis of the fetal spine, chest, and limbs is possible using the transparent, maximum mode (X-ray-like mode). With the use of the maximum mode, starting at 13 weeks, the medullar channel and each vertebra and rib can be visualized, and even the intervertebral disks can be measured (Figures 2.91–2.94). This opens unexpected possibilities for early diagnosis of skeletal malformations.[1,3,4]

The face can be identified with 3D transvaginal sonography by the 10th week of gestation (Figures 2.58–2.60). Detailed observation and evaluation of the fetal face can be obtained between the 19th and 24th weeks (Figures 2.61–2.66). 3D ultrasound enables spatial reconstruction, especially with the surface rendering mode. Integration of data obtained

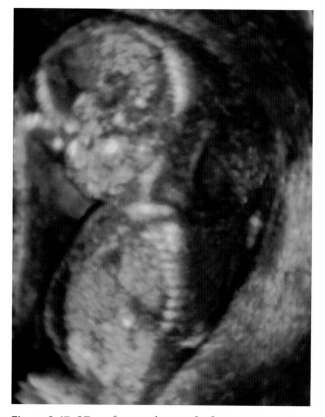

Figure 2.47 3D surface rendering of a fetus at 12 weeks of gestation complicated by cystic hygroma

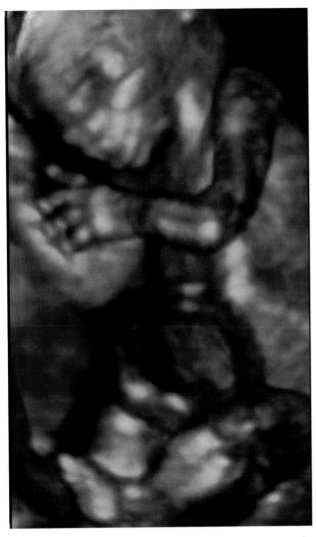

Figure 2.49 Normal appearance of the fetus at 13–14 weeks of gestation. Fetal morphologic development has already been completed

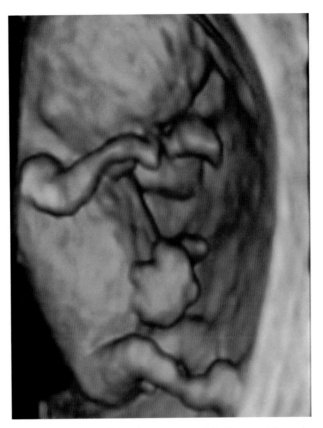

Figure 2.50 Normal hand structures of the fetus at 11 weeks of gestation, as seen by 3D ultrasound

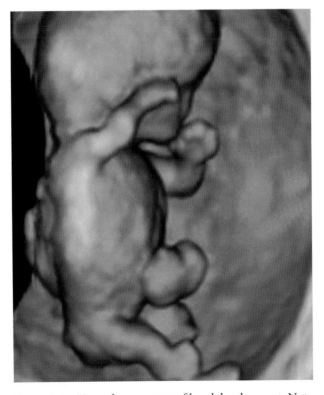

Figure 2.51 Normal appearance of hand development. Note the rotation of the head from the fetus at 11 weeks of gestation. The umbilical cord and feet are also discernible

by volume scanning can be used to depict a 3D plastic ('sculpture-like') reconstruction of the region of interest. Visualization of the fetal face has become one of the main applications of 3D ultrasound scanning. More details of normal and abnormal facial anatomy become available. The surface-rendered image depicts the entire face and the relationship between facial structures (e.g. nostrils, eyelids, and mouth) on a single image (Figures 2.67–2.72). Depiction and observation of the orbital region and the status of fetal eyelids (open versus closed), can easily be performed in this mode. Assessment of facial structures may be useful to detect common abnormalities such as unilateral/bilateral cleft lip (Figures 2.70 and 2.71).[1,3–5] Multiplanar imaging allows detailed examination of fetal shape and anatomic structure. Any lack of cranial

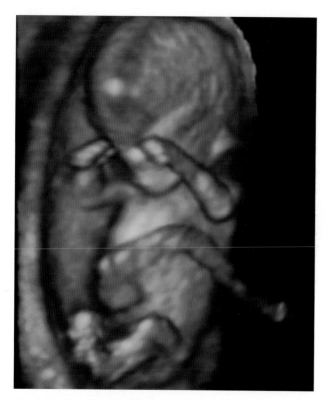

Figure 2.52 Hand-to-face movement of the fetus at 12 weeks of gestation. Spatial reconstruction of the face and hand enables determination of the end of the movement in a 3D perspective

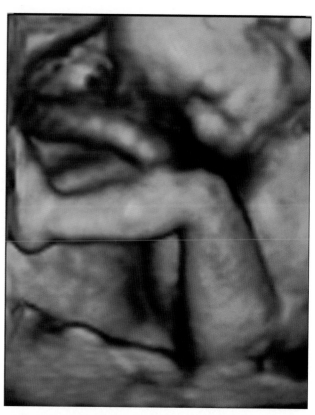

Figure 2.54 Normal morphologic anatomy of the fetus at 20 weeks of gestation as seen by 3D imaging

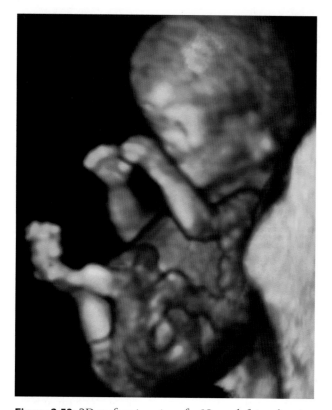

Figure 2.53 3D surface imaging of a 13-week fetus showing hand-to-face movement

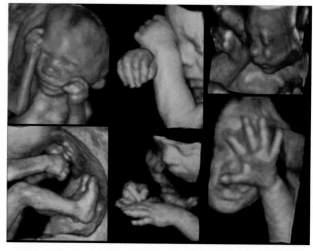

Figure 2.55 Normal appearance of the fetal face at 20–25 weeks of gestation. Note the distinct morphologic structure of the face and extremities

development can be discovered. Surface or maximum rendering can depict an abnormal form of the cranium or the complete absence of development of calvarian bones (Figure 2.72). Other anomalies such as holoprosencephaly, are frequently connected with

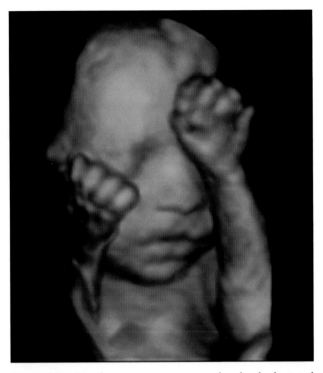

Figure 2.56 Hand-to-eye movement can be clearly depicted by 3D surface rendering

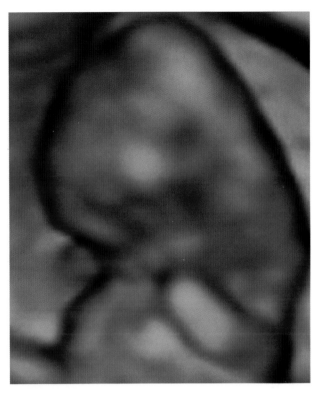

Figure 2.58 Normal appearance of early development of the fetal face on 3D surface rendering

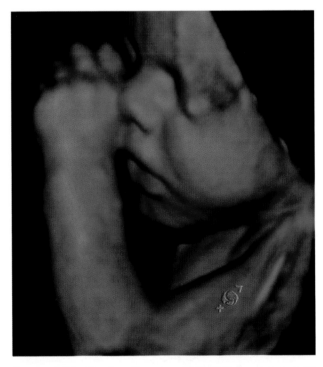

Figure 2.57 Hand-to-face movement of the fetus at 25 weeks of gestation can be seen by 3D imaging. Note the clear visualization of facial structure using 3D surface imaging

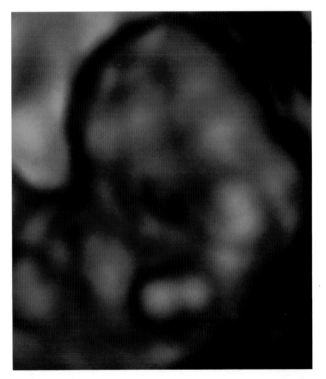

Figure 2.59 Face of an 8-week embryo: the cerebral hemispheres, the mesencephalon, the eye, the nose, the mouth, and the external ear with adjacent otic capsule are depicted. The hand exhibits early digital tubercles demonstrated by 3D surface rendering

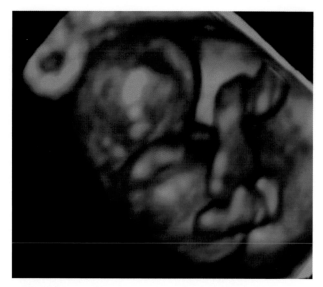

Figure 2.60 Early development of the facial anatomy of the fetus at 8 weeks of gestation. We cannot observe a clear facial structure in this period using 3D imaging

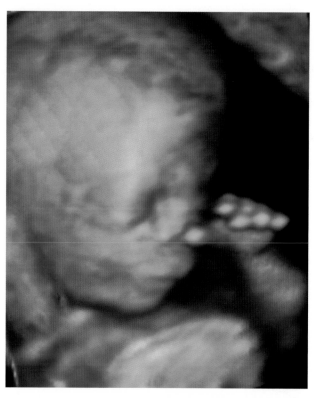

Figure 2.62 Fetus at 13–14 weeks of gestation demonstrating clear visualization of all facial structures

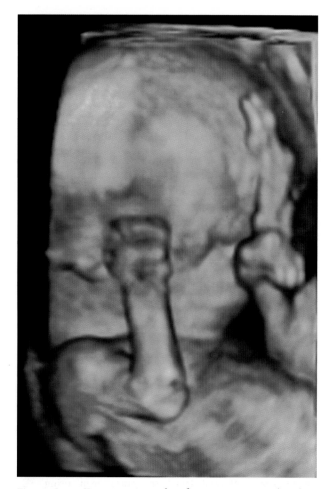

Figure 2.61 Fetus at 13 weeks of gestation. Note the clear visualization of facial structures, including nose, eyes, ear, and cranial sutures

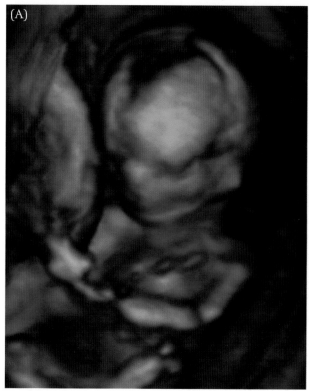

Figure 2.63 Normal appearances of facial structures of the fetus at (A) 15 weeks of gestation

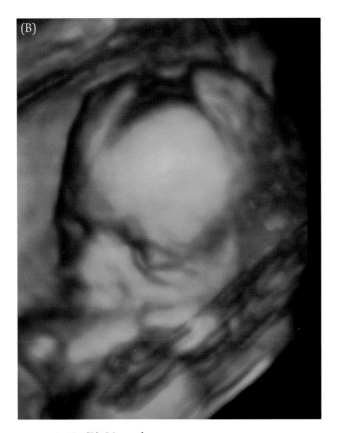

Figure 2.63 (B) 20 weeks

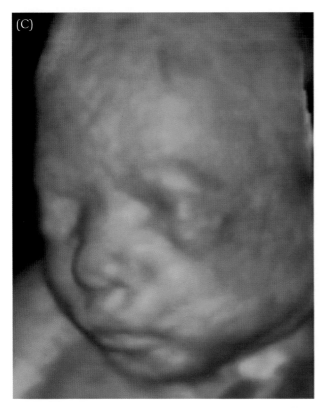

Figure 2.63 (C) 27 weeks. Note that the major fontanel can be clearly seen by 3D imaging

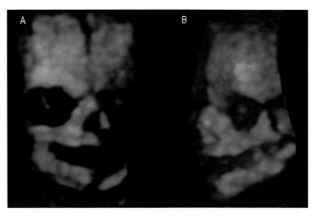

Figure 2.64 By using 3D maximum mode, we can observe the complete bone structure distinctly. This technique provides the possibility of a complete assessment of early anomalies in structural development

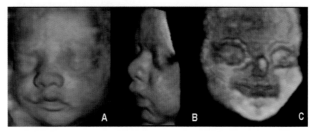

Figure 2.65 Assessment of fetal facial structures using two different techniques of 3D imaging. (A) Fetal facial anatomy from the surface mode. (B) Semiprofile anatomy. (C) Fetal facial anatomy from the inverse mode – we can assess the internal structure behind the external facial structure using this technique

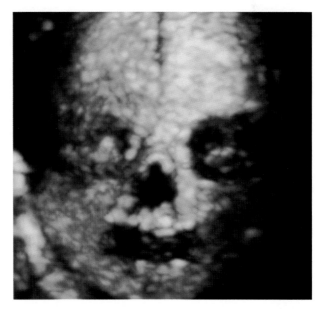

Figure 2.66 Normal facial structures seen using 3D maximum mode. This mode gives an 'X-ray' impression of the bony structures without any exposure of the fetus to radiation

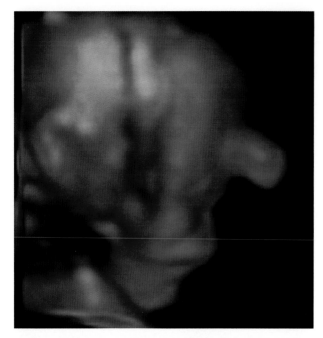

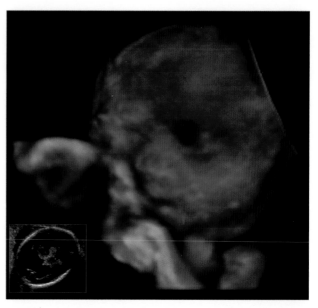

Figure 2.69 Abnormal visualization of the face in a fetus affected by holoprosencephaly (inset). Note that the hypertelorism and rounded fetal face due to scalp edema can be clearly depicted by 3D surface imaging

Figure 2.67 Fetus at 16 weeks of gestation demonstrating proboscis related to trisomy 13 depicted by 3D surface rendering

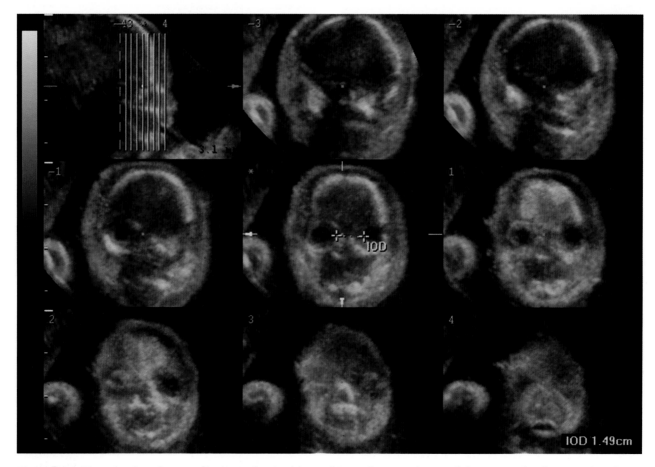

Figure 2.68 Tomographic ultrasound imaging demonstrating abnormal measurement of the intraocular diameter (IOD) in a case of holoprosencephaly. Note the hypertelorism and the scalp edema in this fetus

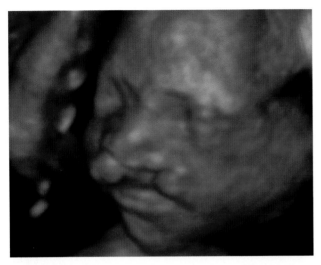

Figure 2.70 Bilateral cleft lip present in a 25-week fetus depicted by 3D surface rendering

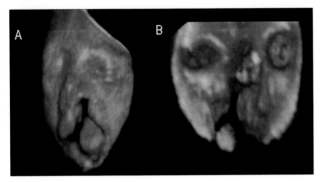

Figure 2.71 Assessment of fetal facial structures using two different techniques of 3D imaging. (A) Fetal facial anatomy from the surface mode in a case of unilateral cleft palate. (B) Fetal facial anatomy of the same fetus using the inverse mode

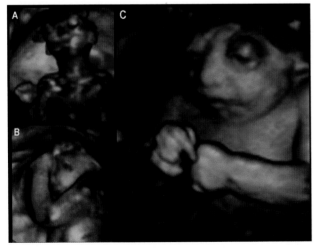

Figure 2.72 Abnormal appearances from an anencephalic fetus seen at (A) 16 weeks of gestation; (B) 26 weeks; (C) 30 weeks. Note that the destruction of the head structure can be seen clearly using 3D imaging

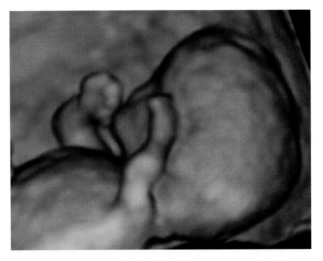

Figure 2.73 Anterior limb of the fetus at 11 weeks of gestation depicted by 3D imaging

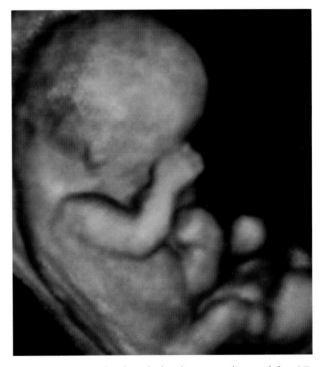

Figure 2.74 Early digital development depicted by 3D imaging at 10 weeks of gestation

serious facial malformations (e.g., cleft lip and palate, severe hypotelorism and cyclopia, and arrhinia with proboscis), and also can be found in some aneuploidies (usually trisomies 13 and 18) (Figures 2.67–2.71). A frontal monoventricle is present in semilobar holoprosencephaly, and there is posterior partial formation of the occipital lobes. In lobar holoprosencephaly, the hemispheres may be fused and the lateral ventricles may communicate extensively because of

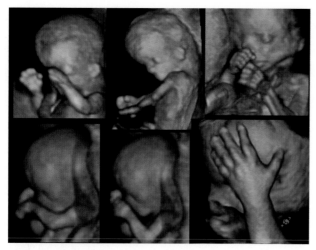

Figure 2.75 Several hand positions clearly depicted by 3D imaging. The anatomy of each digit can be seen clearly using this technique

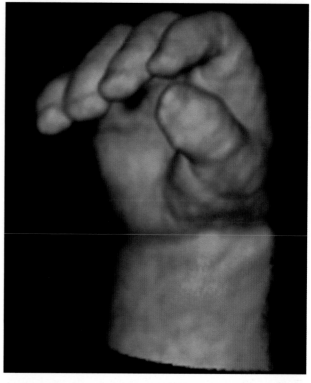

Figure 2.77 3D imaging demonstrating the anatomic structure of the fetal fingers

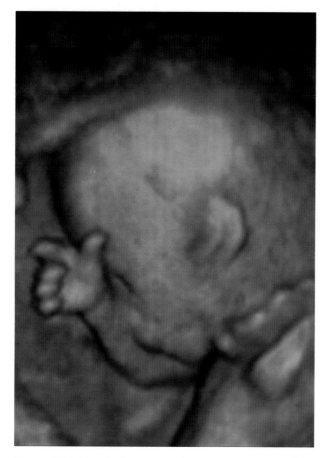

Figure 2.76 Clearly differentiated anatomic structure of the fingers at 14 weeks of gestation shown by 3D imaging

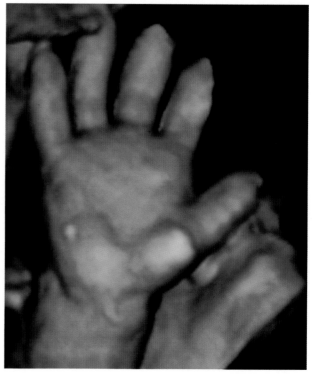

Figure 2.78 Fetal hand with differentiated fingers seen by 3D imaging

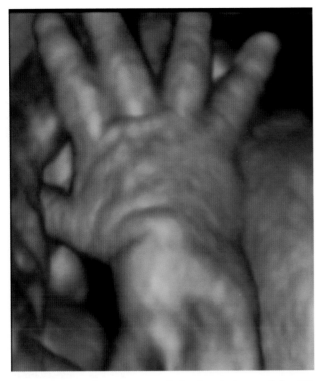

Figure 2.79 The anatomy of the hand depicted by 3D imaging from a fetus at 30 weeks of gestation

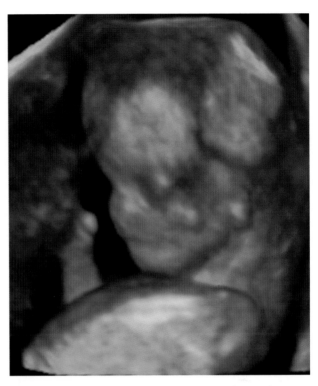

Figure 2.81 Details of the head skeleton and cranial sutures can be depicted by 3D surface imaging

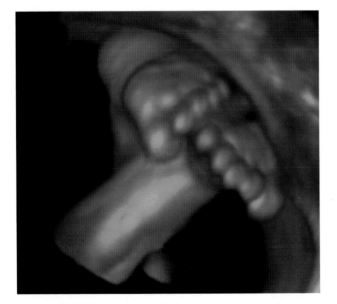

Figure 2.80 The anatomy of the fetal toes can be depicted clearly by 3D imaging

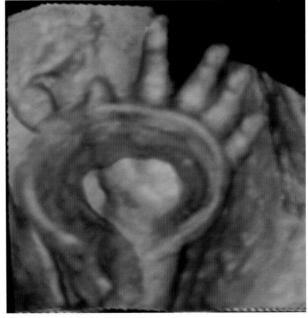

Figure 2.82 Hand structures with fingers can be seen clearly by 3D imaging. Note that the umbilical cord is lying side to side with the palm

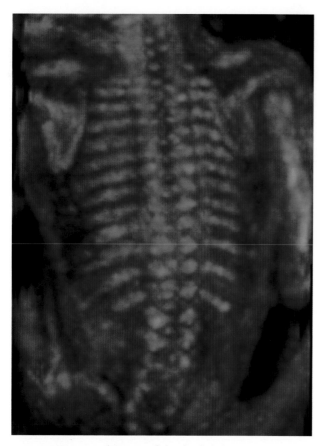

Figure 2.83 Visualization of the fetal skeleton at 20 weeks of gestation by 3D maximum mode

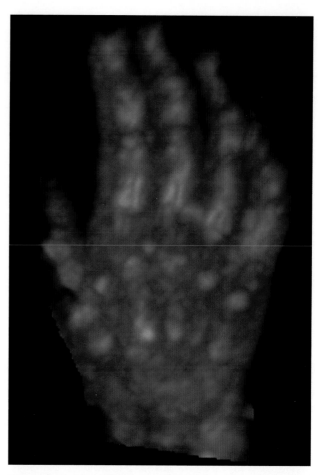

Figure 2.85 Normal appearance of an ossifying fetal hand seen by 3D maximum mode

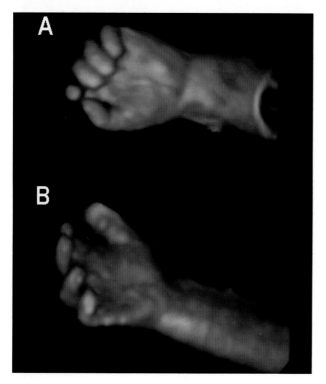

Figure 2.84 Normal anatomy of the fetal hand at 20 weeks of gestation

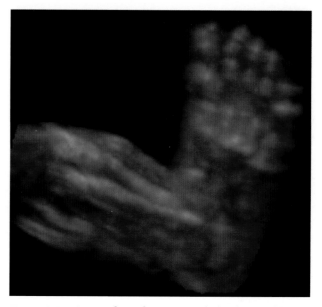

Figure 2.86 An ossifying foot can easily be depicted by 3D maximum mode. At the same time, we can observe the normal appearance of the structures of the extremities

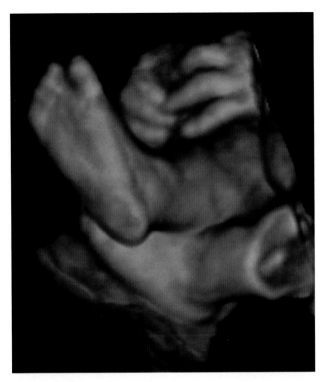

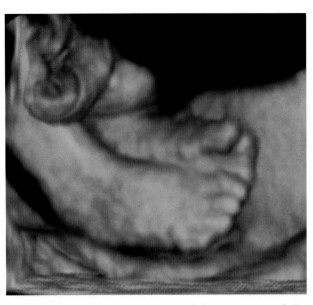

Figure 2.89 Normal appearance of the structures of the lower extremities from a fetus at 25 weeks of gestation

Figure 2.87 Normal appearances of upper and lower extremities from a fetus at 25 weeks of gestation

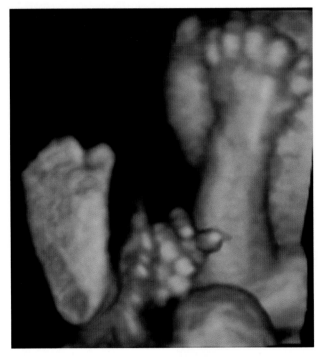

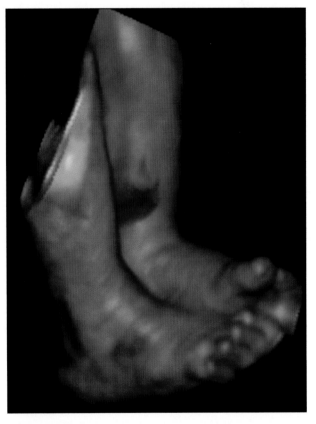

Figure 2.88 All structures from the hands, fingers, and foot are clearly visualized by 3D imaging

Figure 2.90 Normal appearance of the fetal foot at 25 weeks of gestation

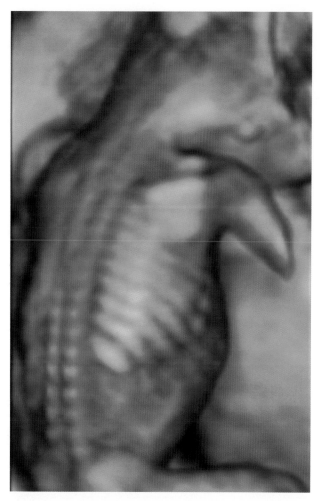

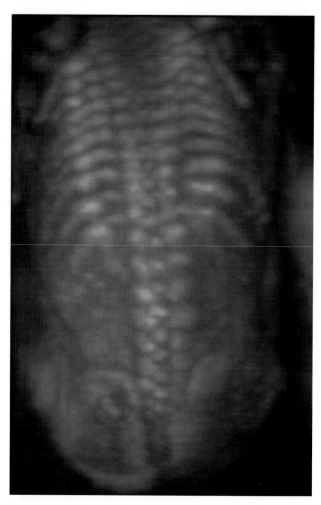

Figure 2.91 3D surface rendering of the dorsal side of the fetus showing the whole structure of the vertebrae

Figure 2.92 The fetal vertebrae as seen by 3D maximum mode

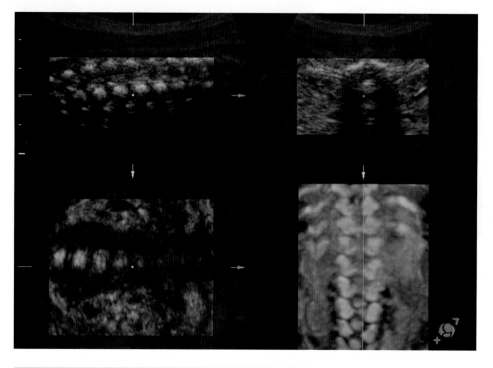

Figure 2.93 Normal structure of the fetal vertebrae at 28 weeks of gestation

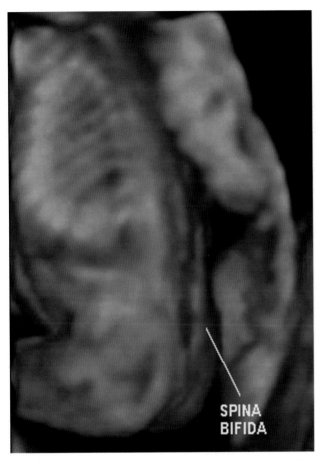

Figure 2.94 Fetal vertebral structure complicated by spina bifida from a fetus at 28 weeks of gestation

the absence of the septum pellucidum. Due to severe interruption of the normal intracranial anatomy, ultrasound diagnosis of holoprosencephaly can be made at the end of the 1st trimester. Absence of a normally developed telencephalon including hyperechoic choroid plexi, frontally positioned monoventricle, and facial anomaly (severe hypotelorism) are characteristics that should be sufficient for diagnosis. 3D sonography enables careful and precise analysis of anatomic features in very early pregnancy, making the diagnostic process accurate and fast.[1,3-5]

FETAL BLOOD CIRCULATION (FIGURES 2.95–2.101)

3D imaging can be used to diagnose abnormal and normal anatomy. Newer techniques for examination of the fetal heart have allowed the problem of shadowing and motion artifacts to be overcome through real-time 3D imaging. It is likely that dynamic multiplanar

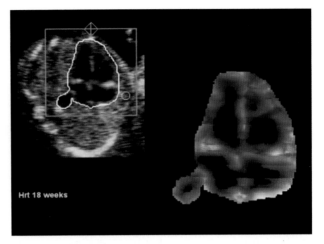

Figure 2.95 Simultaneous 2D and 3D rendering of the atria, ventricles, mitral valve, tricuspid valve, foramen ovale, and right ventricular moderator band. Gestational age is 18 weeks. Segmentation allows removal of surrounding structures (from: Kurjak A, Jackson D, eds. An Atlas of Three- and Four-Dimensional Sonography in Obstetrics and Gynecology. London: Taylor and Francis, 2004, with permission)

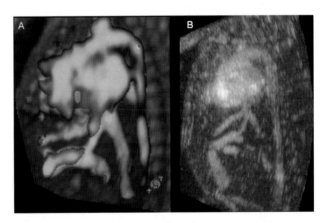

Figure 2.96 Visualization of cardiac anatomy using two different techniques: (A) glassbody mode; (B) B-flow mode. Note that the whole length of the aortic arch can be visualized clearly

and volume surface rendering of the fetal heart will be the technical future of fetal echocardiography. Fetal heart volumes are acquired with a single automated sweep of a mechanical transducer, and the cardiac cycle frames are merged into one volume dataset. Each represents the fetal heart during a single beat.[3,4] For further details, see Chapter 10.

Doppler ultrasound using a 3D technique enables visualization of the great vessels. Whether this information adds significantly to management is under investigation. This technique has been found to be

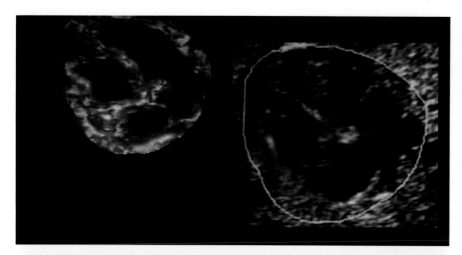

Figure 2.97 A 29-week four-chamber view with 3D rapid volume assessment. No gating was involved. Motion artifacts are minimized when thin slices are utilized for volume rendering (from: Kurjak A, Jackson D, eds. An Atlas of Three- and Four-Dimensional Sonography in Obstetrics and Gynecology. London: Taylor and Francis, 2004, with permission)

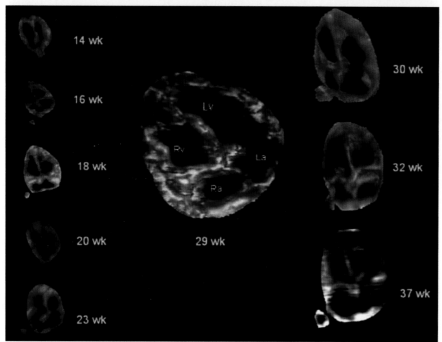

Figure 2.98 Transabdominal 3D rendering of the four-chamber view is feasible. LV, left ventricle; RV, right ventricle; La, left atrium; Ra, right atrium (from: Kurjak A, Jackson D, eds. An Atlas of Three- and Four-Dimensional Sonography in Obstetrics and Gynecology. London: Taylor and Francis, 2004, with permission)

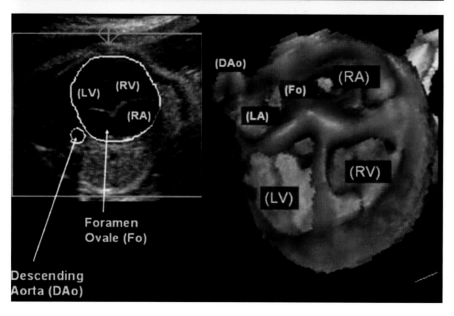

Figure 2.99 Four-chamber view. The acquisition of information regarding valves and outflow tract orientation becomes easier with practice. LV, left ventricle, RV, right ventricle; LA, left atrium; RA, right atrium (from: Kurjak A, Jackson D, eds. An Atlas of Three- and Four-Dimensional Sonography in Obstetrics and Gynecology. London: Taylor and Francis, 2004, with permission)

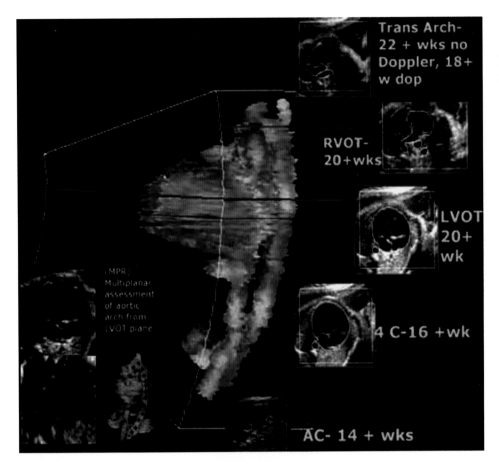

Figure 2.100 Gestational ages with near-100% visualization of each component plane using 3D and 4D technology. The five primary axial planes that provide the information necessary for the axial cardiac screening index (abdominal circumference, four-chambers, left ventricular outflow tract (LVOT), right ventricular outflow tract (RVOT), transverse arches) are augmented by multiplanar sagittal rendering of the aortic arch (from: Kurjak A, Jackson D, eds. An Atlas of Three- and Four-Dimensional Sonography in Obstetrics and Gynecology. London: Taylor and Francis, 2004, with permission)

rapid, and capable of producing elegant images of the heart and great vessels – even the prenatal diagnosis of the right aortic arc with vascular ring can be clearly depicted (Figure 2.101).[3,4]

SEX DIFFERENTIATION (FIGURES 2.102–2.115)

Prenatal determination of fetal gender by ultrasound during the 2nd and 3rd trimesters of pregnancy is based on demonstration of the presence and size of a penis in the male and of labial folds in the female. However, there is no appreciable difference in the size of the penis and the clitoris until after 14 weeks of gestation. There is some evidence that in the early 2nd trimester, fetal gender can be accurately predicted by assessment of the direction in which the genital tubercle points (cranial for males and caudal for females) and also by the sagittal sign, whereby examination of the genital region in the midline sagittal plane demonstrates a caudal notch in females and a cranial notch in males.

The structural precursors of the external genitalia are present, but are not sufficiently differentiated to

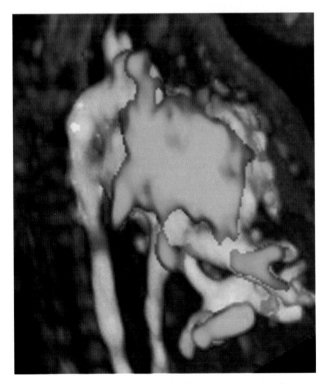

Figure 2.101 3D power Doppler fetal angiography demonstrating complete vascularization from the heart to the upper and lower parts of the body

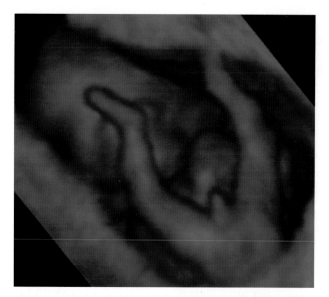

Figure 2.102 Visualization of an early male fetus at 15 weeks of gestation

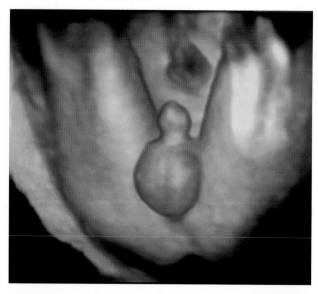

Figure 2.104 Male external genitalia can be depicted clearly by 3D imaging

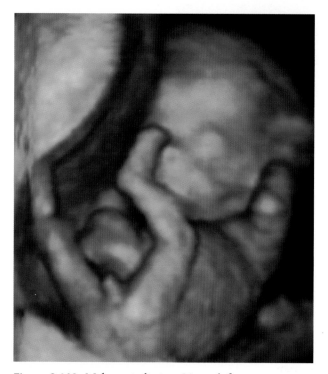

Figure 2.103 Male genitalia in a 20-week fetus

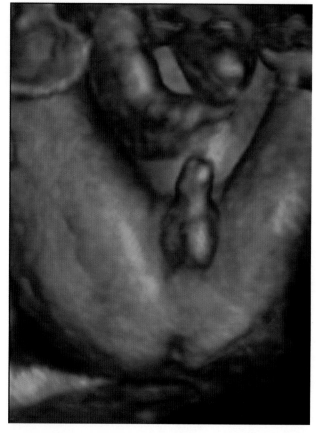

Figure 2.105 Anatomy of male external genitalia depicted by 3D imaging at 28 weeks of gestation

make a clear distinction on examination of the genitalia until after 10 weeks of gestation. However, from 12 weeks, there are distinct changes in the structure of the urogenital sinus. A process of gender-specific changes takes place. In males, the urogenital sinus is replaced by the scrotal and urethral raphe; closure of the urogenital sinus takes place in a zip-like

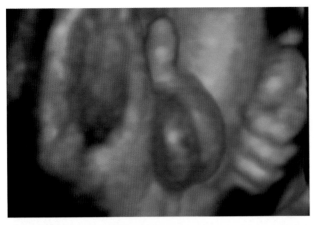

Figure 2.106 3D surface rendering of the external male genitalia demonstrating the anatomic structures at 30 weeks of gestation

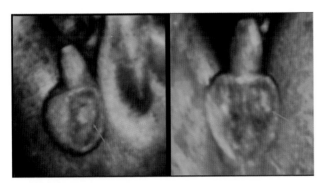

Figure 2.107 3D surface rendering of testicular structures (red arrow)

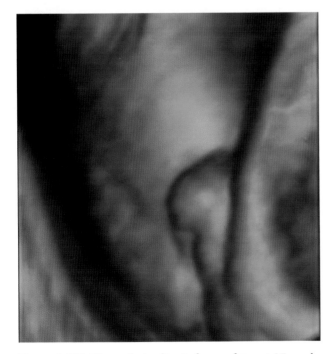

Figure 2.108 Hyperplasia clitoris from a fetus at 27 weeks of gestation as seen by 3D surface imaging

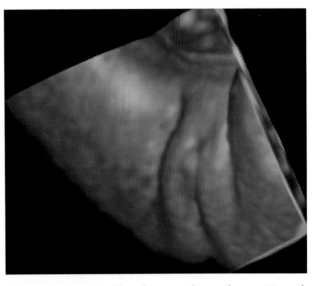

Figure 2.109 Normal female external genitalia in a 26-week fetus depicted by 3D imaging

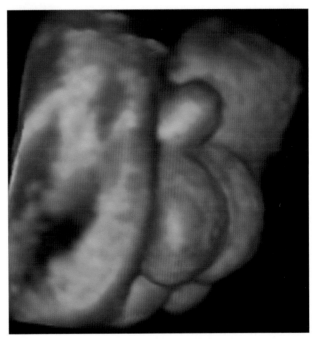

Figure 2.110 External male genitalia at 26 weeks of gestation. Note the clear anatomic structure of the penis and scrotum

fashion, starting from the caudal end of the embryo. This process, combined with elongation of the genital tubercle, gradually displaces the phallus in a rostral direction. In the female, the urogenital sinus remains open and ultimately becomes the vestibule of the vagina. Significant differences in the rate of penile and clitoral growth become evident in the 2nd trimester;

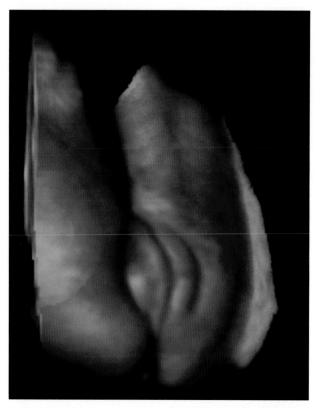

Figure 2.111 Normal appearance of the labial fold from a female fetus at 27 weeks of gestation seen by 3D imaging

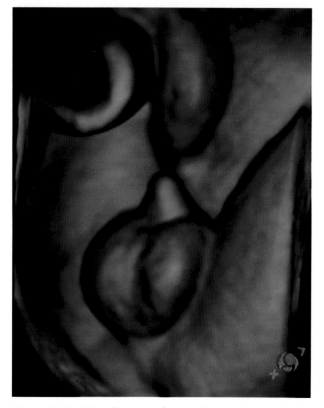

Figure 2.112 Visualization of normal external genitals of a male fetus by 3D imaging

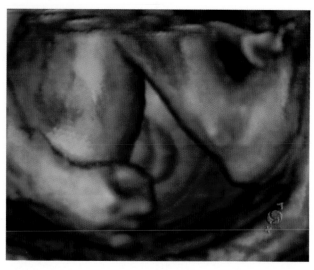

Figure 2.113 Visualization of normal external genitalia of a female fetus by 3D imaging

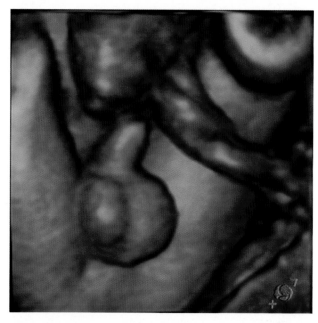

Figure 2.114 Visualization of external male genitalia by 3D surface imaging

the majority of prenatal growth of the penis occurs after 14 weeks of gestation at an almost linear rate.

One of the advantages of 3D ultrasound is that information can be extracted from the stored volume of data in innumerable planes, regardless of the fetal position during acquisition. 3D ultrasound allows saved volume data to be displayed in a multiplanar array, which can be rotated in order to display the image in standard anatomic orientations. These advantages of 3D give us the possibility to assess fetal genitalia in order to determine whether fetal gender

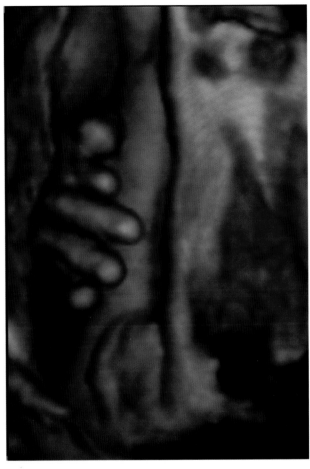

Figure 2.115 Normal appearance of external female genitalia by 3D surface rendering

could be determined from volumes that were not obtained specifically for that purpose.[1,3,4]

CONCLUSIONS

Recent improvements in 3D ultrasound permit detailed observation of the morphology of the early conceptus in utero as clearly as seen by embryofetoscopy and from microscopic specimens. It is possible to use the term 'sonoembryology' for the delineation and observation of all fetal structures as early as at the beginning of the 6th week of gestation. 3D ultrasound has produced more objective and accurate information on embryonic and early fetal development, predominantly for non-invasive assessment of fetal anatomy. Presenting volume data in a standard anatomic orientation gives valuable assistance in recognition of anatomic details. 3D ultrasound is helpful in studying normal embryonic and fetal development, as well as in providing information for families at risk for specific congenital anomalies by confirming normality. This method offers advantages in assessing the embryo in the 1st trimester due to its ability to obtain multiplanar images through volume acquisition.

REFERENCES

1. Benoit B, Hafner T, Kurjak A, et al. Three-dimensional sonoembryology. J Ultrasound Med 2002; 21: 1063–7.

2. Kupesic S. The first three weeks assessed by transvaginal color Doppler. J Perinat Med 1996; 24: 301–17.

3. Andonotopo W, Kurjak A, Azumendi G. Early normal pregnancy. In: Carrera JM, Kurjak A, eds. Atlas of Clinical Application of Ultrasound in Obstetrics and Gynecology. New Delhi: Jaypee Brothers Medical Publishers, 2006: 25–50.

4. Azumendi G, Kurjak A, Andonotopo W, Arenas JB. Three dimensional sonoembriology. In: Kurjak A, Arenas JB, eds. Donald School Textbook of Transvaginal Sonography. London: Taylor and Francis, 2005: 396–407.

5. Kurjak A, Pooh RK, Merce LT, et al. Structural and functional early human development assessed by three-dimensional and four-dimensional sonography. Fertil Steril 2005; 84: 1285–99.

3 Early pregnancy failure

Asim Kurjak, Wiku Andonotopo, and Bernat Serra

INTRODUCTION

Early pregnancy failure is defined as a pregnancy that ends spontaneously before the embryo has reached a viable gestational age detectable by ultrasound. The most common pathologic symptom of early pregnancy failure is vaginal bleeding. When vaginal bleeding occurs, any clinician should ask several questions that can radically alter the management: Is the patient pregnant? Is the embryo viable or not? What is the gestational age? Is there any evidence to suggest that the pregnancy is ectopic? If a miscarriage occurs, is it complete or incomplete? Is there any associated pelvic mass? Accurate estimation of the embryo/fetus status make it possible to apply appropriate therapeutic measures to cases where a normal outcome of the pregnancy can be expected. At present, sonography is considered to be the best diagnostic method for detection of early pregnancy complications. For these patients, the skill of the sonographer is very important, since accurate diagnosis of pregnancy failure will often result in surgical intervention.

Clinical presentation of symptoms such as vaginal bleeding and abdominal pain, with or without expulsion of the products of conception, arouse suspicion of a spontaneous miscarriage. For ultrasound evaluation, it is important to distinguish between threatened, complete, and incomplete miscarriage.

Ultrasound has revolutionized our knowledge of early human development due to its superb depicting capability. Development of modern sensitive two-dimensional (2D) color Doppler ultrasound systems has enabled the assessment and investigation of hemodynamic changes related to the process of placentation.[1–17]

Three-dimensional (3D) power Doppler depicts an integral 3D image of the placenta and embryo and their vascular network.[18] Additionally, it is possible to quantify and numerically express data related to vascular signals in the investigated volume. In this chapter, we present our data on 3D power Doppler assessment of placental, yolk sac, and embryonic/fetal circulation in early pregnancy failure.

ANATOMY OF EARLY PREGNANCY

For a better understanding of early pregnancy, it is useful to summarize some anatomic and physiologic issues in early pregnancy. The exocelomic cavity (ECC) is the largest anatomic space inside the gestational sac between 5 and 9 weeks of gestation[19,20] (Figure 3.1). Development of the ECC is intimately

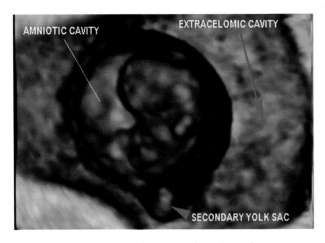

Figure 3.1 Transvaginal image of an 8-week pregnancy demonstrating the exocelomic cavity, amniotic cavity, and secondary yolk sac

linked with that of the secondary yolk sac (SYS), for which it provides a stable environment. The SYS degenerates spontaneously at around 9–10 weeks, when fetal metanephros starts functioning and producing urine, which is passed into the amniotic cavity.[19,20] Subsequently, with accumulation of this fluid, the amniotic membrane moves towards the fetal plate of the placenta, and the ECC will almost entirely disappear by 12–13 weeks of gestation.

The development of transvaginal sonography (TVS)-guided sampling procedures has allowed direct access to the embryonic fluid cavities. Protein electrophoresis has shown that the celomic fluid results from an ultrafiltrate of maternal serum with the addition of specific placental and SYS bioproducts.[21] The higher concentrations of human chorionic gonadotropin (hCG), estradiol, estriol, and proges-terone[22] in the celomic fluid than in maternal serum strongly suggest the presence of a direct pathway between the trophoblast and the ECC. Morphologically, this may be via the villous stromal channels and the loose mesenchymal tissue of the ECC. These findings suggest that the ECC is a physi-ologic liquid extension of the early placenta, and an important interface in fetal nutritional pathways.[19–21]

Uteroplacental circulation

Doppler ultrasound has been extensively used to study the normal development of the placental circulation. The various branches of the uterine circulation can be differentiated by means of color Doppler imaging, and the overall Doppler mapping features correlate well with the anatomic findings.[14,15] In non-pregnant women and during the first half of a normal pregnancy, flow velocity waveforms (FVWs) from the main uterine arteries are characterized by a well-defined protodiastolic 'notch'. End-diastolic frequencies increase in the main uterine arteries and their branches during the second half of the menstrual cycle, and this increase continues as pregnancy advances.[14,15] In 85% of pregnancies, the protodiastolic notch disappears before 20 weeks of gestation, probably reflecting the end of the implantation process and its associated physiologic changes. Blood flow in the radial and spiral arteries is characterized in pregnancy by a low-imped-ance irregular flow pattern that shows no significant changes in shape throughout pregnancy (Figure 3.2).

Overall changes in FVWs reflect a progressive decrease in the downstream resistance to blood flow in the uterine circulation from implantation to term.[23,24] This decrease can be observed in all segments of the uterine circulation. Impedance to blood flow through the spiral arteries in the 2nd trimester is lower in the central area of the placental bed than in peripheral areas. These Doppler data are in agreement with anatomic data that have demonstrated that the uterine vascular network elongates and dilates steadily throughout pregnancy.[25] These changes are required to allow the spiral arteries to increase their rate of blood flow from a few milliliters per minute in the non-pregnant state to approximately 700 ml/min at term.[26]

The most striking of the anatomic transformations related to placentation is observed at the level of the maternal spiral arteries. This transformation results in the metamorphosis of small-caliber, vasoreactive spiral vessels into flaccid, distended uteroplacental arteries. The architecture of their decidual and myometrial segments is disrupted by the loss of myocytes from the media and the internal elastic lamina, which are progressively replaced by fibrinoid.[27,28] These physio-logic changes only occur in the presence of trophoblast cells,[29] and can first be found both within and around the spiral arteries in the placental area. They gradually extend laterally, reaching the periphery of the placenta around midgestation, corroborating the Doppler findings. Depthwise, the changes normally extend as far as the inner third of the myometrium within the central region of the placental bed, but the extent of invasion is progressively shallower towards the periphery. Therefore, even in normal pregnancies, not all the arteries are completely transformed.[30]

ULTRASOUND AND THE PATHOPHYSIOLOGY OF EARLY PREGNANCY FAILURE

Human placentation is more complex than that of other mammalian species, including the higher primates. Abnormalities of placentation are associated with diseases that are almost unique to the human species, such as pre-eclampsia or hydatidiform mole, or are rare in other species, such as miscarriage.[19]

Abnormally high or rapidly fluctuating concentra-tions of oxygen have potentially harmful effects on tissue and in particular on trophoblastic tissue. There is increasing evidence to indicate that failure of placen-tation is associated with an imbalance in reactive oxygen species (ROS), which will further affect

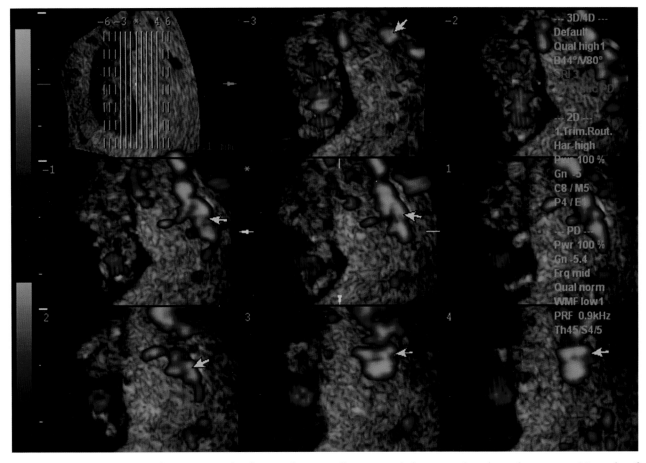

Figure 3.2 Demonstration of power Doppler flow in the intervillous space (white arrow) and spiral arteries at 10 weeks of gestation using tomographic ultrasound imaging (TUI)

placental development and function and may subsequently have an influence on both the fetus and the mother. Maternal metabolic disorders, such as diabetes, which are associated with an increased production of ROS, are also known to be associated with a higher incidence of miscarriage and fetal structural defects.[31] Furthermore, the teratogenicity of drugs such as thalidomide has been shown to involve ROS-mediated oxidative damage,[32] indicating that the human fetus can be irreversibly damaged by oxidative stress. These findings suggest that fetal development is highly sensitive to disruption by ROS, and hence maintaining a low-oxygen environment inside the human uterus during early pregnancy may confer protection.

Implantation

There is increasing evidence showing an association between miscarriage and an anomaly of one of the enzymes involved in the metabolism of ROS.[33,34] These findings suggest that early pregnancy failure can be due to a primary defect of placentation involving a genetic anomaly of the enzymes or cofactor involved in the oxygen metabolism. Data on the role of uterine glands in early fetal nutrition[35,36] suggest that insufficient decidualization could also have an impact on placentation. These glands remain active until at least the 10th week of gestation, and their secretions are delivered freely into the placental intervillous space. An endometrial thickness of 8 mm or more is considered to be favorable for embryo implantation.[37] Both adequate endometrial thickness and vascularization are needed for implantation, and women with adequate endometrial thickness on ultrasound but poor intraendometrial blood flow tend to have poor reproductive outcome.[38] It has been suggested that uterine arterial impedance plays an important role in endometrial receptivity prior to implantation. Delay in decrease of the uterine arterial resistance may result in impaired endometrial function and recurrent

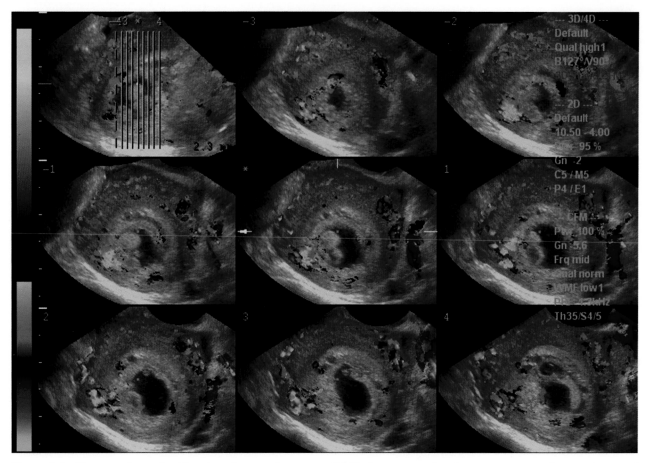

Figure 3.3 Tomographic color Doppler ultrasound imaging (TUI) demonstrated early miscarriage with premature and widespread maternal blood flow

miscarriage.[39–41] Doppler assessment of the uterine vasculature may be useful in determining optimal endometrial receptiveness in assisted reproduction cycles.[42]

Miscarriage and placental blood flow

There is substantial anatomic evidence that in the majority of pregnancy complications (i.e., spontaneous miscarriage and pre-eclampsia) a defect in early trophoblast invasion and a failure to convert the spiral arteries into low-resistance channels occur.[42–47] In about two-thirds of early pregnancy failures, there is anatomic evidence of defective placentation, which is mainly characterized by a thinner and fragmented trophoblast shell, and reduced cytotrophoblast invasion of the lumen at the tips of the spiral arteries.[45] This is associated with premature onset of the maternal circulation throughout the placenta in most cases of miscarriage.[43,48,49] These defects are similar in euploid and most aneuploid miscarriages, but are more pronounced in triploid partial moles. In complete hydatidiform mole, the extravillous trophoblast invasion into the decidua and superficial myometrium is almost entirely absent.[50] The syncytiotrophoblast degeneration/regeneration is probably most extensive in cases of miscarriage, in which maternal blood flow is premature and widespread (Figure 3.3).

The excessive entry of maternal blood into the intervillous space has a direct mechanical effect on the villous tissue and an indirect oxidative stress effect, which contributes to cellular dysfunction and/or damage. Complete loss of syncytiotrophoblast function through oxidative stress would, of course, lead to a precipitate fall in hCG concentration, and hence to early pregnancy failure. Oxidative stress is well known to initiate the caspase cascade leading to cell death in other systems. Generation of ROS in large quantities, such as in maternal diabetes, in the 1st-trimester placenta, which has limited antioxidant defenses, may cause DNA damage and oxidation of proteins and lipids, resulting in extensive cell death. Apoptosis has been found to be intensified in cases of miscarriage, and concentrations of lipid peroxides increase in the decidua of women undergoing early pregnancy loss.[51,52]

The celomic fluid in miscarriages has also been investigated, but has only provided limited information on the mechanisms of early pregnancy failure.[53–55] The fluid collected in anembryonic pregnancies is of exocelomic origin, and its biochemical characteristics reflect a failure of placental metabolic function, transport mechanism, and endocrine activity. These findings support the concept that embryonic and placental development are closely related in the 1st trimester of pregnancy, placental biologic functions persisting only for a limited period of time after embryonic demise. Normal or high maternal serum α-fetoprotein (AFP) levels and AFP molecules (predominantly of yolk sac origin) in the celomic fluid of anembryonic pregnancies on ultrasonography provide further evidence that the most likely explanation for this feature is the early death of the embryo, with persistence of the placental tissue.[55]

The uteroplacental circulation is a dynamic model in which the magnitude of blood flow through the segments may vary significantly. Therefore, the evaluation of blood flow in a single uteroplacental unit is often difficult to interpret and is of limited value in understanding the pathophysiology of placental-related disorders of pregnancy. Recent work has suggested that Doppler sonography in early pregnancy has not been found to be a useful screening tool for placental-related disorders such as pre-eclampsia and growth restriction.[56] These findings clearly need further investigation, as the discovery of a non-invasive screening test for disorders of placental function early in pregnancy remains elusive.

Threatened miscarriage

Threatened miscarriage occurs in 15–20% of viable pregnancies[57] and is one of the commonest gynecologic emergencies. In the past, much emphasis has been placed on the volume of an intrauterine hematoma (IUH)[58–60] or the presence of vaginal bleeding,[59] but not on the location of the hemorrhage. If the bleeding occurs at the level of the definitive placenta (under the cord insertion), it may result in placental separation and subsequent miscarriage. Conversely, an

IUH that only detaches the membrane a distance away from the cord insertion can probably reach a significant volume before it affects normal pregnancy development by a direct volume pressure effect. The presence of a hematoma may also be associated with a chronic inflammatory reaction in the decidua, resulting in persistent myometrial activity and expulsion of the pregnancy.[61] As mentioned previously, in about two-thirds of early pregnancy failures there is defective placentation that is mainly characterized by a thinner and fragmented trophoblast shell and reduced cytotrophoblast invasion of the lumen at the tips of the spiral arteries.[45]

The development of a hematoma may be the first sign of an incomplete placentation associated with an acute oxidative stress, which may impair subsequent placental and membrane development. A delicate balance is probably achieved between the production of free radicals and protective antioxidant activity in early pregnancy. Any change in this equilibrium, resulting in an increase in free-radical formation, such as a premature influx of oxygenated maternal blood, the presence of substances that form free radicals, or a reduction in local antioxidant levels, may result in an impairment of placentation, and subsequent pregnancy complications – from miscarriage at one end of the spectrum, preterm premature rupture of membranes (PPROM)[62] and pre-eclampsia at the other. There is already mounting evidence of a role for free-radical damage in PPROM and pre-eclampsia; however, its role in miscarriage has only recently emerged.[51] The excessive entry of maternal blood inside the membranes, if located near the placenta, may have a direct mechanical effect on the villous tissue and an indirect oxidative stress effect that contributes to cellular dysfunction and/or damage.

Incomplete and complete miscarriage

As a definition, incomplete miscarriage is the passage of some but not all fetal or placental tissue through the cervical canal. In complete miscarriage, all products of conception are expelled through the cervix.[63] In incomplete miscarriage, the uterine debris may consist of a combination of products of conception, blood, and decidua.[64]

TVS plays an important role in evaluating the uterine cavity in spontaneous miscarriage due to detection of the retained products of conception. Retained products of conception after miscarriage may

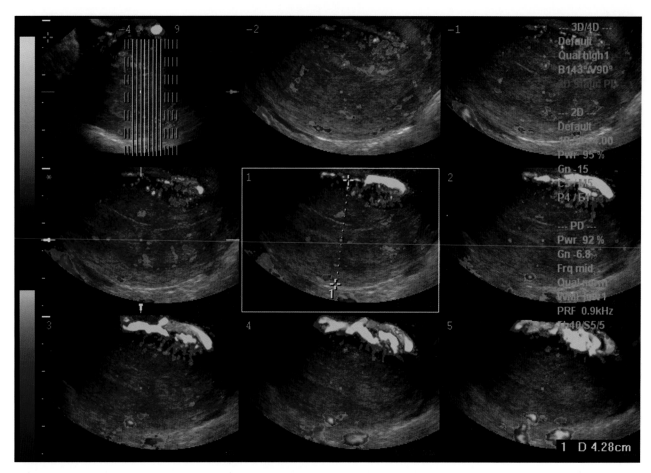

Figure 3.4 A case of incomplete miscarriage with vaginal bleeding demonstrated using tomographic ultrasound imaging (TUI). Abundant color flow is easily detected by power Doppler and represents the response of the dilated spiral arteries and venous system to the active trophoblastic tissue. Note that the endometrial thickness were 4.28 cm

cause bleeding or chorioamnionitis.[65] An echogenic and vascularized mass within the uterine cavity supports the diagnosis of retained products of conception.[66] Wong et al[67] reported 100% sensitivity and 80% specificity of TVS examination in differentiation of complete from incomplete spontaneous miscarriages. The sonographic definition of incomplete miscarriage is a bilayer endometrial thickness of more than 8 mm. In 29% of patients with incomplete miscarriage, transvaginal sonography obviated the need for surgical intervention, but in 30% of patients with complete miscarriage, it detected retained products of conception. Adding color Doppler examination to basic transvaginal 2D ultrasound examination increases the detection rate for the retained trophoblastic tissue.[68–70] Alcázar and Ortiz[71] suggested that transvaginal color Doppler is a helpful method for detecting retained trophoblastic tissue in patients with 1st-trimester spontaneous miscarriage. They analyzed 62 patients with a positive urine pregnancy test and a history of heavy vaginal bleeding whose gestational age was less than 14 weeks. In each patient, transvaginal ultrasound and β-hCG serum measurements were performed at the time of admission to the hospital. Retained trophoblastic tissue was suspected in the presence of low resistance index (RI <0.45) within the myometrium or just beneath the endometrial–myometrial interface. In 29% of women, retained trophoblastic tissue was suspected, and in 88.9% of these patients pathologic analysis was positive for retained trophoblastic tissue. The authors suggested performing B-mode and color Doppler examination when there is suspicion of retained trophoblastic tissue (Figure 3.4).

Recent studies have demonstrated that the risk of repeated spontaneous miscarriage depends exclusively on the number of previous spontaneous miscarriages and their cause. Even though many different risk factors have been thoroughly researched, around 60% of unsuccessful pregnancies remain a 'causa ignota'.[72]

The important criteria for evaluation of pregnancy loss are:[73]

- Always keep in mind that the risk of spontaneous miscarriage is higher in older women.
- Try to uncover causes for repetitive 1st-trimester miscarriages. Karyotyping of couples will reveal that 3–8% have some abnormality, most frequently a balanced chromosomal rearrangement or translocation (other abnormalities include sex chromosome mosaicism, chromosome inversions, or ring chromosomes). Besides spontaneous miscarriages, these abnormalities are associated with a high risk of malformations and mental retardation. Karyotyping is especially vital if the couple have had a malformed infant or fetus in addition to miscarriages in previous pregnancies.
- Smoking, alcohol, and heavy coffee consumption have been reported to be associated with an increased risk of recurrent pregnancy loss.[74]
- Patients with thyroid disease or uncontrolled diabetes mellitus may suffer spontaneous miscarriages, although these diseases are not causes of recurrent miscarriages.
- Uterine abnormalities can result in impaired vascularization, limited space for a fetus due to distortion of the uterine cavity, and incoordinate uterine contractility.
- Looking at 1st trimester miscarriages, a firm correlation with bacterial vaginosis-associated microorganisms was found in the study by Donders et al.[75]
- The major cause of thrombosis in pregnancy is an inherited predisposition for clotting, especially the factor V Leiden mutation.

Immunologic problems can be classified into two groups: autoimmunity (self antigens), and alloimmunity (foreign antigens). In autoimmunity, a humoral or cellular response is directed against a specific component of the host. The lupus anticoagulant and anticardiolipin antibodies are antiphospholipid antibodies, which arise as the result of an autoimmune disease. Several series have demonstrated that 10–16% of women with recurrent miscarriages have had antiphospholipid antibodies.[76] These antibodies are also associated with growth retardation and fetal death in addition to recurrent miscarriages. The preferred treatment for significant titers of antiphospholipid antibodies consists of the combination of low-dose aspirin (80 mg daily) and low-dose heparin as soon as pregnancy is diagnosed.[77,78] Unfortunately, treatment is not always successful. Alloimmunity refers to all causes of pregnancy losses related to an abnormal maternal immune response to antigens on placental or fetal tissues.

Delayed miscarriage (previously anembryonic or missed abortion)

First-trimester bleeding occurs in up to 15–25% of all pregnancies, and is associated with an increased risk of miscarriage and other complications.[79] TVS is the technique of choice in these patients. Demonstration of a large gestational sac without a demonstrable embryo is a well-established indicator of a non-viable pregnancy, although some controversies exist with regard to the optimal size cut-off.[80] When the gestational sac is small, however, it is impossible to establish whether or not the pregnancy is viable, and follow-up sonography is suggested.[81]

The diagnosis of previous missed abortion is determined by the ultrasound identification of an embryo/fetus without any heart activity. It is relatively easy to make this diagnosis by means of transvaginal color Doppler ultrasound. The main parameter is the absence of heartbeats and the lack of color flow signals at its expected position after the 6th week of gestation (Figure 3.5). With the aid of sensitive color Doppler equipment, it is possible to demonstrate two types of blood flow velocity waveforms from the intervillous space (pulsatile arterial-like and continuous venous-like patterns) in both, normal and abnormal early pregnancies.[82] Studies did not show any difference in terms of resistance index and pulsatility index of the intervillous arterial blood flow between women with missed abortion and those with normally developing pregnancy. In long-standing demise, the cessation of the embryonic portion of the placental circulation leaves the fluid pumping action of the trophoblast unaffected, as it remains nourished by the maternal side of the circulation. As a consequence, the embryonic circulation no longer drains a trophoblast-conveyed fluid in the villous stroma. Progressive accumulation of the fluid may result in a significant reduction of the intervillous blood flow impedance. Lower impedance to blood flow, observed in the spiral arteries, indicates that a massive and continuous infiltration of maternal blood without effective drainage causes further disruption of the maternal embryonic interface, resulting in miscarriage. These changes can be effectively studied by 2D and 3D power Doppler.

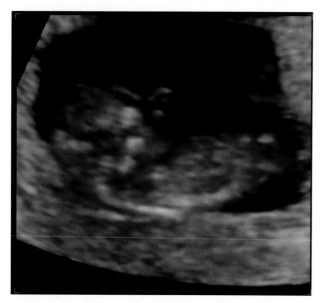

Figure 3.5 Absence of heart activity is noted by power Doppler in the case of delayed miscarriage

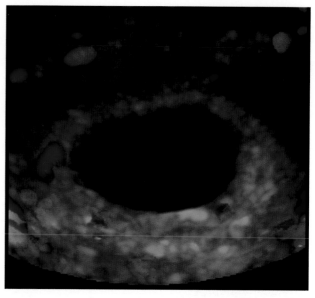

Figure 3.6 3D transvaginal color Doppler scan demonstrating an anembryonic pregnancy. Color signals are obtained from the maternal vessels and intervillous space

Diagnosis of blighted ovum (anembryonic pregnancy) refers to a gestational sac in which the embryo either failed to develop or died at a stage too early to visualize (Figure 3.6). The diagnosis of anembryonic pregnancy is based on the absence of embryonic echoes within the gestational sac, large enough for such structures to be visualized, independent of clinical data or menstrual cycle. Advances in transvaginal sonography allow us to detect this kind of abnormality at a mean sac diameter of 1.5 cm.[83] If the volume of the sac is less than 2.5 ml and does not increase in size by at least 75% over a period of 1 week, the definition of this pathological condition in early pregnancy is blighted ovum. A large empty sac usually measures between 12 and 18 mm in mean diameter. To confirm the diagnosis, these findings should be correlated with other clinical and sonographic data, including the presence of a yolk sac.

It is commonly accepted that in pregnant patients with 1st-trimester bleeding, the documentation of an intrauterine gestational sac 16 mm or smaller without an embryo may be compatible with a viable pregnancy. Falco et al[79] suggested that this finding is associated with a poor outcome, as miscarriage will occur in about two-thirds of cases. Clinical, laboratory, and sonographic findings at the time of admission of the patients were found to have an influence on the probability of miscarriage. An advanced sac, as previously suggested, is a further risk factor for pregnancy failure. Conversely, subchorionic hematomas were not found to be of prognostic significance.[84]

Falco et al[79] suggested that the size of the gestational sac was the most powerful, as well as the only independent, risk factor in predicting the outcome of the pregnancy. When a gestational sac smaller than −1.34 standard deviations (SDs) of the mean is identified, the risk of miscarriage is greatly increased (93%). Conversely, when the gestational sac is greater than −1.34 SDs of the mean, the risk of miscarriage is considerably decreased (27%). Although these results will not change the management of pregnancies with 1st-trimester bleeding, it is believed they will prove useful in patient counseling, as well as in deciding the time and type of follow-up.

Intrauterine hematomas

The shape of the gestational sac, the echogenicity of the placenta, the thickness of the trophoblast,[75] and the presence of an IUH (Figure 3.7) have all been proposed as sonographic markers associated with early spontaneous miscarriage.[85–89] Many of these studies, however, highlight problems with experimental design rather than providing unequivocal answers.

IUHs are crescent-shaped, echo-free areas between the chorionic membrane and the myometrium. Understanding of the resolution of these hematomas

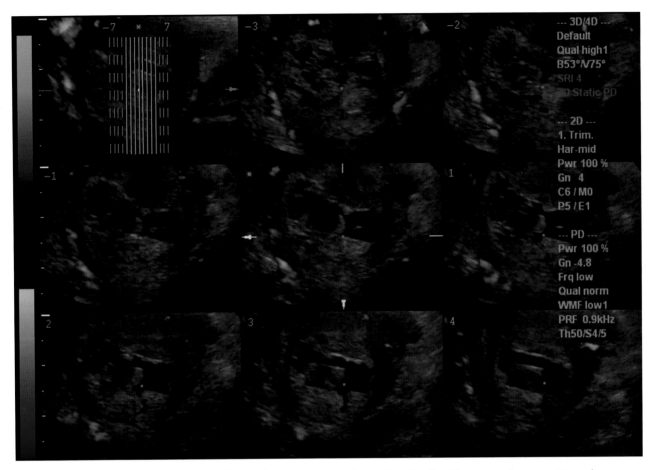

Figure 3.7 Transvaginal sonogram of a large-volume hematoma located in the fundal–corporeal region. Note the uterine blood flow signals on the side of the hematoma

and the prognostic relevance of this ultrasound finding are limited. Many authors have focused on an association between the size of the hematoma and subsequent obstetric complications.[76] The most common causes of IUH are disturbed trophoblast invasion and a defect in spiral artery transformation, infection, mechanical factors, autoimmune factors, and hematologic factors. Overall, the presence of an IUH has been associated with a 4–33% rate of miscarriage, depending on the gestational age at which the complication was described.[77] Vaginal bleeding in very early pregnancy (i.e., before 6 weeks of gestation) does not seem to be associated with any immediate or long-term consequences.[78] Conversely, threatened miscarriage symptoms at 7–12 weeks, even in the presence of detectable fetal cardiac activity, are not only associated with a 5–10% miscarriage rate before 14 weeks of gestation but also with adverse pregnancy outcome later in gestation.[79] In particular, women with bleeding in the 2nd half of the 1st trimester are at higher risk of PPROM and preterm labor. These risks are independent of the presence or absence of an IUH on the initial ultrasound examination, and would suggest that threatened miscarriage in the 1st trimester is a risk factor for adverse pregnancy outcome regardless of the ultrasound findings.

Prognostically, there are two main elements that determine pregnancy outcome. The first is the location of the hematoma. According to Kurjak and associates, the location is a more predictive sign than the volume of the hematoma. It is likely that if the bleeding occurs at the level of the definitive placenta (under the cord insertion), it may result in placental separation and subsequent miscarriage.[90] Conversely, a subchorionic hematoma detaching only a membrane opposite to the cord insertion could probably reach a significant volume before it affects normal pregnancy development.[91] A supracervical hematoma has a much better prognosis, because it is easily drained into the vagina and for this reason does not represent a mechanical factor causing compression of the utero-placental vessels. A higher incidence of spontaneous miscarriages has been reported in cases where the hematoma has been localized in the fundal or corporeal region, which could be attributed to placental location in that area.[92] Retroplacental or central hematomas have the worst prognosis, because they cause the largest effect on the uteroplacental circulation and placental tissue[93] (Figure 3.7). The pathologic mechanism is probably placental abruption, in which retroplacental clots are located between the placenta and myometrium, and preplacental clots are found between the amniotic fluid and the placenta later in the second trimester.

Kurjak et al[92] reported on increased resistance to blood flow and decrease in velocity through the spiral arteries on the side of a subchorionic hematoma, which is a consequence of mechanical compression of the hematoma itself. With progression of pregnancy and growth of trophoblastic tissue, most hematomas gradually disappear, and circulation normalizes, but the pregnancy remains in the high-risk group, with a necessity for intensive monitoring.

The second element in the diagnosis of an IUH is its size. Modern sonographic machines with a transvaginal approach enable accurate evaluation of the size of an IUH. An IUH should be analyzed in relation to the trophoblast tissue and its distance from the internal cervical os.[79] Furthermore, 3D machines can produce 3D images of hematomas and surrounding structures,

as well as measuring their volume and allowing dynamic follow-up of biometric changes (Figure 3.8). At the same time, Doppler measurements can evaluate the compression effect on the adjacent uteroplacental circulation.

ULTRASOUND AND THE DIAGNOSIS OF MISCARRIAGE

The use of TVS has clearly revolutionized the management of early pregnancy problems. The development of highly sensitive urinary hCG assays and greater awareness of early pregnancy ultrasound among healthcare professionals and women alike has resulted in ever earlier presentation. This has led to an increase in the number of inconclusive scans, and as a result an increase in the requirement for repeat assessments to determine both pregnancy location and viability. Knowledge of the typical ultrasound appearances of normal early pregnancy development and a good understanding of the pitfalls involved is essential for the diagnosis and management of early pregnancy failure.[94]

Gestational sac

The deciduo–placental interface and the exocelomic cavity are the first sonographic evidence of a pregnancy that can be visualized with TVS from around 4.4–4.6 menstrual weeks (32–34 days), when they together reach a size of 2–4 mm. In normal intrauterine pregnancies between the 5th and 6th weeks, the gestational sac grows in mean diameter at a rate of approximately 1 mm/day.[95,96] Gestational sac growth has been documented on serial ultrasound examinations to be slower in women who subsequently miscarry;[94] however, it has long been recognized that there is wide scatter in gestational sac volume measurements in 'normal' early pregnancy.[97]

Once a gestational sac has been documented on ultrasound, subsequent loss of viability in the embryonic period remains around 11%.[98] A smaller than expected gestational sac can be a predictor of poor pregnancy outcome, both alone and in combination with other parameters, even in the presence of embryonic cardiac activity.[99–103] In very early pregnancy, there appears to be no difference in gestational sac diameter (GSD) when compared with pregnancy outcome,[104] the difference only becoming apparent

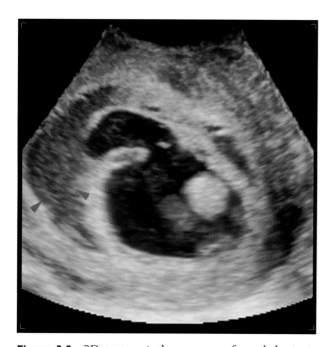

Figure 3.8   3D transvaginal sonogram of a subchorionic hematoma (red arrowheads) in close proximity to the gestational sac

from 5 weeks onwards. Unfortunately, the predictive value of GSD in isolation is variable and highly dependent upon other presenting factors. Interpretation of pregnancy outcome data for any variable in early pregnancy is hampered by significant differences in study design and entry criteria.

Studies involving women undergoing assisted conception are likely to be most accurate in terms of precise dating of the pregnancy, particularly as miscarriage rates for such pregnancies are now believed to be comparable to those in the fertile population.[105,106] Overall, multivariate analyses appear to provide the most sensitive predictors of pregnancy outcome, and GSD features strongly in combination with one or two other parameters in all of these models.[105,107] Small gestational sac size can also be associated with chromosomal abnormality. Triploidy and trisomy 16 are more often associated with a small chorionic sac before 9 weeks of gestation than other chromosomal abnormalities.[18,108]

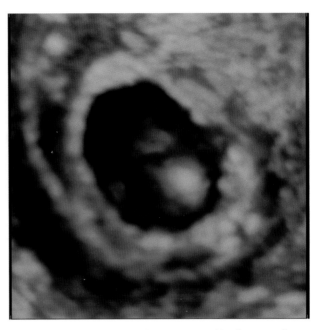

Figure 3.9 3D transvaginal sonogram of hydropic yolk sac showing early pregnancy failure

Crown–rump length

Robinson and Fleming[109] stated that crown–rump length (CRL) is still the main reference for the assessment of gestational age in early pregnancy. Because TVS provides superior resolution and more accurate identification of embryonic structures than abdominal ultrasound, new charts have been developed for the period of gestation before 7 weeks.[110] If an embryo has developed up to 5 mm in length, subsequent loss of viability occurs in 7.2% of cases.[102] Loss rates drop to 3.3% for embryos of 6–10 mm and to 0.5% for embryos over 10 mm.[102] There is conflicting evidence for an association between early growth restriction, as defined by a deficit between the CRL and that predicted by the last menstrual period, and karyotypic abnormalities.[108–114] A smaller than expected CRL has been associated with subsequent miscarriage.[115]

Mean GSD:CRL ratios have also been used to predict pregnancy outcome, with varying degrees of accuracy.[116] Unfortunately, as is the case for GSD measurements, this technique is of limited clinical utility.[19]

Secondary yolk sac

The secondary yolk sac (SYS) can be observed from the beginning of the 5th week of gestation or when the gestational sac reaches 10 mm in diameter.[117] The SYS diameter increases slightly between 6 and 10 weeks of gestation and then decreases.[117] Comparison of ultrasound features with morphologic findings indicates that when the SYS reaches its maximum sonographic size, it already shows important degenerative changes.[118] This suggests that the disappearance of the SYS in normal pregnancies is a spontaneous event in embryonic development rather than the result of mechanical compression by the expanding amniotic cavity. The predictive value of SYS measurements in determining the outcome of an early pregnancy is limited.[119] Most pregnancies that miscarry during the third month of pregnancy have normal SYS measurements at their initial scan before 8 weeks of gestation (Figure 3.9).[118] It is usually the yolk sac that is found to persist inside the gestational sac after embryonic demise.[53] This would suggest that variations in SYS size and sonographic appearance in most abnormal pregnancies are probably the consequence of poor embryonic development or embryonic death rather than being the primary cause of early pregnancy failure.

Fetal heart pulsation

Extensive research has been published examining the predictive value of fetal heart activity on pregnancy outcome.[19] Studies can be broadly divided into those

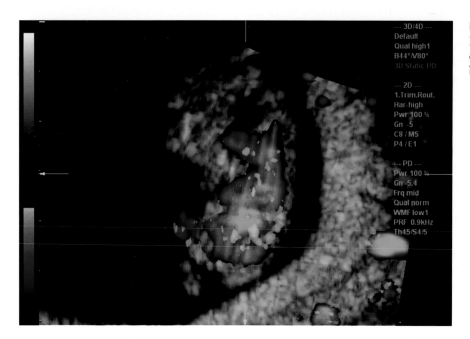

Figure 3.10 3D transvaginal power Doppler scan of a fetus at 7 weeks of gestation showing active heart beating

examining fetal loss after confirmed fetal cardiac activity, and those examining fetal heart rate (FHR) in relation to outcome. Fetal heart activity is the earliest proof of a viable pregnancy, and it has been documented in utero by TVS as early as 36 days of menstrual age, approximately at the time when the heart tube starts to beat (Figure 3.10).[116] Theoretically, cardiac activity should always be evident when the embryo is over 2 mm.[120] However, in around 5–10% of embryos between 2 and 4 mm, it cannot be demonstrated, although the corresponding pregnancies will have a normal outcome.[120] From 5 to 9 weeks of gestation, there is a rapid increase in the mean heart rate from 110 to 175 beats/min (bpm). The heart rate then gradually decreases to around 160–170 bpm.[121]

Abnormal developmental pattern of FHR and/or bradycardia have been associated with subsequent miscarriage.[121] In particular, a slow FHR at 6–8 weeks appears to be associated with subsequent fetal demise.[122] A single observation of an abnormally slow heart rate does not necessarily indicate subsequent embryonic death, but a continuous decline in embryonic heart activity is inevitably associated with miscarriage. With regard to women with recurrent spontaneous miscarriage (defined as three or more consecutive losses in the 1st trimester), there has been much debate concerning whether there is an increased likelihood that fetal heart pulsations will be seen on TVS when compared with idiopathic spontaneous miscarriages,[123] suggesting a different pathophysiology leading to pregnancy loss in these cases. Evidence

would suggest, however, that fetal loss patterns are no different between these groups.[124]

Color Doppler imaging

The ability of transvaginal color Doppler imaging to detect FVWs from small vessels such as the terminal part of the uteroplacental circulation has given rise to much enthusiasm from clinicians interested in predicting early and late pregnancy complications related to abnormal placentation.[11,14,19] Overall, the predictive value of Doppler measurements of resistance to blood flow in early pregnancy is limited.[11,14,19] All Doppler studies in the 1st trimester have failed to demonstrate abnormal blood flow indices in the uteroplacental circulation of pregnancies that subsequently ended in miscarriage.[125] Histologic assessment of decidual endovascular trophoblast invasion in 1st-trimester pregnancies about to undergo therapeutic evacuation, with low- and high-resistance umbilical artery Doppler measurements, has shown that although the proportion of vessels invaded is increased in women with low-resistance Dopplers, invasion is normal in both groups.[126]

ULTRASOUND AND THE MANAGEMENT OF EARLY PREGNANCY LOSS

The routine use of TVS in the investigation and diagnosis of early pregnancy problems has also led to improvements in the management of early pregnancy loss. Improved access to early pregnancy units and increasing awareness among women of their choices in the management of early pregnancy problems has led to an increasing demand for more conservative management of early miscarriage. Up to 70% of women will choose expectant management of miscarriage if given the choice.[127] The diagnosis of a complete miscarriage is generally accepted as an endometrial thickness less than 15 mm with no evidence of retained products of conception, and TVS is a sensitive tool for detecting residual trophoblastic tissue.[128]

The finding of blood flow in the intervillous space in cases of 1st-trimester miscarriage using color Doppler imaging also appears to be useful in the prediction of success of expectant management. Miscarriages with blood flow within the intervillous space are up to four times more likely to complete with expectant management.[129]

The success of expectant management is variable across studies, with a completion rate of 80–96% within 2 weeks in women with incomplete miscarriage and a low complication rate.[130]

It is generally accepted that the likelihood of completion after 2 weeks of missed abortions and anembryonic pregnancies is low, and evacuation of the retained products of conception (ERPC) should be offered.[130] In cases of incomplete miscarriage, where subsequent completion rates are high, it has been shown that other ultrasound parameters such as endometrial thickness and the presence or absence of a gestational sac did not add any further information to the likely outcome.[129] Expectant management of miscarriage, using ultrasound parameters to determine eligibility, could significantly reduce the number of unnecessary ERPCs, depending on the criteria used.

3D TRANSVAGINAL SONOGRAPHY ASSESSMENT IN SPONTANEOUS MISCARRIAGE

As part of the use of ultrasound in diagnostic assessment, measurements play a significant role in defining normal limits for gestation. Measurements of the gestational sac and embryonic size have been used to assess gestational age and evaluate pregnancy failure.[131,132] On-screen distance measurements using electronic calipers on the image obtained by conventional 2D scanning are sufficiently accurate to be useful in routine clinical practice. However, volume estimates are more difficult to achieve. 3D volumetry of 1st-trimester gestational sacs was reported to be superior to 2D volumetry in the study.[133,134] Volume measurements using 2D sonographic methods are known to be less accurate than 3D methods for irregularly shaped objects.[135,136] As the gestational sacs and retained products of conception are irregularly shaped entities in cases of failed pregnancies, the routinely applied methods of assessment by 2D measurement may not be accurate.

Measurements of yolk sac diameter, mean GSD (MSD) in relation to gestational age, and the ratio between CRL and GSD have all been used in an attempt to predict pregnancy outcome in the first trimester.[13,134] 3D ultrasound volumetry has been reported to be accurate and reproducible both in vitro[137] and in vivo in a clinical setting.[134] The ability to obtain accurate volume measurements may permit better diagnostic and prognostic possibilities in early pregnancy.

3D sonography has been demonstrated to improve spatial vision of the surfaces, anatomic boundaries, and contours of the embryonic organs.[138] This, together with accurate volumetric measurements, may provide us with a clearer picture in the evaluation of early pregnancy complications. It is believed that the amount of tissue retained within the uterine cavity is an important predictor of success in non-surgical management of incomplete spontaneous miscarriage. Maximum anterior–posterior diameter of the retained intrauterine tissue has been reported to have significant predictive ability of the success of expectant management of spontaneous miscarriage.[134] Calculation of the volume of intrauterine retained products of conception by 2D sonography is difficult and associated with considerable procedural errors because of their irregular shape. It is also sometimes difficult to accurately define longitudinal diameter of the retained products in a sagittal plane.[139] More accurate assessment of the amount of retained products of conception may be useful while deciding upon the appropriate management regime and objectively determining whether an expectant, medical, or surgical approach is best for individual patients. However, Acharya and Morgan[131] showed that there is a good correlation between the 2D measurements conventionally used for the evaluation of 1st-trimester pregnancy failure and 3D volumetry.

Data from a series of 33 cases of termination of pregnancy where specimens with intact amniotic sacs

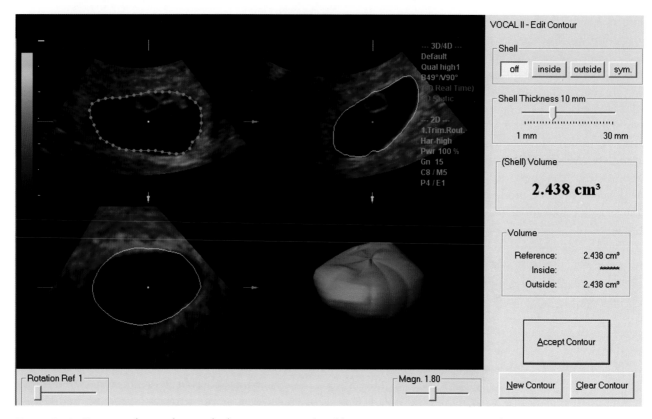

Figure 3.11 Gestational sac volume calculation in a normal viable pregnancy using VOCAL software

were obtained by hysterotomy showed a positive correlation between amniotic fluid volume, CRL, and weight of the fetus.[140] The gestational sac volume (GSV) is closely related to amniotic fluid volume and may reflect uteroplacental function in the 1st trimester.[141] Acharya and Morgan[131] had confirmed that there was a strong correlation between CRL and GSV in normal ongoing pregnancies. A weak correlation between CRL and GSV in cases of missed miscarriage may be due to the reduction in embryonic size following embryonic demise. The 1st-trimester amniotic fluid is an ultrafiltrate of maternal plasma and constitutes the major component of the GSV.[138] Larger GSVs in relation to embryonic size in missed miscarriage suggest that the fetal contribution to the production of amniotic fluid is insignificant before 10–12 weeks of gestation.

The gestational sac is composed of an amniotic and a celomic cavity in the 1st trimester and reflects the environment of embryonic development. Although it is possible to distinguish a viable empty gestational sac from a non-viable one using already-established sonographic criteria, in a significant proportion of cases this cannot be achieved during a single examination.[142] Accurate measurement of GSV may be useful

in predicting the outcome of early pregnancy. It has been suggested that embryos with heart motion but unusually large or small GSVs may represent the presence of abnormal pregnancies.[143] In a preliminary study, a normal GSV in the 1st trimester was reported to predict a successful pregnancy outcome in 97% of cases.[138] However, one study reported no differences between the GSVs of pregnancies with normal or adverse outcome (Figure 3.11).[134] In a retrospective study of 539 patients, a small gestational sac was present before embryonic death only in 10.7% of all cases.[144] An enlarged amniotic cavity relative to the CRL is reported to be a sign of early embryonic demise.[137] In our study, the women with missed miscarriage had larger MSD and GSV in relation to CRL and embryonic volume in comparison with those with ongoing pregnancy, suggesting that volumetry may have some diagnostic value (Figure 3.12).[13] Once an embryo is seen by endovaginal sonography, the absence of cardiac activity usually indicates embryonic demise.

Although chromosomal abnormalities are common in 1st-trimester miscarriages, some of them are karyotypically normal. Small initial chorionic sac diameter has been reported to be more commonly

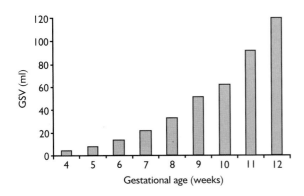

Figure 3.12 Gestational sac volume (GSV) measured by 3D sonography in normal pregnancy[13]

associated with an abnormal karyotype.[145] Karyotypes are difficult to obtain on the abortus due to culture failures, but it would be interesting to investigate whether there is any relationship between GSV or embryonic volume and abortus karyotype in cases of failed pregnancies. However, even established parameters predictive of early pregnancy failure may potentially result in misdiagnosis of non-viability when applied to a large unselected patient population. It is advised to refrain from a diagnosis of embryonic demise based on a single sonogram if the CRL is less than 6 mm.[144] A large MSD : CRL or GSV : embryonic volume ratio is more likely to represent a missed miscarriage. This may be an important finding to consider when diagnosing early fetal demise if the size of the fetal pole is less than 6 mm and no fetal heart motion is demonstrable. Whether such a finding is predictive of poor pregnancy outcome even when fetal heart motion is present needs to be investigated further.

REFERENCES

1. Hafner T, Kurjak A, Funduk-Kurjak B, Bekavac I. Assessment of early chorionic circulation by three-dimensional power Doppler. J Perinat Med 2002; 30: 33–9.

2. Matijevic R, Kurjak A. Early pregnancy loss. In: Kurjak A, Chervenak FA, Carrera JM, eds. The Embryo as a Patient. London: Parthenon, 2001: 70–80.

3. Kurjak A, Zalud I, Predanic M. Transvaginal color Doppler in early pregnancy: rational and clinical potential. J Perinat Med 1994; 22: 475–82.

4. Kurjak A, Kupesic S, Kostovic L. Vascularization of yolk sac and vitelline duct in normal pregnancies studied by transvaginal color Doppler. J Perinat Med 1994; 22: 433–40.

5. Kurjak A, Kupesic S, Predanic M, Salihagic A. Transvaginal color Doppler assessment of the uteroplacental circulation in normal and abnormal early pregnancy. Early Hum Dev 1992; 29: 385–9.

6. Kupesic S, Hafner T, Bjelos D. Events from ovulation to implantation studied by three-dimensional ultrasound. J Perinat Med 2002; 30: 84–98.

7. Kurjak A, Hafner T, Kupesic S, Kostovic L. Three-dimensional power Doppler in study of embryonic vasculogenesis. J Perinat Med 2002; 30: 18–25.

8. Kurjak A, Kupesic S, Banovic I, Hafner T, Kos M. The study of morphology and circulation of early embryo by three-dimensional ultrasound and power Doppler. J Perinat Med 1999: 27: 145–57.

9. Kurjak A, Kupesic S. Parallel Doppler assessment of yolk sac and intervillous circulation in normal pregnancy and missed abortion. Placenta 1998; 19: 619–23.

10. Kurjak A, Hafner T, Kupesic S. Doppler evidence of intervillous circulation during the first trimester of pregnancy. Placenta 1998; 19: 445.

11. Kurjak A, Kupesic S, Kos M. Three-dimensional sonography for assessment of morphology and vascularization of the fetus and placenta. J Soc Gynecol Investig 2002; 9: 186–202.

12. Kupesic S, Kurjak A. Predictors of IVF outcome by three-dimensional ultrasound. Hum Reprod 2002; 17: 950–5.

13. Kupesic S, Kurjak A, Ivancic-Kosuta M. Volume and vascularity of the yolk sac studied by three-dimensional ultrasound and color Doppler. J Perinat Med 1999; 27: 91–6.

14. Kurjak A, Predanic M, Kupesic-Urek S. Transvaginal color Doppler in the assessment of placental blood flow. Eur J Obstet Gynecol Reprod Biol 1993; 49: 29–32.

15. Kurjak A, Zudenigo D, Funduk-Kurjak B, et al. Transvaginal color Doppler in the assessment of the uteroplacental circulation in normal early pregnancy. J Perinat Med 1993; 21: 25–34.

16. Kurjak A. Are color and pulsed Doppler sonography safe in early pregnancy? J Perinat Med 1999; 27: 422–30.

17. Kurjak A, Kupesic S, Hafner T, et al. Conflicting data on intervillous circulation in early pregnancy. J Perinat Med 1997; 25: 225–36.

18. Benoit B, Hafner T, Kurjak A, et al. Three-dimensional sonoembryology. J Perinat Med 2002; 30: 63–73.

19. Jauniaux E, Johns J, Burton GJ. The role of ultrasound imaging in diagnosing and investigating early pregnancy failure. Ultrasound Obstet Gynecol 2005; 25: 613–24.

20. Jauniaux E, Gulbis B. Fluid compartments of the

embryonic environment. Hum Reprod Update 2000; 6: 268–78.

21. Jauniaux E, Gulbis B. Embryonal physiology. In: Jauniaux E, Barnea ER, Edwards R, eds. Embryonic Medicine and Therapy. Oxford: Oxford University Press, 1997: 223–43.

22. Jauniaux E, Gulbis B, Jurkovic D, et al. Protein and steroid levels in embryonic cavities in early human pregnancy. Hum Reprod 1993; 8: 782–7.

23. Jauniaux E, Jurkovic D, Campbell S. In vivo investigations of anatomy and physiology of early human placental circulations. Ultrasound Obstet Gynecol 1991; 1: 435–45.

24. Jauniaux E, Jurkovic D, Campbell S. Current topic: in vivo investigation of the placental circulations by Doppler echography. Placenta 1995; 16: 323–31.

25. Harris JWS, Ramsey EM. The morphology of human uteroplacental vasculature. Contrib Embryol 1966; 260: 43–58.

26. Ramsey EM, Donner NW. Placental Vasculature and Circulation. Stuttgart: Georg Thieme, 1980.

27. Pijnenborg R, Dixon G, Robertson WB, Brosens I. Trophoblastic invasion of human decidua from 8 to 18 weeks of pregnancy. Placenta 1980; 1: 3–19.

28. Pijnenborg R, Bland JM, Robertson WB, Brosens I. Uteroplacental arterial changes related to interstitial trophoblast migration in early human pregnancy. Placenta 1983; 4: 397–414.

29. Kam EPY, Gardner L, Loke YW, King A. The role of trophoblast in the physiological change in decidual spiral arteries. Hum Reprod 1999; 14: 2131–8.

30. Meekins JW, Pijnenborg R, Hanssens M, McFayden IR, van Asshe A. A study of placental bed spiral arteries and trophoblast invasion in normal and severe pre-eclamptic pregnancies. Br J Obstet Gynaecol 1994; 101: 669–74.

31. Wiznitzer A, Furman B, Mazor M, Reece EA. The role of prostanoids in the development of diabetic embryopathy. Semin Reprod Endocrinol 2004; 17: 175–81.

32. Parman T, Wiley MJ, Wells PG. Free radical-mediated oxidative damage in the mechanism of thalidomide teratogenicity. Nat Med 1999; 5: 582–5.

33. Nicol CJ, Zielenski J, Tsui LC, Wells PG. An embryoprotective role for glucose-6–phosphate dehydrogenase in developmental oxidative stress and clinical teratogenesis. FASEB J 2000; 14: 111–27.

34. Tempfer C, Unfried G, Zeillinger R, et al. Endothelial nitric oxide synthase gene polymorphism in women with idiopathic recurrent miscarriage. Hum Reprod 2001; 16: 1644–7.

35. Burton GJ, Watson AL, Hempstock J, Skepper JN, Jauniaux E. Uterine glands provide histiotrophic nutri-

tion for the human fetus during the first trimester of pregnancy. J Clin Endocrinol Metab 2002; 86: 2954–9.

36. Jauniaux E, Hempstock J, Teng C, Battaglia FC, Burton GJ. Polyol concentrations in the fluid compartments of the human conceptus during the first trimester of pregnancy; maintenance of redox potential in a low oxygen environment. J Clin Endocrinol Metab 2005; 90: 1171–5.

37. Basir GS, O WS, So WW, Ng EH, Ho PC. Evaluation of cycle-to-cycle variation of endometrial responsiveness using transvaginal sonography in women undergoing assisted reproduction. Ultrasound Obstet Gynecol 2002; 19: 484–9.

38. Yang JH, Wu MY, Chen CD, et al. Association of endometrial blood flow as determined by a modified colour Doppler technique with subsequent outcome of in-vitro fertilization. Hum Reprod 1999; 14: 1606–10.

39. Rogers PAW. Structure and function of endometrial blood vessels. Hum Reprod Update 1996; 2: 57–62.

40. Habara T, Nakatsuka M, Konishi H, et al. Elevated blood flow resistance in uterine arteries of women with unexplained recurrent pregnancy loss. Hum Reprod 2002; 17: 190–4.

41. Nakatsuka M, Habara T, Noguchi S, Konishi H, Kudo T. Impaired uterine arterial blood flow in pregnant women with recurrent pregnancy loss. J Ultrasound Med 2003; 22: 27–31.

42. Chien LW, Lee WS, Au HK, Tzeng CR. Assessment of changes in utero–ovarian arterial impedance during the periimplantation period by Doppler sonography in women undergoing assisted reproduction. Ultrasound Obstet Gynecol 2004; 23: 496–500.

43. Jauniaux E, Zaidi J, Jurkovic D, Campbell S, Hustin J. Comparison of colour Doppler features and pathological findings in complicated early pregnancy. Hum Reprod 1994; 9: 2432–7.

44. Meekins JW, Pijnenborg R, Hanssens M, McFayden IR, van Asshe A. A study of placental bed spiral arteries and trophoblast invasion in normal and severe pre-eclamptic pregnancies. Br J Obstet Gynaecol 1994; 101: 669–74.

45. Hustin J, Jauniaux ER, Schapps JP. Histological study of the materno–embryonic interface in spontaneous abortion. Placenta 1990; 11: 477–86.

46. Robertson WB, Brosens I, Landells WN. Abnormal placentation. Obstet Gynecol Annu 1985; 14: 411–26.

47. Khong TY, De Wolf F, Robertson WB, Brosens I. Inadequate maternal vascular response in pregnancies complicated by preeclampsia and by small for gestational age infants. Br J Obstet Gynaecol 1986; 93: 1049–59.

48. Jauniaux E, Hempstock J, Greenwold N, Burton GJ. Trophoblastic oxidative stress in relation to temporal

and regional differences in maternal placental blood flow in normal and abnormal early pregnancies. Am J Pathol 2003; 162: 115–25.

49. Schaaps JP, Hustin J. In vivo aspects of the maternal–trophoblastic border during the first trimester of gestation. Troph Res 1988; 3: 39–48.

50. Jauniaux E, Hustin J. Histological examination of first trimester spontaneous abortions: the impact of maternoembryonic interface features. Histopathology 1992; 21: 409–14.

51. Hempstock J, Bao YP, Bar-Issac M, et al. Intralobular differences in antioxidant enzyme expression and activity reflect the pattern of maternal arterial bloodflow within the human placenta. Placenta 2003; 24: 517–23.

52. Sugino N, Kakata M, Kashida S, et al. Decreased superoxide dismutase expression and increased concentrations of lipid peroxide and prostaglandin $F^{2\alpha}$ in the decidua of failed pregnancy. Mol Hum Reprod 2000; 6: 642–7.

53. Jauniaux E, Gulbis B, Nagy AM, et al. Coelomic fluid chorionic gonadotrophin and protein concentrations in normal and complicated first trimester pregnancies. Hum Reprod 1995; 10: 214–20.

54. Jauniaux E, Jurkovic D, Gulbis B, et al. Biochemical composition of the coelomic fluid in anembryonic pregnancy. Am J Obstet Gynecol 1994; 171: 849–53.

55. Jauniaux E, Gulbis B, Jurkovic D, Gavriil P, Campbell S. The origin of alpha-fetoprotein in first trimester anembryonic pregnancies. Am J Obstet Gynecol 1995; 173: 1749–53.

56. Hollis B, Prefumo F, Bhide A, Rao S, Thilaganathan B. First trimester uterine artery blood flow and birth weight. Ultrasound Obstet Gynecol 2003; 22: 376.

57. Jouppila P. Clinical consequences after ultrasonic diagnosis of intrauterine hematoma in threatened abortion. J Clin Ultrasound 1985; 13: 107–11.

58. Mantoni M, Pedersen JF. Intrauterine haematoma – an ultrasonic study of threatened abortion. Br J Obstet Gynaecol 1981; 88: 47–51.

59. Ball RH, Ade CM, Schoenborn JA, Crane JP. The clinical significance of ultrasonographically detected subchorionic hemorrhages. Am J Obstet Gynecol 1996; 174: 996–1002.

60. Abu-Yousef MM, Bleicher JJ, Williamson RA, Weiner CP. Subchorionic hemorrhage: sonographic diagnosis and clinical significance. AJR Am J Roentgenol 1987; 149: 737.

61. Salafia CM, Lopez-Zeno JA, Sherer DM, et al. Histologic evidence of old intrauterine bleeding is more frequent in prematurity. Am J Obstet Gynecol 1995; 173: 1065–70.

62. Johns J, Hyett J, Jauniaux E. Obstetric outcome after threatened miscarriage with and without a hematoma on ultrasound. Obstet Gynecol 2003; 102: 483–7.

63. Kurtz AB, ShIansky-Goldberg BB. Detection of retained products of conception following spontaneous abortion in the first trimester. J Ultrasound Med 1991; 10: 387–95.

64. Chung TKH, Cheung LR, Sahota DS, Haines CJ, Chang AM. Evaluation of the accuracy of transvaginal sonography for the assessment of retained products of conception after spontaneous abortion. Gynecol Obstet Invest 1998; 45: 190–3.

65. Kaakaji Y, Nghiem HV, Nodel C. Sonography of obstetric and gynecologic emergencies. AJR Am J Roentgenol 2000; 174: 641.

66. Moore L, Wilson SR. Ultrasonography in obstetric and gynecologic emergencies. Radiol Clin North Am 1994; 32: 1005.

67. Wong SR, Lam MO, Ho LC. Transvaginal sonography in the detection of retained products of conception after first-trimester spontaneous abortion. J Clin Ultrasound 2002; 30: 428–32.

68. Achiron R, Goldenberg M, Lipitzs, Mashiach S. Transvaginal duplex Doppler sonography in bleeding patients suspected on having residual trophoblastic tissue. Obstet Gynecol 1993; 81: 507–11.

69. Dillon EH, Case CQ, Ramos IM, Holland CK, Taylor KJW. Endovaginal ultrasound and Doppler findings after first-trimester abortion. Radiology 1993; 186: 87–91.

70. Tal J, Timor-Tritsch I, Degani S. Accurate diagnosis of postabortial placental remanant by sonohysterography and color Doppler sonographic studies. Gynecol Obstet Invest 1997; 43: 131–4.

71. Alcázar JL, Ortiz CA. Transvaginal color Doppler ultrasonography in the management of first-trimester spontaneous abortion. Eur J Obstet Gynecol Reprod Biol 2002; 102: 83–7.

72. Kos M, Kupesic S, Latin V. Diagnostics of spontaneous abortion. In: Kurjak A, ed. Ultrasound in Gynecology and Obstetrics. Zagreb: Art Studio Azinovic, 2000: 314–21.

73. Speroff L, Glass RH, Kase NG. Recurrent early pregnancy loss. In: Speroff L, Glass RH, Kase NG, eds. Clinical Gynecologic Endocrinology and Infertility. London: Williams & Wilkins, 1999: 1043–55.

74. Windham GC, von Behren J, Fenster L, Schaefer C, Swan SH. Moderate maternal alcohol consumption and risk of spontaneous abortion. Epidemiology 1997; 8: 509–14.

75. Donders GGG, Odds A, Veercken A, et al. Abnormal vaginal flora in the first trimester, but not full blown bacterial vaginosis, is associated with preterm birth. Prenat Neonat Med 1998; 3: 558–93.

76. Kupesic S, Kurjak A, Chervenak FA. Doppler studies of subchorionic hematomas in early pregnancy. In: Chervenak R, Kurjak A, eds. The Fetus as a Patient. Carnforth, UK: Parthenon, 1996: 33–9.

77. Cowchock FS, Reece EA, Balaban D, Branch DW, Plouffe L. Repeated fetal losses associated with antiphospholipid antibodies: a collaborative randomized trial comparing prednisone with low-dose heparin treatment. Am J Obstet Gynecol 1992; 166: 1318–23.

78. Rai R, Cohen H, Dave M, Regan L. Randomized controlled trial of aspirin and aspirin plus heparin in pregnant women with recurrent miscarriage associated with phospholipid antibodies. BMJ 1997; 314: 253–7.

79. Falco P, Zagonari S, Gabrielli S, et al. Sonography of pregnancies with first-trimester bleeding and a small intrauterine gestational sac without a demonstrable embryo. Ultrasound Obstet Gynecol 2003; 21: 62–5.

80. Levi CS, Lyons EA, Lindsay DJ. Early diagnosis of nonviable pregnancy with endovaginal US. Radiology 1988; 167: 383–5.

81. Hately W, Case J, Campbell S. Establishing the death of the embryo by ultrasound: report of a public inquiry with recommendations. Ultrasound Obstet Gynecol 1995; 5: 353–7.

82. Kurjak A, Kupesic S. Doppler assessment of the intervillous blood flow in normal and abnormal early pregnancy. Ultrasound Obstet Gynecol 1997; 89: 252–6.

83. De Crepigni L. Early diagnosis of pregnancy failure with transvaginal sonography. Am J Obstet Gynecol 1988; 159: 408.

84. Pedersen JF, Mantoni M. Prevalence and significance of subchorionic hemorrhage in threatened abortion: a sonographic study. AJR Am J Roentgenol 1990; 154: 535–7.

85. Bajo J, Moreno-Calvo FJ, Martinez-Cortes L, Haya FJ, Rayward J. Is trophoblastic thickness at the embryonic implantation site a new sign of negative evolution in first trimester pregnancy? Hum Reprod 2004; 15: 1629–31.

86. Bennett GL, Bromley B, Lieberman E, Benacerraf BR. Subchorionic haemorrhage in first trimester pregnancies: prediction of pregnancy outcome with sonography. Radiology 1996; 200: 803–6.

87. Pearlstone M, Baxi L. Subchorionic hematoma: a review. Obstet Gynecol Surv 1993; 48: 65–8.

88. Harville EW, Wilcox AJ, Baird DD, Weinberg CR. Vaginal bleeding in very early pregnancy. Hum Reprod 2003; 18: 1944–7.

89. Tongsong T, Srisomboon J, Wanapirak C, et al. Pregnancy outcome of threatened abortion with demonstrable fetal cardiac activity: a cohort study. J Obstet Gynecol Tokyo 1995; 21: 331–5.

90. Jauniaux E, Gavril P, Nicolaides KH. Ultrasonographic assessment of early pregnancy complication. In: Jurkovic D, Jauniaux E, eds. Ultrasound and Early Pregnancy. Carnforth, UK: Parthenon, 1995: 53–64.

91. Kurjak A, Kupesic S. Blood flow studies in normal and abnormal pregnancy. In: Kurjak A, Kupesic S, eds. An Atlas of Transvaginal Color Doppler. London: Parthenon, 2000: 41–51.

92. Kurjak A, Schulman H, Kupesic S, et al. Subchorionic hematomas in early pregnancy: clinical outcome and blood flow patterns. J Matern Fetal Med 1996; 5: 41–4.

93. Laurini RN. Abruptio placentae: from early pregnancy to term. In: Chervenak FA, Kurjak A, eds. The Fetus as a Patient. Carnforth, UK: Parthenon, 1996: 433–44.

94. The Management of Early Pregnancy Loss (Clinical Green Top Guidelines 25). London: Royal College of Obstetricians and Gynaecologists Press, 2000.

95. Nyberg DA, Mack LA, Laing FC, Patten RM. Distinguishing normal from abnormal gestational sac growth in early pregnancy. J Ultrasound Med 1987; 6: 23–7.

96. Jauniaux ER, Jurkovic D. The role of ultrasound in abnormal early pregnancy. In: Grudzinskas JG, O'Brien PMS, eds. Problems in Early Pregnancy: Advances in Diagnosis and Management. London: Royal College of Obstetricians and Gynaecologists Press, 1997: 137.

97. Robinson HP. 'Gestational sac' volumes as determined by sonar in the first trimester of pregnancy. Br J Obstet Gynaecol 1975; 82: 100–7.

98. Goldstein SR. Embryonic death in early pregnancy: a new look at the first trimester. Obstet Gynecol 1994; 84: 294–7.

99. Bromley B, Harlow BL, Laboda LA, Benacerraf BR. Small sac size in the first trimester. A predictor of poor fetal outcome. Radiology 1991; 178: 375.

100. Dickey RP, Gasser R, Olar TT, et al. Relationship of initial chorionic sac diameter and abortion and abortus karyotype based on new growth curves for the 16th to 49th post-ovulation day. Hum Reprod 1994; 9: 559–65.

101. Elson J, Salim R, Tailor A, et al. Prediction of early pregnancy viability in the absence of an ultrasonically detectable embryo. Ultrasound Obstet Gynecol 2003; 21: 57–61.

102. Falco P, Zagonari S, Gabrielli S, et al. Sonography of pregnancies with first trimester bleeding and a small intrauterine gestational sac without a demonstrable embryo. Ultrasound Obstet Gynecol 2003; 21: 62–5.

103. Makrydimas G, Sebire N, Lolis D, Vlassis N, Nicolaides KH. Fetal loss following ultrasound diagnosis of a live fetus at 6–10 weeks of gestation. Ultrasound Obstet Gynecol 2003; 22: 368–72.

104. Oh JS, Wright G, Coulam CB. Gestational sac diameter in very early pregnancy as a predictor of fetal outcome. Ultrasound Obstet Gynecol 2002; 20: 267.

105. Pregnancies and births resulting from in vitro fertilization: French National Registry, analysis of data 1986 to 1990. FIVNAT (French In Vitro National). Fertil Steril 1995; 64: 746–56.

106. Society for Assisted Reproductive Technology. Assisted reproductive technology in the United States and Canada: 1993 results generated from the American Society for Reproductive Medicine/Society for Assisted Reproductive Technology Registry. Fertil Steril 1995; 64: 13–21.

107. Choong S, Rombauts L, Ugoni A, Meagher S. Ultrasound prediction of risk of spontaneous miscarriage in live embryos from assisted conception. Ultrasound Obstet Gynecol 2003; 22: 571–7.

108. Jauniaux E, Greenwold N, Hempstock J, Burton GJ. Comparison of ultrasonographic and Doppler mapping of the intervillous circulation in normal and abnormal early pregnancies. Fertil Steril 2003; 79: 100–6.

109. Robinson HP, Fleming JEE. A critical evaluation of sonar crown rump length measurements. Br J Obstet Gynaecol 1975; 82: 702–10.

110. Hadlock FP, Shah YP, Kanon DJ, Lindsey JV. Fetal crown–rump length: re-evaluation of relation to menstrual age (5–18 weeks) with high resolution real time US. Radiology 1992; 182: 501–5.

111. Bahado-Singh RO, Lynch L, Deren O, et al. First-trimester growth restriction and fetal aneuploidy: the effect of type of aneuploidy and gestational age. Am J Obstet Gynecol 1997; 176: 976–80.

112. Drugan A, Johnson MP, Isada NB, et al. The smaller than expected first trimester fetus is at increased risk for chromosome anomalies. Am J Obstet Gynecol 1992; 167: 1525–8.

113. Benacerraf BR. Intrauterine growth restriction in the first trimester associated with triploidy. J Ultrasound Med 1988; 7: 153–4.

114. Goldstein SR, Kerenyi T, Scher J, Papp C. Correlation between karyotype and ultrasound findings in patients with failed early pregnancy. Ultrasound Obstet Gynecol 1996; 8: 314–17.

115. Reljic M. The significance of crown–rump length measurement for predicting adverse pregnancy outcome of threatened abortion. Ultrasound Obstet Gynecol 2004; 17: 510–12.

116. Tadmor OP, Achiron R, Rabinowiz R, et al. Predicting first trimester spontaneous abortion. Ratio of mean sac diameter to crown–rump length compared to embryonic heart rate. J Reprod Med 1994; 39: 459–62.

117. Bree LR, Marn CS. Transvaginal sonography in the first trimester: embryology, anatomy and hCG correlation. Semin Ultrasound CT MR 1990; 11: 12–21.

118. Jauniaux E, Jurkovic D, Henriet Y, Rodesch F, Hustin J. Development of the secondary human yolk sac: correlation of sonographic and anatomic features. Hum Reprod 1991; 6: 1160–6.

119. Reece EA, Scioscia AL, Pinter E, et al. Prognostic significance of the human yolk sac assessed by ultrasonography. Am J Obstet Gynecol 1988; 159: 1191–4.

120. Levi CS, Lyons EA, Zheng XH, Lindsay DJ, Holt SC. Endovaginal US: demonstration of cardiac activity in embryos of less than 5.0 mm in crown–rump length. Radiology 1990; 176: 71–4.

121. Tezuka N, Sato S, Kanasugi H, Hiroi M. Embryonic heart rates: development in early first trimester and clinical evaluation. Gynecol Obstet Invest 1991; 32: 210–12.

122. Stefos TI, Lolis DE, Sotiriadis AJ, Ziakas GV. Embryonic heart rate in early pregnancy. J Clin Ultrasound 1998; 26: 33–6.

123. Goto S. Ultrasonographic detection of a live fetus in recurrent spontaneous abortion during the first trimester. Hum Reprod 1993; 8: 627–30.

124. Brigham SA, Conlon C, Farquharson RG. A longitudinal study of pregnancy outcome following idiopathic recurrent miscarriage. Hum Reprod 2002; 14: 2868–71.

125. Bennett GL, Bromley B, Lieberman E, Benacerraf BR. Subchorionic haemorrhage in first trimester pregnancies: prediction of pregnancy outcome with sonography. Radiology 1996; 200: 803–6.

126. Prefumo F, Sebire N, Thilaganathan B. Decreased endovascular trophoblast invasion in first trimester pregnancies with high resistance uterine artery Doppler indices. Hum Reprod 2004; 19: 206–9.

127. Luise C, Jermy K, May C, et al. Outcome of expectant management of spontaneous first trimester miscarriage: observational study. BMJ 2002; 324: 873–5.

128. Alcazar JL, Baldonado C, Laparte C. The reliability of transvaginal ultrasonography to detect retained tissue after spontaneous first-trimester abortion, clinically thought to be complete. Ultrasound Obstet Gynecol 1995; 6: 126–9.

129. Schwarzler P, Holden D, Nielsen S, et al. The conservative management of first trimester miscarriages and the use of colour Doppler sonography for patient selection. Hum Reprod 1999; 14: 1341–5.

130. Luise C, Jermy K, Collins WP, Bourne T. Expectant management of incomplete, spontaneous first trimester miscarriage: outcome according to initial ultrasound criteria and value of follow-up visits. Ultrasound Obstet Gynecol 2002; 19: 580–2.

131. Acharya G, Morgan H. First-trimester, three-dimensional transvaginal ultrasound volumetry in normal pregnancies and spontaneous miscarriages. Ultrasound Obstet Gynecol 2002; 19: 575–9.

132. Hatley W, Case J, Campbell S. Establishing death of an embryo by ultrasound: report of a public inquiry with recommendations. Ultrasound Obstet Gynecol 1995; 5: 353–7.

133. Müller T, Sütterlin M, Pöhls U, Dietl J. Transvaginal volumetry of first trimester gestational sac: a comparison of conventional with three-dimensional ultrasound. J Perinat Med 2000; 28: 214–20.

134. Stampone C, Nicotra M, Muttinelli C, Cosmi EV. Transvaginal sonography of the yolk sac in normal and abnormal pregnancy. J Clin Ultrasound 1996; 24: 3–9.

135. Riccabona M, Nelson TR, Pretorius DH. Three-dimensional ultrasound: accuracy of distance and volume measurements. Ultrasound Obstet Gynecol 1996; 7: 429–34.

136. Gregg AR, Steiner H, Staudach A, Weiner CP. Accuracy of 3D sonographic volume measurements. Am J Obstet Gynecol 1993; 168: 348.

137. Harrow MM. Enlarged amniotic cavity: a new sonographic sign of early embryonic death. AJR Am J Roentgenol 1992; 158: 359–62.

138. Blaas HG, Eik-Nes SH, Berg S, Torp H. In-vivo three-dimensional reconstruction of embryos and early fetuses. Lancet 1998; 352: 1182–6.

139. Nielsen S, Halin M, Oden A. Using a logistic model to identify women with first-trimester spontaneous miscarriage suitable for expectant management. Br J Obstet Gynaecol 1996; 103: 1230–5.

140. Abramovich DR. The volume of amniotic fluid in early pregnancy. J Obstet Gynaecol Br Commonw 1968; 75: 728–31.

141. Steiner H, Gregg AR, Bogner G, et al. First trimester three-dimensional ultrasound volumetry of the gestational sac. Arch Gynecol Obstet 1994; 255: 165–70.

142. Tongsong T, Wanapirak C, Srisomboom J, et al. Transvaginal ultrasound in threatened abortions with empty gestational sacs. Int J Gynecol Obstet 1994; 46: 297–301.

143. Goldstein SR, Subramanyam BR, Snyder JR. Ratio of gestational sac volume to crown–rump length in early pregnancy. J Reprod Med 1986; 31: 320–1.

144. Report of the RCOG Working Party on Early Pregnancy Assessment. London: Royal College of Obstetricians and Gynaecologists Press, 1996.

145. Dickey RP, Olar TT, Taylor SN, Curole DN, Matulich EM. Relationship of small gestational sac–crown–rump length differences to miscarriage and abortus karyotypes. Obstet Gynecol 1992; 79: 554–7.

4 Ultrasound imaging of early extraembryonic structures

Tibor Fekete, Zoran Belics, and Zoltan Papp

INTRODUCTION

An estimated 60% of pregnancy loss occurs during the 1st trimester of pregnancy. Between 15% and 20% of all clinically recognized pregnancies end in miscarriage. The first visible structures in pregnancy are extraembryonic structures. In order to predict the outcome of pregnancy, we need to fully appreciate the development and pathologic conditions of early extraembryonic structures.

GESTATIONAL SAC

Seven days after conception, the blastocyst reaches the uterine cavity. It embeds into the secretory-phase endometrium, and begins to implant. The trophoblast cells penetrate the endometrium, erode the maternal capillaries, and make contact with the maternal circulation. The trophoblast and the decidua cells form the gestational sac, which is the first visible structure in early pregnancy: it can be detected by transvaginal sonography after the 4th week of gestation.

The gestational sac is a ring-shaped structure with a double-layered wall, embedded eccentrically into the endometrium. It is important to differentiate it from the pseudogestational sac of ectopic pregnancy (Table 4.1). The pseudogestational sac is in fact a fluid-filled cavity between the layers of the enlarged endometrium. It has a thin simple wall, and is usually in a central position. Peritrophoblastic activity is never visible in the underlying layers.[1]

Volumetry of the gestational sac

Using three-dimensional (3D) ultrasound, Kupesic and Kurjak[2] found a positive correlation between gestational age and the volume of the gestational sac and yolk sac until the 10th week of gestation. At the end of the 1st trimester, the yolk sac volume remains constant, while the gestational sac volume continues to grow.

Along with crown–rump length (CRL) the volume of the gestational sac and yolk sac may have prognostic value for embryonic development. Regression analysis revealed a strong correlation between gestational sac volume and gestational age. Logarithmic relationship was observed when yolk sac volumes were plotted against gestational age. Both gestational sac volumetry and CRL measurements proved to have statistically significant predictive value for adverse outcome ($p < 0.05$). Mean yolk sac/gestational sac ratios also had good predictive values ($p < 0.05$).[3]

Table 4.1 The difference between the gestational and pseudogestational sac

	Gestational sac	Pseudogestational sac
Localization	Lateral	Central
Shape	Spheroid	Ovoid
Contour	Thick, double-layered wall	Thin, monolayered wall
Peritrophoblastic circulation	Exists	Non-existent

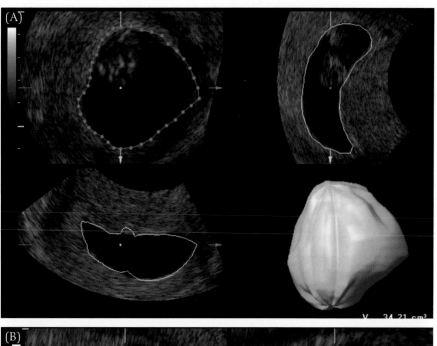

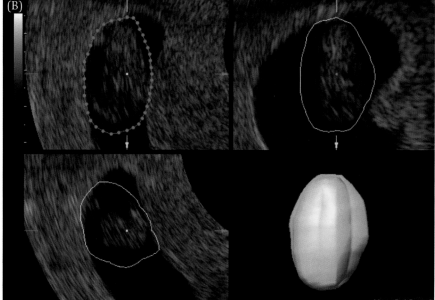

Figure 4.1 (A, B) Volumetry of gestational and amniotic sacs

Our group found that the volumes of the gestational and amniotic sacs grow exponentially during the 1st trimester (Figures 4.1 and 4.2). We found no difference between male and female embryos with regard to gestational or amniotic sac volumes (Figure 4.3). In the case of midtrimester abortions, the growth rate of the gestational and amniotic sacs was slower than in a normnal pregnancy (Figure 4.4).

In the case of chromosomal aberration, the mean gestational sac volume for gestational age is not significantly different from normal in fetuses with trisomy 21, trisomy 18, or Turner syndrome, but it is smaller in those with triploidy or trisomy 13. However, the mean gestational sac volume for CRL is significantly larger in trisomy 18, smaller in triploidy and trisomy 13, and not different from normal in trisomy 21 and Turner syndrome. The mean CRL for gestational age is significantly smaller than normal in trisomy 18, triploidy, and trisomy 13.[4]

BLIGHTED OVUM (FIGURE 4.5)

In an anembryonic pregnancy, a fertilized ovum develops into a blastocyst without inner cell mass development. Trophoblast cells invade the endometrium and form the gestational sac. They produce human chorionic

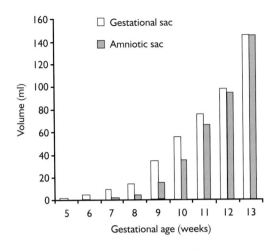

Figure 4.2 Volumes of gestational and amniotic sacs in normal pregnancy

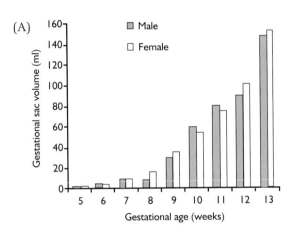

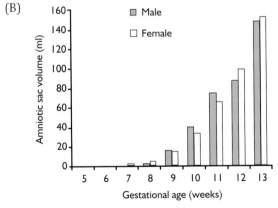

Figure 4.3 Volumes of gestational sac (A) and amniotic sac (B) in male and female embryos

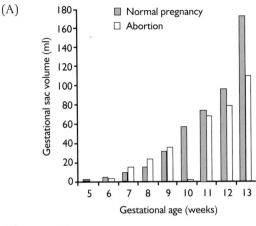

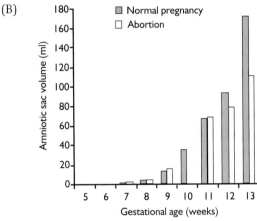

Figure 4.4 Volumes of gestational sac (A) and amniotic sac (B) in normal pregnancy and midtrimester abortion

With ultrasound examination, the mean sac diameter is the most useful criterion for determining non-viability. If the mean sac diameter is more than 17 mm and no embryo is detected or if it is more than 13 mm without a visible yolk sac, the probability for non-viable gestation is close to 100%. A deformed shape and thin wall of the gestational sac and position close to the cervix are strong indicators of non-viable gestation, but are not 100% accurate.[5]

When no accurate distinction between viable and non-viable gestation can be made at a single examination, serial examinations should be carried out before active management is advocated.

CHORIONIC PLATE

By the 8th day of development, the blastocyst is partially embedded in the endometrial stroma. In the area over the embryoblast, the trophoblast differentiates into two

gonadotropins; therefore, a pregnancy test will be positive and clinical signs of pregnancy are present.

The ultrasound diagnosis is based on the absence of embryonic echoes within the gestational sac, large enough for such structures to be visualized.

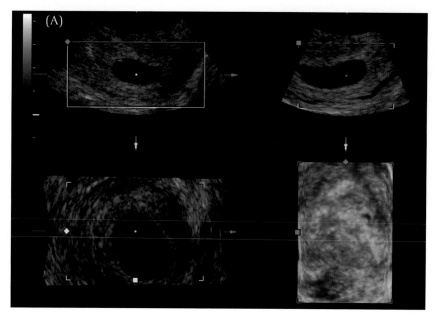
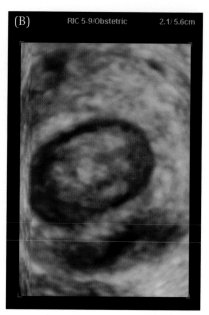

Figure 4.5 (A,B) Blighted ovum

layers: an inner layer – the cytotrophoblast – and an outer zone – the syncytiotrophoblast. The syncytiotrophoblast penetrates the stroma and erodes the endothelial lining of the maternal capillaries. These congested and dilated capillaries are known as sinusoids. The syncytial lacunae then become continuous with the sinusoids, and maternal blood enters the lacunar system. As the trophoblast continues to erode more sinusoids, maternal blood begins to flow through the trophoblastic system, thus establishing the utero-placental circulation.

Regular placentation supposes a progressive trophoblast invasion of spiral arteries. Normally, this process is finished by the 20th week. In the majority of abortions and in pre-eclampsia, this process is disturbed: the evolving chorionic plate becomes thin and fragile, and the trophoblast cork, which hinders the maternal flow in the first trimester, is missing.

Usually, there is no significant maternal flow in the intervillous space until the 12th week.[6] If the maternal blood floods into the intervillous space in advance, it increases the pressure and mechanically injures and lifts the thin chorionic plate, which leads to abortion. In fact, regardless of its etiology, this process is in the background of the majority of 1st trimester abortions.

Subchorionic hemorrhage (Figure 4.6)

In contrast to subchorionic hemorrhage of the chorion laeve, hemorrhage of the chorion frondosum indicates

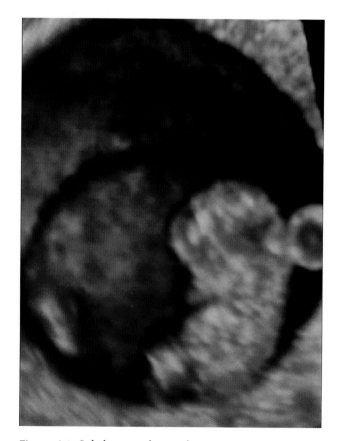

Figure 4.6 Subchorionic hemorrhage

a bad prognosis. Subchorionic hemorrhage can be visualized as a fluid-filled cavity of variable size and echogenicity under the chorionic plate. The incidence of subchorionic hemorrhage in a normal early pregnancy is 2–4% and doubles the probability of abortion. In every second case of threatened abortion, subchorionic hemorrhage can be detected.

According to the literature, it is not the volume but the position of the hematoma that determines the prognosis. A subchorionic hemorrhage under the chorion laeve can reach large dimensions without any serious consequence, while even a small hematoma at the insertion site of the umbilical cord can lead to abortion. Subchorionic hemorrhage near the cervix can clear spontaneously – thus, the prognosis is good in most cases. In these cases, fresh vaginal bleeding indicates immediate clearing, while brown spotting indicates previous hemorrhage. A hematoma near the fundus can significantly increase the intrauterine volume, causing spontaneous termination of the pregnancy.[7–9]

Makikallio et al[10] measured the pulzatility index of uterine, arcuate, spiral, umbilical, and chorionic arteries in the 1st trimester of pregnancies complicated by vaginal bleeding or subchorionic hematomas. They found that vaginal bleeding with or without a subchorionic hematoma is associated with increased radial artery impedance at the 7th week of gestation. Persistence of the subchorionic hematoma does not affect uterine and umblicoplacental circulation.

Subchorionic hemorrhage is iso-echogenic with the endometrium, and slow blood flow can be detected inside it. During the process of absorption, the hematoma becomes hypoechogenic, and finally the area will be anechoic. If the hemorrhage does not lead to an abortion, there is an increased risk of placental complications in the 2nd and 3rd trimesters. The risk of pre-eclampsia, intrauterine growth retardation, and the need for cesarean section increases significantly, probably due to placental complications. The pathologic mechanism is still undetermined.[11] The relative risks of complications in cases of retroplacental hematomas are as follows:

- cesarean delivery   2.1
- hypertension   2.1
- pre-eclampsia   4.0
- placental abruption   5.6
- placental separation abnormalities   3.2
- preterm delivery   2.3
- fetal growth restriction   2.4
- fetal distress   2.6

In practice, it is advisable to consider every pregnancy complicated by subchorionic hemorrhage as a high-risk pregnancy. Repeated ultrasound examination is not advisable, due to the lack of therapeutic consequence.

YOLK SAC (TABLE 4.2)

Development of the yolk sac

Between the 22nd and 28th postmenstrual days, the embryo consists of only two layers: the embryonal ectoderm and the primary endoderm. These two layers form two cavities around the embryo: the amniotic cavity (ectoderm) and the primary yolk sac (endoderm). The secondary yolk sac evolves from the primary yolk sac by the 5th postmenstrual week (29–36 days). By this time, the primary yolk sac is absorbed and the secondary yolk sac has completely developed. The extraembryonic mesoderm, which fills the cavity of the blastocyst, is converted into a thin layer, covering both the amnion and the yolk sac, forming the somato- and splanchnopleura. These two shields communicate only by the body stalk.

Compared with the amniotic cavity, the growth rate of the yolk sac is higher. On ultrasound examination, the yolk sac is the first visible structure in the chorionic cavity and can usually be detected at the beginning of the 5th week. It is a round structure with an echogenic rim and a hypoechoic center. At this

Table 4.2 Normal and abnormal yolk sac characteristics

	Normal findings	**Abnormal findings**
Characteristic	Echogenic rim, hypoechoic center	Hyperechoic
Shape	Round	Distorted
Size	3–4 mm in the 5th week 5–6 mm in the 10th week	<2 mm or >6 mm
Doppler	Non-continuous, absence of diastolic flow	Irregular blood flow, permanent diastolic flow, venous blood flow

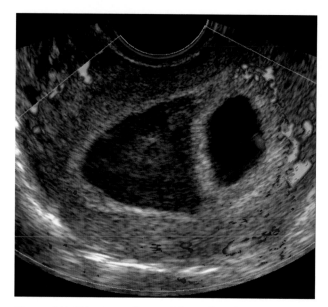

Figure 4.7 3D picture from a 9th week embryo

intestinal duct. There is no basal membrane between the inner and middle layers.

The external layer is the *mesothelial layer* containing 5–10 μm high cells with 2–5 μm microvilli on the surface. The cells are full of intracellular vacuoles.

After the 9th week, the structure of the yolk sac changes. The microvilli and the inner cell structure dissolves, and the process of degeneration begins.

Function of the yolk sac

Due to its structure and position, the yolk sac plays an important role in transport of nutrition. The following facts support this role:

- The wall and the cavity of the yolk sac are in direct contact with the primitive mid-gut.
- Its histologic structure is very similar to that of the the liver.
- The composition of the celomic fluid is significantly different from the amnionic fluid: it contains proteins, creatinine, and human chorionic gonadotropin (hCG) in a higher concentration.[13]
- The yolk sac synthesizes numerous proteins (α-fetoprotein (AFP), $α_1$-antitrypsin, albumin, prealbumin, and transferrin), which, after the 10th postmenstrual week, are produced by the liver.[14,15]

time, the diameter is 3–4 mm. The secondary yolk sac is the unambiguous evidence of intrauterine gravidity. Until there is a detectable yolk sac inside the uterine cavity, we should always take ectopic pregnancy into account.

Around 36–38 postmenstrual days, the embryo becomes visible between the amniotic cavity and the yolk sac as a 2–3 mm long, linear, hyperechoic structure. At this stage, we can detect the embryo's heart activity, although until the 6th week of gestation there is no detectable circulation in the yolk sac.

By the 9th week (Figure 4.7), the yolk sac grows to a diameter of 5–6 mm, but it begins to degenerate soon after, and disappears by the 12th week.[12]

Structure of the yolk sac

The yolk sac consists of three layers: the inner endoderm, the middle mesenchymal layer, and the external mesothelial layer.

The *inner endodermal layer* contains 10–20 μm wide columnar cells, with 0.5–1.0 μm long cilia on the surface. Inside the cells, there are mitochondria, a highly developed Golgi apparatus, lysosomes, glycogen, and intracellular vacuoles. These cells are very similar to liver cells, due to their similar functions. The canalicular network of these cells also resembles that of the liver.

The middle layer is the *mesenchymal layer*. It contains blood vessels, red blood cells, and macrophages. The vessels spring from the vitello-

Circulation of the yolk sac (Figure 4.8)

At the end of the 5th week, mesodermal cells of the yolk sac walls differentiate into blood cells and blood vessels. Centrally located cells then give rise to primitive blood cells, while those on the periphery flatten and form endothelial cells lining blood islands. These blood islands approach each other rapidly by sprouting of endothelial cells, and, after fusion, give rise to small vessels. At the same time, blood cells and capillaries develop in the extraembryonic mesoderm of the villous stems and the connecting stalk. Inside the embryo, extraembryonic vessels establish contact with each other by continuous budding. Intraembryonic blood vessels, including the heart tube, are established in exactly the same manner as extraembryonic vessels.

By rhythmic contractions of the heart, the primitive blood is pumped from the connecting stalk towards the cranial portion of the embryo. Meanwhile, the intraembryonic blood vessels protrude into the

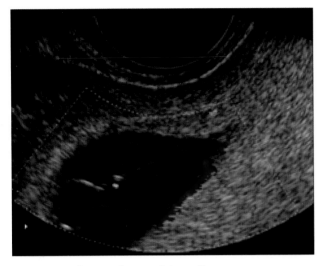

Figure 4.8 The circulation of the yolk sac

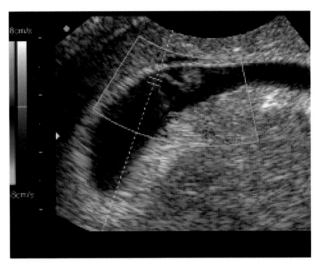

Figure 4.9 The normal waveform of the yolk sac circulation

chorion through the body stalk, and form capillary loops at the axis of the villi, giving rise to the placental circulation.

The intraembryonic circulation precedes blood flow in the intervillous space. Normal placental circulation starts only after the end of organogenesis around the 13th week, which confirms the significant role of the yolk sac in nutritive and transport functions.

Kupesic and Kurjak examined the circulation of the yolk sac and vitelline duct in early pregnancy.[16,17] Before the 6th week, no circulation in the body stalk or the yolk sac was detectable on ultrasound Doppler examination. Between the 6th and 12th weeks, a non-continuous, low-velocity waveform could be detected, with an absence of diastolic flow (Figure 4.9). The overall visualization rate for yolk sac vessels was 80%. The highest visualization rates were obtained in the 7th and 8th weeks of gestation, reaching values of 90%. In the same period, the visualization rates of the vitelline duct arteries were 87% and 91%. The characteristic waveform profile showed a low velocity (5.8 ± 1.7 cm/s) and an absence of diastolic flow, which was obtained from all examined yolk sacs. The pulsatility index had a mean value of 3.24 ± 0.94. Vitelline vessels showed similar values of velocity (5.4 ± 1.8 cm/s) and pulsatility index (3.14 ± 0.91).[2]

Abnormalities of yolk sac development

From the formation and function of the yolk sac, it is evident that any deviation in these complicated processes can disturb the development of the embryo.

The yolk sac plays an important role in the nutritive, metabolic and hematopoietic processes of the 1st trimester.[18] Any abnormality in the shape, size, structure, or circulation of the yolk sac (e.g., a double yolk sac: Figure 4.10) indicates a major abnormality in development.[19,20]

Absence of the yolk sac is the first sonographic indicator of early maldevelopment. These cases are defined as blighted ovum, but differential diagnosis with a pseudogestational sac is important.

Abnormal yolk sac size can also be an indicator of maldevelopment. According to Lyons[21] the yolk sac diameter should be less than 4 mm in a gestational sac less than 10 mm in diameter. A large yolk sac (Figure 4.11) can indicate a poor pregnancy outcome. In surviving embryos, the relative risk of chromosomal aberrations is increased.

A small yolk sac can also predict a poor pregnancy outcome,[22] as reported by Green and Hobbins.[23] Kucuk et al[24] found that a yolk sac diameter bigger or smaller than 2 standard deviations of the mean at a certain gestational age allowed prediction of an abnormal pregnancy outcome with a sensitivity of 65%, a specificity of 97%, a positive predictive value of 71%, and a negative predictive value of 95%. An abnormal yolk sac shape allowed prediction of an abnormal pregnancy outcome with a sensitivity of 29%, a specificity of 95%, a positive predictive value of 47%, and a negative predictive value of 90.5%.

Changes in echogenicity can also be predicting factors. The presence of a hyperechogenic yolk sac is strongly associated with chromosomal aneuploidy between the 9th and 11th gestational weeks.[25]

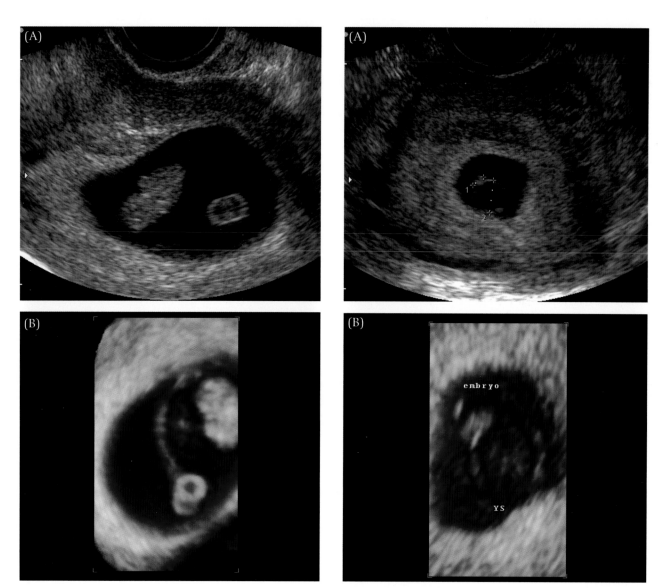

Figure 4.10 (A,B) Double yolk sac

Figure 4.11 Large yolk sac

Kupesik and Kurjak[2] demonstrated the characteristics of the yolk sac circulation. They found a non-continuous low-velocity waveform with absent diastolic flow. They also detected three different types of abnormal waveform of the yolk sac circulation signals in patients with missed abortions: irregular blood flow, permanent diastolic flow, and venous blood flow (Figure 4.12).

Makikallio et al[26] examined the Doppler parameters of uterine, spiral, intraplacental, chorionic, umbilical, and yolk sac hemodynamics in early pregnancy. They found that at the 8th week of gestation, the maternal intraplacental resistance index was higher in patients who later had pre-eclampsia. A week later, the yolk sac resistance index and umbilical artery mean velocity were lower. In the late 1st trimester, increased

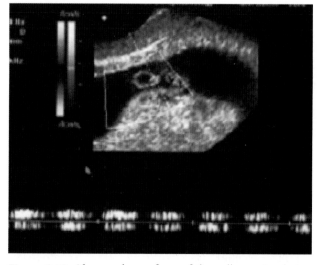

Figure 4.12 Abnormal waveform of the yolk sac circulation

velocities and resistance index were observed in the chorionic arteries. No differences in uterine and spiral artery hemodynamics or in umbilical artery pulsatility index were observed.

In diamniotic twin pregnancies, the number of embryos equals the number of yolk sacs. In monochorionic monoamniotic twin pregnancies, a single yolk sac may be a normal finding. However, cases of a single yolk sac are strongly associated with conjoined twins.[27]

REFERENCES

1. Nyberg DA, Laing FC, Filly RA. Ultrasonographic differentiation of gestational sac of early intrauterine pregnancy from the pseudogestational sac of ectopic pregnancy. Radiology 1983; 146: 755.

2. Kupesic S, Kurjak A. Volume and vascularity of the yolk sac assessed by three-dimensional and power Doppler ultrasound. Early Pregnancy 2001; 5: 40–1.

3. Babinszki A, Nyari T, Jordan S, et al. Three-dimensional measurement of gestational and yolk sac volumes as predictors of pregnancy outcome in the first trimester. Am J Perinatol 2001; 18: 203–11.

4. Falcon O, Wegrzyn P, Faro C, Peralta CF, Nicolaides KH. Gestational sac volume measured by three-dimensional ultrasound at 11 to 13 + 6 weeks of gestation: relation to chromosomal defects. Ultrasound Obstet Gynecol 2005; 25: 546–50.

5. Tongsong T, Wanapirak C, Srisomboon J, et al. Transvaginal ultrasound in threatened abortions with empty gestational sacs. Int J Gynecol Obstet 1994; 46: 297–301.

6. Kurjak A, Laurini R, Kupesic S, et al. A combined Doppler and morphopathological study of intervillous circulation. Ultrasound Obstet Gynecol 1995; 6: 116.

7. Kurjak A, Schulman H, Zudenigo D, et al. Subchorionic hematomas in early pregnancy: clinical outcome and blood flow patterns. J Matern Fetal Med 1996; 5: 41–4.

8. Ball RH, Ade CM, Schoenborn JA, Crane JP. The clinical significance of ultrasonographically detected subchorionic hemorrhages. Am J Obstet Gynecol 1996; 174: 996–1002.

9. Pearlstone M, Baxi L. Subchorionic hematoma: a review. Obstet Gynecol Surv 1993; 48: 65–8.

10. Makikallio K, Tekay A, Jouppila P. Effects of bleeding on uteroplacental and yolk-sac hemodynamics in early pregnancy. Ultrasound Obstet Gynecol 2001; 18: 352–6.

11. Nagy S, Bush M, Stone J, Lapinski RH, Gardo S. Clinical significance of subchorionic and retroplacental hematomas detected in the first trimester of pregnancy. Obstet Gynecol 2003; 102: 94–100.

12. Jauniaux E, Jurkovic D, Henriet Y. Development of the secondary yolk sac: correlation of sonographic and anatomic features. Hum Reprod 1991; 6: 1160–6.

13. Jauniaux E, Jurkovic D, Gulbis B. Biochemical composition of exocoelomic fluid in early human pregnancy. Obstet Gynecol 1991; 78: 1124–8.

14. Gitlin D, Perricelli A, Gitlin GM. Synthesis of alpha-fetoprotein by the liver, yolk sac and gastrointestinal tract of the human conceptus. Cancer Res 1972; 32: 979–82.

15. Gitlin GM, Perricelli A. Synthesis of serum albumin, prealbumin, alpha-fetoprotein, alpha-1–antitrypsin and transferrin by the human yolk sac. Nature 1970; 228: 995–7.

16. Kurjak A, Kupesic S, Kostovi LJ. Vascularisation of yolk sac and vitelline duct in normal pregnancies studied by transvaginal color and pulsed Doppler. J Perinat Med 1994; 22: 433–40.

17. Kurjak A, Kupesic S. Color Doppler in Obstetrics, Gynecology and Infertility. London: Parthenon, 1999.

18. Brent RL, Beckmann BM, Koszalka TR. Experimental yolk sac dysfunction as a model for studying nutritional disturbances in the embryo during early organogenesis. Teratology 1990; 41: 405–13.

19. Lindsay DJ, Lovett IS, Lyons EA, et al. Endovaginal appearance of the yolk sac in pregnancy: normal growth and usefulness as a predictor of abnormal pregnancy outcome. Radiology 1992; 183: 115–18.

20. Ferrazzi E, Brambati B, Lanzani A et al. The yolk sac in early pregnancy failure. Am J Obstet Gynecol 1988; 159: 137–42.

21. Lyons EA. Endovaginal sonography of the first trimester of pregnancy. In: Proceedings of the 3rd International Perinatal and Gynecologycal Ultrasound Symposium, Ottawa, Ontario, 1994: 1–25.

22. Bromley B, Harlow BL, Laboda LA, Benacerraf BR. Small sac size in the first trimester: a predictor for poor fetal outcome. Radiology 1991; 178: 375–7.

23. Green JJ, Hobbins JC. Abdominal ultrasound examination of the first trimester fetus. Am J Obstet Gynecol 1988; 159: 165–75.

24. Kucuk T, Duru NK, Yenen MC, et al. Yolk sac size and shape as predictors of poor pregnancy outcome. J Perinat Med 1992; 27: 316–20.

25. Szabo J, Gellen J, Szemere G, Farago M. Significance of hyper-echogenic yolk sac in the first-trimester screening for chromosome aneuploidy. Orv Hetil 1996; 137: 2313–15.

26. Makikallio K, Jouppila P, Tekay A. First trimester uterine, placental and yolk sac haemodynamics in preeclampsia and preterm labour. Hum Reprod 2004; 19: 729–33.

27. Levi CS, Lyons EA, Dashefsky SM, Lindsay DJ, Holt SC. Yolk sac number, size and morphologic features in monodhorionic monoamniotic twin pregnancy. Can Assoc Radiol J 1996; 47: 98–100.

5 Normal and abnormal early human structural development

Ritsuko K Pooh and Asim Kurjak

INTRODUCTION

Since the introduction of high-frequency transvaginal transducers, sonographic visualization of embryos and fetuses in early stages has progressed remarkably and the field of sonoembryology has become well established. Furthermore, recent advances in three- and four-dimensional (3D/4D) ultrasound combined with the transvaginal approach have produced more objective and accurate information on early embyonic and fetal development and the natural history of fetal abnormalities.

YOLK SAC

The yolk sac plays an important role in embryonic hematopoiesis and fetomaternal transport of nutritive properties before the establishment of fetoplacental circulation. The primary yolk sac forms at around 3 weeks of menstrual age; then, following the formation of the extraembryonic celom, the secondary yolk sac is formed. From the 6th week of gestation, it appears as a spherical cystic structure covered by numerous superficial small vessels merging at the basis of the vitelline duct. This connects the yolk sac to the ventral part of the embryo, the gut, and the main blood circulation. During the 10th week of gestation, the yolk sac begins to degenerate and rapidly ceases to function.[1]

It has been reported that an abnormal size and/or shape of the yolk sac may be associated with an ominous outcome of pregnancy.[2] A large yolk sac is defined as being more than 2 standard deviations above the mean, which indicates over 5.6 mm of diameter at less than 10 weeks of menstrual age.[2,3] A large yolk sac is associated with a chromosomal aberration, namely autosomal trisomy (Figures 5.1 and 5.2). An echogenic yolk sac (Figure 5.3) is also related to an adverse outcome of pregnancy, with autosomal trisomy.

NUCHAL TRANSLUCENCY (FIGURES 5.4 AND 5.5)

Nuchal translucency is a fluid collection under the skin behind the neck of fetuses at 10 or 11–13 weeks that can be measured by ultrasound examination. In fetuses with chromosomal abnormalities, cardiac defects, and many genetic syndromes, nuchal tranclucency is increased.

The measurement of nuchal tranclucency suggested by Nicolaides[4] is as follows:

- The fetal crown–rump length (CRL) should be between 45 and 84 mm.
- A good sagittal section of the fetus must be obtained, with the fetus horizontal on the screen. The correct view is a clearly visualized fetal profile.
- The fetus should be in a neutral position, with the head in line with the spine, not hyperextended or flexed.
- Ideally, only the fetal head and upper thorax should be included. The magnification should be as large as possible and *always* such that each slight movement of the calipers produces only a 0.1 mm change in the measurement.
- The widest part of the translucency must always be measured.

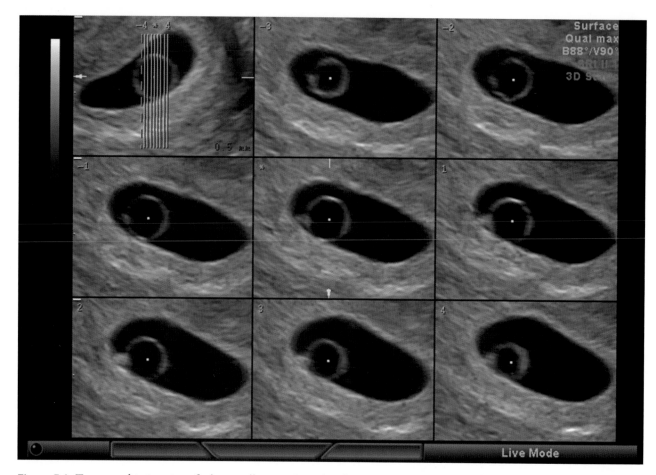

Figure 5.1 Tomographic imaging of a large yolk sac at 6 weeks of gestation. A large yolk sac with normal fetal heartbeat was observed. Fetal demise was confirmed at 8 weeks. A villous chromosome examination showed 47, XY, +22

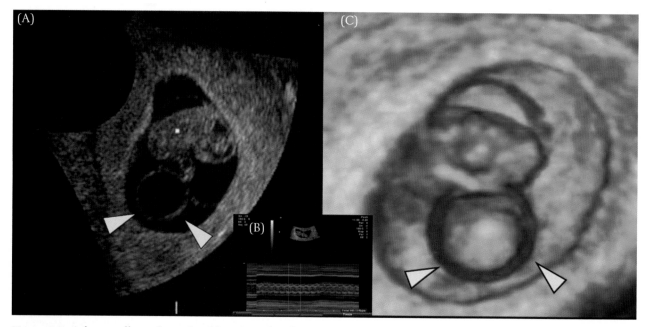

Figure 5.2 A large yolk sac (arrowheads) at 8 weeks of gestation. (A) 2D sagittal section of the fetus. A normal-appearing 8-week fetus and amniotic membrane are visible, but a large yolk sac with diameter 12 mm is demonstrated. (B) A regular fetal heart rate of 174 bpm is confirmed. (C) 3D image. Intrauterine fetal demise was confirmed 30 hours later. A villous chromosome examination showed a double trisomy: 48, XY, +15, +21

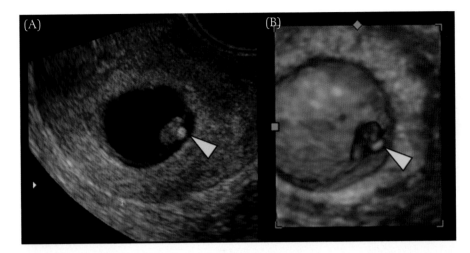

Figure 5.3 Highly echogenic yolk sac. (A) 2D ultrasound image of yolk sac (arrowhead) at 9 weeks and 1 day. A small embryo, compatible with 7 weeks of gestation, was visible, with regular heartbeats, in the abnormally large amniotic sac. (B) 3D ultrasound image. Intrauterine fetal demise was confirmed 3 days later, and villous chromosome examination showed trisomy 15

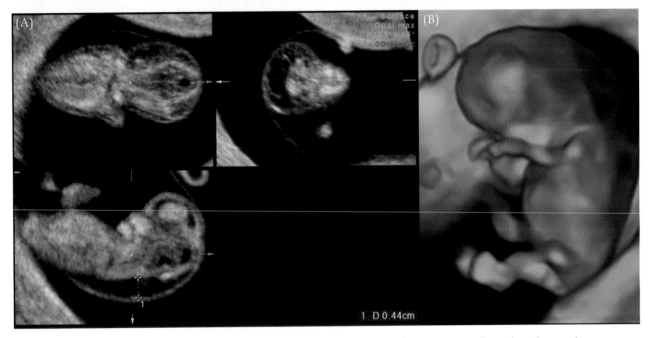

Figure 5.4 Nuchal translucency at 10 weeks of gestation. (A) 3D orthogonal views. Coronal, axial, and sagittal sections are shown. A multidimensional approach to nuchal translucency is useful to distinguish it from amniotic membrane and to measure translucency thickness on an accurate midsagittal section. (B) 3D imaging of the fetus with nuchal translucency

- Measurements should be taken with the inner border of the horizontal line of the calipers placed *on* the line that defines the nuchal translucency thickness – the crossbar of the calipers should be such that it is hardly visible as it merges with the white line of the border, not in the nuchal fluid:

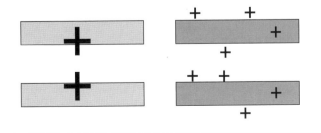

- In magnifying the image (pre or post freeze zoom), it is important to turn down the gain. This avoids the mistake of placing the calipers on the fuzzy edge of the line, which leads to underestimation of the nuchal measurement. Tissue harmonic imaging should not be used for measurement of nuchal translucency, because this thickens the lines and underestimates the measurement.
- Care must be taken to distinguish between fetal skin and amnion.
- During the scan, more than one measurement must be taken, and the maximum one that meets

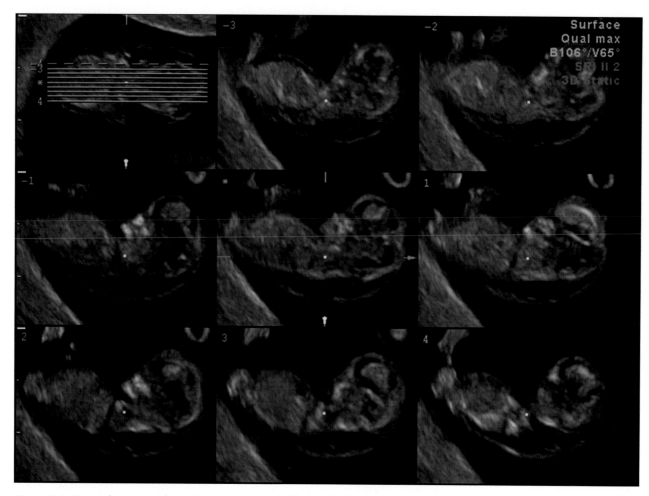

Figure 5.5 Sagittal tomographic ultrasound imaging of nuchal translucency. Parallel slices of a sagittal cutting section are demonstrated. The slicing width can easily be altered. The picture shows a median section of the fetus with nuchal translucency

all of the above criteria should be recorded in the database. It is good practice to retain at least one image for the patient records.

Prospective studies in a total of 200 868 pregnancies, including 871 fetuses with trisomy 21, have demonstrated that increased nuchal translucency can identify 76.8% of fetuses with trisomy 21, which represents a false-positive rate of 4.2%. However, by screening for trisomy 21 by a combination of sonography for the measurement of fetal nuchal translucency, the assessment of fetal nasal bone, and measurement of maternal serum for free β human chorionic gonadotropin (β-hCG) and pregnancy-associated plasma protein A (PAPP-A), it was estimated that, for a false-positive rate of 5%, the detection rate of trisomy 21 would be 97% and, for a false-positive rate of 0.5%, the detection rate would be 91%.[4]

CYSTIC HYGROMA

Cystic hygromas are multiloculated cystic structures that are benign in nature. They may occur anywhere in the body, although they are most frequently encountered in the neck (75%) and axilla (20%). Concerning the origin of cystic hygroma, it was suggested that an early jugular–lymphatic obstructive sequence could cause hydrops fetalis, pterigium colli, and cystic hygroma.[5] This obstruction impedes communication between the jugular lymphatic sacs and the internal jugular vein. There are two other theories: one is that cystic hygroma is caused by an abnormal embryonic sequestration of lymphatic tissue and its subsequent failure to join normal lymphatic channels;[6,7] the other is that abnormal budding of the lymphatics occurs between the 6th and 9th weeks of gestation.[8] More than 50% of cases of cystic hygroma

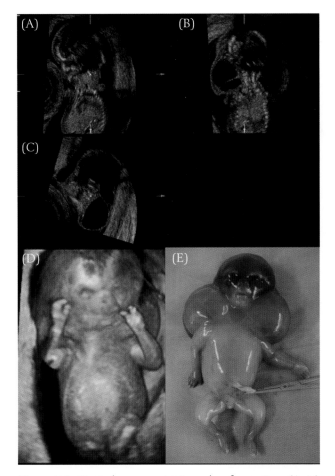

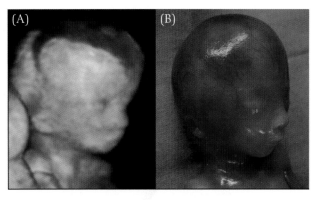

Figure 5.7 Micrognathia and low-set ears at 15 weeks of gestation. (A) 3D ultrasound image of the fetal face at 15 weeks. Micrognathia and low-set ear are demonstrated. Amniocentesis showed trisomy 18. (B) Macrosopic picture of the face of the aborted fetus[12]

Figure 5.6 Cystic hygroma at 14 weeks of gestation. (A–C) 3D orthogonal views of cystic hygroma in the sagittal (A), coronal (B), and axial (C) planes. Multicystic hygroma is demonstrated. (D) 3D imaging of the fetus. (E) Macrosopic picture of the aborted fetus. Chromosomal examination showed 45,X, Turner syndrome

demonstrated aneuploidy, with Turner syndrome being the most common (Figure 5.6). Howarth et al[9] reported that the 'normal outcome' rate from pregnancies complicated by prenatally diagnosed cystic hygroma is less than 10%.

FACIAL ABNORMALITIES

Congenital facial abnormalities that can be detected in the 1st and early 2nd trimesters includes hypotelorism, cyclopia, nasal bone dysplasia, cleft lip, low-set ears (Figure 5.7), micrognathia, and agnathia (Figure 5.8). Facial abnormality is occasionally associated with abnormal structure of the central nervous

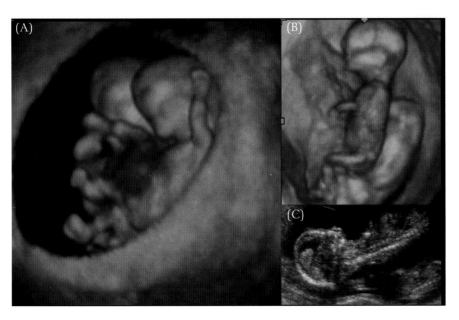

Figure 5.8 Agnathia in the 1st trimester. (A) 3D imaging. Agnathia was suspected in one of monochorionic monoamniotic twins at 11 weeks. (B) 3D imaging at 14 weeks. (C) 2D sagittal imaging of the fetal face[12]

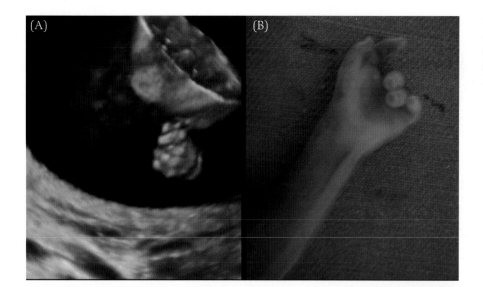

Figure 5.9 Overlapping fingers in a case of trisomy 18 at 17 weeks of gestation. (A) 3D ultrasound imaging. (B) Macrosopic picture of the aborted fetus[12]

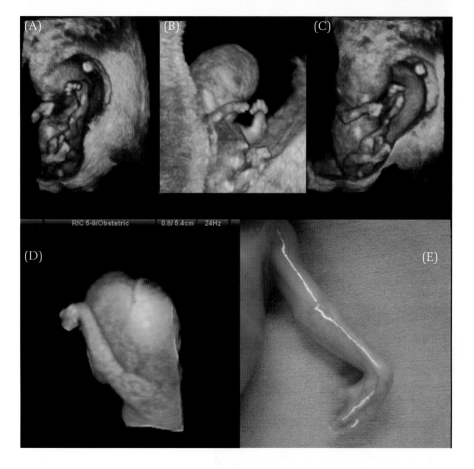

Figure 5.10 Left wrist contracture in a case of trisomy 18. (A–C) 3D ultrasound images of left wrist contracture at 11 weeks of gestation. The right wrist is normal. (D) 3D image at 16 weeks. (E) Macroscopic picture of the aborted fetus[12]

system, syndromic diseases, and/or chromosomal aberrations.[12]

LIMB ABNORMALITIES

Limb abnormality occurs as an isolated finding or as part of a set of syndromic or chromosomal abnormal-ities. Only 5% of congenital hand anomalies occur as part of a recognized syndrome. Overlapping fingers (Figure 5.9), wrist contracture (Figure 5.10), and forearm deformity are often associated with trisomy 18. Skeletal dysplasias such as dwarfism (Figure 5.11) gradually became detectable during pregnancy. Congenital skeletal abnormality in early pregnancy as shown in Figure 5.12 is rare. Polydactyly (Figure 5.13)

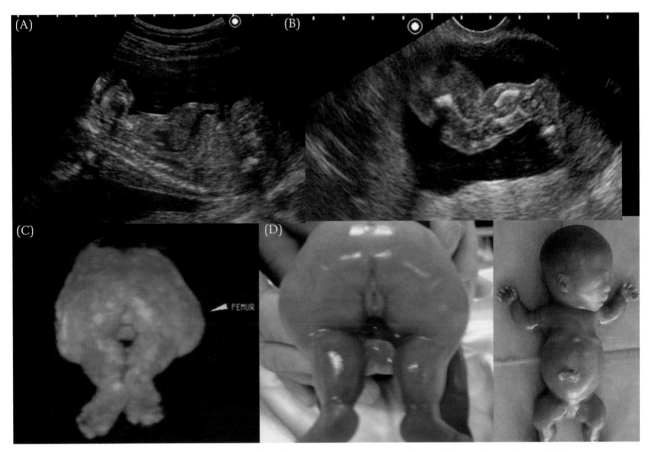

Figure 5.11 Thanatophoric dwarfism at 19 weeks of gestation. (A) Narrow chest and hypoplastic lung. (B) Lower extremities. Short and curved long bones are demonstrated. (C) 3D imaging of the lower extremities. (D) Macroscopic pictures of the aborted fetus[12]

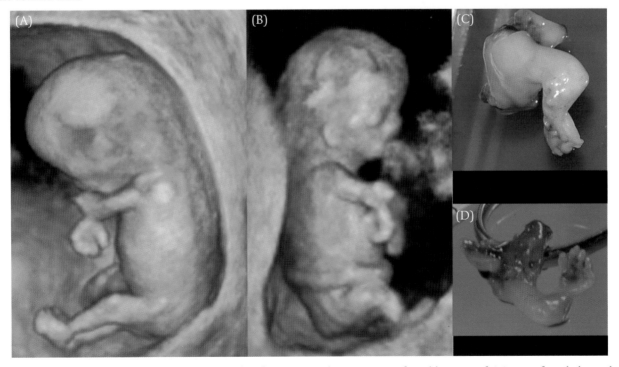

Figure 5.12 Upper limb abnormality at 11 weeks of gestation. This case was referred because of 4.4 mm of nuchal translucency at 11 weeks of gestation. (A,B) 3D ultrasound revealed skeletal dysplasia of the bilateral upper extremities. (C,D) Macroscopic appearance of the upper limbs of the aborted fetus[12]

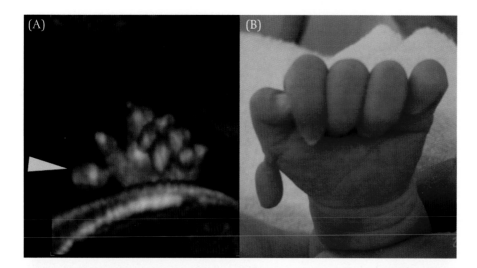

Figure 5.13 Polydactyly. (A) 3D ultrasound image at 19 weeks of gestation. (B) Postnatal appearance[12]

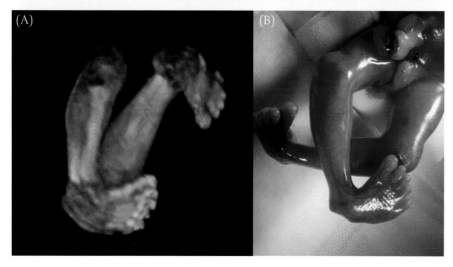

Figure 5.14 Clubfoot at 19 weeks of gestation. (A) 3D imaging of the lower extremities. (B) Macroscopic picture of the aborted fetus[12]

is the most common congenital anomaly of the upper limb. Preaxial polydactyly most often presents as a triphalangeal thumb. Syndactyly is also a common congenital anomaly. The third and then the fourth web in the hand and the second web in the foot are the most commonly affected. Syndactyly is occasionally associated with syndromes such as Apert syndrome. Congenital clubfoot (Figure 5.14) often occurs with unknown etiology. Chromosomal aberration, spina bifida, and oligohydramnios may result in clubfoot.

CHEST ABNORMALITY

Congenital diaphragmatic hernia (CDH) occurs in 1 of every 2000–4000 live births and accounts for 8% of all major congenital anomalies. There are three types of CDH; posterolateral Bochdalek hernia (occurring at approximately 6 weeks of gestation), anterior Morgagni hernia, and hiatus hernia. Left-sided Bochdalek hernia (Figure 5.15) occurs in approximately 90% of cases. Left-sided hernias allow herniation of both small and large bowel as well as intra-abdominal solid organs into the thoracic cavity. In right-sided hernias, only the liver and a portion of the large bowel tend to herniate. Bilateral hernias are uncommon; however, we have had a case with congenital diaphragmatic defect in early pregnancy (Figure 5.16).

In many cases with thoracic fluid collection, pleural effusion with floating lungs (Figure 5.17) is demonstrated. Pleural effusion is seen in many hydropic fetuses, but in some cases it is an isolated or transient finding.

Pericardial effusion with floating heart with normal beats (Figure 5.18) is a rare condition. Successful treatment in utero with aspiration of the pericardial fluid in the 1st and 2nd trimesters has been reported.[10]

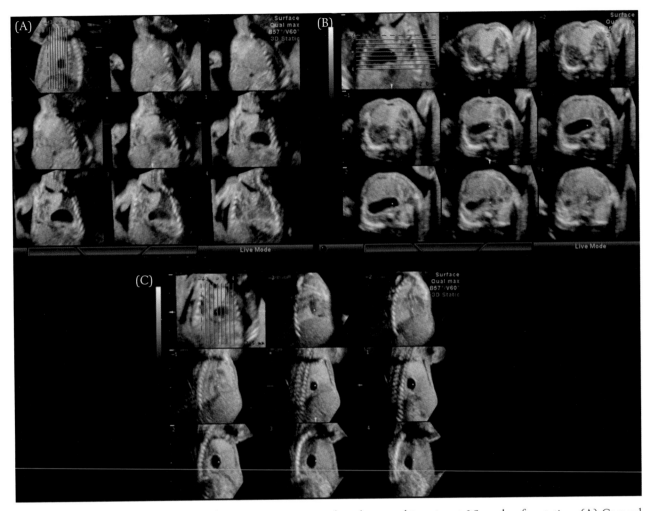

Figure 5.15 Congenital diaphragmatic hernia on 3D tomographic ultrasound imaging at 16 weeks of gestation. (A) Coronal sections. The stomach bubble and liver are visible inside the chest. (B) Axial sections. (C) Sagittal sections[12]

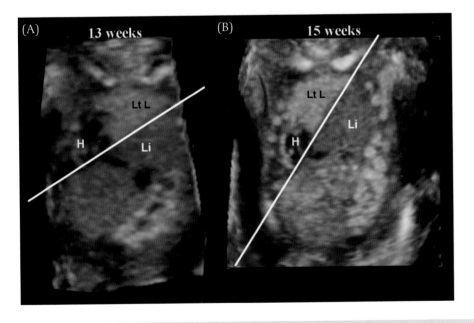

Figure 5.16 Congenital diaphragmatic defect at 13 and 15 weeks of gestation. This case was referred because of nuchal translucency of 3 mm at 11 weeks of gestation. (A) Frontal view at 13 weeks. Dextrocardia (H), liver-up (Li) and oppressed left lung (Lt L) are demonstrated. (B) Frontal view at 15 weeks. The line of the lung–liver border is at an acute angle due to progressive liver-up[12]

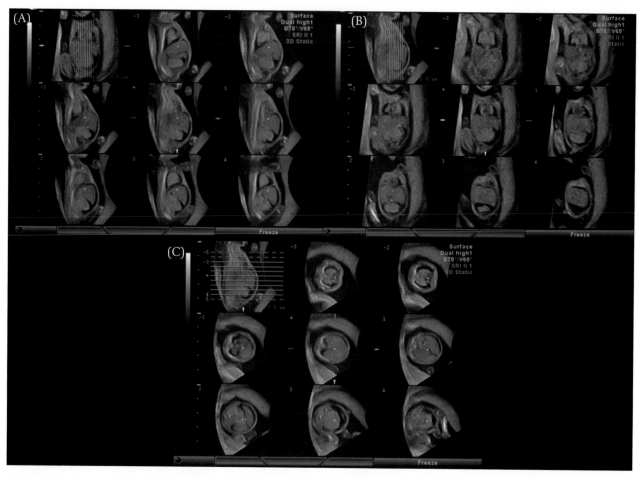

Figure 5.17 Tomographic ultrasound scan of bilateral pleural effusion and ascites at 19 weeks of gestation. Sagittal (A), coronal (B), and axial (C) tomographic images. Amniocentesis showed a low-frequency mosaicism of 45,X/46,XY[12]

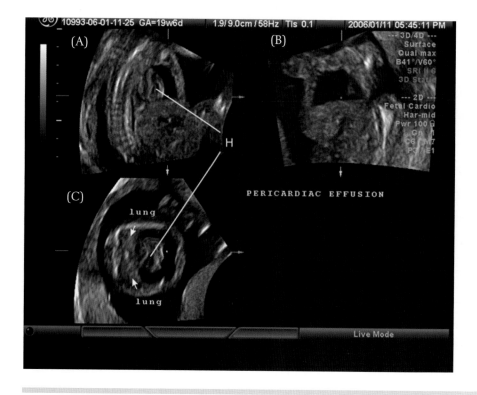

Figure 5.18 Pericardial effusion at 19 weeks of gestation. 3D orthogonal views. Sagittal (A), coronal (B), and axial (C) sections. Because of a large amount of pericardial effusion, the heart (H) moved like a pendulum and the bilateral lungs are oppressed backwards[12]

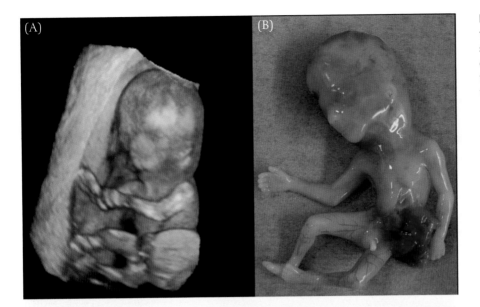

Figure 5.19 Omphalocele at 12 weeks of gestation. (A) 3D ultrasound image at 12 weeks and 5 days. (B) Macroscopic picture of the aborted fetus. The hernial sac was ruptured at delivery[12]

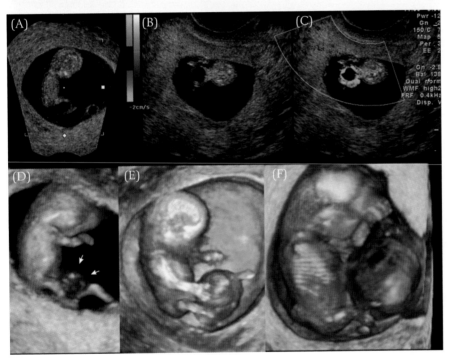

Figure 5.20 Bladder exstrophy in the 1st trimester. (A–C) Cystic formation between bilateral umbilical arteries. No bladder is visible inside the fetus. (D–F) 3D ultrasound images of 10 (D), 11 (E), and 12 (F) weeks. A rapid increase in the size of the external bladder is clearly demonstrated[12]

ABNORMALITY OF ABDOMINAL WALL

Around 10 weeks of gestation, physiologic umbilical hernia can occur. However, after 12 weeks of gestation, extra-abdominal masses indicate omphalocele or gastroschisis. An omphalocele (Figure 5.19) is covered by a membrane (consisting of an outer layer of amnion and an inner layer of peritoneum), with the cord inserting through this covering. In cases of omphalocele, there is a strong association with other malformations and chromosomal abnormalities. Gastroschisis is a paraumbilical defect involving all the layers of the abdominal wall, with

evisceration of abdominal organs, usually the small bowel and on occasion the large bowel and stomach. Between 7% and 30% of fetuses with gastroschisis can have an associated malformation. In general, the survival rate is more than 95% because of the absence of associated anomalies and improvements in neonatal care.

URINARY TRACT ABNORMALITIES

Bladder extrophy (Figure 5.20) is a rare abnormality, which may be associated with cloaca malformation or

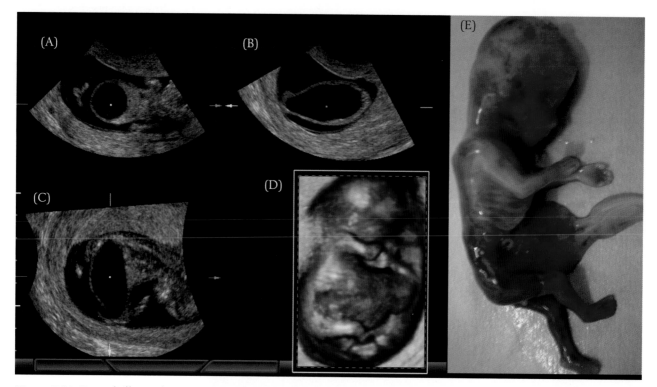

Figure 5.21 Prune-belly syndrome at 11 weeks of gestation. (A–C) 3D orthogonal views of coronal (A), axial (B), and sagittal (C) sections. A huge bladder and fragile abdominal wall are visible. (D) 3D imaging of the fetus. (E) Macroscopic picture of the aborted fetus[12]

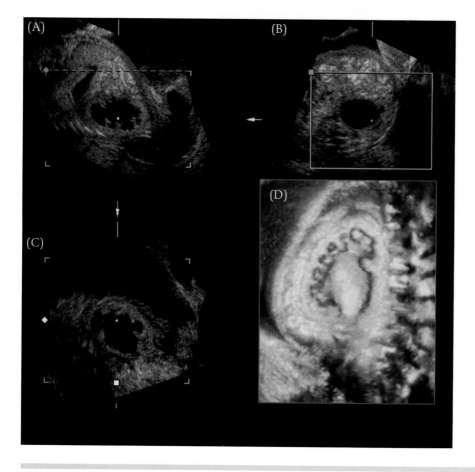

Figure 5.22 Unilateral hydronephrosis at 18 weeks of gestation. (A–C) 3D orthogonal views of a unlateral kidney. (D) Inside of the kidney. Renal parenchyma, an enlarged renal pelvis, and calicectasis are clearly demonstrated[12]

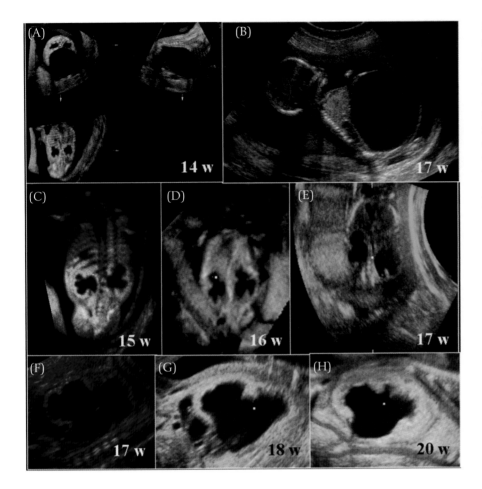

Figure 5.23 Huge bladder before and after a vesicoamniotic shunt (VAS) operation. (A) 3D orthogonal view at 14 weeks of gestation. A huge bladder and bilateral hydronephrosis are demonstrated. The abdominal wall is not fragile as in prune-belly syndrome. (B) Sagittal image at 17 weeks before VAS. The bladder volume is 137.7 ml. (C–E) Changing appearance of the kidneys at 15 (C), 16 (D), and 17 (E) weeks. Rapid thinning of the renal parenchyma with progressive hydronephrosis is clearly demonstrated. (F–H) Changing appearance of the renal parenchyma (at 17 (F), 18 (G), and 20 (H) weeks) after a VAS operation performed at 17 weeks. The renal parenchyma thickness recovered rapidly after the VAS procedure, with improvement of hydronephrosis[12]

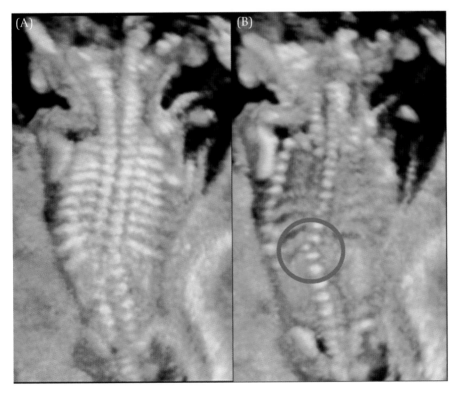

Figure 5.24 T11 hemivertebra at 19 weeks of gestation. There was 11 mm of nuchal translucency at 11 weeks; chromosomes were normal. (A) Scoliosis; left 11 ribs and right 10 ribs are demonstrated. (B) T11 vertebral body shows a hemivertebra, which is the cause of scoliosis[12]

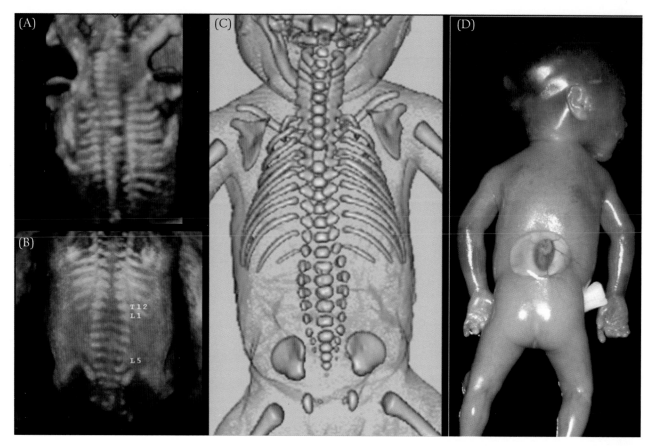

Figure 5.25 L4, L5 vertebral body defect and spina bifida. (A) 3D imaging of vertebral body defect at 15 weeks of gestation. (B) 3D imaging of spina bifida lower than T11 at 17 weeks. (C) 3D computed tomographic imaging of the aborted fetus at 21 weeks. The L4,L5 vertebral body defect, spina bifida, and 11 rubs are clearly demonstrated. (D) Macroscopic picture of the aborted fetus. Rupture of a myelomeningocele is demonstrated[12]

the OEIS (omphalocele, bladder extrophy, imperforate anus, spine defect) complex. Prune-belly syndrome (Figure 5.21) describes the triad of dilatation of the urinary tract, a deficiency of the abdominal wall musculature, and failure of testicular descent. Hydronephrosis (Figure 5.22) is the most common pathologic finding in the urinary tract on prenatal sonographic screening. Fetal obstructive uropathy has become detectable earlier, and fetal therapy using vesicoamniotic shunting (VAS) is the accepted procedure in well-defined cases. It has been reported that the long-term outcomes indicate that VAS at 18–30 weeks may not change the prognosis of renal function and that fetal surgery for obstructive uropathy should be performed only for the carefully selected patient who has severe oligohydramnios and 'normal'-appearing kidneys.[11] To preserve renal function, however, earlier VAS may be preferable (Figure 5.23).

VERTEBRAL ABNORMALITIES

Hemivertebra (Figure 5.24) is a rare congenital spinal anomaly where only a unilateral vertebral body develops, resulting in a deformed spine, such as scoliosis or kyphosis. Partial vertebral body dysplasia (Figure 5.25) and vertebral body dysplasia (Figure 5.26) are rare conditions of the spine. Complete vertebral body dysplasia is associated with spondylocostal dysplasia, spondylothoracic dysplasia, type II collagenopathies, and other skeletal dysplasias.

REFERENCES

1. Jaumiaux E, Gulbis B, Burton GJ. The human first trimester gestational sac limits rather than facilitates oxygen transfer to the foetus – a review. Placenta 2003; 24: S86–93.

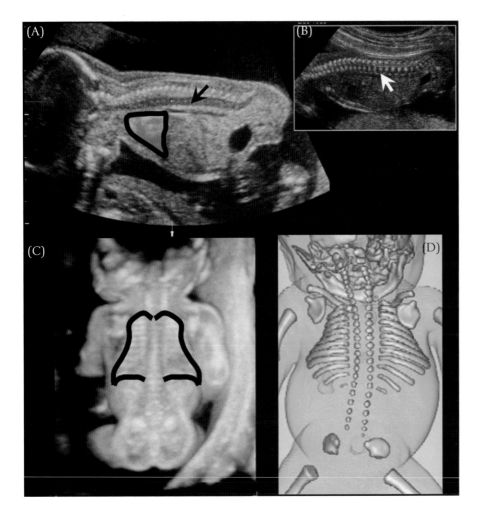

Figure 5.26 Congenital vertebral body dysplasia at 20 weeks of gestation. (A) Short truncus with short thorax (enclosure) with vertebral body dysplasia (black arrow) are demonstrated. (B) Normal sagittal image at the same gestational age. Vertebral bodies are detected in normal cases as echogenic dots (white arrow). (C) 3D image of the ribs. A hypoplastic lung was suspected. (D) 3D computed tomographic image. Vertebral bodies and sacral vertebra are completely invisible

2. Kucuk T, Duru NK, Yenen MC, et al. Yolk sac size and shape as predictors of poor pregnancy outcome. J Perinat Med 1999; 27: 316–20.

3. Lindsay DJ, Lovett IS, Lyons EA, et al. Yolk sac diameter and shape at endovaginal US: predictors of pregnancy outcome in the first trimester. Radiology 1992; 183: 115–18.

4. Nicolaides KH. Nuchal translucency and other first-trimester sonographic markers of chromosomal abnormalities. Am J Obstet Gynecol 2004; 191: 45–67.

5. Smith DW, Graham JM. Jugular lymphatic obstruction sequence. In: Jones K, ed. Recognizable Patterns of Human Malformation: Genetic Embryologic and Clinical Aspects. Philadelphia, PA: WB Saunders, 1982: 472.

6. Goetsch E. Hygroma colli cysticum and hygroma axillae: pathologic and clinical study and report of twelve cases. Arch Surg 1938; 394: 36.

7. Phillips H, McGaham J. Intrauterine fetal cystic hygroma: sonographic detection. AJR Am J Roentgenol 1981; 136: 799.

8. Lee K, Klein T. Surgery of cysts and tumors of the neck. In: Paparella M, Snunriek D, eds. Otolaryngology. Philadelphia, PA: WB Saunders, 1980: 2987.

9. Howarth ES, Draper ES, Budd JL, et al. Population-based study of the outcome following the prenatal diagnosis of cystic hygroma. Prenat Diagn 2005; 25: 286–91.

10. McAuliffe FM, Hornberger LK, Johnson J, Chitayat D, Ryan G. Cardiac diverticulum with pericardial effusion: report of two new cases treated by in-utero pericardiocentesis and a review of the literature. Ultrasound Obstet Gynecol 2005; 25: 401–4.

11. Holmes N, Harrison MR, Baskin LS. Fetal surgery for posterior urethral valves: long-term postnatal outcomes. Pediatrics 2001; 108: 1–7.

12. Kurjak A, Chervenak F, Carrera JM (eds). Donald School Atlas of Fetal Anomalies. Jaypee Brothers, New Delhi: 2006.

6 Markers of chromosomal anomalies studied by 3D sonography

Asim Kurjak, Wiku Andonotopo, and Elena Scazzocchio

INTRODUCTION

The value of ultrasonic markers in the detection of chromosomopathies is now very well established. Various sonographic markers have been proposed for detecting fetuses with aneuploidy, including a thickened nuchal fold, shortened long-bone measurements, and the ratio of biparietal diameter (BPD) to femur length.[1,2] A combination of sonographic aneuploidy markers has been shown to increase sensitivity and to decrease the number of unnecessary invasive diagnostic procedures.[3,4] Therefore, it is reasonable to continue searching for further sonographic markers in an attempt to further increase the prenatal detection rate of chromosomal abnormalities. In this way, in a population of high-risk women, when one or more of these markers are visualized by sonography, the sensitivity for the detection of aneuploidy may be increased. Conversely, in high-risk women who want this information, the absence of such markers can decrease the a priori risk of aneuploidy to levels low enough to avoid amniocentesis and its possible complications. In this chapter, we will review the use of three-dimensional (3D) sonography in this important field.

Some observational studies have described surface rendering of external embryonic features in singleton and twin pregnancies,[5–8] including reconstructions performed with a 20 MHz catheter-based high-resolution transducer before therapeutic abortion,[9] further detailed characterization of the development of the embryonic brain,[7] and improved differentiation between cystic hygroma and nuchal translucency (NT) thickness,[10] as well as the possibility of completing a 1st-trimester study that included NT measurements in less time than 2D sonography, and with the same degree of reliability.[11]

FIRST-TRIMESTER GESTATIONAL SAC VOLUME

Kupesic et al[4] reported on the visualization of the gestational sac, yolk sac, embryo, and amniotic sac by 3D sonography performed at the 1st trimester. They suggested that 3D sonography can provide a highly reproducible measurement of the gestational sac volume (GSV) (Figure 6.1); that in normal pregnancies the GSV increases with gestation. In another study, Falcon et al[12] reported that in fetuses with some chromosomal defects, the GSV is altered. The observed doubling in GSV during the 1st trimester can be attributed to the simultaneous doubling in fetal size and an increase in amniotic fluid volume (Figure 6.2).[4,12] In the 1st trimester of pregnancy, the electrolyte composition and osmolality of amniotic fluid are essentially the same as those of maternal blood, and the most likely mechanism for the formation of amniotic fluid is an active transport of solute by the amnion into the amniotic space, with water moving passively down the chemical potential gradient.[13] Subsequently, with the onset of fetal urination and swallowing, these are the two major pathways for the formation and clearance of amniotic fluid. Sonographic studies have demonstrated the presence of the fetal bladder and stomach from as early as 8 weeks and in nearly all fetuses by 11 weeks.[14]

In their study, Falcon et al[12] found normal fetal karyotype in 417 pregnancies and abnormal in 83. In the chromosomally normal group, the mean GSV

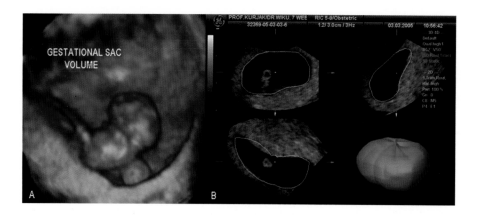

Figure 6.1 (A) 3D surface rendering showing gestational sac volume. (B) VOCAL measurement of gestational sac

increased significantly with gestational age from a mean of 69 ml at 11 weeks to 144 ml at 14 weeks (the standard deviation was 27 ml). In the chromosomally abnormal group, the mean GSV for gestational age was not significantly different from normal in fetuses with trisomy 21, trisomy 18, or Turner syndrome, but it was smaller in those with triploidy and trisomy 13. However, the mean GSV for crown–rump length (CRL) was significantly larger in trisomy 18, smaller in triploidy and trisomy 13, and not different from normal in trisomy 21 and Turner syndrome. The mean CRL for gestational age was significantly smaller than normal in trisomy 18, triploidy, and trisomy 13.

According to Falcon et al,[12] in trisomy 21, the GSVs both for gestational age and for fetal CRL are not significantly different from normal, and therefore measurement of the GSV does not provide useful prediction of this chromosomal defect. The same is also true for Turner syndrome. In contrast, trisomy 13 and triploidy are associated with a significantly smaller GSV than normal. In both of these chromosomal defects, there was early-onset fetal growth restriction, but the GSV for CRL was significantly reduced, suggesting that the decrease in GSV is not a mere consequence of small fetal size but also of a decrease in amniotic fluid volume. Such a decrease in amniotic fluid volume may reflect impaired placental function, acting either directly in the production of the ultrafiltrate and/or through a decrease in fetal urination.

In trisomy 18, as in trisomy 13 and triploidy, there was early-onset fetal growth restriction.[12] However, contrary to the findings in trisomy 13 and triploidy, where the GSV was decreased, in trisomy 18 the GSV was normal for gestational age but increased for CRL. These findings suggest that in fetuses with this chromosomal defect, the amniotic fluid volume is actually increased. This increase is unlikely to be a consequence of improved placental function, because

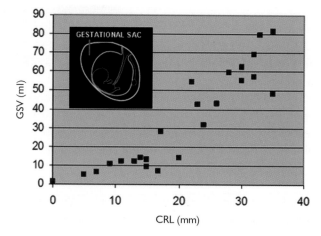

Figure 6.2 Reference range of gestational sac volume (GSV) with crown–rump length (CRL) in normal pregnancies at 11–14 weeks of gestation (adapted from reference 4 with permission)

a common finding in all three of these chromosomal defects is an impaired production of free β-human chorionic gonadotropin (β-hCG) and pregnancy-associated plasma protein A (PAPP-A).[15] Consequently, the increase in GSV in trisomy 18 pregnancies is probably due to the presence of associated fetal defects that interfere with fetal swallowing, such as diaphragmatic hernia, esophageal atresia, or central nervous system abnormalities.

Falcon et al[12] confirmed that measurement of the GSV at 11–14 weeks of gestation is unlikely to provide useful prediction of major chromosomal defects. Although there are alterations in the GSV in trisomy 18, trisomy 13, and triploidy, in the vast majority of cases the values are within the normal ranges. Furthermore, effective screening for these defects is provided by a combination of fetal nuchal translucency thickness and free β-hCG and PAPP-A maternal serum.

FETAL NUCHAL TRANSLUCENCY THICKNESS

Nuchal translucency measurement has become a standard technique in many obstetric units for the risk assessment of chromosomal abnormality.[11] Although nuchal translucency measurement can be completed without difficulty in most cases, the success rates vary between different centers.[11,16,17] These variations have been attributed mainly to differences in sonographers' training. Other possible factors affecting the success in obtaining the measurements are variations in quality of the ultrasound equipment, route of examination (transabdominal or transvaginal), and the gestational age at which the measurement is attempted.[17] However, even under optimal conditions, the examination may occasionally take a long time to complete when the fetus is lying in an unfavorable position.

It has been suggested that 3D sonography may help to overcome some of these problems.[17,18] This technique enables a fast acquisition of a large number of 2D sections using a scanner that monitors the spatial orientation of the images. The scans are then stored in the machine's computer memory in the form of a volume set. The stored ultrasound data may be resliced in any desired plane, thus providing the views of the organ of interest that could not be seen on a conventional 2D scan. Theoretically, this may enable measurements of nuchal translucency to be performed regardless of fetal position, which could significantly shorten the examination time. In addition, by displaying three orthogonal planes at the same time, the use of 3D sonography may ensure that the measurements are always performed in the true midsagittal plane (Figure 6.3).

Paul et al[17] showed that nuchal translucency measurements could be accurately replicated on stored 3D sonographic volumes. Therefore, theoretical concerns that subtle movement artifacts caused by maternal heart pulsations could distort 3D volumes and affect the accuracy of nuchal translucency measurements were not substantiated by our results. We also showed that the majority of 2D nuchal translucency measurements were not performed in the

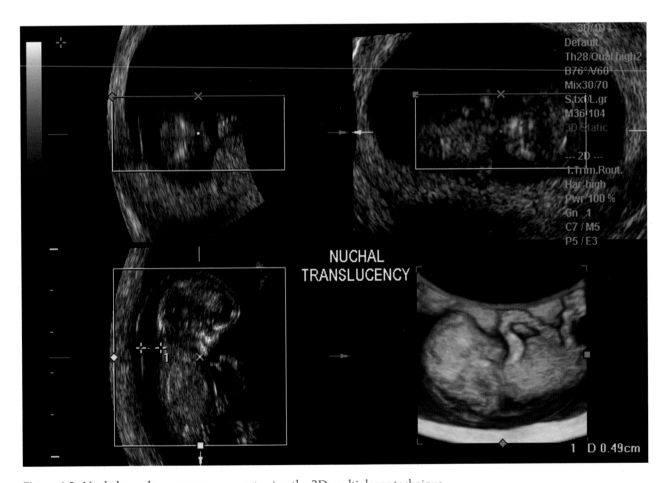

Figure 6.3 Nuchal translucency measurement using the 3D multiplanar technique

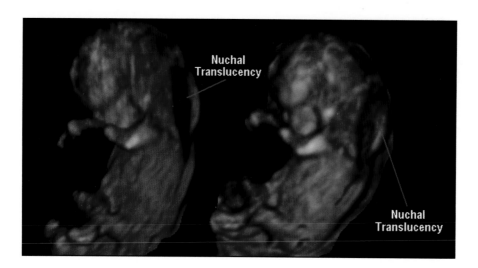

Figure 6.4 3D surface rendering showing nuchal translucency thickness at 11 weeks of gestation

true midsagittal plane. However, the mean difference between measurements in the true midsagittal and in other planes was very small; it would therefore be possible to calculate the risk for trisomy 21 with 3D sonography by using the same approach to risk assessment as with conventional 2D scanning.[11]

It has to be emphasized that 3D measurements can be performed successfully only by examination of sagittal volumes containing a clear view of the nuchal translucency in the initial plane. In this situation, the measurement can also be completed without difficulty on 2D scans. Fetal movements, which often occur at this stage of gestation, facilitate differentiation between the nuchal skin fold and the amniotic membrane on real-time 2D scans. A 3D scan, on the contrary, can only be performed successfully when the fetus is resting. This prolongs the examination time and decreases the success rate for obtaining a clear view of the nuchal fold, as has happened in two of our cases.[11,17]

Failure to obtain measurements regularly occurred with the fetal long axis lying parallel to the ultrasound beam. The measurements were also unsuccessful when the fetal sagittal plane was lying perpendicular to the ultrasound beam. In both positions, the skin covering the cervical spine was positioned parallel to the ultrasound beam, which prevented clear visualization of the nuchal translucency on both 2D and 3D scans.

The main theoretical advantage of using 3D sonography would be in cases when nuchal translucency measurement cannot be completed due to an unfavorable fetal position. The ability to overcome this problem by rotating and reslicing 3D volumes would be of great help in clinical practice. Unfortunately, the quality of a 3D sonographic examination is determined by the clarity of the 2D images constituting the volume, which cannot be improved by subsequent manipulation.[17]

Kurjak et al[11] suggested that 3D sonography is likely to improve the accuracy of nuchal translucency measurements in the future. They examined the reproducibility of nuchal translucency measurements using the transvaginal approach. They obtained satisfactory views of the nuchal region in 85% of examinations performed by 2D sonography and in 100% when 3D sonography was used (Figures 6.3 and 6.4).

Chung et al[19] could also record 3D volumes only when a clear view of the nuchal fold was seen on the initial 2D scan. They did not attempt to compare the results of 3D scans with measurements obtained on 2D scans. Therefore, their study does not provide any information on the accuracy or repeatability of nuchal translucency thickness measurements by 3D sonography; nor does it assess the potential role of 3D sonography in situations when measurements cannot be completed on 2D scans. Furthermore, 2D and 3D examinations performed by different operators may have influenced the success rate. In addition, 3D volumes were recorded only when a clear view of the nuchal translucency was obtained on 2D scans, rather than using the technique of random volume as in the study by Paul et al.[17] They confirmed that reslicing of stored 3D sonographic volumes can be used to replicate nuchal translucency measurements when nuchal skin can be clearly seen on 2D scans as well. However, when the fetus is lying in a position that precludes clear visualization of the nuchal fold, 3D sonography is unlikely to be of help. This severely limits the potential role of this technique in screening for Down syndrome in the 1st trimester of pregnancy.

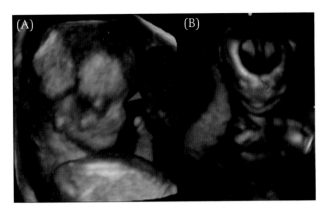

Figure 6.5 (A) Midsagittal view of a fetus demonstrating nasal bone using 3D maximum mode. (B) The same fetus in a frontal view by 3D surface rendering

FIRST-TRIMESTER FETAL NASAL BONE

Trisomy 21 is associated with absence of the fetal nasal bone at 11–14 weeks of gestation.[20] It has been estimated that in screening for trisomy 21 using a combination of maternal age and fetal nuchal translucency, inclusion of examination of the fetal profile for the presence or absence of the nasal bone could increase the sensitivity from 75% to 93% for a fixed false-positive rate of 5%.[20–22] For examination of the nasal bone, the fetus should preferably be facing up towards the transducer, the image should be magnified so that only the head and the upper thorax are included in the screen, and a midsagittal view of the fetal profile must be obtained.

3D sonography makes it possible to obtain a perfect midsagittal view of the fetal face and to rotate the fetal profile to any desired angle (Figures 6.5 and 6.6). However, the extent to which the nasal bone can be demonstrated to be present in a given reconstructed section is entirely dependent on the 2D start section of the volume acquisition. This is not surprising, since the 3D volumes are obtained while the probe is sweeping 2D scans between the margins of the volume to be acquired. In this way, each pixel (the smallest 2D picture unit) is placed in its correct position in the voxel (the smallest 3D picture unit).

When the 2D start section is transverse or coronal, the percentage of cases in which it is possible to demonstrate the nasal bone in the reconstructed true

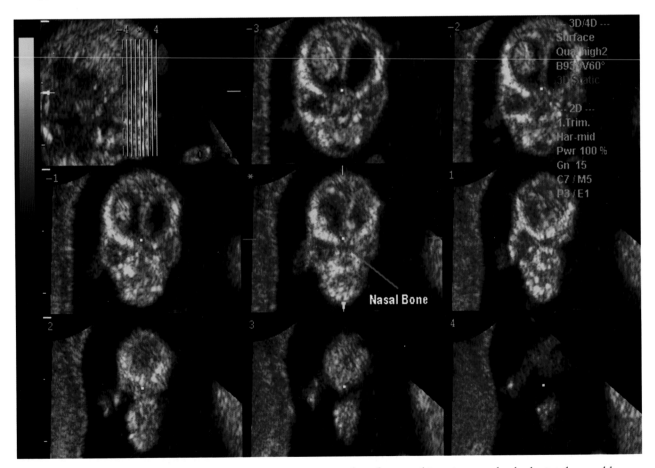

Figure 6.6 Visualization of fetal surface structure using tomographic ultrasound imaging can clearly depict the nasal bone

midsagittal section is very low. Similarly, in cases in which the 2D start section is midsagittal but the angle between the ultrasound transducer and an imaginary line passing through the fetal profile is less than 30° or more than 60°, it is not possible to demonstrate the nasal bone in the reconstructed image achieved by rotation of the fetal profile around its vertical axis to achieve the desired 45°. It is important to appreciate that the quality of the static image in any reconstructed section does not improve by mere rotation on its vertical axis. Consequently, the inability to examine the nasal bone by 2D scanning because the fetal head is hyperextended or very flexed cannot be overcome by obtaining a 3D volume.[20]

The same is true when the fetus is facing down and away from the transducer. In this situation, it is possible to visualize the nasal bone both by 2D and by 3D imaging only if a perfect midsagittal section is obtained and the angle between the transducer and the fetal profile is between 30° and 60°. However, it is always preferable to wait for fetal movements and rotation to the upward-facing position, because this avoids the shadowing caused by the occipital bones. In addition, when the fetus faces posteriorly, there is often no intervening amniotic fluid to separate the fetal face from the uterine wall or placenta. Such technical problems cannot be overcome by a mere 180° rotation of either a 2D or a 3D image.[20]

The main value of 3D scanning in the assessment of the fetal nasal bone is in achieving a satisfactory reconstructed midsagittal section when the 2D start section is parasagittal or slightly oblique. However, this is possible only if in the 2D start section the angle between the ultrasound transducer and an imaginary line passing through the fetal profile is between 30° and 60°. An alternative to the use of 3D scanning in such situations is to wait for spontaneous fetal movements that within a few minutes would alter the fetal position, making it possible to examine the fetal profile by conventional 2D imaging.[20]

According to Rembouskos et al,[20] it is possible to obtain a perfect midsagittal section using 3D sonography because of the ability to display three orthogonal planes simultaneously. Consequently, 3D scanning may be useful in cases where the nasal bone cannot be visualized in 2D scanning and there is uncertainty as to whether this is the consequence of a true absence of the bone or of failure to obtain a perfect midsagittal view. However, in their study, Rembouskos et al[20] examined the usefulness or the possible limits of 3D technology in the assessment of the fetal nasal bone

after previous confirmation of its presence by 2D scanning. Their findings suggest that routine application of 3D scanning for the nasal bone in screening for trisomy 21 is likely to be associated with a very high false-positive rate. Essentially, if the sonographer does not appreciate that the ability to examine the nasal bone is critically dependent on obtaining a good 2D image, then the nasal bone will be classified as being absent in many cases in which the 2D start section is transverse or coronal and when the angle between the ultrasound transducer and the fetal profile is less than 30° or more than 60°.[20]

FIRST-TRIMESTER PLACENTAL VOLUME

The early detection of pregnancies with chromosomal anomalies is one of the current aims of fetal medicine. Markers such as increased nuchal translucency thickness,[23,24] altered biochemical parameters in maternal serum,[25] or combinations of both,[26] help to determine who might benefit most from prenatal chromosomal analysis. Nevertheless, other factors should also be evaluated, especially those that could lead to diagnosis in the 1st trimester.

Wegrzyn et al[27] stated that in normal pregnancy there is a doubling in placental volume between 11 and 14 weeks of gestation, which is accompanied by a simultaneous doubling in fetal size and gestational sac volume. In previous studies investigating placental volume in early pregnancy by 3D sonography, a series of parallel sections of approximately 1 cm in thickness were used.[28] In a recent study, placental volume was estimated using 12 sections obtained using the rotational VOCAL technique.[27] There is some evidence from in vitro studies that in the estimation of volumes of an irregular object, such as the placenta, the VOCAL technique may be more accurate (Figure 6.7).[27]

Placental size has been described as being different in pregnancies with aneuploidies. Stoll et al[29] examined nearly 400 Down syndrome fetuses and reported that their placentas at term were considerably smaller than those of unaffected pregnancies. In a somewhat contradictory Japanese study, a tendency for a heavy placenta in trisomy 21 and a light placenta in trisomies 13 and 18 was mentioned.[30] Furthermore, undervascularization has been described in pregnancies with trisomies 13, 18, or 21.[31] Hypotrophy was also mentioned as being typical in a series of 30 trisomic pregnancies.[32]

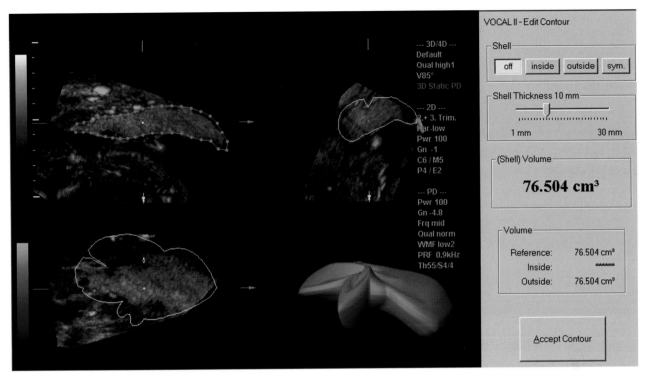

Figure 6.7 3D VOCAL measurement of placental volume during the 1st trimester

The identification of smaller placental volumes in the majority of aneuploid fetuses at the end of the 1st trimester could lead to an improvement in 1st-trimester screening for chromosomal anomalies. Placental volumetry can be performed fairly quickly (acquisition of volume and measurement takes approximately 3 minutes) and the technique is easy to learn. Nuchal translucency thickness measurement is generally regarded as the gold standard in 1st-trimester risk assessment by ultrasound, with a sensitivity of 75% for a false-positive rate of 5%.[33] Its combination with biochemical serum screening gives a detection rate of nearly 90% at a false-positive rate of 5%. Metzenbauer et al,[23] found in their study that nine cases of trisomy 21 had nuchal translucency thickness less than 2.5 mm, but of these 50% had a small placenta.

According to Wegrzyn et al,[27] the mean placental volume was significantly smaller than normal in trisomies 13 and 18 and was below the 5th centile of the normal range in 39% of cases. This is consistent with the finding that in these chromosomal defects at 11–14 weeks the maternal serum concentrations of both free β-hCG and PAPP-A are on average about one-third of the normal concentrations.[34] In terms of 1st-trimester screening for trisomies 13 and 18, it is unlikely that the detection rate will be improved by the measurement of placental volume. First, the detection rate of these trisomies by a program combining maternal age with fetal nuchal translucency and free β-hCG and PAPP-A in maternal serum is more than 90%. Second, there is a significant association between placental volume and free β-hCG and PAPP-A in maternal serum and therefore measurement of placental volume may have little to add to maternal serum testing.[35,36] Third, these trisomies are often associated with other easily detectable 1st-trimester sonographic markers such as exomphalos and small CRL in trisomy 18 and megacystis, holoprosencephaly and tachycardia in trisomy 13.[27]

Wegrzyn et al[27] also found that in trisomy 21 pregnancies, the placental volume, both for gestation and for fetal CRL, is not significantly different from normal, and was below the 5th centile of the normal range in only 2 of 45 cases. Consequently, measurement of placental volume is not useful in screening for trisomy 21. Similarly, in Turner syndrome, placental volume was not significantly different from normal. For triploidy, the finding that in some cases the placental volume is substantially increased while in others it is substantially decreased presumably reflects the two different origins of this chromosomal abnormality. Thus, in diandric triploidy, with a double paternal chromosomal constitution, there is a large molar placenta and a 10-fold increase in free β-hCG in maternal serum, whereas digynic triploidy is associated with a very small placenta and a 10-fold reduction in the concentration of placental products in the maternal circulation.[36]

FIRST-TRIMESTER UMBILICAL CORD DIAMETER AS A MARKER OF FETAL ANEUPLOIDY

Early identification of women at increased risk of fetal chromosomal abnormalities remains one of the most important challenges in prenatal medicine.[37] The most extensively studied early sonographic feature of chromosomal defects is fetal nuchal translucency, which is also a marker for cardiac defects and for some genetic syndromes.[38–42] A structure that is always easily visible on ultrasound in the late 1st trimester is the umbilical cord (Figure 6.8).

Ghezzi et al[43] have previously reported that the umbilical cord diameter in the 1st trimester is correlated with the growth of the embryo and that its measurement might be useful for identifying a subset of fetuses at risk of spontaneous abortion and preeclampsia. Morphologic alterations of the umbilical cord structure and composition have been found at delivery in a variety of pathologic conditions, such as hypertensive disorders,[44] gestational diabetes,[45,46] fetal distress,[47] and growth restriction.[48] Umbilical cords with single artery,[49] uncoiled cords,[50] and short umbilical cords[51] have been described in cases with adverse pregnancy outcome and other genetic syndromes. Moreover, it has been reported that fetuses with Down syndrome have significantly shorter umbilical cords compared with normal infants.[52]

Ghezzi et al[37] showed that a relationship exists between fetal chromosomal abnormalities and the morphology of the umbilical cord. They analyzed 784 patients who met the inclusion criteria (fetuses with a CRL of 45–85 mm). Of these, a fetal or placental chromosomal abnormality was present in 17 cases. The mean umbilical cord diameter increased with gestational age ($r = 0.41$, $p <0.001$). The proportion of fetuses with an umbilical cord diameter above the 95th centile was higher in the presence of fetal or placental chromosomal abnormalities than in normal fetuses (5/17 vs 39/767; $p <0.01$). Among fetuses with an abnormal fetal or placental karyotype, nuchal translucency was above the 95th centile for gestational age in 10 cases. When only fetal chromosomal abnormalities were considered ($n = 14$), the combined detection rate was 85.7% (12/14).

Although the underlying pathophysiologic mechanism leading to an increased umbilical cord diameter in fetuses with chromosomal abnormalities remains to be explored, certain etiologic mechanisms might explain the increases in both nuchal translucency and umbilical cord diameter.[37]

A number of studies have demonstrated that alterations of the extracellular matrix are present in fetuses affected by trisomies 21, 13, or 18.[53–58] In fetuses with trisomy 21, the extracellular matrix of the nuchal skin is much richer in glycosaminoglycans, especially hyaluronan, compared with chromosomally normal fetuses.[57,59] This appears to be the consequence of a decreased degradation of hyaluronan in fetuses with trisomy 21. In the nuchal skin of trisomy 18 fetuses, the distribution and organization of collagen types I and III are different from those in normal fetuses, resembling the modifications occurring with aging.[59] Finally, in trisomy 18, most dermal fibroblasts have

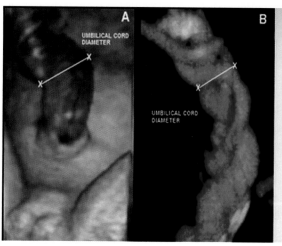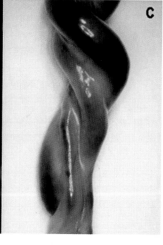

Figure 6.8 (A) 3D surface rendering of umbilical cord. (B) 3D power Doppler mode demonstrating the umbilical cord. (C) Normal anatomy of the umbilical cord

been found to be laminin-positive, and in trisomy 13, most dermal fibroblasts are collagen type IV-positive.[57] In gestational age-matched control normal fetuses, this was never found to be the case.[57]

Therefore, overexpression, as well as underexpression, of different structural proteins, polysaccharides, and proteoglycans of the extracellular matrix, which might result in abnormal accumulation of fluid, could explain both the increased nuchal translucency and increased umbilical cord diameter.[37]

Another interesting question is why fetuses with Turner syndrome might have a thicker than normal umbilical cord.[60] The most plausible mechanism to explain the hygroma colli generally present in fetuses with Turner syndrome is lymphatic vessel hypoplasia in the upper dermis.[60] This does not explain the increased umbilical cord diameter in fetuses affected by Turner syndrome, because lymphatic vessels are completely absent from the umbilical cord and the placenta.[61] However, alterations of proteoglycan expression have been found in the skin of fetuses with Turner syndrome. It has been reported that in fetuses with Turner syndrome, biglycan, which is encoded on chromosome X, is underexpressed and chondroitin-6-sulfate is overexpressed.[62] Thus, it is reasonable to assume that similar extracellular matrix modifications might also affect the Wharton's jelly, which for a large part is composed of proteoglycans.

Another mechanism that might explain the increased umbilical cord size is venous congestion.[60] Considering that the amount of Wharton's jelly in the 1st and early 2nd trimesters is lower than that in the 3rd trimester,[61] the increase in umbilical cord size in early gestation could be the consequence of a progressive enlargement of the umbilical cord vessels or an overrepresentation of Wharton's jelly, or both. Cardiac defects and abnormalities of the great arteries are common findings in fetuses with increased nuchal translucency.[63] Moreover, an absent or reversed flow during atrial contraction at the level of the ductus venosus has been reported in a very high proportion of chromosomally abnormal fetuses between 11 and 14 weeks of gestation.[64] As a consequence, umbilical vein congestion may cause umbilical vein dilatation, transudation of fluid into the Wharton's jelly, and enlargement of the umbilical cord. It is noteworthy that it has been demonstrated that Wharton's jelly is a metabolically active tissue involved in the exchanges between amniotic fluid and the blood in umbilical vessels.[65] Hence, it is possible that venous congestion, frequently seen in trisomic fetuses, might cause an alteration in the transfer of fluid normally present in the 1st trimester of gestation[13] between Wharton's jelly and the umbilical vessels. The sonographic counterpart of the abnormal accumulation of fluid in the Wharton's jelly is an increased umbilical cord size.

Ghezzi et al[37] proved that umbilical cord size early in gestation is different between normal and chromosomally abnormal fetuses. They hypothesized that the underlying pathophysiologic mechanisms leading to an increase in umbilical cord diameter might be those that also explain the increased nuchal translucency in fetuses with abnormal karyotype, such as alterations of the extracellular matrix components or fetal venous congestion. However, larger studies should aim to explore the possible clinical application of routine sonographic evaluation of the umbilical cord in early gestation.[37]

ASSOCIATED ANOMALIES IN FETUSES WITH CLEFT LIP AND PALATE

Facial clefting is attributed to failure of the nasal and maxillofacial processes to fuse during embryologic development.[66] Cleft lip with or without cleft palate may be isolated, with no other congenital abnormalities being present (Figures 6.9 and 6.10),[66,67] or it may be one component of a more global fetal abnormality. Approximately 350 syndromes have been linked with facial clefting, some of which may result in death or severe morbidity.[68] Previous studies have shown that the rate of associated anomalies for cleft lips with or without cleft palate range between 35% and 63%.[69,70]

Ultrasound has played a key role in prenatal identification of cleft lip with or without cleft palate.[71,72] Chmait et al[72] found that 2D sonography with adjunct 3D sonography of the fetal face detected all of the fetuses with a cleft lip and 90% of those with a cleft primary palate. Although the location and extent of cleft lip with or without cleft palate are important with regard to prognosis, the presence or absence of an associated anomaly is equally if not more critical to the outcome of the fetus. The prenatal identification of facial clefting with or without associated anomalies is essential for prenatal counseling and planning obstetric and neonatal management.[66]

Previous studies have noted a varying rate of associated anomalies in prenatally detected cleft lip with or without cleft palate. In a retrospective review of 4180 cases, multiple anomalies were found in 35% of those with a cleft lip with or without cleft palate and 54%

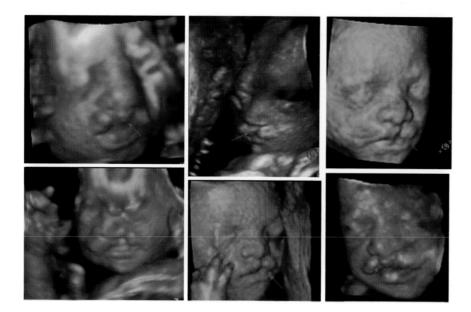

Figure 6.9 3D surface rendering showing cleft palate and cleft lip with no other congenital abnormalities present

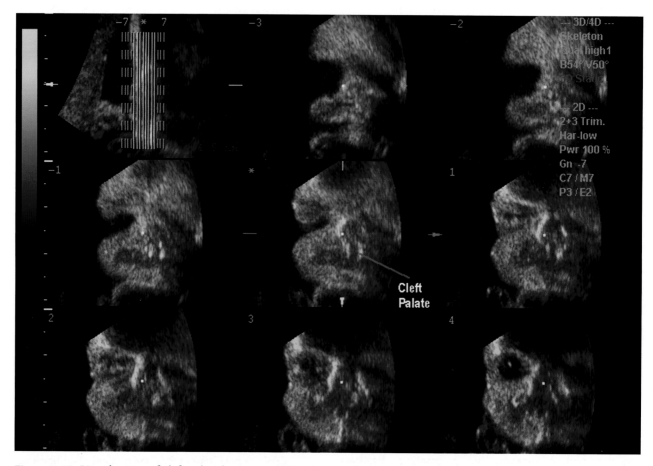

Figure 6.10 Visualization of cleft palate by tomographic ultrasound imaging

of those with a cleft palate.[69] Similarly, in a study of 238 942 consecutive deliveries in northeastern France between 1979 and 1996, 460 infants had clefts. Of the total cleft cases, 36.7% had associated defects.[73] The rate of associated malformation was 13.6% for cleft lip, 36.8% for cleft lip and palate, and 46.7% for cleft palate alone.[73–75]

Chmait et al[66] found the rate of associated anomalies to be around 35.6% in their study group. They reported that all cases in their study that had an additional abnormality had both a cleft lip and a primary cleft palate. It is of some concern that in half of these fetuses, the additional malformation was not detected prenatally, despite the fact that these fetuses were examined on multiple occasions with 2D sonography. Furthermore, in this study, 3D sonography was used to visualize the fetal face only. Thus, of the 37 cases of presumed 'isolated' cleft lip with or without cleft palate, 8 (21.6%) were found to have an associated anomaly after delivery.[66]

The 21.6% rate of undiagnosed associated anomalies in cases with a cleft lip with or without cleft palate is in line with previous studies that have shown the relative insensitivity of ultrasound in prenatal diagnosis.[74,75] This finding warrants guarded optimism when counseling patients regarding the prognosis of prenatally diagnosed cleft lip with or without cleft palate. The natural history of fetuses with a cleft lip with or without cleft palate and an additional anomaly is unfavorable both in utero and in the neonatal period.[66]

Chmait et al[66] stated that the diagnoses of several of the associated anomalies may have been obtainable prenatally under optimal conditions. This is especially true regarding the twins with trisomy 21, in whom an amniocentesis would have elucidated the karyotypic abnormality. However, the realities of prenatal diagnosis may preclude the prenatal identification of severe yet diagnosable abnormalities. In the case with transposition of the great vessels, prenatal evaluation of the fetus did not occur until 34 weeks of gestation and views of the fetal heart were limited by fetal position. Understanding these limitations and conveying them to the parents is imperative.[66]

In three of the eight cases in the study by Chmait et al[66] with presumed 'isolated' cleft lip with or without cleft palate, the pregnancy was terminated. Pathologic evaluation of these three cases revealed the additional abnormalities. This has important implications regarding reproductive counseling. Postnatal follow-up may help discriminate between etiologic and syndromic diagnoses. The empiric recurrence risk for non-syndromic fetal cleft lip with or without primary cleft palate is approximately 4% if the family history is negative for an oral cleft. The recurrence risk for syndromic causes is specific to the diagnosis.[66]

Chmait et al[66] found that 21.6% of fetuses with a presumed 'isolated' cleft lip with or without cleft palate had an additional anomaly; this has important implications regarding prenatal diagnosis and counseling of patients. All efforts should be made to assess the entire fetus for an additional anomaly if a cleft lip with or without cleft palate is detected. Although associated anomalies were only seen in fetuses with cleft lip and palate in this study, fetal chromosomal evaluation should be considered for cleft lip only as well as cleft lip and palate, since both anomalies are part of the same developmental spectrum. The patient should also be instructed of the limitations of current diagnostic capabilities, and that additional malformations may be discovered postnatally.[66] Chmait et al[66] also suggested that the patient should be informed of the inability of the prenatal sonogram to reliably evaluate the secondary palate. The presence of an additional malformation may significantly alter the prognosis. Referral to a dysmorphologist is prudent in order to assess associated anomalies and to establish the recurrence risk.[66]

REFERENCES

1. Benacerraf BR, Neuberg D, Frigoletto FD. Humeral shortening in second-trimester fetuses with Down syndrome. Obstet Gynecol 1991; 77: 223–7.

2. Benacerraf BR, Gelman R, Frigoletto FD. Sonographic identification of second-trimester fetuses with Down syndrome. N Engl J Med 1987; 317: 1371–6.

3. Bromley B, Shipp T, Benacerraf BR. Genetic sonogram scoring index: accuracy and clinical utility. J Ultrasound Med 1999; 18: 523–8.

4. Kupesic S, Kurjak A, Ivancic-Kosuta M. Volume and vascularity of the yolk sac studied by three-dimensional ultrasound and color Doppler. J Perinat Med 1999; 27: 91–6.

5. Blaas HG, Eik-Nes SH, Kiserud T, et al. Three-dimensional imaging of the brain cavities in human embryos. Ultrasound Obstet Gynecol 1995; 5: 228–32.

6. Hata T, Aoki S, Manabe A, Hata K, Miyazaki K. Three dimensional ultrasonography in the first trimester of human pregnancy. Hum Reprod 1997; 12: 1800–4.

7. Blaas HG, Eik-Nes SH, Berg S, Torp H. In-vivo three dimensional ultrasound reconstructions of embryos and early fetuses. Lancet 1998; 352: 1182–6.

8. Benoit B, Hafner T, Kurjak A, et al. Three-dimensional sonoembryology. J Perinat Med 2002; 30: 63–73.

9. Hata T, Manabe A, Aoki S, et al. Three-dimensional intrauterine sonography in the early first-trimester of human pregnancy: preliminary study. Hum Reprod 1998; 13: 740–3.

10. Bonilla-Musoles F, Raga F, Villalobos A, Blanes J, Osborne NG. First-trimester neck abnormalities: three dimensional evaluation. J Ultrasound Med 1998; 17: 419–25.

11. Kurjak A, Kupesic S, Ivancic-Kosuta M. Three-dimensional transvaginal ultrasound improves measurement of nuchal translucency. J Perinat Med 1999; 27: 97–102.

12. Falcon O, Wegrzyn P, Faro C, Peralta CFA, Nicolaides KH. Gestational sac volume measured by three-dimensional ultrasound at 11 to 13 + 6 weeks of gestation: relation to chromosomal defects. Ultrasound Obstet Gynecol 2005; 25: 546–50.

13. Gilbert WM, Brace RA. Amniotic fluid volume and normal flows to and from the amniotic cavity. Semin Perinatol 1993; 17: 150–7.

14. Blaas HG, Eik-Nes SH, Kiserud T, Hellevik LR. Early development of the abdominal wall, stomach and heart from 7 to 12 weeks of gestation: a longitudinal ultrasound study. Ultrasound Obstet Gynecol 1995; 6: 240–9.

15. Nicolaides KH. Nuchal translucency and other first-trimester sonographic markers of chromosomal abnormalities. Am J Obstet Gynecol 2004; 191: 45–67.

16. Economides DL, Whitlow BJ, Kadir R, Lazanakis M, Verdin SM. First trimester sonographic detection of chromosomal abnormalities in an unselected population. Br J Obstet Gynaecol 1998; 105: 58–62.

17. Paul C, Krampl E, Skentou C, Jurkovic D, Nicolaides KH. Measurement of fetal nuchal translucency thickness by three-dimensional ultrasound. Ultrasound Obstet Gynecol 2001; 18: 481–4.

18. Gregg AR, Steiner H, Staudach A, Weiner CP. Accuracy of 3D sonographic volume measurements. Am J Obstet Gynecol 1993; 168: 348.

19. Chung BL, Kim HJ, Lee KH. The application of three-dimensional ultrasound to nuchal translucency measurement in early pregnancy (10–14 weeks): a preliminary study. Ultrasound Obstet Gynecol 2000; 15: 122–5.

20. Rembouskos G, Cicero S, Longo D, Vandecruys H, Nicolaides KH. Assessment of the fetal nasal bone at 11–14 weeks of gestation by three-dimensional ultrasound. Ultrasound Obstet Gynecol 2004; 23: 232–6.

21. Cicero S, Longo D, Rembouskos G, Sacchini C, Nicolaides KH. Absent nasal bone at 11–14 weeks of gestation and chromosomal defects. Ultrasound Obstet Gynecol 2003; 22: 31–5.

22. Cicero S, Dezerega V, Andrade E, Scheier M, Nicolaides KH. Learning curve for sonographic examination of the fetal nasal bone at 11–14 weeks. Ultrasound Obstet Gynecol 2003; 22: 135–7.

23. Metzenbauer M, Hafner E, Schuchter K, Philipp K. First-trimester placental volume as a marker for chromosomal anomalies: preliminary results from an unselected population. Ultrasound Obstet Gynecol 2002; 19: 240–2.

24. Nicolaides KH, Azar G, Byrne D, Mansur C, Marks K. Fetal nuchal translucency: ultrasound screening for chromosomal defects in first trimester of pregnancy. BMJ 1992; 304: 867–9.

25. Wald NJ, George L, Smith D, Densem JW, Petterson K. Serum screening for Down's syndrome between 8 and 14 weeks of pregnancy. International Prenatal Screening Research Group. Br J Obstet Gynaecol 1996; 103: 407–12.

26. Spencer K, Souter V, Tul N, Snijders R, Nicolaides KH. A screening program for trisomy 21 at 10–14 weeks using fetal nuchal translucency, maternal serum free beta-human chorionic gonadotropin and pregnancy-associated plasma protein-A. Ultrasound Obstet Gynecol 1999; 13: 231–7.

27. Wegrzyn P, Faro C, Falcon O, Peralta CFA, Nicolaides KH. Placental volume measured by three-dimensional ultrasound at 11 to 13 + 6 weeks of gestation: relation to chromosomal defects. Ultrasound Obstet Gynecol 2005; 26: 28–32.

28. Hafner E, Schuchter K, van Leeuwen M, et al. Three-dimensional sonographic volumetry of the placenta and the fetus between weeks 15 and 17 of gestation. Ultrasound Obstet Gynecol 2001; 18: 116–20.

29. Stoll C, Alembik Y, Dott B, Roth MP. Study of Down syndrome in 238,942 consecutive births. Ann Genet 1998; 41: 44–51.

30. Arizawa M, Nakayama M. Pathological analysis of the placenta in trisomies 21, 18 and 13. Nippon Sanka Fujinka Gakkai Zasshi 1992; 44: 9–13.

31. Rochelson B, Kaplan C, Guzman E, et al. A quantitative analysis of placental vasculature in the third-trimester fetus with autosomal trisomy. Obstet Gynecol 1990; 75: 59–63.

32. Labbe S, Copin H, Choiset A, Girard S, Barbet JP. The placenta and trisomies 13, 18, 21. J Gynecol Obstet Biol Reprod 1989; 18: 989–96.

33. Snijders RJ, Noble P, Sebire N, Souka A, Nicolaides KH. UK multicentre project on assessment of risk of trisomy 21 by maternal age and fetal nuchal-translucency thickness at 10–14 weeks of gestation. Fetal Medicine Foundation First Trimester Screening Group. Lancet 1998; 352: 343–6.

34. Snijders RJ, Sebire NJ, Nayar R, Souka A, Nicolaides KH. Increased nuchal translucency in trisomy 13

fetuses at 10–14 weeks of gestation. Am J Med Genet 1999; 86: 205–7.

35. Metzenbauer M, Hafner E, Hoefinger D, et al. Three-dimensional ultrasound measurement of the placental volume in early pregnancy: method and correlation with biochemical placenta parameters. Placenta 2001; 22: 602–5.

36. Spencer K, Liao AW, Skentou H, Cicero S, Nicolaides KH. Screening for triploidy by fetal nuchal translucency and maternal serum free beta-hCG and PAPP-A at 10–14 weeks of gestation. Prenat Diagn 2000; 20: 495–9.

37. Ghezzi F, Raio L, Di Naro E, et al. First-trimester umbilical cord diameter: a novel marker of fetal aneuploidy. Ultrasound Obstet Gynecol 2002; 19: 235–9.

38. Nicolaides KH, Azar G, Byrne D, Mansur C, Marks K. Fetal nuchal translucency: ultrasound screening for chromosomal defects in the first trimester of pregnancy. BMJ 1992; 304: 867–9.

39. Pandya PP, Brizot ML, Kuhn P, Snijders RJ, Nicolaides KH. First trimester fetal nuchal translucency thickness and risk for trisomies. Obstet Gynecol 1994; 101: 782–6.

40. Hyett J, Perdu M, Sharland G, Snijders R, Nicolaides KH. Using fetal nuchal translucency to screen for major congenital cardiac defects at 10–14 weeks of gestation: population based cohort study. BMJ 1999; 352: 1662.

41. Zosmer N, Souter VL, Chan CS, Huggon IC, Nicolaides KH. Early diagnosis of major cardiac defects in chromosomally normal fetuses with increased nuchal translucency. Br J Obstet Gynaecol 1999; 106: 829–33.

42. Souka AP, Krampl E, Bakalis S, Heath V, Nicolaides KH. Outcome of pregnancy in chromosomally normal fetuses with increased nuchal translucency in the first trimester. Ultrasound Obstet Gynecol 2001; 18: 9–17.

43. Ghezzi F, Raio L, Di Naro E, et al. First-trimester umbilical cord diameter and the growth of the human embryo. Ultrasound Obstet Gynecol 2001; 18: 348–51.

44. Bankowski E, Sobolewski K, Romanowicz L, Chyczewski L, Jawosrski S. Collagen and glycosaminoglycans of Wharton's jelly and their alterations in EPH-gestosis. Eur J Obstet Gynecol Reprod Biol 1996; 66: 109–17.

45. Singh SD. Gestational diabetes and its effect on the umbilical cord. Early Hum Dev 1986; 14: 89–98.

46. Weissman A, Jakobi P. Sonographic measurements of the umbilical cord in pregnancies complicated by gestational diabetes. J Ultrasound Med 1997; 16: 691–4.

47. Raio L, Ghezzi F, Di Naro E, et al. Prenatal diagnosis of a lean umbilical cord: a simple marker for fetuses at risk of being small for gestational age at birth. Ultrasound Obstet Gynecol 1999; 13: 176–80.

48. Bruch JF, Sibony O, Benali K, et al. Computerized microscope morphometry of umbilical vessels from pregnancies with intrauterine growth retardation and abnormal umbilical artery Doppler. Hum Pathol 1997; 28: 1139–45.

49. Predanic M, Perni SC, Friedman A, Chervenak FA, Chasen ST. Fetal growth assessment and neonatal birth weight in fetuses with an isolated single umbilical artery. Obstet Gynecol 2005;105: 1093–7.

50. Predanic M, Perni SC, Chasen ST, Baergen RN, Chervenak FA. Ultrasound evaluation of abnormal umbilical cord coiling in second trimester of gestation in association with adverse pregnancy outcome. Am J Obstet Gynecol 2005; 193: 387–94.

51. Gilbert-Barness E, Drut RM, Drut R, Grange DK, Opitz JM. Developmental abnormalities resulting in short umbilical cord. Birth Defects 1993; 29: 113–40.

52. Moessinger AC, Mills JL, Harley EE, et al. Umbilical cord length in Down's syndrome. Am J Dis Child 1986; 140: 1276–7.

53. Takechi K, Kuwabara Y, Mizuno M. Ultrastructural and immunohistochemical studies of Wharton's jelly umbilical cord cells. Placenta 1993; 14: 235–45.

54. Vizza E, Correr S, Goranova V, et al. The collagen skeleton of the human umbilical cord at term. A scanning electron microscopy study after 2N-NaOH maceration. Reprod Fertil Dev 1996; 8: 885–94.

55. Klein J, Meyer F. Tissue structure and macromolecular diffusion in umbilical cord immobilization of endogenous hyaluronic acid. Biochim Biophys Acta 1983; 22: 400–11.

56. Nanaev AK, Kohnen G, Milovanov AP, Domogatsky SP, Kaufmann P. Stromal differentiation and architecture of the human umbilical cord. Placenta 1997; 18: 53–64.

57. Von Kaisenberg CS, Krenn V, Ludwig M, Nicolaides KH, Brand-Saberi B. Morphological classification of nuchal skin in human fetuses with trisomy 21, 18 and 13 at 12–18 weeks and in a trisomy 16 mouse. Anat Embryol (Berl) 1998; 197: 105–24.

58. Von Kaisenberg CS, Brand-Saberi B, Christ B, et al. Collagen type VI gene expression in the skin of trisomy 21 fetuses. Obstet Gynecol 1998; 91: 319–23.

59. Brandt-Saberi B, Epperlein HH, Romanos GE, Christ B. Distribution of extracellular matrix components in nuchal skin from fetuses carrying trisomy 18 and trisomy 21. Cell Tissue Res 1994; 277: 465–75.

60. Von Kaisenberg CS, Nicolaides KH, Brand-Saberi B. Lymphatic vessel hypoplasia in fetuses with Turner syndrome. Hum Reprod 1999; 14: 823–6.

61. Benirschke K, Kaufman P. Pathology of the Human Placenta, 3rd edn. New York: Springer-Verlag, 1995: 323.

62. Von Kaisenberg C, Hyett J. Pathophysiology of increased nuchal translucency. In: Nicolaides KH, Sebire NJ, Snijders RJM, eds. The 11–14-Week Scan. The Diagnosis of Fetal Abnormalities. London: Parthenon, 1999: 95–114.

63. Pandya P. Nuchal translucency thickness. In: Nicolaides KH, Sebire NJ, Snijders RJM, eds. The 11–14-Week Scan. The Diagnosis of Fetal Abnormalities. London: Parthenon, 1999: 14–18.

64. Matias A, Gomes C, Flack N, Montenegro N, Nicolaides K. Screening for chromosomal abnormalities at 11–14 weeks: the role of ductus venosus blood flow. Ultrasound Obstet Gynecol 1998; 12: 380–4.

65. Gilbert WM, Cheung CY, Brace RA. Rapid intramembranous absorption into the fetal circulation of arginine vasopressin injected intraamniotically. Am J Obstet Gynecol 1991; 164: 1013–18.

66. Chmait R, Pretorius D, Moore T, et al. Prenatal detection of associated anomalies in fetuses diagnosed with cleft lip with or without cleft palate in utero. Ultrasound Obstet Gynecol 2006; 27: 173–6.

67. Jones MC. Facial clefting. Etiology and developmental pathogenesis. Clin Plast Surg 1993; 20: 599–606.

68. Gorlin RJ, Cohen MM, Hennekam RCM. Syndromes of the Head and Neck, 4th edn. New York: Oxford University Press, 2001; 859.

69. Rollnick BR, Prusansky S. Genetic services at a center for craniofacial anomalies. Cleft Palate J 1981; 18: 304–13.

70. Shprintzen RJ, Siegel-Sadewitz VL, Amato J, Goldberg RB. Anomalies associated with cleft lip, cleft palate, or both. Am J Med Genet 1985; 20: 585–95.

71. Clementi M, Tenconi R, Bianchi F, Stoll C. Evaluation of prenatal diagnosis of cleft lip with or without cleft palate and cleft palate by ultrasound: experience from 20 European registries. EUROSCAN Study Group. Prenat Diagn 2000; 20: 870–5.

72. Chmait R, Pretorius D, Jones M, et al. Prenatal evaluation of facial clefts with two dimensional and adjunctive three-dimensional ultrasonography: a prospective trial. Am J Obstet Gynecol 2002; 187: 946–9.

73. Stoll C, Alembik Y, Dott B, Roth MP. Associated malformations in cases with oral clefts. Cleft Palate Craniofac J 2000; 37: 41–7.

74. Crane JP, Lefevre ML, Winborn RC, et al. A randomized trial of prenatal ultrasonographic screening: impact on the detection, management, and outcome of anomalous fetuses. Am J Obstet Gynecol 1994; 171: 392–9.

75. Porter HJ, Weston M, Andrews J, Berry PJ. Is ultrasound scanning an adequate antenatal diagnostic and screening technique: review of 150 abnormal fetuses. Pediatr Pathol 1992; 12: 897–8.

7 Assessment of fetal movements in the 1st trimester

Wiku Andonotopo, Asim Kurjak, and Sanja Kupesic

INTRODUCTION

Development of the central nervous system (CNS) begins as early as the 2nd postconceptional week, proceeds throughout gestation, and continues long after birth. Although some histogenetic processes are not finished until puberty, motor development and motor behavior events are very active in early pregnancy.[1–4] During the 1st trimester of gestation, the most intensive histogenetic process is neurogenesis. Neuronal migration and synaptogenesis begin almost simultaneously with proliferation, although their intensity increases during the 2nd trimester. The intensity of developmental processes, as well as their complexity, designates this period as the period of high vulnerability for the developing brain. Harmful events occurring during the 1st trimester of pregnancy can result in a variety of abnormalities of the CNS, from life-threatening morphologic anomalies of neural tube formation to a reduction in the number of neurons and consequently reduced developmental potential.[3]

The development of real-time two-dimensional (2D) sonography was one of the milestones in the studying of embryonic and fetal neural development, because it offered for the first time the possibility of studying prenatal activity and motility in real time. The classic studies by de Vries et al[5,6] have shown that motor activity begins as early as the late embryonic period. The number and complexity of fetal motor patterns increases rapidly during the 1st trimester of gestation, and the major development and motor behavior events are precisely followed by the appearance of new motor patterns or by significant changes in the existing patterns.[5,6] Numerous studies have been undertaken since this pioneer research, resulting in a precise and detailed description of various movement patterns, the temporal sequence of their appearance during pregnancy, and their correlation with structural motor development and motor behavior events.[7,8] It has been shown that even in early pregnancy, embryonic and fetal motor activity appears as spontaneous patterned activity, rather than a chaotic, random motion. Major movement patterns, observable during pregnancy, develop and appear most frequently during the 1st trimester, which also reflects the intensity of the motor development and motor behavior processes in this period.[5,6] The 2nd and 3rd trimesters are characterized by the progressive organization of fetal motor activity and its integration with other parameters of fetal activity into well-organized fetal behavioral states.[8–10] Furthermore, it has been shown that alterations in the quality of fetal movements may reveal any structural and functional impairment of the fetal CNS, as seen in studies on anencephalic fetuses.[11,12] However, the criteria for intrauterine diagnosis of cerebral dysfunctions have not yet been established, mainly due to the technical limitations of the imaging techniques.

Recently, the development of three-dimensional (3D) and four-dimensional (4D) sonography has provided new opportunities for the investigation of embryonic and fetal morphology and behavior.[2,3,13,14] Our 4D sonographic research has shown that this technique allows the visualization of fetal motility in all trimesters of pregnancy.[15–19] It also allows visualization of subtle fetal movements such as facial mimics and facial expressions in the 3rd trimester of pregnancy, which has not been possible with 2D ultrasound.[18,20] The application of 4D sonography in the examination of fetal facial movements has revealed the existence of a full range of facial expressions, similar to emotional expressions in adults, but the significance of this finding remains to be determined in future investigations.[17,18] 4D sonography also seems to be superior to 2D sonography in studying the fine motor behavior of the upper limbs, because it provides more details on the dynamics of small anatomic structures.[18,21]

During the 1st trimester of pregnancy, 3D sonography provides additional morphologic information that could facilitate the early detection of serious motor development and motor behavior malformations, such as spina bifida.[22] However, the possible benefits of 4D over 2D sonography in the assessment of embryonic and fetal movements in the 1st trimester of pregnancy have not yet been evaluated systematically. The aim of the study reported here was to compare the assessment of embryonic and early fetal motor development and motor behavior in the 1st trimester of normal pregnancy using 2D and 4D sonography. The study was designed to determine if the 4D sonographic assessment of early embryonic and fetal motility provides any additional information on early normal neural activity in comparison with classic 2D sonography. To the best of our knowledge, this is the first report on this important topic.

2D AND 4D SONOGRAPHIC SCANNING METHOD

In our study, we enrolled pregnant women who had been referred to the outpatient clinic for regular ultrasound examination in early pregnancy.[1] The inclusion criteria were singleton pregnancy and a gestational age of 6–14 weeks confirmed by the first 2D ultrasound examination. The exclusion criteria were embryonic and fetal abnormalities detected by morphologic 2D ultrasound examination, complications of pregnancy (vaginal bleeding, reported pain in the lower abdomen, or verified bacterial infection of the lower genital tract), maternal pathologic conditions (i.e., hypertension, diabetes mellitus, cardiac or pulmonary diseases, or severe anemia). After the regular 2D morphologic examination, those who met the inclusion criteria were offered 2D and 4D examination of fetal movements. The regular morphologic assessment was followed by 2D recording of fetal movements over a duration of 15 minutes. After standard assessment with 2D B-mode ultrasound, the 4D mode was turned on and a live 3D image was built by selecting the ideal representative 2D image placed in the region of interest (ROI) to visualize the whole fetus. The crystal array of the transducer was moved mechanically over the defined ROI. The volume was automatically scanned every 2 seconds, and 4D images were displayed on screen and recorded on videotape during the 15-minute observation period. 2D and 4D examinations were performed on a Voluson 730 machine (Kretztechnik, Zipf, Austria) with a transvaginal 8 MHz transducer and a Sonoline Antares machine (Siemens AG, USA) with a transabdominal 5 MHz transducer. 2D and 4D sonographic examinations were performed by one trained and experienced sonographer. During the examination period, the women were placed in a semirecumbent position, in a quiet room, at room temperature. Investigations were performed in the morning and the women abstained from food 2 hours prior to the beginning of the investigation. Both 2D and 4D records were analyzed by two investigators independently, and a consensus reading was subsequently performed. The observed movements were classified according to the description given by de Vries et al.[5]

Table 7.1 Correlation of median frequencies of movement patterns and bias in the 1st trimester using 2D and 4D sonography between 7 and 8 weeks of gestation

Movement pattern	Frequency of movement patterns per 15 min (min–median–max)		R_s	p	Bias
	2D	**4D**			
General movements	0–3–15	0–1–12	0.92	<0.05	0.15
Startle	0–1–15	0–1–15	0.89	<0.05	−0.05
Isolated arm movements	0–0–2	0–0–1	0.59	<0.05	−0.10
Isolated leg movements	0–0–1	0–0–2	0.43	<0.05	0.21

R_s, Spearman rank order coefficient

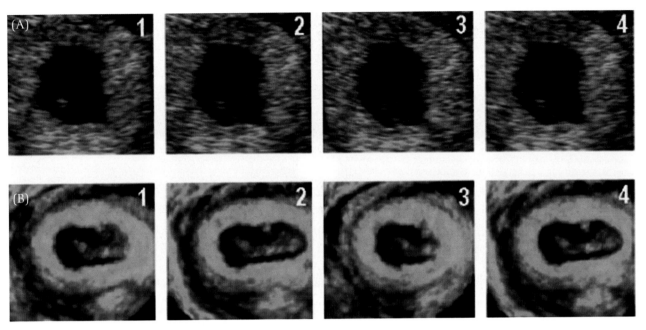

Figure 7.1 (A) 2D ultrasound sequence demonstrating an embryo at 6 weeks of gestation, showing no movements. (B) 4D imaging sequence of the same embryo, without any visible movements

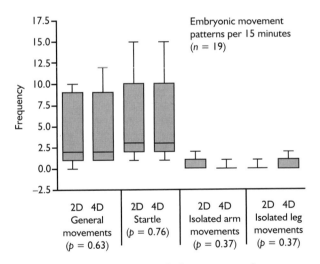

Figure 7.2 Comparison of frequencies of movement patterns between 7 and 8 weeks of gestation, observed by 2D and 4D sonography. $\mathbf{I}$, minimum–maximum; $\square$, 25%–75%; —, median value; p-values according to Wilcoxon sum rank test

CLASSIFICATION OF MOVEMENT PATTERN

We classified the embryos and fetuses into three groups according to their gestational ages in order to obtain a more precise analysis of the motor patterns. In four embryos assessed at 6 weeks of gestation, no signs of motor activity could be observed, by either 2D or 4D ultrasound. Despite the immobility, embryos were clearly visible by 2D and 4D ultrasound and could easily be distinguished from the adjacent yolk sac (Figure 7.1).

We detected the earliest embryonic movements at 7 weeks of gestation. The motor activity of embryos studied between 7 and 8 weeks of gestation ($n = 19$) was clearly recognizable and consisted of several movement patterns, observed by both 2D and 4D sonography (Figure 7.2).[1]

Movements involving the whole body, such as general movements (Figure 7.3) and startles, occurred most frequently, although in 8-week-old embryos, isolated arm and leg movements could also be observed. There was no difference in the median frequencies of movements observed by 2D and 4D sonography (Figure 7.2), and Spearman rank order correlation reached statistical significance for all compared movement patterns (Table 7.1). A positive bias was found in general movements and isolated leg movements between 7 and 8 weeks of gestation, showing that 4D sonography produced higher observations than 2D sonography (Table 7.1).

All of the movement patterns described above were also recognizable by both imaging methods in fetuses studied between 9 and 14 weeks of gestation ($n = 27$). However, the median frequencies of those movement patterns increased and several other motor patterns

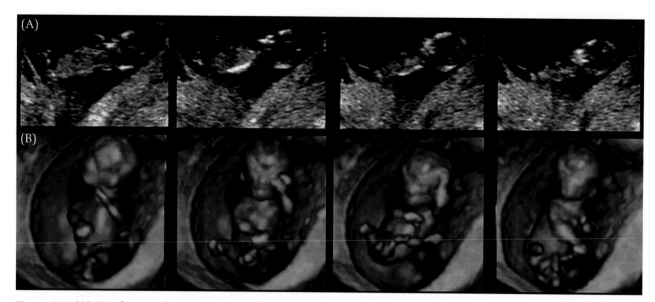

Figure 7.3 (A) 2D ultrasound sequence demonstrating an embryo at 12 weeks of gestation, showing general movements. (B) 4D imaging sequence showing the same pattern

appeared. The stretching movement pattern, observed from the 9th week onwards, could be added to a group of body movements (Figure 7.4). There were no differences in the median frequencies of general movements, stretching, startles, and isolated leg movements (Figure 7.5), although the Wilcoxon sum rank test detected a significant difference ($p = 0.02$) between the median frequencies of isolated arm movements (Figure 7.6). Nevertheless, the Spearman rank order correlation test reached statistical significance for all observed movement patterns (Table 7.2).

From 9 weeks onwards, it was possible to detect the direction of hand movements (Figures 7.4 and 7.7).

Some hand movements were directed towards the fetal face, although those movements appeared less frequently than the random arm movements. From 10 weeks onwards, head anteflexion, retroflexion, and rotation could easily be observed by both 2D and 4D sonography. There were no differences in their median frequencies detected by the two imaging techniques (Figure 7.8). The Spearman rank order correlation between the 2D and 4D techniques reached statistical significance for all observed movement patterns (Table 7.2).

A positive bias was found in isolated leg movement, stretching, and head retroflexion between 9 and 14

Table 7.2 Correlation of median frequencies of movement patterns and bias in the 1st trimester using 2D and 4D sonography between 9 and 14 weeks of gestation

Movement pattern	Frequency of movement patterns per 15 min (min–median–max)		R_s	p	Bias
	2D	4D			
General movements	8–25–15	9–22–80	0.95	<0.05	−0.18
Startle	10–25–45	10–22–45	0.96	<0.05	−0.22
Isolated arm movements	5–24–45	3–22–38	0.93	<0.05	−1.48
Isolated leg movements	1–6–20	1–7–18	0.94	<0.05	0.33
Stretching	0–2–12	0–3–15	0.97	<0.05	0.33
Hand-to-face	0–14–40	0–15–38	0.96	<0.05	−0.44
Head retroflection	0–6–50	0–6–45	0.98	<0.05	0.11
Hand anteflection	0–4–10	0–3–13	0.94	<0.05	−0.11
Head rotation	0–2–15	0–2–15	0.95	<0.05	−0.29

R_S, Spearman rank order correlation

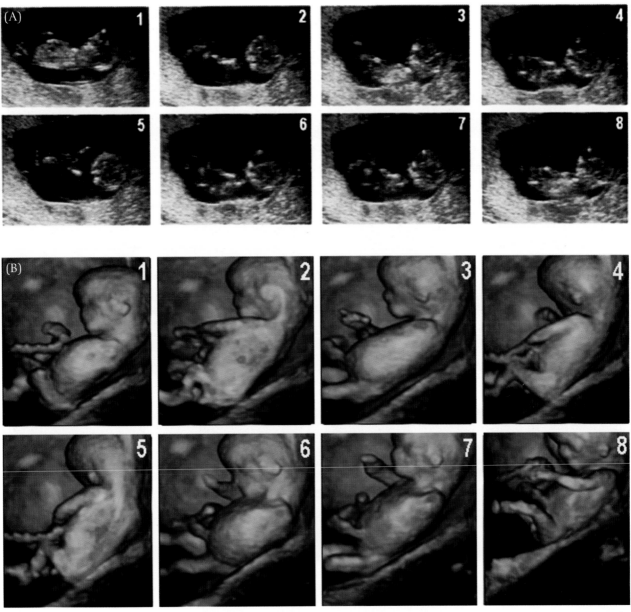

Figure 7.4 (A) 2D imaging sequence of a fetus at 11 weeks of gestation showing hand-to-head movement and stretching pattern. (B) The same fetus observed by 4D sonography

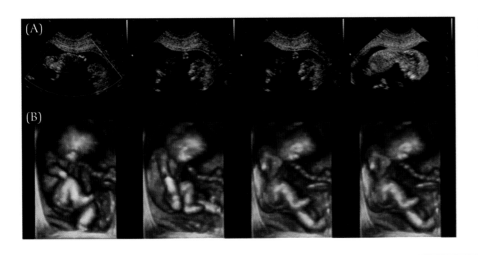

Figure 7.5 (A) 2D sonography demonstrating a fetus at 12 weeks of gestation, showing isolated leg movement. (B) The same fetus observed by 4D sonography

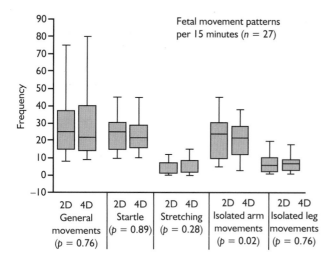

Fetal movement patterns per 15 minutes (n = 27)

Figure 7.6 Comparison of frequencies of body movement patterns and isolated limb movements between 9 and 14 weeks of gestation, observed by 2D and 4D sonography. I, minimum–maximum; □, 25%–75%; —, median value; *p*-values according to Wilcoxon sum rank test

weeks of gestation, showing that 4D sonography produced higher observations than 2D sonography (Table 7.2).

Several movement patterns, such as sideways bending, hiccup, and swallowing, could not be observed by 4D sonography, although they were clearly visible by 2D sonography (Figures 7.9–7.11). The frequencies of these movements are shown in Figure 7.12. Sideways bending, which occurred with the lowest frequency, was notable only in 7-week-old embryos. Breathing movements and hiccups, which appeared in the 9th week, were the most frequent movement patterns. Facial movements, swallowing, mouth opening, and yawning appeared in the 10th week and occurred less frequently, but were clearly distinguishable on 2D sonography. Although our previous studies have shown that the full range of facial movements can be recognized by 4D sonography in the 3rd trimester of pregnancy, this investigation failed to find the same results in the 1st trimester.[16–18]

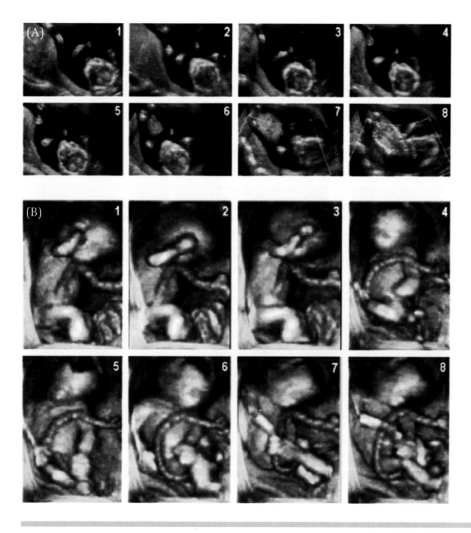

Figure 7.7 (A) 2D sonography demonstrating a fetus at 12 weeks of gestation, showing hand-to-head movement. (B) The same fetus observed by 4D sonography showing hand-to-head movement and isolated leg movement

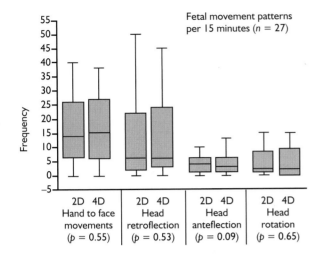

Figure 7.8 Comparison of frequencies of hand-to-face movements and head movement patterns between 9 and 14 weeks of gestation, observed by 2D and 4D sonography. ⊥, minimum–maximum; □, 25%–75%; —, median value; p-values according to Wilcoxon sum rank test

COMPARISON OF 2D AND 4D SCANNING

The 1st trimester of pregnancy is a period of very intensive progressive motor development and motor behavior processes, such as proliferation and migration of neurons. Major structures of the fetal brain are formed in this period, although the maturational processes continue long after delivery.[23–25] Although movements in this early stage of gestation can be elicited by tactile stimulation, and by other sensory stimuli as the pregnancy progresses, the major proportion of intrauterine motor activity is endogenously generated by the CNS.[9,26] The intensity of structural and functional motor development and motor behavior processes in the 1st trimester of pregnancy and the subsequent vulnerability of the nervous system make fetal neurologic assessment a very challenging issue.

Our study included embryos and fetuses between 6 and 14 weeks of gestation.[1] The chronologic appearance of the complex and specific movement patterns was in agreement with the pioneering research by de Vries et al.[5] At 6 weeks of gestation embryonic movements could not be observed by either 2D or 4D sonography (Figure 7.1). The embryo appeared immobile, although heart action was present. The first spontaneous embryonic movements were observed by 2D and 4D ultrasound at 7 weeks of gestation. This is in accordance with the 2D studies by de Vries et al,[5,6] who registered the earliest patterns of spontaneous embryonic motor activity at 7.5–8 weeks of gestation. Two motor patterns – general movements and startles – were observed with similar accuracy and in the same period of gestation by 2D and 4D sonography. Sideways bending could be observed only by 2D sonography, probably due to its higher resolution. This discrete movement pattern was notable only in the 7th week of gestation, and appeared less frequently than the other movement patterns. It should be noted that the earliest embryonic movements appeared as organized patterned activity. This is in accordance with in vitro studies, which have shown that neurons

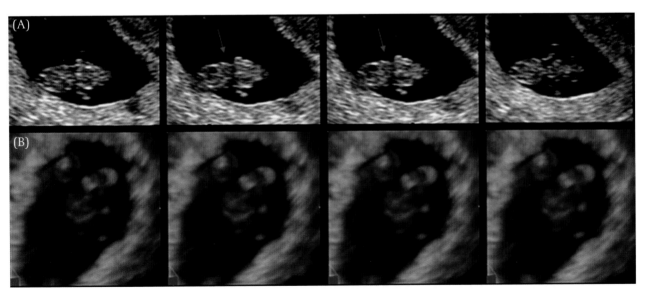

Figure 7.9 (A) 2D imaging of a fetus at 7 weeks of gestation showing sideways bending (red arrow). (B) 4D imaging could not visualize this type of movement pattern

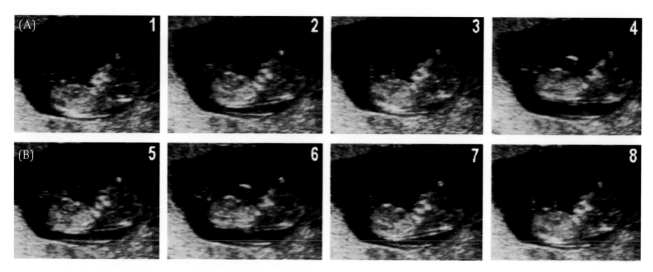

Figure 7.10 (A) Swallowing movement pattern as observed by 2D sonography. (B) 4D sonography could not observe this movement pattern due to the rapid movements

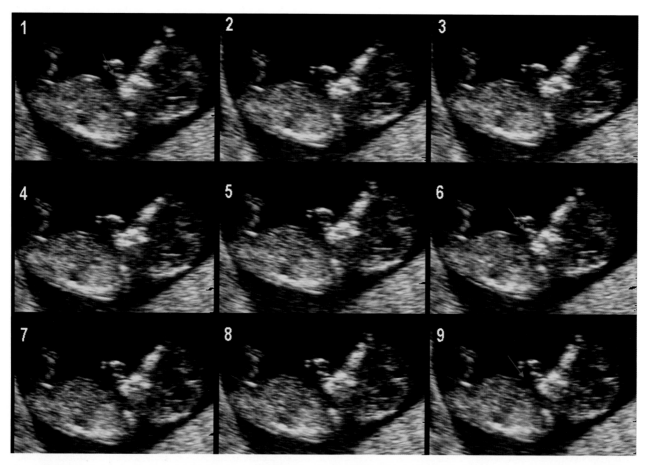

Figure 7.11 Hiccup movement pattern, which can only be observed by 2D sonography due to the rapid movements. Note the rapid repertoire of flexion and extension of the head to the chest (red arrow)

begin to generate and propagate the patterned bursts of action potentials as soon as they interconnect.[27] Generally, it seems that patterned activity emerges in networks of interacting neurons, due to intrinsic membrane properties and synaptic interactions.[27] However, during the 1st trimester, the brainstem,

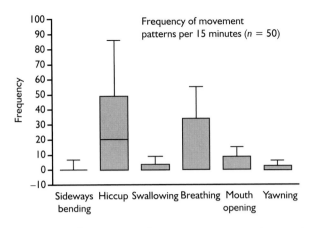

Figure 7.12 Frequencies of movement patterns that can be observed only by 2D sonography. ⊥, minimum–maximum; □, 25%–75%; —, median value

which begins to develop and mature at 7 weeks of gestation, gradually begins to take the control over fetal movements and behavioral patterns. Until delivery, subunits of the brainstem will remain the main regulators of all fetal behavioral patterns.[28] Development of the brainstem proceeds in a caudal-to-rostral direction, which means that its phylogenetically older structures, such as the medulla oblongata, will form and mature earlier in gestation.[3,28]

In our study, general movements were present from the 8th week of gestation onwards and were one of the most frequent movement patterns observed by both 2D and 4D sonography (Figure 7.3).[1] According to the literature, general movements can be recognized from 8–9 weeks of gestation onwards, and remain present until 16–20 weeks after birth.[6,29] Qualitative alterations in general movements have been reported in fetuses with various neurologic disorders, such as anencephaly, and fetuses from pregnancies complicated with maternal diabetes mellitus.[7,11,12,30] Their movements seem to lose any elegance and become erratic and jerky.[7,11,12]

Spatial imaging using 4D sonography, which allows simultaneous visualization of all fetal extremities, head, and trunk, could significantly improve the qualitative assessment of general movements.[13] However, the fact that 4D imaging occurs in near real time might represent a potential limitation on such an assessment. The results of our study show that, even at present, quantitative analysis of general movements by 4D sonography is not limited by the sampling time for data acquisition and can be performed with the same accuracy as 2D sonography.

Several features of fetal body and limb movements between 9 and 14 weeks could be observed by 4D sonography, and quantitative analysis of these movement patterns could be performed with almost the same accuracy as when using 2D sonography. We found no difference in the frequency of body movement patterns or the isolated leg movements. However, isolated arm movements could be observed less frequently on 4D sonography – probably due to the lower resolution and discordance between the velocity of movement and sampling time for data acquisition. Nevertheless, there was a significant correlation between the frequencies of these movements observed by the two techniques. Furthermore, 4D sonography appeared to be equally potent in the assessment of specific hand movements such as hand-to-face contacts, which occurred less frequently than isolated arm movements, and there was a positive correlation between the movements recorded by the two techniques. Head movement patterns, head rotation, anteflexion, and retroflexion could be observed from 10 weeks onwards by both imaging methods, and there were no statistically significant differences in their frequencies.

In our study, fetal breathing and hiccups (Figure 7.11), present from 9 weeks onwards, as well as swallowing (Figure 7.10) and yawning, recognizable from 10 weeks onwards, could be observed only by 2D ultrasound (Figures 7.9–7.12).[1] Facial movements, such as yawning and mouth opening, are controlled by pontine structures (the Vth–VIIth cranial nerves). The pons, which also contains structures important for arousal and sleep–wake cycles, begins to form almost simultaneously with the medulla oblongata, but its maturation is more prolonged.[28] Our previous studies have shown that a full range of subtle facial expressions as well as swallowing and yawning movements are clearly recognizable by 4D sonography in the 3rd trimester, and their qualitative characteristics as well as frequency are almost the same as in the neonate.[16–18,31] In the 1st trimester, however, the structures of the fetal face are not easily distinguishable. The complicated development of the face, the curled composition of the fetus, and the low resolution of 4D images complicate the scanning of the facial structures in the 1st trimester. Rapid fetal movements (lasting 1–2 seconds) or discrete movements, such as chest movements during fetal breathing or hiccups, may not be evaluated using the 4D technique due to the relatively slow sampling time for data acquisition to obtain an image of satisfactory quality. Breathing and hiccups are produced by movements of the diaphragm, whereas the movements of the chest wall are mostly very discrete. Characteristic oscillations of the diaphragm can easily be recognized on 2D sonography, whereas 4D sonography allows only superficial scanning of the fetal body, which limits the possibility of detecting these movements. At present, real-time 2D sonography remains the gold standard for the evaluation of these types of movement.

The clinical utility of 4D sonography has not been clearly established, and only a few publications on this topic are available at present. In previous studies, we aimed to evaluate the utility of 4D sonography in the 2nd and 3rd trimesters. Those studies showed the advantages of this technique in the qualitative assessment of fetal hand movements, and particularly in the evaluation of fetal facial expressions.[15–17,31] This study has shown that, at present, real-time 2D and 4D sonography could be used as complementary methods for the evaluation of fetal movement patterns in early pregnancy. Although quantitative analysis of most movement patterns can be performed using either technique, 2D sonography appears to be superior in the evaluation of certain movement patterns, such as hiccup, mouth opening, yawning, and breathing movements. However, the evolution of the 4D technique may lead to faster acquisition of images and allow true real-time 3D evaluation of fetal motility in the future. From the present results, it is reasonable to expect that such technological improvement may provide some new information about intrauterine motor activity. Thus, it could contribute to a better understanding of early fetal motor development and motor behavior, and facilitate the prenatal detection of some neurologic disorders.

CONCLUSIONS

Presently, both 2D and 4D methods are required for the assessment of early fetal motor development and motor behavior. It is reasonable to expect that technological improvements may provide some new information about intrauterine motor activity and facilitate the prenatal detection of some neurologic disorders.

REFERENCES

1. Andonotopo W, Medic M, Salihagic-Kadic A, et al. The assessment of fetal behavior in early pregnancy: comparison between 2D and 4D sonographic scanning. J Perinat Med 2005; 33: 406–14.

2. Kurjak A, Carrera JM, Stanojevic M, et al. The role of 4D sonography in the neurological assessment of early human development. Ultrasound Rev Obstet Gynecol 2004; 4: 148–59.

3. Pomeroy SL, Volpe JJ. Development of the nervous system. In: Polin RA, Fow WW, eds. Fetal and Neonatal Physiology. Philadelphia, PA: WB Saunders, 1992: 1491.

4. Salihagic-Kadic A, Medic M, Kurjak A. Neurophysiology of fetal behavior. Ultrasound Rev Obstet Gynecol 2004; 4: 2–11.

5. de Vries JIP, Visser GHA, Prechtl HFR. The emergence of fetal behavior I: Qualitative aspects. Early Hum Dev 1982; 7: 301–22.

6. de Vries JIP, Visser GHA, Prechtl HFR. The emergence of fetal behavior II: Quantitative aspects. Early Hum Dev 1985; 12: 99–120.

7. Prechtl HFR. Qualitative changes of spontaneous movements in fetus and preterm infant are a marker of neurological dysfunction. Early Hum Dev 1990; 23: 151–8.

8. Roodenburg PJ, Wladimiroff JW, van Es A, Prechtl HFR. Classification and quantitative aspects of fetal movements during the second half of normal pregnancy. Early Hum Dev 1991; 25: 19–35.

9. Nijhuis JG. Neurobehavioral development of the fetal brain. In: Nijhuis JG, ed. Fetal Behavior: Developmental and Perinatal Aspects. Oxford: Oxford University Press, 1992: 489.

10. Wheeler T, Gennser G, Lindvall R, Murrils AJ. Changes in the fetal heart rate associated with fetal breathing and fetal movement. Br J Obstet Gynecol 1980; 12: 1068–79.

11. Andonotopo W, Kurjak A, Ivancic-Kosuta M. Behavior of anencephalic fetus studied by 4D ultrasound. J Matern Fetal Neonatal Med 2005; 17: 165–8.

12. Visser GHA, Laurini RN, Vries JIP, Beckedam DJ, Prechtl HF. Abnormal motor behavior in anencephalic fetuses. Early Human Dev 1985; 12: 173–82.

13. Andonotopo W, Stanojevic M, Kurjak A, Azumendi G, Carrera JM. Assessment of fetal behavior and general movements by four-dimensional sonography. Ultrasound Rev Obstet Gynecol 2004; 4: 103–14.

14. Kurjak A, Vecek N, Hafner T, et al. Prenatal diagnosis: what does four-dimensional ultrasound add? J Perinat Med 2002; 30: 57–62.

15. Kurjak A, Vecek N, Kupesic S, Azumendi G, Solak M. Four-dimensional ultrasound: How much does it improve perinatal practice? In: Carrera JM, Chervenak FA, Kurjak A, eds. Controversies in Perinatal Medicine: Studies on the Fetus as a Patient. New York: Parthenon, 2003: 222.

16. Kurjak A, Stanojevic M, Andonotopo W, et al. Behavioral pattern continuity from prenatal to postnatal life – a study by four dimensional (4D) ultrasonography. J Perinat Med 2004; 32: 346–53.

17. Kurjak A, Stanojevic M, Azumendi G, Carrera JM. The potential of four-dimensional (4D) ultrasonography in the assessment of fetal awareness. J Perinat Med 2005; 33: 46–53.

18. Kurjak A, Azumendi G, Vecek N, et al. Fetal hand movements and facial expression in normal pregnancy studied by four-dimensional sonography. J Perinat Med 2003; 31: 496–508.

19. Lightman SL, Insel TR, Ingram CD. New genomic avenues in behavioral neuroendocrinology. Eur J Neurosci 2002; 16: 369–72.

20. Azumendi G, Kurjak A. Three-dimensional and four-dimensional sonography in the study of the fetal face. Ultrasound Rev Obstet Gynecol 2003; 3: 1–6.

21. Pooh RK, Ogura T. Normal and abnormal fetal hand positioning and movement in early pregnancy detected by three- and four-dimensional ultrasound. Ultrasound Rev Obstet Gynecol 2004; 4: 46–51.

22. Kurjak A, Pooh RK, Merce LT, et al. Structural and functional early human development assessed by three-dimensional (3D) and four-dimensional (4D) sonography. Fertil Steril 2005; 84: 1285–99.

23. Kostovic I, Judas M, Petanjek Z, Simic G. Ontogenesis of goal-directed behavior: anatomo–functional considerations. Int J Psychophysiol 1995; 19: 85–102.

24. Kostovic I, Judas M. Transient patterns of organization of the human fetal brain. Croat Med J 1998; 2: 107–14.

25. Kostovic I, Judas M, Rados M, Hrabac P. Laminar organization of the human fetal cerebrum revealed by histochemical markers and magnetic resonance imaging. Cerebral Cortex 2002; 12: 536–44.

26. Morokuma S, Fukushima K, Kawai N, et al. Fetal habituation correlates with functional brain development. Behav Brain Res 2004; 31: 459–63.

27. Stafstrom CE, Johnston D, Wehner JM, Sheppard JR. Spontaneous neural activity in fetal brain reaggregate culture. Neuroscience 1980; 10: 1681–9.

28. Joseph R. Fetal brain and cognitive development. Dev Rev 1999; 20: 81–5.

29. Prechtl HF. State of the art of a new functional assessment of the young nervous system. An early predictor of cerebral palsy. Early Hum Dev 1997; 50: 1–11.

30. Visser GH, Mulder EJ, Bekedam DJ, van Ballegooie E, Prechtl HF. Fetal behavior in type-1 diabetic women. Eur J Obstet Gynecol Reprod Biol 1986; 21: 315–20.

31. Kurjak A, Stanojevic M, Andonotopo W, et al. Fetal behavior assessed in all three trimesters of normal pregnancy by four dimensional (4D) sonography. Croat Med J 2005; 46: 772–80.

8 Maternal, placental, and fetal circulation: What does 3D power Doppler add?

Luis T Mercé, María J Barco, and Asim Kurjak

INTRODUCTION

Three-dimensional (3D) power Doppler angiography is an emerging technique in the field of ultrasound and Doppler diagnostics in obstetrics and gynecology. Since 1996, there have been around 400 publications on 3D ultrasound, although no more than 100 deal specifically with the diagnostic problems arising with this technique.

A more precise evaluation of the maternal, placental and fetal circulations throughout the course of a normal pregnancy can be achieved with this technique. 3D power Doppler angiography can provide new data on the physiology of placentation and normal fetal vascular development. This is essential to allow establishment of new diagnostic criteria and indications in the management of fetal growth anomalies and vascular pathology during the course of pregnancy.

ESSENTIALS OF 3D POWER DOPPLER

In 1996, Ritchie et al[1] reported a new technique for producing 3D angiograms from slices obtained by 2D power Doppler. They suggested that this technique would be useful for the assessment of vascular anatomy and blood flow perfusion of organs such as the kidney and placenta.

The development of 3D power Doppler sonography and power Doppler angiography is closely linked to the diagnostic abilities of power Doppler and the design of the software capable of representing and properly evaluating the vascularization of different organs.

3D power Doppler sonography is essentially characterized by its high sensitivity to depict any vessel – the great vessels as well as microvascularization.[2] This is possible because, unlike conventional color Doppler, images are obtained from the ultrasound amplitude instead of the Doppler frequency. The color map acquired is not affected by the insonation angle and does not show dark zones or aliasing.[3]

VOCAL ('virtual organ computer-aided analysis') is software developed from a rotational method for the automated or manual assessment of 3D volumes.[4] This program allows surface definition and characterization by the 'surface' or 'skin' mode, automatic or manual calculation of the volumes of different structures, production of a virtual 'shell' of different thickness, and automated calculation of 3D Doppler indices for the assessment of organ vascularization.[5]

By means of a histogram, the VOCAL program performs an automated calculation of the grayscale and color values from the acquired volume. The 3D volume is made up of units termed 'voxels', which store all the information about the grayscale and color expressed in an intensity scale from 0 to 100. In this way, a gray index and three color indices are obtained for the quantitative assessment of vascularization.[4,5]

The mean gray (MG) represents the mean gray value among all the gray voxels from the acquired volume. The vascularization index (VI) estimates the number of color voxels inside the volume, thus expressing the number of blood vessels as a percentage. The flow index (FI) is the average color value from all the color voxels, depicting the mean intensity of blood flow. The vascularization flow index (VFI) is the average color value out of all the color and gray

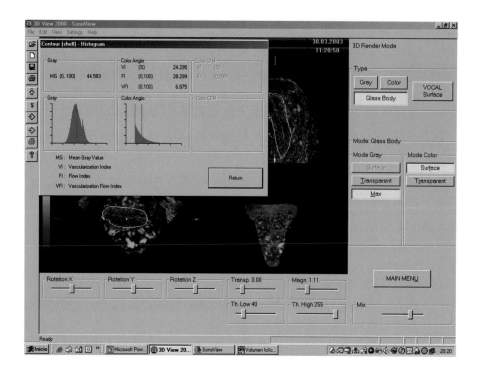

Figure 8.1 The VOCAL imaging program allows calculation of 3D Doppler indices to evaluate vascularity

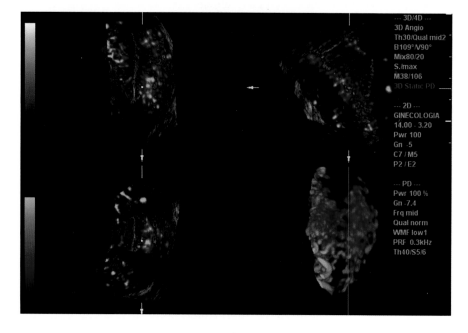

Figure 8.2 Endometrial and subendometrial vascular network rendered by 3D power Doppler

voxels (vascularization as well as blood flow) – in other words, the perfusion inside the region of interest (Figure 8.1).[4,5]

VOCAL is a useful tool for the quantitative evaluation of 3D power Doppler angiography, especially given that 3D power Doppler can depict in a precise way the whole tree network. The determination of the morphology and architecture of the vascular networks can clearly contribute to the diagnosis of vascular anomalies.

MATERNAL AND PLACENTAL CIRCULATION

Endometrial blood flow reflects uterine receptivity because the endometrium is the place where embryonic implantation is going to take place.[6] In a scan, the absence of color at the endometrial and subendometrial levels implies a significant decrease in implantation rate,[7,8] whereas the pregnancy rate increases when vessels reach the subendometrial halo and the endometrium.[7,9]

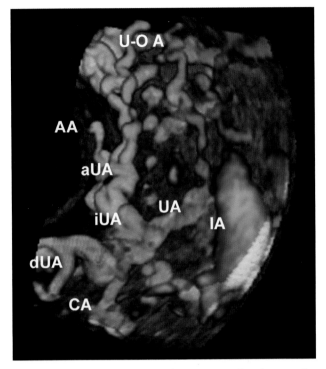

Figure 8.3 3D power Doppler angiography depicts the uterine artery and the trajectories of its main branches during early pregnancy. IA, iliac artery; UA, uterine artery; aUA, ascendent branch of the uterine artery; iUA, isthmic part of the uterine artery; dUA, descendent branch of the uterine artery; CA, cervical artery; U-O A, utero-ovarian artery

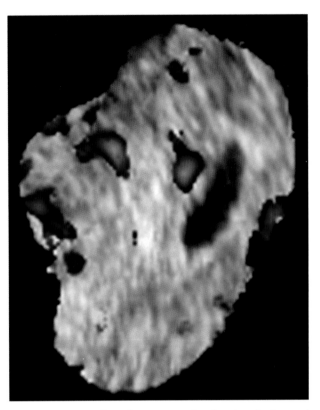

Figure 8.4 Power Doppler angiography showing the 'comet' sign produced by early placentation, with transformation of the spiral arteries closer to the gestational sac into uteroplacental arteries in a 4 week plus 4 day pregnancy

Ultrasonography and 3D power Doppler have the advantage of simultaneously assessing endometrial volume and subendometrial and endometrial blood flow. For all the 3D vascular indices from the endometrium and subendometrium, excellent intra- and interobserver reproducibility has been observed, with intraclass correlation coefficients greater than 0.90.[10,11]

3D Doppler indices vary significantly with the menstrual cycle, and are characterized by a pre-ovulatory peak and a post-ovulatory nadir.[12] The subendometrial flow index on the day of embryo transfer is greater among those patients who become pregnant,[13] and the subendometrial vascularization flow index on the day of human chorionic gonadotropin (hCG) administration is better than the endometrial volume for predicting a pregnancy in in vitro fertilization (IVF) cycles.[14] It has also been shown that those patients with a high response to the hCG treatment show lower endometrial and subendometrial 3D vascular indices (Figure 8.2).[15]

In one recent study, it was not possible to demonstrate significant differences in the endometrial and subendometrial indices of vascularization after the follicle-stimulating hormone (FSH) stimulation and on the oocyte recovery day between conceptional and nonconceptional cycles.[16] Nevertheless, as we proposed some time ago,[6] uterine receptivity should be assessed in the midluteal phase, when implantation occurs. Only this way could new strategies be defined to avoid implantation failure and enhance pregnancy rates with assisted-reproduction technology.[17]

Power Doppler angiography allows representation of the whole uterine circulation with its several branches throughout gestation – although more precisely during early pregnancy (Figure 8.3).

Around the 4th to 5th weeks in normal gestations, it is possible to observe how the spiral arteries approach the gestational sac producing the picture of a comet – the 'comet sign' (Figure 8.4). Invasion of the radial and spiral arteries by the cytotrophoblast is the mechanism leading to a progressive increase in uteroplacental perfusion. These arteries lose their self-regulative ability and grow in diameter, becoming the uteroplacental arteries.[18]

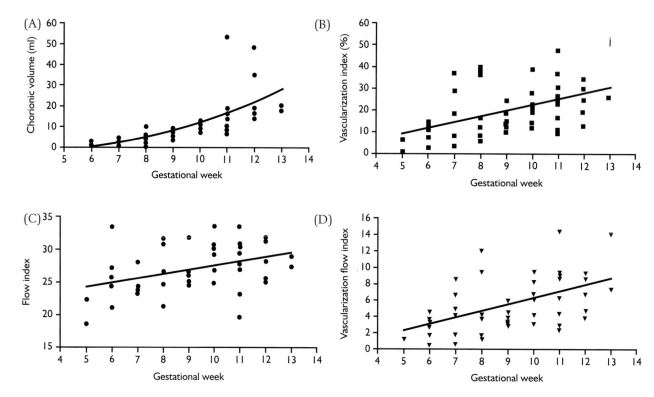

Figure 8.5 Chorionic volume and intervillous blood flow throughout early normal pregnancy, from 46 normal pregnancies: (A) chorionic volume; (B) vascularization index; (C) flow index; (D) vascularization flow index

During the 1st trimester of gestation, the size of the placenta allows it to be completely included inside the examination field of a 3D transvaginal probe. From the 6th week onwards, we can differentiate the uterochorionic circulation (essentially constituted by the spiral and radial arteries), from the intrachorionic circulation or, in other words, the intervillous blood flow.

Although the VOCAL software is able to assess independently the uterochorionic and intervillous circulations, we have initially studied the intervillous circulation alone by excluding the retrochorionic one. 3D Doppler indices increase gradually but significantly between the 6th and 12th weeks in a normal gestation. These findings confirm the previous results obtained by transvaginal color Doppler[19–21] demonstrating the appearance of intervillous blood flow from the 6th week of gestation and no later, at the end of the 1st trimester, as supported by other authors.[22,23] The progressive disappearance of the trophoblastic plugs from the spiral arteries during the 1st trimester leads to increases in the color Doppler signal from the chorion frondosum (vascularization index) and in its intensity (flow index) – which imply an increase in intervillous blood flow (Figure 8.5).

In cases of miscarriage, increases as well as decreases in the uterochorionic circulation have been reported, depending on the natural evolution of the process.[24] The intervillous flow is usually increased – pointing also to a failure in early placentation.[25] Recently, we have observed that the flow index is greater in those early pregnancies ending in miscarriage than in normal ongoing pregnancies.[26] This supports our previous findings demonstrating an increased intervillous velocity in cases of spontaneous abortion.[24]

In 1998, 3D power Doppler sonography was proposed as a means to discriminate placental vessels from the fetal circulation as well as from the maternal circulation (Figure 8.6).[27] Some years later, this method was proven to be superior to 2D power Doppler to detect the terminal vascular branches of the fetal circulation in the placental tree.[28] It has been demonstrated that 3D power Doppler angiography can evaluate normal placental development and investigate placental anomalies in real time, and it has now become a diagnostic method of surveillance and care during gestation.[29]

From the 1st trimester onward, the scanning field of a 3D probe cannot include the whole placental volume. To overcome this problem, we have

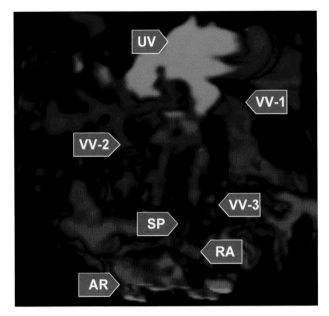

Figure 8.6 3D power Doppler angiography of the placental circulation during a normal 3rd-trimester pregnancy. UV, umbilical vessels; VV-1, 1st-order villous vascular branch; VV-2, 2nd-order villous vascular branch; VV-3, 3rd-order villous vascular branch; SP, spiral vessels; RA, radial vessels; AR, arcuate vessels.

developed the 'placental biopsy' method.[30,31] In summary, the aim is the acquisition of a representative sample from the placental vascular tree by application of the VOCAL program and calculation of vascular power Doppler indices. The placental sample is usually taken from the central part, where villous vascularization is most dense. Maternal and fetal movement should be avoided during the procedure. Using a multiplanar system, the placental zone with the best color map from the stored region of interest is selected offline. Finally, in the A-plane as a working image, the limits of a virtual reference axis between the basal and chorionic plates (both of which are excluded) are set, and the volume of a sphere is automatically obtained by rotation to calculate volume and Doppler indices (Figure 8.7).

The 'placental biopsy' method has good reproducibility and intraobserver agreement for 3D Doppler indices. The intraclass correlation coefficient is greater than 0.85 for all indices studied.[30,31]

The placental vascular tree shows progressive growth during normal gestation. Up to week 20, the vessels from the chorionic and basal plates are usually depicted, with the exception of the vascular branches of the fetal villous tree (Figure 8.8A). From 20 weeks up to 30–32 weeks, first- and second-order vascular villous branches develop. During the 3rd trimester, the vascular villous tree is fully developed and the third-order villous vessels can be rendered with growing thickness and density of their branches (Figure 8.8B).[29,30] This pattern of vascular development is very similar to that described in the classic histologic studies and by electronic microscopy.[32]

Placental blood flow as assessed by the 'placental biopsy' method through 3D Doppler indices is significantly related to gestational age (Figure 8.9). The flow index shows a linear and significant increase from 14 to 40 weeks ($r = 0.58$, $p < 0.01$) (Figure 8.9C). On the contrary, the vascularization index ($r = 0.29$, $p < 0.05$)

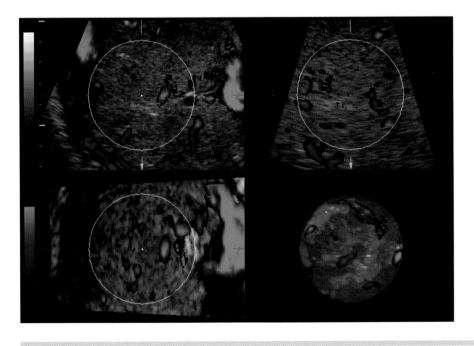

Figure 8.7 Placental biopsy by 3D power Doppler. A sphere of placental tissue between the chorionic and basal plates is obtained

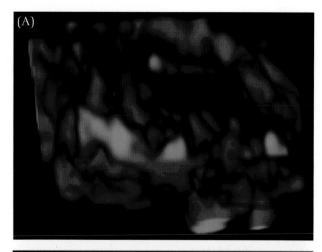

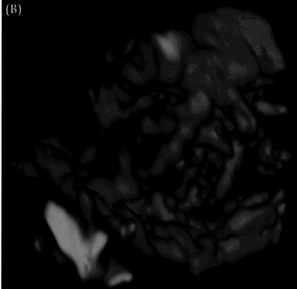

Figure 8.8 Power Doppler angiography of the placental vascular tree in the 2nd (A) and 3rd (B) trimesters of normal gestation

and vascularization flow index (r = 0.32, p <0.01) show a curve flattening from 30 weeks and a decrease at term gestation (Figure 8.9B,D). These results are slightly different from those of Yu et al.[33] These authors showed progressive increases in vascularization, flow and vascularization flow indices with gestational age, although no explanation was given as to the source of the placental sample.

Study of the placental circulation by 3D power Doppler is of great interest mainly for two reasons. Abnormal and deficient development of the placental vascular tree is closely associated with the fetal growth restriction.[34] Moreover, a decrease in intraplacental blood flow may precede an increase in umbilical resistance.[35] The blood flow through the intraplacental

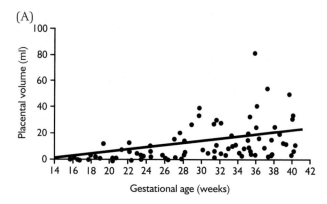

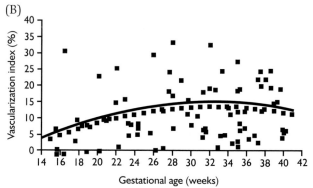

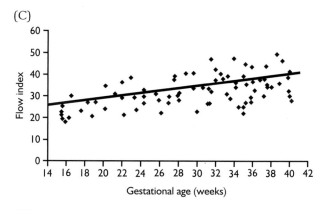

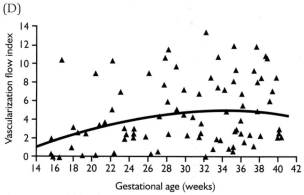

Figure 8.9 Placental volume from 'placental biopsy' and placental blood flow through an early normal pregnancy from 86 normal pregnancies: (A) chorionic volume; (B) vascularization index; (C) flow index; (D) vascularization flow index

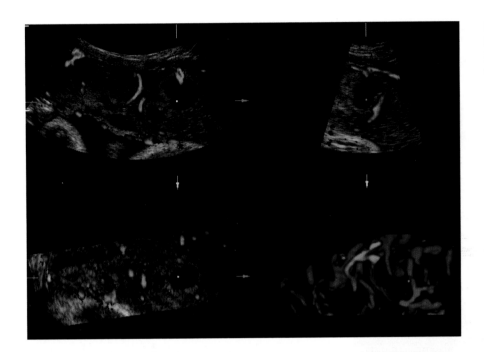

Figure 8.10 Villous vascular tree in a growth-restricted fetus confirmed after birth and with normal umbilical artery Doppler

vascular tree could be affected in some cases with a normal umbilical Doppler scan.[32] In fact, the intraplacental vascular resistance obtained by multigate spectral Doppler is more sensitive, and changes in its value precede the umbilical Doppler changes that allow detection of fetal growth restriction.[35] It has also been shown that the number of villous arteries is significantly decreased in growth-retarded gestations (Figure 8.10).[32]

Finally, this technique should play an essential role in the assessment and prediction of the outcome of placental vascular tumors such as chorioangiomas.[36]

EMBRYONIC AND FETAL CIRCULATION

Power Doppler angiography can depict the circulations in the embryo and fetus.[37]

At the 6th and 7th weeks, we can only see the cardiac signal, but progressively the fetoplacental and fetal circulations are rendered by 3D power Doppler. At the 8th week, it is possible to differentiate between the vessels in the uteroplacental circulation and the uterine non-placental vessels. The intervillous blood flow, the fetoplacental circulation, and the heart can also be observed (Figure 8.11).

At 10 weeks of gestation, the development of the embryo/fetal circulation is completed. By means of power Doppler angiography, the cerebral vessels and the ductus venosus can be detected (Figure 8.12). At the end of the 1st trimester, the majority of fetal vessels can be visualized (Figure 8.13).

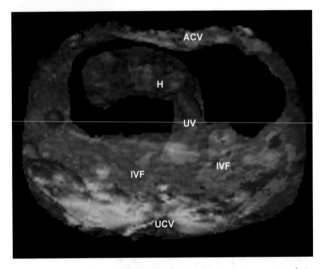

Figure 8.11 Placental and fetal circulations in a normal 8-week-pregnancy. UCV, uterochorionic vessels; IVF, intervillous flow; ACV, antichorionic vessels; UV, umbilical vessels; H, heart

3D power Doppler angiography can depict the whole umbilical cord from the placental to the fetal insertion. It is hampered by the same problems as conventional color Doppler – basically, the cord location and its trajectory, which is usually hidden by the fetus.

It has been suggested that this technique provides more information than conventional ultrasound and color Doppler to detect the nuchal cord (Figure 8.14).[38] Some authors believe that it has some value in the assessment of cord insertion,[39] and it may help to

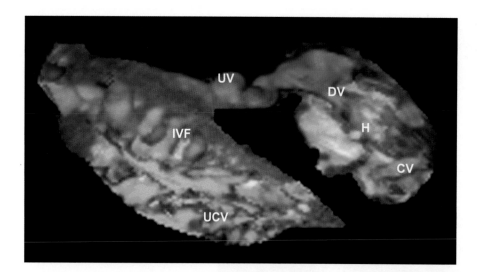

Figure 8.12 Placental and fetal circulations in a normal 10-week pregnancy. UCV, uterochorionic vessels; IVF, intervillous flow; UV, umbilical vessels; DV, ductus venosus; H, heart; CV, cerebral vessels

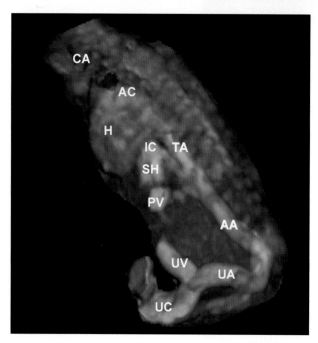

Figure 8.13 Fetal circulation at 15 weeks of amenorrhea. UC, umbilical cord; UV, umbilical vein; UA, umbilical artery; PV, portal vein; SH, suprahepatic veins; IC, inferior vena cava; AA, abdominal aorta; TA, thoracic aorta; H, heart; AC, aortic arch; CA, carotid artery

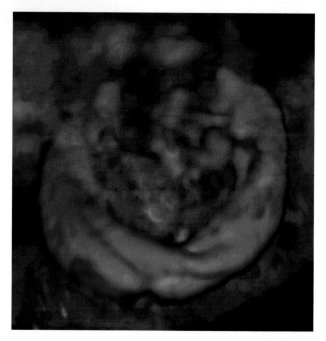

Figure 8.14 Nuchal cord on power Doppler angiography

diagnose some anomalies of insertion, such as vasa previa.[40]

Every fetal vascular territory can be rendered by 3D power Doppler angiography, but we shall focus here only on those that have attracted attention up to now.

This technique was suggested early on as a very promising approach to the evaluation of cerebral circulation and its vascular malformations.[41] Pooh et al[42] pointed out that multiplanar analysis and the potential to rotate the cerebral volume with the

vessels included provide the same diagnostic possibilities as magnetic resonance imaging.

More recently, it has been reported that fetal cerebral vascularization and blood flow increase significantly during pregnancy[43] and that 3D power Doppler can optimally detect aneurysms of the vein of Galen and its connections (Figure 8.15).[44,45]

Fetal heart examination by 3D sonography was initially faced with the technical problem that the heart is an organ that is in constant motion. This has been solved by the application of the STIC (spatio-temporal image correlation) mode. Using this technique, the cardiac volume is first determined by

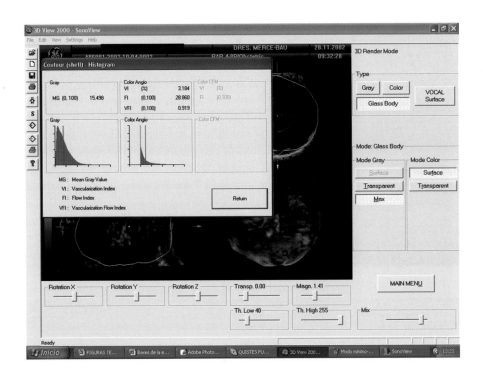

Figure 8.15 Histogram of the cerebral vascular network in a 25-week fetus using VOCAL program imaging

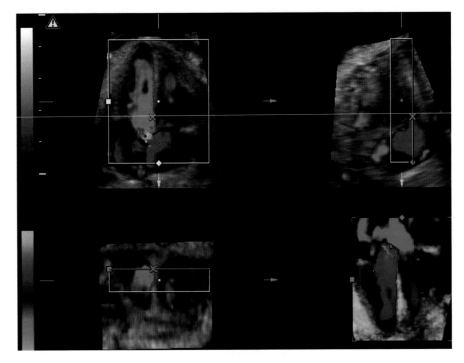

Figure 8.16 Power Doppler angiography of the fetal heart using the STIC modality

automated scanning. The image is then analyzed according to its spatial and temporal characteristics to achieve a 3D dynamic sequence online and a 'surface' reconstruction of the heart.[46]

The advantages of this technique are good resolution in B-mode, with an unlimited number of images, a short examination time, and 3D reconstruction.[46] Visualization of the outflow tracts and its main connections is easily achieved by rotation of the heart around the X- and Y-axes from the four-chamber view as basal image (Figure 8.16).[47,48] The only limitations appear to be the presence of large hearts in term gestations and the low discrimination of the signal in early pregnancy.[49]

Another advantage of this technique is the storage of the volumes and the possibility to send them for

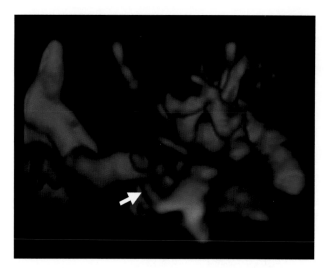

Figure 8.17 3D power Doppler angiography of the hepatic circulation. The arrow indicates the ductus venosus

3D power Doppler is very useful for the visualization of fetal hepatic and portal circulations and for identification of vascular anomalies of the umbilical and portosystemic venous systems (Figure 8.17). These malformations have a prevalence of 2.6%: ductus venosus absence and direct connection between the umbilical and cava veins or the right atrium.[52] Through calculation of 3D Doppler indices, it has been shown that hepatic vascularization and blood flow increase significantly during normal pregnancy.[53]

Even though it is not always easy to depict fetal renal vascularization,[51] it has been demonstrated by means of 3D power Doppler indices that renal vascularization and blood flow increase significantly with gestational age during normal gestations (Figure 8.18).[54]

remote analysis in a looped movie sequence.[46] Thus, the STIC data could be acquired by a general obstetrician, but examined by a fetal echocardiologist, who could confirm the normality of the cardiac structures or rule out major cardiac malformations.[47]

The percentage of 3D power Doppler representations of great vessels has increased considerably from the first publications.[50] Different detection rates have been reported for different vessels: umbilical 100%, abdominal and placental 84%, pulmonary 64%, and renal 51%. Failures in fetal vessel rendering are mainly due to a unfavorable fetal position and fetal movements.[51]

REFERENCES

1. Ritchie CJ, Edwards WS, Mack LA, Cyr DR, Kim Y. Three-dimensional ultrasonic angiography using power-mode Doppler. Ultrasound Med Biol 1996; 22: 277–86.

2. Rubin JM, Bude RO, Carson PL, Bree RL, Adler RS. Power Doppler US: a potentially useful alternative to mean frequency-based color Doppler US. Radiology 1994; 190: 853–6.

3. Maulik D. Sonographic color flow mapping: basic principles. In: Maulik D, ed. Doppler Ultrasound in

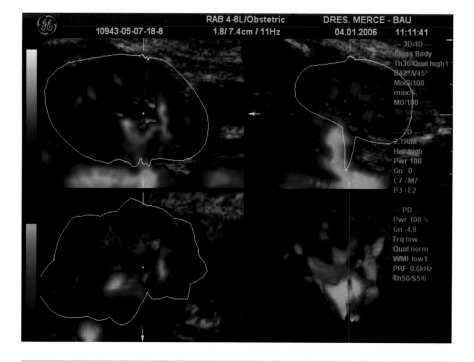

Figure 8.18 3D power Doppler angiography of the renal vessels

Obstetrics and Gynecology. New York: Springer-Verlag, 1997; 68–87.

4. VOCAL (Virtual Organ Computer-aided Analysis). In: VOLUSON 730. Operation Manual. Vienna: Kretztechnik AG, 2001: 10/98–109.

5. Mercé LT, Barco MJ, Alcázar JL, Falcón O. Mediciones con la ecografía tridimensional y el programa VOCAL. Cálculo de volúmenes e índices de la angiografía power Doppler tridimensional. En: Mercé LT, ed. Manual MISUS. Teoría y Práctica de la Ecografía y Angiografía Power Doppler Tridimensional en Obstetricia y Ginecología. Madrid: HABE, 2006; 43–57.

6. Mercé LT. Ultrasound markers of implantation. Ultrasound Rev Obstet Gynecol 2002; 2: 110–23.

7. Chien LW, Au HK, Chen PL, Xiao J, Tzeng CR. Assessment of uterine receptivity by the endometrial-subendometrial blood flow distribution pattern in women undergoing in vitro fertilization–embryo transfer. Fertil Steril 2002; 78: 245–51.

8. Maugey-Laulom B, Commenges-Ducos M, Jullien V, et al. Endometrial vascularity and ongoing pregnancy after IVF. Eur J Obstet Gynecol Reprod Biol 2002; 104: 137–43.

9. Zaidi J, Campbell S, Pittrof R, Tan SL. Endometrial thickness, morphology, vascular penetration and velocimetry in predicting implantation in an in vitro fertilization program. Ultrasound Obstet Gynecol 1995; 6: 191–8.

10. Raine-Fenning NJ, Campbell BK, Clewes JS, Kendall NR, Johnson IR. The reliability of virtual organ computer-aided analysis (VOCAL) for the semiquantification of ovarian, endometrial and subendometrial perfusion. Ultrasound Obstet Gynecol 2003; 22: 633–9.

11. Raine-Fenning NJ, Campbell BK, Clewes JS, Kendall NR, Johnson IR. The interobserver reliability of three-dimensional power Doppler data acquisition within the female pelvis. Ultrasound Obstet Gynecol 2004; 23: 501–8.

12. Raine-Fenning NJ, Campbell BK, Kendall NR, Clewes JS, Johnson IR. Quantifying the changes in endometrial vascularity throughout the normal menstrual cycle with three-dimensional power Doppler angiography. Hum Reprod 2004; 19: 330–8.

13. Kupesic S, Bekavac I, Bjelos D, Kurjak A. Assessment of endometrial receptivity by transvaginal color Doppler and three-dimensional power Doppler ultrasonography in patients undergoing in vitro fertilization procedures. J Ultrasound Med 2001; 20: 125–34.

14. Wu HM, Chiang CH, Huang HY, et al. Detection of the subendometrial vascularization flow index by three-dimensional ultrasound may be useful for predicting the pregnancy rate for patients undergoing in vitro fertilization–embryo transfer. Fertil Steril 2003; 79: 507–11.

15. Ng EH, Chan CC, Tang OS, Yeung WS, Ho PC. Endometrial and subendometrial blood flow measured during early luteal phase by three-dimensional power Doppler ultrasound in excessive ovarian responders. Hum Reprod 2004; 19: 924–31.

16. Järvelä IY, Sladkevicius P, Kelly S, et al. Evaluation of endometrial receptivity during in-vitro fertilization using three-dimensional power Doppler ultrasound. Ultrasound Obstet Gynecol 2005; 26: 765–9.

17. Lédée N. Uterine receptivity and the two and three dimensions of ultrasound. Ultrasound Obstet Gynecol 2005; 26: 695–8.

18. Mercé LT, Barco MJ, de la Fuente F. Doppler velocimetry measured in retrochorionic space and uterine arteries during early human pregnancy. Acta Obstet Gynecol Scand 1989; 8: 603–7.

19. Mercé LT, Barco MJ, Bau S. Color Doppler sonographic assessment of placental circulation in the first trimester of normal pregnancy. J Ultrasound Med 1996; 15: 135–42.

20. Valentin L, Sladkevicius P, Laurini R, Söderberg H, Marsal K. Uteroplacental and luteal circulation in normal first-trimester pregnancies: Doppler ultrasonographic and morphologic study. Am J Obstet Gynecol 1996; 174: 768–75.

21. Kurjak A, Kupesic S. Doppler assessment of the intervillous blood flow in normal and abnormal early pregnancy. Obstet Gynecol 1997; 89: 252–6.

22. Jauniaux E, Jurkovic D, Campbell S, Hustin J. Doppler ultrasonographic features of the developing placental circulation: correlation with anatomic findings. Am J Obstet Gynecol 1992; 166: 585–7.

23. Jaffe R, Woods JR. Color Doppler imaging and in vivo assessment of the anatomy and physiology of the early uteroplacental circulation. Fertil Steril 1993; 60: 293–7.

24. Mercé LT, Barco MJ, Bau S. Color Doppler sonography of the retrochorionic and intervellous circulation: predictive value in small gestational sacs. Med Imag Int 1997; 7: 16–19.

25. Jaffe R, Dorgan A, Abramowicz JS. Color Doppler imaging of the uteroplacental circulation in the first trimester: value in predicting pregnancy failure or complication. Am J Roentgenol 1995; 164: 1255–8.

26. Alcázar JL, Mercé LT, García-Manero M. Two-dimensional and Three-dimensional Doppler assessment of abnormal early intrauterine pregnancy. In: Kurjak A, Chervenak F, eds. Textbook of Perinatal Medicine. London: Informa Healthcare, 2006; 1085–90.

27. Pretorius DH, Nelson TR, Baergen RN, Pai E, Cantrell C. Imaging of placental vasculature using three-dimensional ultrasound and color power Doppler: a preliminary study. Ultrasound Obstet Gynecol 1998; 12: 45–9.

28. Matijevic R, Kurjak A. The assessment of placental blood vessels by three-dimensional power Doppler ultrasound. J Perinat Med 2002; 30: 26–32.

29. Konje JC, Huppertz B, Bell SC, Taylor DJ, Kaufmann P. 3-Dimensional colour power angiography for staging human placental development. Lancet 2003; 362: 1199–201.

30. Mercé LT, Bau S. 'Biopsia vascular placentaria' mediante mapa de amplitud tridimensional: validación de la técnica. Rev Es Ultra Obs Gin 2003; 1: 1–5.

31. Mercé LT, Barco MJ, Bau S. Reproducibility of the study of placental vascularization by three-dimensional power Doppler. J Perinat Med 2004; 32: 228–33.

32. Mu J, Kanzaki T, Tomimatsu T, et al. Investigation of intraplacental villous arteries by Doppler flow imaging in growth-restricted fetuses. Am J Obstet Gynecol 2002; 186: 297–302.

33. Yu CH, Chang CH, Ko HC, Chen WC, Chang FM. Assessment of placental fractional moving blood volume using quantitative three-dimensional power Doppler ultrasound. Ultrasound Med Biol 2003; 29: 19–23.

34. Todros T, Sciarrone A, Piccoli E, et al. Umbilical Doppler waveforms and placental villous angiogenesis in pregnancies complicated by fetal growth restriction. Obstet Gynecol 1999; 93: 499–503.

35. Yagel S, Anteby EY, Shen O, et al. Placental blood flow measured by simultaneous multigate spectral Doppler imaging in pregnancies complicate by placental vascular abnormalities. Ultrasound Obstet Gynecol 1999; 14: 262–6.

36. Shih JC, Ko TL, Lin MC, et al. Quantitative three-dimensional power Doppler ultrasound predicts the outcome of placental chorioangioma. Ultrasound Obstet Gynecol 2004; 24: 202–6.

37. Kurjak A, Kupesic S, Banovic I, Hafner T, Kos M. The study of morphology and circulation of early embryo by three-dimensional ultrasound and power Doppler. J Perinat Med 1999; 27: 145–57.

38. Hanaoka U, Yanagihara T, Tanaka H, Hata T. Comparison of three-dimensional, two-dimensional and color Doppler ultrasound in predicting the presence of a nuchal cord at birth. Ultrasound Obstet Gynecol 2002; 19: 471–4.

39. Sepulveda W, Rojas I, Robert JA, Schnapp C, Alcalde JL. Prenatal detection of velamentous insertion of the umbilical cord: a prospective color Doppler ultrasound study. Ultrasound Obstet Gynecol 2003; 21: 564–9.

40. Oyelese Y, Chavez MR, Yeo L, et al. Three-dimensional sonographic diagnosis of vasa previa. Ultrasound Obstet Gynecol 2004; 24: 211–15.

41. Heling KS, Chaoui R, Bollmann R. Prenatal diagnosis of an aneurysm of the vein of Galen with three-dimen-sional color power angiography. Ultrasound Obstet Gynecol 2000; 15: 333–6.

42. Pooh RK, Pooh K. Transvaginal 3D and Doppler ultra-sonography of the fetal brain. Semin Perinatol 2001; 25: 38–43.

43. Chang CH, Yu CH, Ko HC, Chen CL, Chang FM. Three-dimensional power Doppler ultrasound for the assessment of the fetal brain blood flow in normal gestation. Ultrasound Med Biol 2003; 29: 1273–9.

44. Ruano R, Benachi A, Aubry MC, et al. Perinatal three-dimensional color power Doppler ultrasonography of vein of Galen aneurysms. J Ultrasound Med 2003; 22: 1357–62.

45. Gerards FA, Engels MA, Barkhof F, et al. Prenatal diagnosis of aneurysms of the vein of Galen (vena magna cerebri) with conventional sonography, three-dimen-sional sonography, and magnetic resonance imaging: report of 2 cases. J Ultrasound Med 2003; 22: 1363–8.

46. DeVore GR, Falkensammer P, Sklansky MS, Platt LD. Spatio-temporal image correlation (STIC): new technology for evaluation of the fetal heart. Ultrasound Obstet Gynecol 2003; 22: 380–7.

47. Vinals F, Poblete P, Giuliano A. Spatio-temporal image correlation (STIC): a new tool for the prenatal screen-ing of congenital heart defects. Ultrasound Obstet Gynecol 2003; 22: 388–94.

48. DeVore GR, Polanco B, Sklansky MS, Platt LD. The 'spin' technique: a new method for examination of the fetal outflow tracts using three-dimensional ultrasound. Ultrasound Obstet Gynecol 2004; 24: 72–82.

49. Chaoui R, Hoffmann J, Heling KS. Three-dimensional (3D) and 4D color Doppler fetal echocardiography using spatio-temporal image correlation (STIC). Ultrasound Obstet Gynecol 2004; 23: 535–45.

50. Chaoui R, Kalache KD, Hartung J. Application of three-dimensional power Doppler ultrasound in prena-tal diagnosis. Ultrasound Obstet Gynecol 2001; 17: 22–9.

51. Hartung J, Kalache KD, Chaoui R. Three-dimensional power Doppler ultrasonography (3D-PDU) in fetal diagnosis. Ultraschall Med 2004; 25: 200–5.

52. Kalache K, Romero R, Goncalves LF, et al. Three-dimensional color power imaging of the fetal hepatic circulation. Am J Obstet Gynecol 2003; 189: 1401–6.

53. Chang CH, Yu CH, Ko HC, Chang FM, Chen HY. Assessment of normal fetal liver blood flow using quantitative three-dimensional power Doppler ultra-sound. Ultrasound Med Biol 2003; 29: 943–9.

54. Chang CH, Yu CH, Ko HC, Chen WC, Chang FM. Quantitative three-dimensional power Doppler sonog-raphy for assessment of the fetal renal blood flow in normal gestation. Ultrasound Med Biol 2003; 29: 929–33.

9 3D power Doppler in the diagnosis and assessment of gestational trophoblastic disease

Kazuo Maeda, Asim Kurjak, and Gino Varga

INTRODUCTION

There have been significant improvements in the diagnosis and assessment of gestational trophoblastic diseases following the introduction of 3D power Doppler. We will review this here in some detail.

CLASSIFICATION, DEVELOPMENT, AND PATHOLOGY OF TROPHOBLASTIC DISEASE

Trophoblastic diseases are classified as hydatidiform moles and choriocarcinomas on the basis of pathologic findings.[1] The distinction is important, not least because of the clear differences in outcome between these conditions. There is also a clinical classification due to the US National Cancer Institute/National Institutes for Health (NCI/NIH), as well as a staging system due to the International Federation of Gynecology and Obstetrics (Fédération Internationale de Gynécologie et d'Obstétrique, FIGO).

Complete hydatidiform mole

This is an abnormal pregnancy, with placental villi changing into molar vesicles, with no embryo, fetus, placenta or umbilical cord (Figure 9.1). An amnion is, however, found in some complete mole cases.[2] No capillary vessels are found in molar vesicles covered by proliferated trophoblasts. An intravascular mole occurs when the vesicles spread into blood vessels. Metastases to distant organs are rare. The karyotype is usually diploid, 46,XX, with the XX both of male

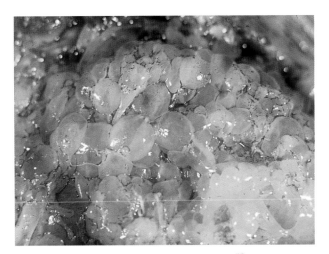

Figure 9.1 The whole uterine cavity is occupied by the vesicles of a complete hydatidiform mole in this case. The patient chose to have a hysterectomy because she was afraid of postmolar choriocarcinoma

origin. A vacant ovum without nucleus is fertilized by a sperm of haploid 23,X then the haploid duplicates in the developmental mechanism (androgenesis).[3,4] Rarely, it is 46,XY, with X and Y being of male origin.[5] A complete hydatidiform mole may also develop in one of twins or triplets. The risk of a repeated mole is less than 1%, and it is not an indication for chemotherapy.[6] Genetic character of the mole is related possibly with the recurrent mole and the progress to choriocarcinoma.[7] Ovarian theca lutein cysts are frequent in developed complete and invasive moles (Figure 9.2). The incidence is low in the 1st trimester.[8] Since a lutein cyst is not a trophoblastic disease and disappears after the remission, surgical removal is not appropriate.

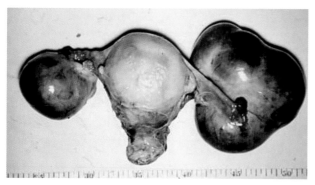

Figure 9.2 Ovarian theca lutein cysts associated with an invasive mole. The cysts were removed at the same time as the hysterectomy in 1960 when the benign nature of the lutein cyst was unknown

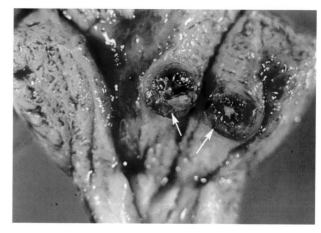

Figure 9.4 Invasive mole found in a hysterectomy specimen (arrows)

Partial hydatidiform mole

This is the partial change of placental villi into molar vesicles, and is associated with the embryo, fetus or fetal parts (Figure 9.3). Fetal anomalies are common.

Chromosomes are usually triploids, including 69,XXX, 69,XXY, or 69,XYY.[9] DNA analysis confirmed the androgenetic mechanism.[10] Capillary vessels are found in the interstitium of molar vesicles.

Invasive hydatidiform mole

This is invasion of molar vesicles into the myometrium, accompanied by its destruction and hemorrhage. The lesion is found in either complete or partial mole, usually after molar evacuation, although the invasion may develop before termination. The change is noted visually and microscopically in surgical specimens (Figure 9.4) where proliferate trophoblasts hemorrhage and necrose in the myometrium (Figure 9.5). Invasive moles rarely metastasize and have low malignant potential; for example, in one case, a pulmonary focus spontaneously disappeared after hysterectomy for an invasive mole. The outcome is more favorable than that of choriocarcinoma.

Choriocarcinoma

This is a solid trophoblastic tumor that develops primarily in the myometrium (Figure 9.6), or in distant organs and tissues,[11-16] usually after the removal of a complete mole and rarely after the partial mole, and further infrequently after abortion and

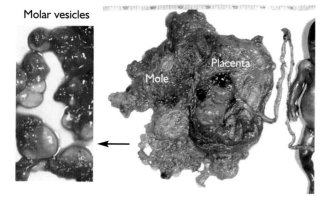

Figure 9.3 Partial hydatidiform mole. An anomalous fetus is shown at the right, a partial change of the placenta into molar tissue in the middle, and enlarged molar vesicles on the left

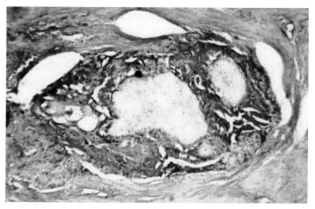

Figure 9.5 Low-power microscopic view of the villous pattern of an invasive mole

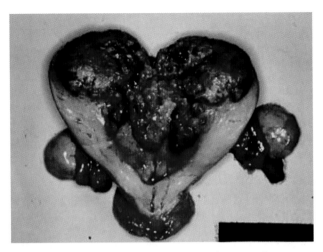

Figure 9.6 Uterine choriocarcinoma. In this case, the patient underwent hysterectomy – this was in the period before the introduction of effective chemotherapy

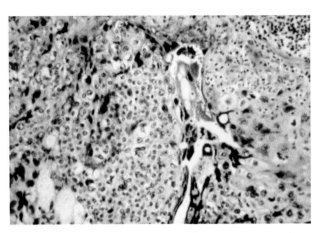

Figure 9.7 Microscopic view of a choriocarcinoma. Note the proliferation of trophoblastic cells and the absence of a villuos pattern where most of the tumor was occupied by the cytotrophoblasts

normal delivery. Choriocarcinomas can be gestational choriocarcinomas or trophoblastic disease (GTD). Non-gestational choriocarcinoma develops from germ cells or other cancer cells in children.[11] Primary choriocarcinomas have been reported in reproductive as well as in non-reproductive organs, including vulva,[12] uterine cervix,[13] lung, stomach and pancreas,[14,15] gallbladder,[16] and urinary bladder.[17] Uterine cervical choriocarcinoma was also experienced.[18]

Choriocarcinoma is divided into three subtypes:

- *Gestational choriocarcinoma* is related to pregnancy, and three categories are further classified:
  - *Uterine choriocarcinoma* is the most common, developing in the uterus after a hydatidiform mole, and rarely after abortion or normal delivery. A choriocarcinoma with an intact pregnancy has been reported.[19]
  - *Extrauterine choriocarcinoma* develops primarily in the location of an ectopic pregnancy, without a choriocarcinoma in the uterus.
  - *Intraplacental choriocarcinoma* is found in the placenta mainly after delivery. Cases have been reported to be associated with viable pregnancy.[20]
- *Non-gestational choriocarcinoma* is divided into two categories:
  - *Choriocarcinoma of germ cell origin* is a subtype of germ cell tumor developing in the ovary of a nulligravid young woman or the testis of an adult male. These tumors are more resistant to chemotherapy than the gestational type.

  - *Choriocarcinoma derived from other carcinoma* is a choriocarcinomatous change of another cancer that can secrete human chorionic gonadotropin (hCG).
- *Unclassified choriocarcinoma* is a choriocarcinoma that cannot be classified as either gestational or non-gestational.

A choriocarcinoma is composed of syncytiotrophoblasts and cytotrophoblasts, and shows no villous pattern at all (Figure 9.7). Since a villous pattern is a characteristic sign of an invasive mole, the outcome of which is less malignant than that of a choriocarcinoma, microscopic studies should be performed on the whole specimen if the uterus is removed.

Widespread distant metastases of choriocarcinoma were common before the introduction of effective chemotherapy. The interval between diagnosis and metastasis was about 6 months to 1 year. Early metastases were dark red tumors on the external genitalia and vaginal wall (Figure 9.8). Subsequent spread was frequently on the lung, where typical foci showed a round shape of various sizes (Figure 9.9A), while a diffuse pulmonary shadow was found in multiple trophoblast emboli in the pulmonary arterioles (Figure 9.9B). Any organs or tissues could be affected after pulmonary metastasis, including the skin,[21] subcutaneous tissue, intestine, liver (Figure 9.10), spleen, kidney, heart,[22,23] and finally the brain (Figure 9.11). Tumor cells were also found in blood vessels (Figure 9.12). Every organ could be damaged by the trophoblasts and hemorrhage. Before the introduction of effective chemotherapy, patients died from the

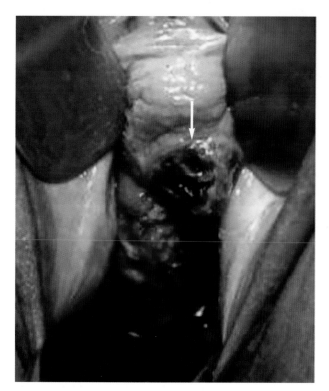

Figure 9.8 Vaginal wall metastasis of choriocarcinoma. Note the dark red tumor (arrow)

brain metastasis and multiple metastases due to the damage and dysfunction of organs.

Placental-site trophoblastic tumor

Placental-site trophoblastic tumor (PSTT) is a rare uterine tumor of proliferative intermediate trophoblasts.[24] The tumor is preceded by hydatidiform mole, abortion, or delivery. The hCG is low and the human placental lactogen (HPL) is higher than β-hCG.[2] Final diagnosis is made by histologic study. Metastasis and recurrence are common.[24–27] PSTT is highly malignant, and can be fatal.[2] A case of PSTT has been reported in a mother and child.[28]

Persistent trophoblastic disease

Persistent trophoblastic disease (PTD) is a postmolar metastatic mole, invasive mole, or choriocarcinoma, where no specimen has been obtained or the pathologic finding is unknown.

- *Postmolar persistent hCG* shows an abnormal type II hCG regression pattern after a hydatidiform

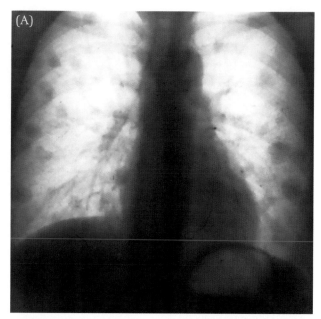

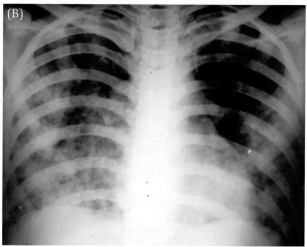

Figure 9.9 (A) Typical pulmonary metastases of a choriocarcinoma which are round 'snowball' type. (B) Diffuse metastatic foci which were pathologically multiple emboli of choriocarcinoma in pulmonary arterioles. Dyspnea was the presenting symptom

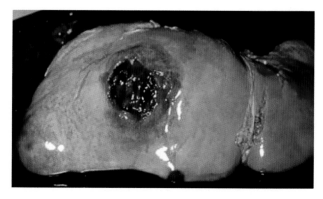

Figure 9.10 Choriocarcinoma metastasis on the right lobe of the liver

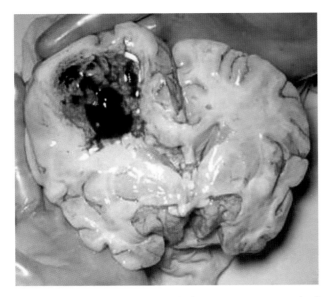

Figure 9.11 Brain metastasis of choriocarcinoma, cerebral hemorrhage and brain edema

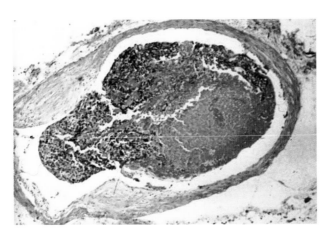

Figure 9.12 Grouped choriocarcinoma cells in the coronary artery found at autopsy. The metastatic foci demonstrated in Figures 9.9(B)–9.12 were postmortem autopsy findings before introduction of effective chemotherapy

mole; i.e., urinary hCG is higher than 1000 mIU/ml after 5 weeks, serum hCG is higher than 100 mIU/ml after 8 weeks, or serum β-hCG is higher than 1.0 mIU/ml β-human chorionic gonadotropin with carboxy-terminal peptide (β-hCG-carbonyl-terminal peptide (CTP) 0.5 mIU/ml) after 20 weeks, where the focus is unknown.

- *A clinical invasive mole or metastatic mole* is estimated by the modified Ishizuka scoring system, or by the suspected focus.
- *Clinical choriocarcinoma* is estimated from the Ishizuka scoring system, the suspected focus, or

the postmolar state, where hCG is elevated again after complete remission confirmed by hCG lower than the cut-off, except for a new pregnancy.

SYMPTOMS OF GESTATIONAL TROPHOBLASTIC DISEASE

Hydatidiform mole

Typical symptoms of well-developed complete hydatidiform mole are hyperemesis, hypertension, no fetal movement, no fetal heartbeat on Doppler, larger uterus than in a normal pregnancy, abdominal pain, hemorrhage after amenorrhea, expelled molar vesicles, and usually urinary hCG higher than 100 000 mIU/ml. These typical symptoms are infrequent at the time of sonographic screening in the 1st trimester of pregnancy, particularly with transvaginal scans, where an early-stage hydatidiform mole can be detected and evacuated before its development. Ovarian theca lutein cysts can also be detected by ultrasound.

Partial hydatidiform mole

The symptoms of a mole associated with a living fetus are similar to those of a normal pregnancy except for hyperemesis, an enlarged uterus, and a high hCG titer. Sonographic screening during pregnancy detects partial molar changes of the placenta, with an embryo, fetus, or fetal particles being present. Twenty percent of complete moles are followed by sequelae, and choriocarcinoma develops in 2% of cases after a complete mole, whereas partial moles show sequelae in only 5% of cases, and rarely progress to choriocarcinoma.[2]

Invasive mole

This is found after a mole, and exhibits vaginal bleeding, enlarged uterus, bilaterally enlarged ovaries, and high urinary or serum hCG. The symptoms resemble those of a choriocarcinoma, and a differential diagnosis is required. The interval from an antecedent molar pregnancy is usually less than 6 months, which is shorter than with a choriocarcinoma. Urinary hCG is continuously elevated after molar curettage, but the titer is lower than with choriocarcinoma. Sonography

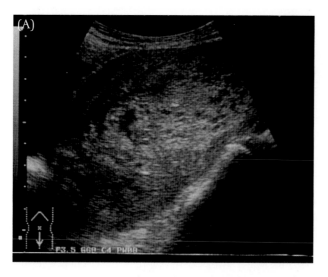
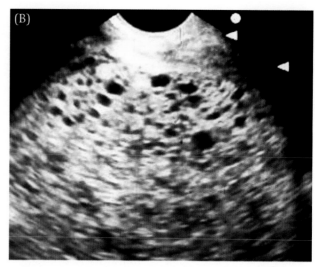

Figure 9.13 (A) Typical complete hydatidiform mole at 11 weeks of gestation (courtesy of Dr M Utsu). (B) Established complete mole (courtesy of Professor S Kupesic)

discloses the presence of molar vesicles in the myometrial mass (see the section below on diagnosis).

Choriocarcinoma

Gestational choriocarcinoma is usually preceded by a molar pregnancy, and rarely by abortion or term delivery. The interval from an antecedent pregnancy can be longer than 1 year – longer than in the case of an invasive mole. There may be a period of partial remission, which can be more than 10 years in the case of extrauterine choriocarcinoma. The symptoms are vaginal bleeding, an enlarged uterus, a high hCG titer, ovarian masses, and irregular basal body temperature (BBT). Choriocarcinoma is strongly suggested by the presence of metastasis. Multiple pulmonary foci indicate progression of malignancy. The hCG titer should be checked even in non-gynecological cases when pulmonary round foci are found in a female patient. Symptoms due to distant metastases suggest choriocarcinoma: for example, abdominal pain and hemorrhage in hepatic lesions, or persistent headache and vomiting followed by unconsciousness and apnea in the case of brain metastases.

PSTT

This is preceded by any gestational process. An enlarged uterus and vaginal bleeding are the clinical symptoms. Metastasis is frequent. The disease often recurs after treatment. PSTT is malignant and can be fatal.[2]

PTD

This includes postmolar hCG persistence, a clinically invasive or metastatic mole, and choriocarcinoma. Although the focus is unknown, all three show persistence of an abnormally high hCG titer.

DIAGNOSIS OF GESTATIONAL TROPHOBLASTIC DISEASE

Complete hydatidiform mole

This is diagnosed by its symptoms, high urinary and serum hCG titer, and particularly by B-mode sonography, color Doppler, and Doppler flowmetry. A transvaginal scan is useful in the first trimester. B-mode sonography detects molar vesicles in the uterine cavity without detecting the fetus or embryo or its particles (Figure 9.13). The amniotic membrane and fluid are, however, occasionally detected by B-mode.

Characteristic changes are found in complete hydatidiform moles by various ultrasonic imaging techniques.

Real-time B-mode

Complete hydatidiform moles are detected in early stages by screening in the 1st trimester. An empty gestational sac, with a wall showing cystic change without an embryo, can be detected sonographically before the typical growth of a complete hydatidiform mole (Figure 9.14). An early complete mole resembles

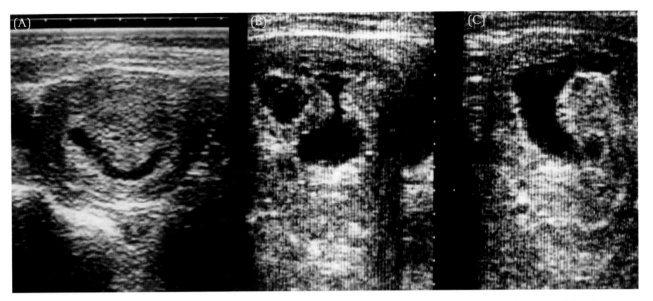

Figure 9.14 (A–C) Real-time B-mode sonograms of three complete hydatidiform moles in the early stage of development. There is no embryo or fetus, the chorionic plate includes only small cysts in the GS wall in their earliest stage, and it is similar to a blighted ovum. The chorionic membrane increases in thickness and clear cysts appear within 1–2 weeks, and an early complete mole is diagnosed

a blighted ovum, although the vomiting and high urinary hCG titer in the case of a mole distinguish it from a blighted ovum. The chorionic plate thickness increases, and typical molar cysts develop within 1–2 weeks in early pregnancy. The characteristic molar pattern is composed of multiple small cysts, but not a snowstorm pattern, on sonographic examination with modern B-mode devices (Figure 9.13). A complete hydatidiform mole can develop in one of a set of twins or triplets. It is diagnosed sonographically by molar tissue separated by a septum originating from the fetus (Figure 9.15). A partial mole in a singleton pregnancy

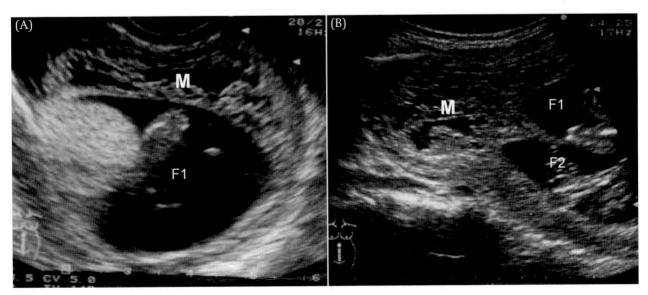

Figure 9.15 Complete moles developing in multiple pregnancies. (A) One twin has changed into a complete hydatidiform mole. F, fetus; M, mole. (B) One triplet has changed into a complete hydatidiform mole. F1, F2, two triplet fetuses; M, mole. Sonographic diagnosis of a complete mole in a twin or triplet is made by the presence of clear septum between the normal fetuses and complete mole. Genetic analysis of the specimens contributes the differentiation, if the diagnosis is difficult. (Courtesy of Dr M Utsu of Seirei Mikatahara Hospital)

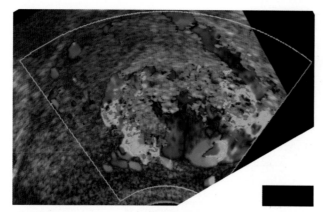

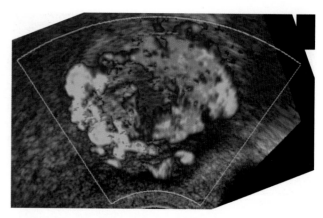

Figure 9.16 Color flow mapping of a complete hydatidiform mole. The full color shows rich blood flow in the uterus which was completely different from the flow of the placenta and that of the fetus. The color flow signals filling whole uterus to show the rich blood flow. Therefore, the color Doppler flow mapping can be a new diagnostic technique of a complete hydatidiform mole

Figure 9.17 2D power Doppler flow image of a complete hydatidiform mole. Small molar vesicles can be seen in the power flow image. The proof of molar vesicles by the color/power Doppler is another new mole diagnosis in the case of difficult imaging of the molar vesicle by the real-time B-mode

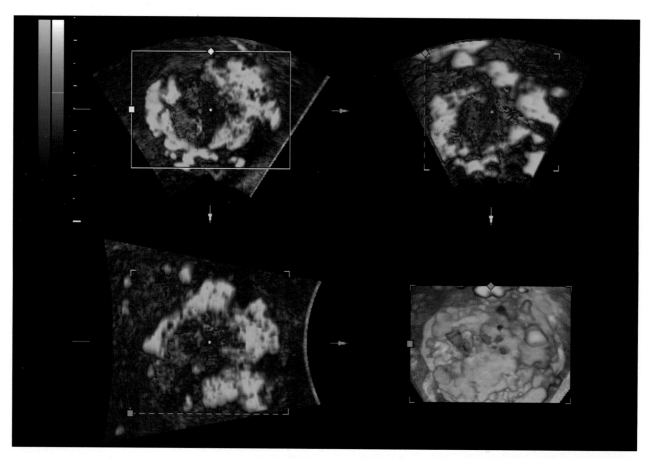

Figure 9.18 Three multiplanes and surface imaging of 3D power Doppler of a complete hydatidiform mole. A rich blood flow fills uterine cavity and conceals molar vesicle

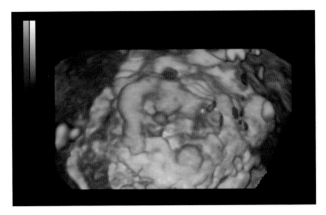

Figure 9.19 3D power Doppler flow image of a complete hydatidiform mole suggesting the existence of rich blood streams of various flow directions in the uterus

can be differentiated from a complete mole in a multiple pregnancy by the partial molar change of the placental villi without the presence of a separating septum, or by the presence of a triploid chromosome.

Color Doppler flow mapping

Complete hydatidiform moles can be studied with two-dimensional (2D) color Doppler, power Doppler, pulsed Doppler flow wave with flow impedance, and 3D power Doppler flow mapping. Color Doppler flow mapping discloses filling of the uterine cavity with color flow signals with various directions in the space between molar vesicles (Figure 9.16).

2D and 3D power Doppler flow images

2D power Doppler of a complete mole discloses molar vesicles in the rich blood flow (Figure 9.17). The three sections of 3D power Doppler images also show rich blood flow (Figure 9.18), and the imaging surface of 3D power Doppler displays blood streams covering the molar vesicles (Figure 9.19). Since the maternal blood flow is not the same in a complete mole as in a normal cotyledon, the blood flow between the vesicles of a complete hydatidiform mole is interesting. The blood stream ejected into the uterine cavity by arterial aperture may flow through the molar vesicles and return to the myometrial vein, because various blood flow directions are shown in 2D color Doppler, and 3D power Doppler also shows intrauterine blood stream lines.

Pulsed Doppler flow wave and flow impedance

Diastolic flow is larger and resistance index (RI) is lower in the uterine, arcuate, radial, and spiral arteries in a mole than in a normal pregnancy.[29] Also, RI is low in the molar flow.[30] In the intervesicular space of a complete mole, the peak systolic velocity of maternal arterial blood can be as low as 14 cm/s and the RI as low as 0.42 (Figure 9.20). Theoretically, fetal blood flow cannot be recorded, since there is no fetal capillary in the complete molar vesicle.

A complete mole can be recognized by the morphologic and functional characteristics detected

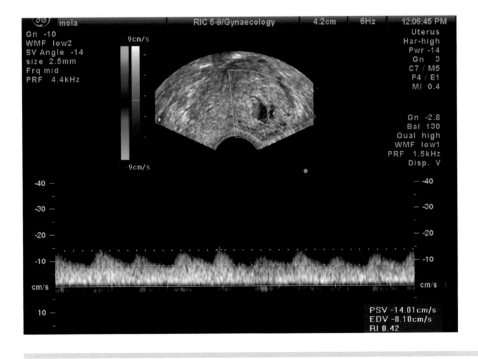

Figure 9.20 The diastolic flow recorded by pulsed Doppler flow velocity wave of a complete mole in the uterus is rich. The peak systolic velocity is 14 cm/s, the resistance index is as low as 0.42 and the heart rate is almost 80 bpm in the maternal arterial blood flow in the inter-molar space

by ultrasound techniques. Further progress is expected in elucidating the flow characteristics of hydatidiform moles by 3D and possibly 4D sonography.

hCG and other diagnostic methods

A complete hydatidiform mole should be suspected when urinary or serum hCG is higher than 100 000 mIU/ml, which is the upper normal limit in early pregnancy. A complete mole cannot, however, be ruled out even if the hCG level is lower. After complete removal of a mole by repeated curettages, the postmolar state is monitored every 1–2 weeks by hCG, sonography, and local condition until the hCG reaches the lower cut-off level. In the case of abnormal regression of hCG or persistent trophoblastic disease chemotherapy should be given for the prophylaxis of choriocarcinoma. Chromosomal diploidy and DNA analysis indicate an androgenic origin.

Partial hydatidiform mole

This is diagnosed by symptoms, high urinary hCG, and sonographic findings in the presence of a fetus, or a partial image of the fetus and partial changes of the placenta into molar vesicles. 3D sonography allows diagnosis of a partial mole in early pregnancy (Figure 9.21). Anomalies are frequent in the fetus. Chromosome of most partial mole is triploidy; complete and partial moles can be differentiated by

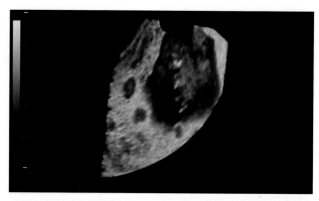

Figure 9.21 3D image of a partial hydatidiform mole in early pregnancy reveals a small fetus with extremities and molar vesicles in the placenta (courtesy of Dr JR Benitez, Clinica Gutenenberg, Spain)

molecular genetic studies in case of difficult diagnosis. Postmolar changes of urinary and serum hCG are the same as those of a complete hydatidiform mole. Chemotherapy in the case of abnormal regression and persistent trophoblastic disease is also the same as for a complete hydatidiform mole.

Invasive hydatidiform mole

This is mainly found within 6 months of termination of a complete or partial molar pregnancy, although the molar tissue can invade the myometrium during pregnancy. Myometrial invasion may be detected by

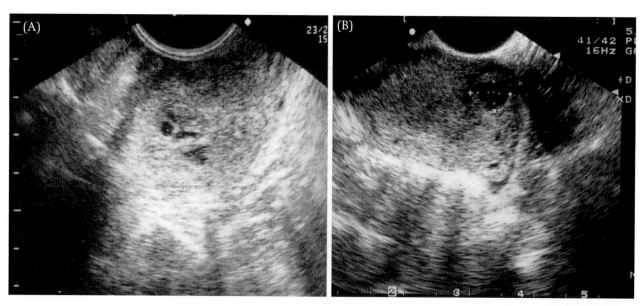

Figure 9.22 (A) Cystic vesicle of an invasive mole recorded by real-time B-mode sonography. (B) The focus size of the villus cyst was 1.23 cm × 0.88 cm in this invasive mole (courtesy of Dr S Yoshida, Tottori University)

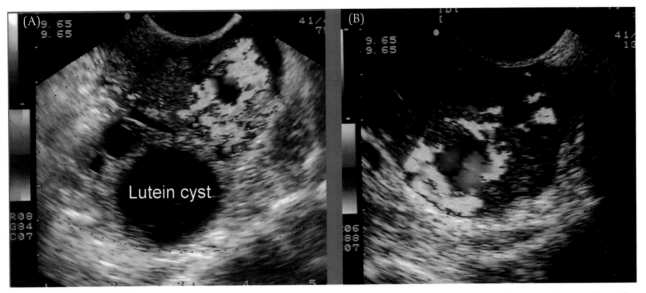

Figure 9.23 (A) Color Doppler image showing rich blood flow and a villous cyst in an invasive mole. (B) Change where the focus was barely detectible by color Doppler after two courses of methotrexate (courtesy of Dr S Yoshida)

detailed study with B-mode and color flow or power Doppler flow mapping on the uterine wall before termination.

The symptoms of an invasive mole resemble those of choriocarcinoma, i.e., postmolar development, vaginal bleeding, an enlarged uterus, and possible metastasis. Urinary or serum hCG are positive, but the level is lower than in the case of choriocarcinoma. B-mode sonography shows a uterine mass. The presence of an invasive mole is clear if molar vesicles are imaged in the tumor (Figure 9.22). Rich blood flow is found on color flow mapping (Figures 9.23 and 9.24) and power Doppler imaging. Flow impedance is low in invasive moles. On the contrary, flow impedance is high in the wall artery of a theca lutein cyst.

Gestational choriocarcinoma

This develops after a hydatidiform mole, abortion, or normal delivery. The clinical symptoms are vaginal bleeding, enlarged uterus, ovarian masses, high hCG titer, and it is similar to an invasive mole when it is at an early stage before metastasis. It develops usually more than 6 months after the mole; this is longer than the interval for an invasive mole, which is usually less than 6 months. Metastases are found in external genitalia, the vaginal wall in the early stage (Figure 9.8), and then in the lung (Figure 9.9). Invasive moles also, but rarely, metastasize.

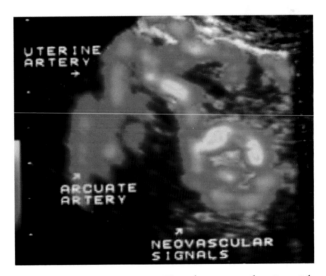

Figure 9.24 Intense power Doppler image showing rich blood flow in an invasive mole (courtesy of Professor S Kupesic)

Differential diagnosis between a choriocarcinoma and an invasive mole is important, because the outcome is ominous in the former and less risky in the latter, in spite of the similarity of the clinical symptoms. Sonographic detection of villous pattern in the focus (Figures 9.22–9.24) is decisive evidence of an invasive mole, while a cystic villous pattern is not detected in choriocarcinoma (Figure 9.25). Color Doppler flow mapping shows rich blood flow (Figure 9.26). Flow impedance is usually low in both diseases, but it is lower in choriocarcinomas than in invasive

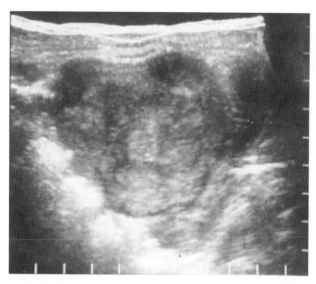

Figure 9.25 Abdominal scan of a choriocarcinoma recorded by B-mode sonography. No molar vesicle is found in the intrauterine tumor (courtesy of Dr Terahara, Imakyurei Hospital)

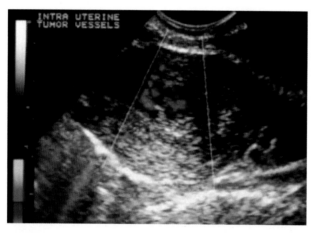

Figure 9.26 Uterine choriocarcinoma with moderate color flow pattern. The RI was as low as 0.3 by the pulsed Doppler flow velocity (courtesy of Dr S Kondo, Saitama University)

moles. The RI of the uterine artery is significantly lower in choriocarcinomas than in hydatidiform moles.[31] A differential gene expression pattern is reported between normal trophoblast and choriocarcinoma cells.[32] Although the risk is given by the FIGO staging, the NIC/NIH classification, and the Ishizuka and World Health Organization (WHO) scoring tables, it is important to examine trophoblastic disease with objective imaging techniques, particularly with various sonographic methods. Pelvic angiography has been used in the past, but sonography is now considered a better approach.

Non-gestational choriocarcinoma

Non-gestational choriocarcinoma of germ cell origin develops in the ovary or testis without gestation having occurred. Urinary and serum hCG are positive; palpation and sonography reveal the tumor. DNA polymorphism analysis has been reported in pure non-gestational choriocarcinoma.[33] *Cancer metamorphosed to choriocarcinoma* is diagnosed by its own symptoms and findings associated with hCG secretion.

PTD

Since PTD patients receive chemotherapy that may lead to complete remission without surgical removal of the foci, no histologic diagnosis is made and the clinical diagnosis is final in the case of complete remission.

PSTT

The long interval after the antecedent gestation, symptoms including vaginal bleeding and an enlarged uterus, and the lack of a high hCG titer suggest the presence of this disease. Differential diagnosis from other malignant trophoblastic disease is required. Also, due to its rarity, the diagnosis is sometimes incorrect. The final diagnosis is made by histology of removed specimens. Other than the usual examinations and B-mode sonography, color Doppler documents a marked uterine vascularity that is characterized by low resistance to flow, persistence after the chemotherapy, and negative plasma β-hCG. Serial transvaginal color Doppler is useful in monitoring chemotherapy and residual tumor.[34]

THERAPY

Hydatidiform moles

Complete hydatidiform mole

This is treated primarily by curettage, where a well-developed massive total mole should be carefully treated; i.e., the cervix is slowly dilated and uterine contraction is induced by prostaglandin before expulsion and curettage, in order to prevent excessive hemorrhage and uterine damage. Evacuation of a sonographically diagnosed early-stage mole is easier than dealing with the developed mole in a later stage. Curettage is repeated for complete evacuation.

Sonographic monitoring of the intrauterine maneuvers is useful for successful curettage and prevention of uterine damage. No surgery is performed unless the disease is refractory to chemotherapy or massive hemorrhage.

Partial hydatidiform mole

Labor is induced by prostaglandin and followed by curettage, to expel the fetus and remove the mole.

Postmolar monitoring

This is indispensable for the detection of any sequelae and prevention of malignant trophoblastic disease. After sonographically confirmed complete evacuation of the uterus, the local state, transvaginal sonography, and urinary or serum hCG are studied every 1–2 weeks until hCG decreases to the normal cut-off level, then every 1–2 months for a year.[2] X-ray images should be examined if there is any concern regarding pulmonary change. Contraception is not essential for as long a period as in the past, because a new pregnancy can easily be diagnosed by ultrasound. Clinical care, however, is necssary for 3 years, because 85% of choriocarcinomas develop, 3 years after a mole.

Regression is classified as being of type I when the postmolar hCG regression pattern is normal, with urinary hCG decreasing to 1000 mIU/ml or less after 5 weeks, serum hCG to 100 mIU/ml or less after 8 weeks, and serum hCG is 1 mIU/ml or less with the β-hCG system and 0.5 mIU/ml or less with the β-hCG–CTP system after 20 weeks. Type II regression is abnormal regression, where the hCG level is higher than in type I regression. Type II or hCG re-elevation after transient remission should be treated by chemotherapy[35] to prevent the development of choriocarcinoma; the use of methotrexate is common. Prophylactic chemotherapy was tried in our controlled study,[36] where significantly less choriocarcinoma (actually zero) developed in the study group than in the control group.

Choriocarcinoma

This is treated by primary chemotherapy. Hysterectomy was formerly a common treatment, but was frequently followed by metastases. Local radiotherapy was also employed. Methotrexate was the first primary chemotherapy, in the 1960s. This was systemic chemotherapy, because choriocarcinoma was recognized as a systemic disease. Results were further improved with the use of combined chemotherapy: EMA (etoposide, methotrexate, and dactinomycin (actinomycin-D)),[37] or in further combination with CO (cyclophosphamide and vincristine), forming the EMA/CO regimen.[38,39] The most intensive therapy may be salvage chemotherapy including etoposide or cisplatin.[40] Chemotherapy-resistant metastasis or recurrence is treated with surgery (e.g. pulmonary lobectomy or craniotomy[41]), and the uterus is removed in the case of severe vaginal bleeding. Combination of hysterectomy[42] or endoscopic surgery[43] with chemotherapy has resulted in favorable remission rates.

The serum hCG level should be lower than the cut-off level for complete remission (defined as disappearance of primary and metastatic foci). Since there is cross-sensitivity of hCG antibody to pituitary luteinizing hormone (LH), a β-hCG or β-hCG–CTP antibody that is more specific for hCG is in common use in trophoblastic diseases, particularly for low levels of hCG. Recent studies have reported, however, the presence of false-positive tests with some hCG antibodies including β-hCG and β-hCG–CTP.[44,45] These reports have suggested the use of repeated tests, urine tests instead of serum tests, serial serum dilution tests, or removal of interfering substances, if there is any discrepancy among clinical conditions and test results.

Systemic side-effects of intensive chemotherapy include stomatitis, skin eruption, alopecia, fever, reduced granulocyte count, bone marrow damage, hepatic lesions, and gastrointestinal tract damage. The most life-threatening of these is the bone marrow damage and consequent leukopenia in the peripheral blood. Mild leukopenia is curable by steroids, while severe damage must be treated by bone marrow transplantation and stem cell support.[42]

Intra-arterial infusion chemotherapy has been tried in liver metastases, which decreased on treatment.[46] Internal iliac arterial MTX infusion was tried in the chemotherapy of uterine cervical choriocarcinoma; this was followed by tumor regression and necrotic change.[18]

Pregnancy outcome after complete remission obtained by intensive chemotherapy was favorable and the treatment showed minimal impact.[47] With regard to further long-term effects of chemotherapy, menopause was earlier by 3 years than in control women.[48]

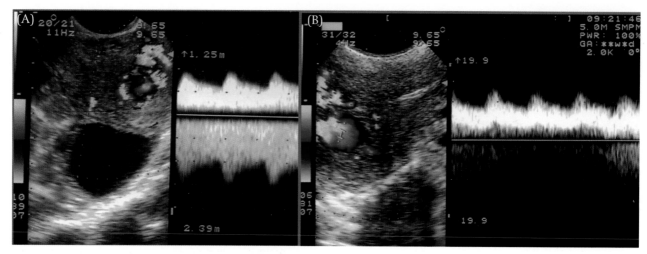

Figure 9.27 Color Doppler images and pulsed Doppler flow waves in an invasive mole. (A) Before chemotherapy. (B) After two courses of methotrexate. RI was 0.23 before chemotherapy and 0.36 after the two courses (courtesy of Dr S Yoshida)

The role of sonography in the chemotherapy of choriocarcinoma

Tumor size and blood flow are effectively monitored in chemotherapy by various sonographic techniques. When chemotherapy is effective, the ultrasound image of a primary or metastatic tumor decreases in size and the tumoral blood flow appears reduced on color or power flow imaging. Early estimation of tumor sensitivity to systemic chemotherapy is necessary.

Pulsed Doppler for the early detection of sensitivity to chemotherapy

Impedance to flow in the tumor, as reflected by RI and pulsatility index (PI), is clearly elevated immediately after initiation of the first course in chemotherapy, when the choriocarcinoma is sensitive to chemotherapy before later reductions in hCG and the size of color Doppler flow image.[49] These changes in flow indices may be caused by tumor shrinkage. In contrast, chemotherapy-resistant invasive moles show no changes in RI and PI[49] or only mild increases in RI at the end of systemic chemotherapy (Figure 9.27). Tumor blood flow impedance can be an indicator of tumor sensitivity in the early period of chemotherapy.

Non-gestational choriocarcinoma

Choriocarcinoma of germ cell origin is usually treated by resection followed by adjuvant chemotherapy. Metastases are removed surgically, with subsequent chemotherapy. Resistant cases receive multiple adjuvant therapy, usually EMA/CO chemotherapy. Cancers metamorphosed to choriocarcinoma may receive their own therapy and chemotherapy.

PTD

Postmolar hCG persistence is treated with prophylactic chemotherapy (usually methotrexate). The treatment is repeated until the hCG reaches a normal level. Choriocarcinoma is treated as described above. Iinvasive moles are treated with chemotherapy, and hysterectomy when refractory.

Invasive mole

This is treated by systemic chemotherapy, although it tends to be refractory. Invasive moles are more highly differentiated than choriocarcinomas, and higher local doses may be needed than for the latter. Tumor resection, laser ablation, or focused hyperthermia induced by ultrasound may be used as local therapy preceding hysterectomy.

PSTT

This has been treated by hysterectomy when limited to the uterus, with chemotherapy being used in the case of spread outside the uterus, although the clinical outcome is poor when preceding pregnancy is more than 2 years before advent of the tumor.[50] Janni et al[51] recommended a cytostatic-surgical approach for metastatic PSTT. Tsuji et al[52] have reported that resection of the tumor and EMA/CO chemotherapy can achieve long-term remission and save the fertility of young patients. Other workers[53–57] have also obtained favorable results, mainly with EMA/CO chemotherapy and further use of etoposide–cisplatin.[57]

The outcome of patients with FIGO stage I–II disease has been excellent after hysterectomy, but stage III–IV patients have a survival rate of only 30%.[55]

Other reported treatment

Watanabe et al[58] have reported the treatment of choriocarcinoma in the pulmorary artery with emergency pulmorary embolectomy under cardiopulmonary bypass. Kohyama et al[59] have reported stereotactic radiotherapy of choriocarcinoma in the cranium, followed by conventional craniospinal irradiation. Bohlmann et al[22] reported intracardiac resection of a metastatic choriocarcinoma. Brain metastasis is usually treated with intensive chemotherapy.[60] We have also used intensive methotrexate chemotherapy in a case of brain metastasis, who has survived for more than 20 years.

REFERENCES

1. Japan Society of Obstetrics and Gynecology and Japanese Pathological Society. The General Rules for Clinical and Pathological Management of Trophoblastic Diseases, 2nd edn. Tokyo: Kanehara Shuppan, 1995.

2. Hassadia A, Gillespie A, Tydy J, et al. Placental site trophoblastic tumor: clinical features and management. Gynecol Oncol 2005; 99: 603–7.

3. Weaver DT, Fisher RA, Newlands ES, Paradinas FJ. Amniotic tissue in complete hydtidiform moles can be androgenetic. J Pathol 2000; 191: 67–70.

4. Kajii T, Ohama K. Androgenetic origin of hydatidiform mole. Nature 1977; 268: 633–4.

5. Ohama K, Kajii T, Okamoto E, et al. Dispermic origin of XY hydatidiform mole. Nature 1981; 292: 551–2.

6. Lorigan PC, Sharma S, Bright N, Coleman RE, Hancock BW. Characteristics of women with recurrent molar pregnancies. Gynecol Oncol 2000; 78: 288–92.

7. Fisher RA, Hodges MD, Newlands ES. Familial recurrent hydatidiform mole: a review. J Reprod Med 2004; 49: 595–601.

8. Lazarus E, Hulka C, Siewert B, Levine D. Sonographic appearance of early complete molar pregnancy. J Ultrasound Med 1999; 18: 589–94.

9. Szulman AE, Philippe E, Boue JG, Boue A. Human triploidy. Association with partial hydatidiform moles and nonmolar conceptuses. Hum Pathol 1981; 12: 1016–21.

10. Hirose M, Kimura T, Mitsuno N, et al. DNA flow cytometric quantification and DNA polymorhism analysis in the case of a complete mole with a coexisting fetus. J Assist Reprod Genet 1999; 16: 263–7.

11. Suita S, Shono K, Tajiri T, et al. Malignant germ cell tumors: Clinical characteristics, treatment, and outcome. A report from the Study Group for Pediatric Solid Malignant Tumors in the Kyushu Area, Japan. J Pediatr Surg 2002; 37: 1703–6.

12. Weiss S, Amit A, Schwartz MR, Kaplan AL. Primary choriocarcinoma of the vulva. Int J Gynecol Cancer 2001; 11: 251–4.

13. Yahata T, Kodama S, Kase H, et al. Primary choriocarcinoma of the uterine cervix: clinical, MRI, and color Doppler ultrasonographic study. Gynecol Oncol 1997; 64: 274–8.

14. Coskun M, Agildere AM, Boyvat F, Tarhan C, Niron EA. Primary choriocarcinoma of the stomach and pancreas: CT findings. Eur Radiol 1998; 8: 1425–8.

15. Liu Z, Mira JL, Cruz-Caudillo JC. Primary gastric choriocarcinoma: a case report and review of the literature. Arch Pathol Lab Med 2001; 125: 1601–4.

16. Wang JC, Angeles S, Chak P, Platt AB, Nimmagadda N. Choriocarcinoma of the gallbladder: treated with cisplatin-based chemotherapy. Med Oncol 2001; 18: 165–9.

17. Sievert K, Weber EA, Herwig R, et al. Pure primary choriocarcinoma of the urinary bladder with long-term survival. Urology 2000; 56: 856.

18. Koga K, Izuchi S, Maeda K, Noutomi Y. Treatment of chorionepithelioma of uterine cervix with hypogastric arterial infusion of amethopterin. J Jpn Obstet Gynecol Soc 1966; 13: 245–9.

19. Steigrad SJ, Cheung AP, Osborn RA. Choriocarcinoma co-existent with an intact pregnancy: case report and review of the literature. J Obstet Gynecol Res 1999; 25: 197–203.

20. Jacques SM, Qureshi F, Doss BJ, Munkarah A. Intraplacental choriocarcinoma associated with viable pregnancy: pathologic features and implications for the mother and infant. Pediatr Dev Pathol 1998; 1: 380–7.

21. Chama CM, Nggada HA, Nuhu A. Cutaneous metastasis of gestational choriocarcinoma. Int J Gynecol Obstet 2002; 77: 249–50.

22. Bohlmann MK, Eckstein FS, Allemann Y, Stauffer E, Carrel TP. Intracardiac resection of a metastatic choriocarcinoma. Gynecol Oncol 2002; 84: 157–60.

23. Gersak B, Lakic N, Gorjup V, et al. Right ventricular metastatic choriocarcinoma obstructing inflow and outflow tract. Ann Thorac Surg 2002; 73: 1631–3.

24. Feltmate CM, Genest DR, Goldstein DP, Berkowitz RS. Advances in the understanding of placental site trophoblastic tumor. J Reprod Med 2002; 47: 337–41.

25. Mangili G, Garavaglia E, De Marzi P, Zanetto F, Taccagni G. Metastatic placental site trophoblastic tumor. Report of a case with complete response to chemotherapy. J Reprod Med 2001; 46: 259–62.

26. Remadi S, Lifschita-Mercer B, Ben-Hur H, Dgani R, Czernobilsky B. Metastasizing placental site trophoblastic tumor: immunohistochemical and DNA analysis. 2 case reports and a review of the literature. Arch Gynecol Obstet 1997; 259: 97–103.

27. Feltmate CM, Genest DR, Wise L, et al. Placental site trophoblastic tumor: a 17–year experience at the New England Trophoblastic Disease Center. Gynecol Oncol 2001; 82: 415–9.

28. Monclair T, Abeler VM, Kren J, Walaas L, Zeller B. Placental site trophoblastic tumor (PSTT) in mother and child: first report of PSTT in infancy. Med Pediatr Oncol 2002; 38: 187–91.

29. Kurjak A, Zalud I, Predanic M, Kupesic S. Transvaginal color and pulsed Doppler study of uterine blood flow in the first and early second trimesters of pregnancy: normal versus abnormal. J Ultrasound Med 1994; 13: 43–7.

30. Kurjak A, Zalud I, Salihagic A, Cervenkovic G, Maijevic R. Transvaginal color Doppler in the assessment of abnormal early pregnancy. J Perinat Med 1991; 19: 155–65.

31. Gungor T, Ekin M, Dumanli H, Gokmen O. Color Doppler ultrasonography in the earlier differentiation of benign hydatidiform mole from malignant gestational trophoblastic disease. Acta Obstet Gynecol Scand 1998; 77: 860–2.

32. Vegan GL, Fulop V, Liu Y, et al. Differential gene expression pattern between normal human trophoblast and choriocarcioma cell lines: downregulation of heat shock protein-27 in choriocarcinoma in vitro and in vivo. Gynecol Oncol 1999; 75: 391–6.

33. Shigematsu T, Kamura T, Arima T, Wake N, Nakano H. DNA polymorphism analysis of a pure non-gestational choriocarcinoma of the ovary: case report. Eur J Gynaecol Oncol 2000; 21: 153–4.

34. Bettencourt E, Pinto E, Abraul E, Dinis M, De Oliveira CF. Placental site tropoblastic tumor: the value of transvaginal colour and pulsed Doppler sonography (TV–CGS) in diagnosis: case report. Eur J Gynecol Oncol 1997; 18: 461–4.

35. Park TK, Kim SN, Lee SK. Analysis of risk factors for postmolar trophoblastic disease: categorization of risk factors and effect of prophlactic chemotherapy. Yonsei Med J 1996; 37: 412–19.

36. Koga K, Maeda K. Prophylactic chemotherapy with amethopterin for the prevention of choriocarcinoma following removal of hydatidiform mole. Am J Obstet Gynecol 1968; 100: 270–5.

37. Soto-Wright V, Goldstein DP, Bernstein MR, Berkowitz RS. The management of gestational trohoblastic tumors with etoposide, methotrexate, and actinomycin D. Gynecol Oncol 1997; 64: 156–9.

38. Newlands ES, Paradinas FJ, Fisher RA. Recent advances in gestational trophoblastic disease. Hematol Oncol Clin North Am 1999; 13: 225–44.

39. Nozue A, Ichikawa Y, Minami R, et al. Postpartum choriocarcinoma complicated by brain and lung metastases treated successfully with EMA/CO regimen. Br J Obstet Gynaecol 2000; 107: 1171–2.

40. Okamoto T, Goto S. Resistance to multiple agent chemotherapy including cisplatin after chronic low-dose oral etoposide administration in gestational choriocarcinoma. Gynecol Obstet Invest 2001; 52: 139–41.

41. Kang SB, Lee CM, Kim JW, Park NH, Lee HP. Chemoresistant choriocarcinoma cured by pulmonary lobectomy and craniotomy. Int J Gynecol Cancer 2000; 10: 165–9.

42. Knox S, Brooks SE, Wong-You-Cheong J, et al. Choriocarcinoma and epithelial trophoblastic tumor: successful treatment of relapse with hysterectomy and high dose chemotherapy with peripheral stem cell support: a case report. Gynecol Oncol 2002; 85: 204–8.

43. Chou HH, Lai CH, Wang PN, et al. Combination of high-dose chemotherapy, autologous bone marrow/peripheral blood stem cell transplantation, and thoracoscopic surgery in refractory nongestational choriocarcinoma of a 45XO/46XY female: a case report. Gynecol Oncol 1997; 64: 521–5.

44. Cole LA, Butler S. Detection of hCG in trophoblastic disease. The USA hCG Reference Service experience. J Reprod Med 2002; 47: 433–44.

45. ACOG Committee Opinion. Avoiding inappropriate clinical decisions based on false-positive human chorionic gonadotropin test results. Am J Obstet Gynecol 2002; 100: 1057–9.

46. Tanase K, Tawada M, Moriyama N, Muranaka K. Intra-arterial infusion chemotherapy for liver metasases of testicular tumors: report of two cases. Hinyokika Kiyo 2000; 46: 823–7.

47. Woolas RP, Bower M, Newlands ES, et al. Influence of chemotherapy for gestational trophoblastic disease on subsequent pregnancy outcome. Br J Obstet Gynaecol 1998; 105: 1032–5.

48. Bower M, Rustin GJ, Newlands ES, et al. Chemotherapy for gestational trophoblastic tumours hastens menopause by 3 years. Eur J Cancer 1998; 34: 1204–7.

49. Maeda K. Gestational trophoblastic disease. Lecture at the Ian Donald Inter-University School of Medical Ultrasound, Dubrovnik, 1995.

50. Newlands ES, Bower M, Fisher RA, Paradinas FJ. Management of placental site trophoblastic tumors. J Reprod Med 1998; 3: 53–9.

51. Janni W, Hantschmann P, Rehbock J, et al. Successful treatment of malignant placental site trophoblastic tumor with combined cytostatic–surgical approach: case report and review of literature. Gynecol Oncol 1999; 75: 164–9.

52. Tsuji Y, Tsubamoto H, Hori M, Ogasawara T, Koyama K. Case of PSTT treated with chemotherapy flowed by open uterine tumor resection to preserve fertility. Gynecol Oncol 2002; 87: 303–7.

53. Twiggs LB, Hartenbach E, Saltzman AK, King LA. Metastatic placental site trophoblastic tumor. Int J Gynecol Obst 1998; 60(Suppl 1): S51–5.

54. Swisher E, Drescher CW. Metastatic placental site trophoblastic tumor: long-term remission in a patient treated with EMA/CO chemotherapy. Gynecol Oncol 1998; 68: 62–5.

55. Chang YL, Chang TC, Hsuen S, et al. Prognostic factors and treatment for placental site trophoblastic tumor – report of 3 cases and analysis of 88 cases. Gynecol Oncol 1999; 73: 216–22.

56. Mangili G, Garavaglia E, De Marzi P, Zanetto F. Taccagni G. Metastatic placental site trophoblastic tumor. Report of a case with complete response to chemotherapy. J Reprod Med 2001; 46: 259–62.

57. Randall TC, Coukos G, Wheeler JE, Rubin SC. Prolonged remission of recurrent, metastatic placental site trophoblastic tumor after chemotherapy. Gynecol Oncol 2000; 76: 115–17.

58. Watanabe S, Shimokawa S, Sakasegawa K, et al. Choriocarcinoma in the pulmonary artery treated with emergency pulmonary embolectomy. Chest 2002; 121: 654–6.

59. Kohyama S, Uematsu M, Ishihara S, et al. An experience of stereotactic radiation therapy for primary intracranial choriocarcinoma. Tumori 2001; 87: 162–5.

60. Landanio G, Sartore-Bianchi A, Giannetta L, et al. Controversies in the management of brain metastases: the role of chemotherapy. Forum (Geneva) 2001; 11: 59–74.

10 3D and 4D sonographic evaluation of the fetal heart

Carmina Comas Gabriel and Guillermo Azumendi

INTRODUCTION

During the past 25 years, two-dimensional (2D) imaging of the fetal heart has evolved into a sophisticated and widely practiced clinical tool, but most heart diseases still go undetected prenatally despite routine fetal ultrasound evaluations. Over the coming years, tremendous advances in fetal cardiac imaging, including 3D imaging, promise to revolutionize both the prenatal detection and diagnosis of congenital heart disease (CHD). Image resolution continues to improve year after year, allowing earlier and better visualization of cardiac structures. This chapter reviews the possibilities of 3D and 4D fetal echocardiography. 3D imaging of the fetal heart may improve the detection of outflow tract abnormalities and facilitate comprehension of complex forms of CHD. This review highlights the potential of acquiring a digital volume dataset of a heart cycle for later offline examination, for an offline diagnosis, for a second opinion (e.g., via Internet link), or for teaching fetal echocardiography to trainees and sonographers. On the other hand, other imaging modalities, such as Doppler tissue imaging and magnetic resonance imaging (MRI), continue to evolve and to complement 2D and 3D sonographic imaging of the fetal heart. As a result of these ongoing advances in prenatal detection and assessment of CHD, this is an exciting and promising time for the field of fetal cardiac imaging.[1]

IMPACT OF CHD: EPIDEMIOLOGY AND POPULATION AT RISK

Prenatal detection of fetal congenital heart defects remains the most problematic issue of prenatal diagno-sis.[2] Major CHDs are the most common severe congenital malformations, with an incidence of about 5 in 1000 live births, whenever complete ascertainment is done and minor lesions are excluded.[2,3] Congenital heart anomalies have a significant effect on affected children's lives, with a mortality rate of up to 25–35% during pregnancy and the postnatal period, and it is during the first year of life when 60% of this mortality occurs. Moreover, major CHDs are responsible for nearly 50% of all neonatal and infant deaths due to congenital anomalies, and this figure is likely to be significantly higher if spontaneous abortions are considered. Although CHDs used to appear isolated, they are frequently associated with other defects, chromosomal anomalies, and genetic syndromes. Their incidence is 6 times greater than that of chromosomal abnormalities and 4 times greater than that of neural tube defects.[2–4] Nonetheless, structural cardiac defects are among the most frequently missed abnormalities by prenatal ultrasound.[5] Although the at-risk population-based approach has been crucial in decreasing disease, prenatal diagnosis of CHD remains largely a scenario of too much effort for too few diagnoses. Clinicians need to re-examine the reasons for this shortfall and redefine new strategies to improve the efficacy of our efforts.

It must be remembered that 90% of congenital heart defects occur in low-risk mothers. The way forward to increase the detection rate of CHD is to improve the effectiveness of screening programs so that a higher number of cases from low-risk populations are referred for a specialized scan. The positive aspect of screening for cardiac defects compared with other anomalies (e.g. Down syndrome and neural tube defects) is that it does not automatically result in termination of pregnancy in most cases. Cardiac defects are among the anomalies where optimizing management of the neonate in the perinatal period could improve outcome. Improved morbidity/mortality has been clearly shown as a result of prenatal diagnosis in the outcome of all forms of CHD that are dependent on the patency of the arterial duct in the immediate postnatal period, with transposition of the great arteries being the single most important lesion to diagnose prenatally.[6]

All of these reasons emphasize the role of sonography in prenatal diagnosis of congenital heart abnormalities.

PRENATAL DIAGNOSIS OF CHD: CURRENT SITUATION

Screening techniques

Most major CHDs can be prenatally diagnosed by detailed transabdominal 2nd-trimester echocardiography at 20–22 weeks of gestation.[2,4,7–9] The identification of pregnancies at high risk for CHD needing referral to specialist centers is of paramount importance in order to reduce the rate of overlooked defects.[9,10] However, the main problem in prenatal diagnosis of CHD is that the majority of cases occur in pregnancies with no identifiable risk factors. Therefore, there is wide agreement that cardiac ultrasound screening should be introduced as an integral part of the routine scan at 20–22 weeks. In the 1990s, the American Institute of Ultrasound in Medicine and the American College of Radiology incorporated the four-chamber view into their formal guidelines for fetal ultrasound screening.[11,12] Although early investigators found the four-chamber view to have a high sensitivity for the prenatal detection of CHD, subsequent studies have found this view to be far less sensitive. Even in the best hands, this plane may fail to detect a significant percentage of major, frequently ductal-dependent, CHD. Many investigators have demonstrated an incremental value of adding outflow tracts to the routine fetal ultrasound screening.[13,14] When applied to a low-risk population, scrutiny of the four-chamber view allows the detection of only 40% of anomalies, while additional visualization of the outflow tracts and the great arteries increases the rate to 60–70%.[4,7,8] The systematic incorporation of the four–chamber view and outflow tracts into routine fetal ultrasound screening represents an important advance in fetal cardiac imaging.

Standard fetal cardiac examination protocol

The basic fetal cardiac screening examination entails an analysis of the four-chamber view, obtained from an axial plane across the fetal thorax. If technically feasible, optional views of the outflow tracts can be obtained as part of an extended cardiac screening examination. Summarizing the data from screening studies, a detection rate of less than 10% can be expected if the heart is not explicitly examined, a rate of 10–40% if the four-chamber view is visualized, and a rate of 40–80% if visualization of the great vessels is added.[4,7,8]

In a high-risk pregnancy, in addition to information provided by the basic screening examination, a detailed analysis of cardiac structure and function may further characterize visceroatrial situs, systemic and pulmonary venous connections, foramen ovale mechanism, atrioventricular connections, ventriculoarterial connections, great vessel relationships, and sagittal views of the aortic and ductal arches. Additional sonographic techniques can be used for this purpose, such as Doppler ultrasonography and M-mode.

Color Doppler is an essential tool for the fetal cardiologist, but is not considered the standard of care for a routine obstetric scan. Color Doppler findings can substantially increase the likelihood of prenatal diagnosis and decrease the incidence of false-positive diagnosis. Spectral power Doppler can also add important information to normal and abnormal color flow patterns.

Recently, a sequential segmental approach for the complete evaluation of fetal heart disease as a screening technique has been described using five or six short-axis views from the fetal upper abdomen to the mediastinum.[15,16] A transverse view of the fetal upper abdomen is obtained to determine the arrangement of the abdominal organs, which, in most cases, provides important clues to the determination of the atrial arrangement. A four-chamber view is obtained to evaluate the atrioventricular junctions. Views of the left and right ventricular outflow tracts are obtained to evaluate the ventriculoarterial junctions. A three-vessel view and aortic arch view are obtained for evaluation of the arrangement and size of the great arteries, which provides additional clues to the diagnosis of abnormalities involving the ventriculoarterial junctions and the great arteries.

Suggestions to improve detection rate of congenital heart defects

Inadequate examination is likely to be the most common cause of heart defects being overlooked in the four-chamber view. Chaoui[17] has provided some hints to improve visualization of the heart. Examination of the fetal heart should be carried out at every 2nd-trimester screening examination. This should ideally be performed at 20–22 weeks of gestation, using a 5 MHz transducer. Optimal analysis of the heart may be achieved by magnification of the image, using the zoom function, so that the heart fills a third to half of the screen, and by the use of the cine-loop to assess the different phases of the cardiac cycle. Established ultrasound screening programs also increase detection rates.[5] They have to focus on equivocal prenatal signs of heart abnormality, so-called borderline findings, that should raise suspicion for referral to a specialist, such as echogenic foci, small pericardial effusions, mild discrepancy in ventricular size, tricuspid regurgitation, or deviation of the cardiac axis. Since heart anomalies developing in utero can be missed at the 2nd-trimester scan, the fetal heart should be examined if 3rd-trimester scanning is performed. The use of color Doppler during cardiac scanning will also improve detection rates, increasing the speed and accuracy of the fetal cardiac scan, although the use of this modality for screening purposes is controversial.

Finally, the introduction of 3D technology in the field of prenatal diagnosis has allowed better evaluation of the static anatomic structures. Nevertheless, its application in the study of the fetal heart has not involved a significant advance up to now, since, because the fetal heart is a structure in rapid movement, the conventional 3D image appears distorted without providing significant diagnostic information.

HISTORY OF FETAL ECHOCARDIOGRAPHY

The birth of fetal echocardiography occurred in the late 1970s, when fetal heart movements were first visualized by primitive A-scan ultrasound or by M-mode techniques. Since then, different technologies and modalities have been incorporated in order to improve the diagnostic accuracy and possibilities in this field. We review the diagnostic tools that are available and the potential roles of fetal echocardiography in the field of fetal medicine.[18]

Real-time ultrasound

This is still the gold standard for the structural evaluation of the fetal heart. In the most sophisticated ultra-sound machines, there is an ideal setting for fetal heart evaluation, which is based on a high image resolution, a high frame rate, and good penetration. Two main features have facilitated the prenatal assessment of the fetal heart: the use of transducers with a high frequency (5–7 MHz transducers) and the incorporation of cine-loop and zoom functions. Tissue harmonic imaging (THI) has recently been introduced to enhance diagnostic performance in individuals with limited acoustic window, mainly due to obesity or abdominal scarring.[19] Its different behavior from fundamental-frequency ultrasound, the energy of which decreases linearly with depth, is the reason why the use of THI has been shown to improve image quality in some circumstances, particularly in obese individuals.

Time motion (M-mode)

This was a revolutionary tool in fetal cardiology when simultaneous real-time visualization became available. First used for cardiac biometry, it was soon relegated to the second line since such measurements became easier using cine-loop techniques to selectively image diastole and systole. Two main fields of interest are still in the domain of M-mode: the assessment and classification of fetal arrhythmias (where this mode can document atrioventricular conduction by putting the cursor simultaneously in an atrial and ventricular structure) and to assess myocardial contractility (calculating indices such as shortening fraction and ejection fraction).

Pulsed and continuous-wave Doppler

The acquisition of flow velocity waveforms from different fetal cardiac structures and vessels by using pulsed or continuous-wave Doppler ultrasound enables non-invasive quantification of perfusion: evaluation of peak velocities in different sites of the circulatory system, measurement of contractility indices and stroke volume, and the recent incorporation of the assessment of coronary and venous system are some examples. The pathologic conditions investigated are no longer confined to fetal heart defects, but have expanded to include other fetal conditions involving the cardiovascular system. Investigation of intracardiac flow in severe intrauterine growth restriction, diabetes, or fetal anemia are some examples of the great potential of this technical modality.

Color Doppler

In addition to grayscale examination of the fetal heart, color Doppler is now considered to be a second-line investigation for cardiac evaluation. This method allows rapid orientation within the fetal heart and completes the evaluation supplied by grayscale information. Once abnormal flow is suspected, quantification by Doppler flow velocity waveforms becomes mandatory.

Color Doppler is an essential tool for the fetal cardiologist, but is not considered the standard of care for a routine obstetric scan.

Power Doppler

This is a technique introduced in the early 1990s using the information from the amplitude of the Doppler signal rather than the frequency shift and direction, opening the possibility of displaying flow independently of its velocity and direction. Since this technique is significantly more sensitive than conventional color Doppler, it has been applied in regions with low flow and small vessels. This technique can be used in fetal cardiology, facilitating the detection of some CHDs (such as small ventricular septal defects) and enabling spatial orientation of the great vessels. On the other hand, it cannot obtain information about blood direction or turbulence. However, its characteristics make it suitable for 3D evaluation of the cardiovascular system.

Tissue Doppler echocardiography

In this technique, color-coding is used to visualize wall movements rather than blood flow. Tissue Doppler echocardiography (TDE) has only recently been applied to the fetus, with promising preliminary results.[20,21] Color and power Doppler mapping can be applied using a regular high-resolution ultrasound machine by sampling the relatively high reflected acoustic energy from the cardiac walls. Fetal TDE is a new technique that can provide additional insights into fetal cardiac function that are not available with the conventional approach.

Three-dimensional imaging

Although fetal 3D imaging currently faces important concerns regarding image resolution, the technique

has the potential to improve markedly both the prenatal detection and diagnosis of CHD. Already demonstrated to improve the diagnosis of CHD in infants, children, and adults, 3D imaging of the fetal heart offers important potential advantages over conventional 2D imaging. By acquiring volumetric data within a few seconds from a single window, 3D imaging may reduce scanning time and operator dependence. For screening the low-risk pregnancy, 3D imaging may facilitate visualization of the four-chamber view and outflow tracts, particularly when 2D imaging fails because of time constraints, limited window, or sonographer inexperience. Volume datasets could be transmitted electronically to experts for further evaluation. For teaching purposes, the volumetric datasets could be sent to a remote virtual scanning station. Finally, quantitative measurements using 3D imaging promise to be more accurate and reproducible than those derived from 2D imaging. Sophisticated volume processing algorithms that allow quantitative measurements of volume and function may offer additional insights into cardiac function and development.

Recently, *spatiotemporal image correlation (STIC)* has been introduced as a new 3D technique allowing the automatic acquisition of a volume of data from the fetal heart, displayed as a cine loop of a single cardiac cycle. This technique allows dynamic multiplanar slicing and surface rendering of heart anatomy. STIC, in combination with color or power Doppler ultrasound, is a promising new tool for multiplanar and 3D/4D rendering of the fetal heart, making possible the assessment of hemodynamic changes throughout the cardiac cycle. Since its commercial introduction in 2002, a number of authors have published their experience in the management and application of this new technology. In a later section of this chapter, we review this topic in depth and present the first study on a nationwide scale with the introduction of the new technology in our environment.

Telemedicine

This represents an emerging but potentially critical advance in prenatal screening for CHD.[22,23] Telemedicine, like 3D ultrasound, may enable fetuses to be scanned at remote sites, with these studies reviewed instantaneously or within minutes at more centrally located, highly specialized centers, avoiding the need to transport a pregnant patient.

NEW PERSPECTIVES IN 3D AND 4D FETAL ECHOCARDIOGRAPHY

Rapid advances in graphics computing and microengineering have offered new techniques for prenatal cardiac imaging. Some of these can be non-invasively applied in both clinical and laboratory settings, including dynamic 3D echocardiography, myocardial Doppler imaging, harmonic ultrasound imaging, and B-flow sonography. Appropriate use of these new tools will not only provide unique information for better clinical assessment of fetal cardiac disease but also offer new ways to improved understanding of cardiovascular development and pathogenesis.[24] This improvement in imaging technology combined with new sophisticated computer processing systems promise to revolutionize both prenatal detection and diagnosis of CHD.[25] Although 2D imaging remains the principal diagnostic modality to confirm normal cardiac development and in cases of congenital heart abnormalities, new techniques (dynamic 3D color Doppler ultrasound, Doppler-gated 3D fetal echocardiography, and 3D multiplanar time–motion ultrasound) are now technically feasible for a wide range of lesions, and may provide additional information of clinical value in some selected cases. New terms have been recently incorporated in our practice, for describing various multidimensional imaging features, including '3D', '4D', 'real-time', 'cardiac gating', 'online' and 'offline'.[26] This chapter reviews the possibilities of 3D and 4D fetal echocardiography, where a volume dataset can be acquired as a static volume, as a real-time 3D volume, or as an offline 4D volume cine using STIC software.[27] STIC is explained and the potentials of this modality are particularly emphasized in the next section.

Fetal cardiac screening

As current methods to screen the fetus for cardiac abnormalities continue to miss most CHDs, a more effective approach to screening the low-risk population for fetal heart disease would represent an important clinical advance. Preliminary results suggest that 3D and 4D technologies applied to prenatal diagnosis have the potential to function as screening tools for fetal heart diseases. Investigators are trying to demonstrate the feasibility and applications of different modalities, such as real-time echocardiography,[28] gated reconstructive 3D imaging,[29] and fetal real-time 3D echocardiography (RT3DE).[30]

Feasibility of obtaining a greater number of cardiac views

3D sonography permits a greater number of cardiac planes to be extracted from volume data than does standard 2D sonography. A study by Bega et al[31] compared the percentage of cardiac planes obtained by conventional 2D or 3D sonography, and demonstrated greater success with the later technique for the left and right outflow tracts and the ductal and aortic arches.

Improvement of basic cardiac views in unfavorable fetal positions

Among the basic cardiac views in fetuses in anterior spine positions, 3D ultrasound improves the visualization of pulmonary outflow tracts and provides a reliable alternate technique for clinical use.[32]

Evaluation of fetal cardiac function

3D echocardiography can provide estimates of ventricular volume and function.[33] In particular, 3D imaging can provide estimates of ventricular volume changes in fetal hearts with abnormal ventricular morphology that cannot easily be obtained by 2D echocardiography.[34] This technique is a promising tool for evaluation of fetuses with CHD and cardiac dysfunction, and it may provide insight into evolving CHDs.

Dynamic 3D color Doppler ultrasound

By using simultaneously two ultrasound machines – one for grayscale and color Doppler echocardiography and the other for spectral Doppler ultrasound – a novel technique has made possible prenatal visualization of the spatial distribution and the true direction of intracardiac flow of blood in four dimensions in the absence of motion artifacts. This technique suggests that diagnosis of cardiac malformations can be made on the basis of morphologic and hemodynamic changes throughout the entire cardiac cycle, offering significant information complementary to that obtained by conventional techniques.[35]

Doppler-gated 3D fetal echocardiography

Although 2D imaging remains the principal diagnostic modality for confirming normal or abnormal cardiac development, Doppler-gated 3D fetal echocardiography is technically feasible for a wide range of lesions, and may provide additional information of clinical value in some selected cases.[36] Gated 3D fetal echocardiography provides significantly better visualization and comprehension of cardiac anatomy than non-gated 3D fetal echocardiography. The superiority of the gated over the non-gated technique appears to come from both improved image quality and the anatomic clues that derive from the ability to view cardiac motion.[29]

Real-time 3D echocardiography

Conventional prenatal screening for CHD involves a time-consuming and highly operator-dependent acquisition of the four-chamber view and outflow tracts. In response, many investigators have demonstrated the potential for gated, reconstructive 3D echocardiography to evaluate the fetal heart. Reconstructive 3D echocardiography has been shown to simplify and shorten the acquisition component of fetal cardiac imaging. However, reconstructive 3D fetal cardiac imaging reconstructs a volume of data following the sequential acquisition of a series of planes. As a result, reconstructive approaches suffer from artifacts related to cardiac gating and random fetal and maternal motion. In contrast, fetal RT3DE acquires a volume of data virtually instantaneously, without the need for cardiac gating, and with less potential for artifacts. By acquiring the entire fetal heart instantaneously as a single volume, RT3DE may facilitate fetal cardiac screening. Preliminary studies suggest a high sensitivity for detecting CHD (93%), although specificity is low (45%), with a high rate of 'cannot determine' responses and false-positive artifacts.[30] These preliminary results suggest that RT3DE has the potential to function as a screening tool for fetal heart disease. However, artifacts must be recognized and minimized, resolution must improve, and substantial training will be necessary prior to widespread clinical use.

3D power Doppler ultrasound

In recent years, a few reports and studies have demonstrated that 3D power Doppler ultrasound (3D-PDU) helps in reconstruction of the vessels of interest and thus improves understanding of the spatial appearance of the vascular tree.[37]

3D multiplanar time–motion ultrasound

This new technique enables the easy acquisition of optimal M-mode traces from different heart structures. Because offline plane positioning is possible on 3D multiplanar reconstruction, M-mode traces can be obtained from different stored cardiac structures independently of fetal position.[38]

STIC

STIC is a new approach for clinical assessment of the fetal heart. This feature offers an easy-to-use technique to acquire data from the fetal heart and its visualization in a 4D sequence. The acquisition is performed in two steps. First, data are acquired by a single, automatic volume sweep. In the second step, the system analyzes the data in their spatial and temporal domains, and processes a 4D sequence. This sequence presents the heart beating in real time in a multiplanar display. The examiner can navigate within the heart, reslice, and produce all the standard planes necessary for comprehensive diagnosis.

New reconstructive approaches

RT3DE with instantaneous volume-rendered displays of the fetal heart represents a new approach to fetal cardiac imaging with tremendous clinical potential.[28] New plans and views, not visualized in conventional fetal 2D echocardiography, can be generated with minimal processing of rendered image displays.

Virtual echocardiography by Internet link

A complete virtual cardiologic examination can be achieved in stored 3D volumes of the fetal heart and transmitted to a tertiary fetal cardiology center via the Internet. Previous experiences have demonstrated that 3D virtual cardiac examination is possible.[39,40] The use of the Internet link has major implications, particularly for situations in which the scanning center is geographically remote from the tertiary center or for facilitating a second-opinion diagnosis.

CLINICAL APPLICATION OF 3D AND 4D SONOGRAPHY IN THE FETAL CARDIOVASCULAR SYSTEM

The clinical application of 3D and 4D sonography in prenatal visualization of the fetal cardiovascular system is closely related to the regions of interest known from the application of color and power Doppler ultrasound: vessels of the placenta, umbilical cord, abdomen, kidneys, lung, and brain, and fetal tumors, as well as the heart and great vessels.[37]

Peripheral vascular systems in 3D

Umbilical cord and placenta

From Chaoui's experience, these seem to be the structures most easily accessible to 3D sonography throughout pregnancy. Intraplacental vessel network architecture can be visualized with this method. Abnormalities such as placenta previa, vasa previa, or velamentous insertion can be demonstrated, as well as single umbilical artery or less important conditions such as connecting vessels in twin pregnancies, nuchal cord, or true or false knot.[37,41]

Intra-abdominal vessels

The vessels of interest are the umbilical vein, the ductus venosus, the portal vein, the hepatic veins, the splenic vessels, the inferior vena cava, and the abdominal aorta. Since the application of color Doppler and the recent intensive study of the ductus venosus, abnormalities of the intrahepatic venous system have been found to be more common than previously expected. Conditions suitable for study by 3D power Doppler could involve abnormal cord insertion on the abdomen (omphalocele and gastroschisis), abnormal umbilical vein size (varix and ectasia), and absence of the ductus venosus or abnormal course of vessels in isomerism conditions.

Renal vessels

Visualization of the renal vessels is known to increase the accuracy of diagnosis of kidney malformations in the fetus. The renal vascular tree is well visualized in a coronal plane, with the descending aorta showing a horizontal course. Conditions possibly benefitting from application of 3D-PDU are agenesis of one or both kidneys, arteries in duplex kidney, horseshoe, and pelvic kidney.

Intracerebral vessels

Transverse insonation allows easy reconstruction of the circle of Willis, whereas a more sagittal approach enables visualization of the pericallosal artery with its ramifications. Choosing a lower-velocity scale flow, the cerebral veins and sagittal sinus can be imaged as well. The main fields of interest are an abnormal anterior cerebral artery in agenesis of the corpus callosum, aneurysm of the vein of Galen, and disturbed vascular anatomy in cerebral malformations.

Lung vessels

Fields of interest are analysis of the 3D vessel architecture in cystic lung malformation, congenital diaphragmatic hernia, and bronchopulmonary sequestration. Color and power Doppler have not been successful in predicting pulmonary hypoplasia and it is not expected that 3D demonstration of the vessels could be of great interest in this field in the near future.[37]

Fetal tumors and aberrant vessels

Aberrant vessels can be visualized in the presence of several malformations such as lung sequestration, chorioangioma, and lymphangioma, and in sacrococcygeal teratoma, acardiac twin, etc. Visualization of fetal tumors could be useful not only because of the risk of cardiac failure due to the presence of arteriovenous fistulas, but also to assess compression or shifting of neighboring organs.

Fetal heart in 3D and 4D

In the last decade, 3D and 4D fetal echocardiography has been investigated intensively in laboratories using external work stations, static volume sweep, and matrix transducers, and recently new ultrasound equipment with integrated software (STIC) has been introduced, allowing reliable 3D and 4D fetal echocardiography.

STIC: A NEW APPROACH TO 3D AND 4D EVALUATION OF THE FETAL HEART

In 2002, the Voluson Expert 730 machine (GE Medical Systems, Kretz Ultrasound, Zipf, Austria) introduced a new technological concept called spatiotemporal image correlation (STIC). This technology enables one to review, handle, and store digitally volume data on the fetal heart in a looped cine sequence. The aim of the development of the STIC technique was to create a useful screening tool that is easy to use and facilitates detection of the fetal heart anomalies during routine obstetric scans. In several studies, 4D fetal echocardiography has proved to offer comprehensive assessment of fetal heart morphology and relationship of the great vessels,[29,36,42] even when the fetus is in an unfavorable scanning position.[32]

STIC basically allows displays in three different imaging modalities: grayscale, color Doppler, and power Doppler (Figure 10.1). Each of these modalities

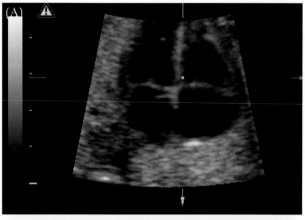

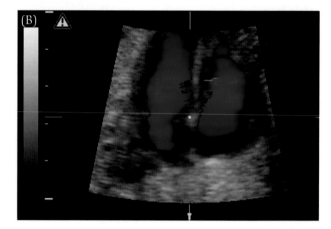

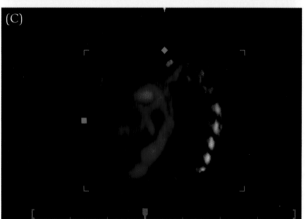

Figure 10.1 The spatio-temporal image correlation (STIC) technique offers different display modalities – in grayscale or combined with color and power Doppler: (A) display format in grayscale; (B) display format in grayscale combined with color Doppler; (C) display format in grayscale combined with power Doppler

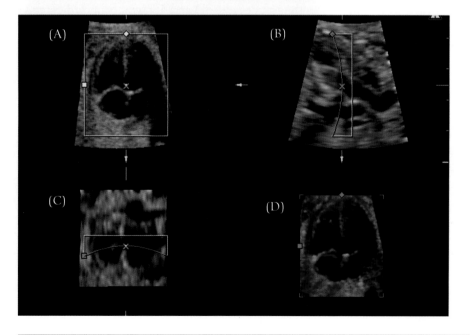

Figure 10.2 The STIC technique offers different display formats: a multiplanar view (three planes perpendicular to each other), a single plane, and volume rendering. Four simultaneous image displays are presented in this figure. (A) The A-plane shows the acquired image obtained during the STIC sweep. (B) The B-plane is the orthogonal plane vertical to the A-plane (sagittal plane). (C) The C-plane is the orthogonal plane horizontal to the A-plane (coronal plane). (D) Volume-rendered image

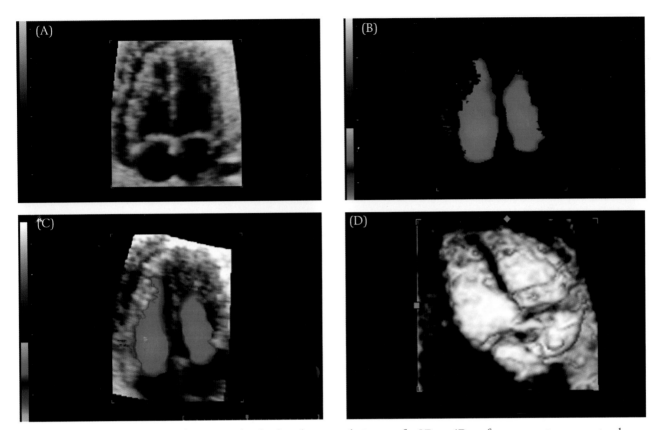

Figure 10.3 The heart volume dataset can be displayed as a single image of a 3D or 4D surface or as a transparent volume, in which grayscale or color Doppler information or both can be demonstrated (the so-called 'glassbody' mode). The inverse mode has been recently described as a new rendering algorithm that transforms echolucent structures into echogenic voxels. (A) Gray rendering volume. (B) Color rendering volume. (C) Glassbody rendering volume. (D) Inverse-mode rendering volume

can display two possible formats: multiplanar (showing planes perpendicular to each other) or volume-rendered (Figure 10.2). The rendered format can be displayed in different algorithms (gray, color, and glassbody) (Figure 10.3). The multiplanar format is the first system to allow simultaneous and dynamic multiplanar evaluation of several 2D planes. The volumetric format is a technique in which the 3D structures of the scanned volume are transferred to a 2D image.

Technical basis

The main aspects that have to be considered when evaluating a 3D imaging system are volume data acquisition and the image rendering display. Acquisition can be achieved either in 3D static mode (a volume consisting of series of still images) or in 4D mode (which reflects the beating character of the heart). The latter can be acquired either in live real-time 3D or as offline 4D, which is possible with the recent advent of the new STIC software. In these acquisitions, heart and vessels can be visualized either in grayscale mode or in combination with color Doppler,[43] power Doppler or B-flow.[37] Image rendering is the process of creating a 3D visual representation of the parameters of interest.

The STIC technology enables the automatic and sequential acquisition of 2D images in a volume that is stored digitally, performing a single sweep in slow motion over a limited area of interest, which provides a high-resolution image (150 frames/s). It is possible to optimize the image by changing the acquisition time (between 7, 5, and 15 seconds, with intervals of 2.5 seconds) and the sweep angle (from 15° to 40°, with intervals of 5°). The steps are as follows.

Acquisition

With automatic volume acquisition, the array inside the transducer housing performs an automatic slow single sweep, recording a single 3D dataset. This volume consists of a high number of sequential 2D frames. Due to the small region of interest, the B-mode frame rate during the volume scan is very high, in the region of 150 frames/s, which means that 2D images are stored at high resolution.

Post-processing

After the volume scan has been acquired, the system performs a spatial and temporal correlation of the recorded data. This technique identifies the rhythmic movements, and, depending on their periodicity, the fetal heart rate can be calculated. Based on the exact timing of the systolic peak and the time interval between one systole and the next, the system rearranges the 2D images, obtaining consecutive volumes presenting a complete and 'synchronized' cardiac cycle (it correlates the images of different cardiac cycles obtained in the slow sweep, rearranging the events into their spatial and temporal domains).

Visualization

These volumes are displayed in an endless cine sequence (showing the heart cycle in real time in a cine loop), which can be played back in different ways (slow motion, frame-by-frame, stopped at any stage during the cycle, rotation in the three spatial planes (x-, y-, and z-planes), multiplanar view, single plane, volumetric reconstruction, etc.). Similarly, it is possible to perform post–processing adjustments, such as gamma curve correction to optimize the contrast resolution, modification of color threshold (balancing to control and modify color intensity over the grayscale) or grayscale threshold, etc.

In summary, thanks to this algorithm, following dynamic acquisition of a volume dataset including the fetal heart, a single cardiac cycle is virtually reconstructed according to heart rate with fundamental sectional planes being displayed in multiplanar fashion or integrated into a moving volume (4D echocardiography). In this sense, STIC can be defined as an 'online' system with an 'indirect volume scan' and 'post-3/4D-acquisition correlation'.[43] Thanks to this technique, a more comprehensive investigation of the fetal heart is feasible, since all structures are amenable to exploration along any angle of view, irrespective of fetal position.

Advantages of STIC

Improved temporal resolution

Because of the increased number of frames acquired for a specific anatomic region using the STIC technique, this method results in improved temporal resolution of the online dynamic 3D image sequence that is displayed in the multiplanar or the rendered display.[44] As a result, cardiac images that are difficult to interpret or that cannot be identified in the conventional 2D mode can be improved with this new approach.

Dynamic evaluation of the four-chamber view

STIC enables dynamic evaluation of the four-chamber view. It does not examine a single static four-chamber plane at a single time-point but allows a dynamic study of this view in three planes – anteroposterior, latero-lateral, and supero-inferior – in this way allowing the planes to rotate 360° around an axis.

Evaluation of the outflow tracts

2D evaluation of the outflow tracts may be difficult due to an inappropriate fetal orientation or to fetal movement. The STIC technique facilitates assessment of the outflow tracts, since it enables rotation of the data volume around a single reference point.[32,43]

Multiplanar dynamic display and navigation

The volume acquired by 3D sonography can be displayed on a monitor in three orthogonal planes, representing the transverse, sagittal, and coronal planes of a representative 2D plane within the volume. Such a display of three orthogonal planes from the 3D volume acquisition is termed a 'multiplanar display'. STIC is the first system with a simultaneous dynamic multiplanar view in the three planes.[44,45] Using multiplanar slicing, examiners can dynamically visualize the heart in three orthogonal planes at the same time. The reference dot can be employed to 'navigate' the volume in any direction, by placing the dot at any location in the A-, B-, and C-planes and observing the corresponding plane changes in the respective images (Figures 10.4–10.6).

Reconstruction of a 3D rendered image

STIC enables reconstruction of a 3D rendered image containing depth and volume, which may provide

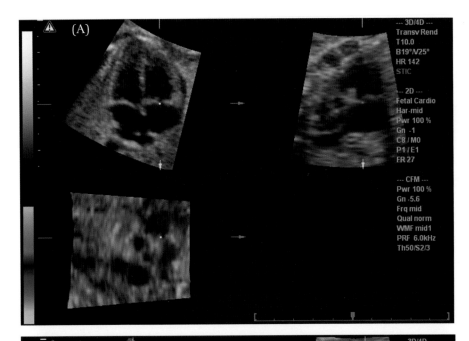

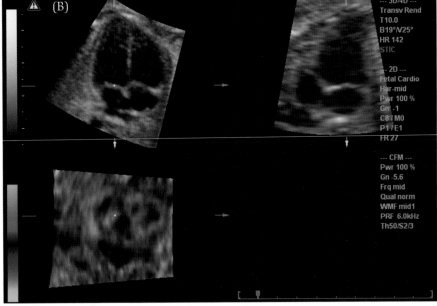

Figure 10.4 3D multiplanar slicing of the four-chamber view. The examiner can place the reference dot at any location in the *a*-, *b*-, or *c*-plane and observe the corresponding planes change their respective images. By using the cine-loop, the examiner can choose within the volume the heart cycle phase of interest. (A) The reference dot is positioned at the level of the tricuspid valve during systole. The valves can be visualized simultaneously in the three orthogonal planes: transverse (left upper panel), sagittal (right upper panel), and coronal (left lower panel). (B) The reference dot is positioned at the level of the mitral valve during systole. The valves can be visualized simultaneously in the three orthogonal planes: transverse (left upper panel), sagittal (right upper panel), and coronal (left lower panel)

continued

additional information that is not available from the multiplanar image slices.[43,45] Thanks to multiplanar volume rendering of the cardiac structures, some CHDs, traditionally difficult to diagnose prenatally, can be accurately documented, such as small ventricular defects[46] and abnormal venous connections.[47]

Online acquisition (patient in the room)

STIC reduces the online exploration time. Moreover, acquisition is less operator-dependent than conventional 2D sonography.

Offline analysis

The STIC technique allows recreation of the cardiac examination. In the 2D mode, static images or videotapes can only be reviewed retrospectively. Undoubtedly, this is one of the most promising applications of this technique, opening up new opportunities for consultation, clinical diagnosis, and screening strategies.[44,48]

Timing

Theoretically, STIC can be applied at any time during gestation. However, some limitations may be found

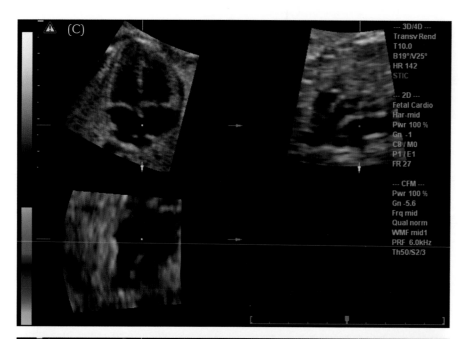

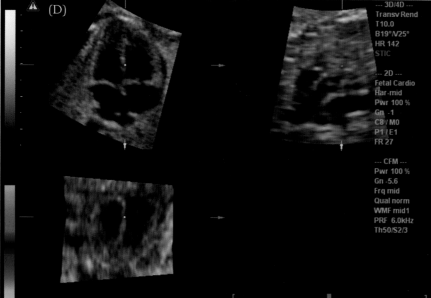

Figure 10.4 (C) The reference dot is positioned at the level of the foramen ovale. Both atria can be visualized in the coronal plane (left lower panel), and a sagittal view of the foramen ovale is provided on the right upper panel. (D) The reference dot is positioned at the level of the interventricular septum. A sagittal view of the interventricular septum can be visualized simultaneously in the right upper panel. TV, tricuspid valve; MV, mitral valve; FO, foramen ovale; IVS, interventricular septum

later in gestation in fetuses with large hearts and early in gestation as a result of low signal discrimination.[43]

New anatomic planes

STIC presents new anatomic planes, which can be difficult or impossible to obtain through the conventional 2D mode. Such views could focus on demonstrating the atrioventricular valves, the so-called 'en face view' of these valves,[43] or the interventricular or interatrial septum. The future will show which views are appropriate for clinical application.

Promising new technology

Promising new technology can be introduced, in combination with the STIC technique, such as a speckle reduction imaging (SRI) or tomographic ultrasound imaging (TUI). SRI allows improved image resolution, particularly in difficult scan conditions (Figure 10.7). TUI allows the diagnosis on one screen of multiple images (Figure 10.8).

Applications in telemedicine (TELESTIC)

STIC lends itself to storage and review of volume data

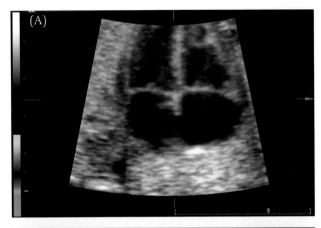

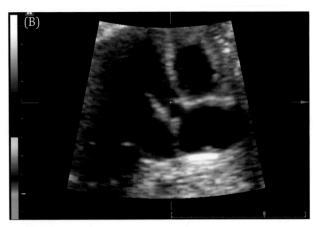

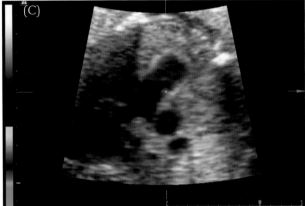

Figure 10.5 The examiner can magnify and visualize the *a*-plane in a single format. By scrolling through the volume, any plane can be visualized. In this case, the most important planes are presented: (A) the four-chamber view; (B) the five-chamber view; (C) the three vessels and trachea view. By using the cine-loop, the examiner can choose within the volume the heart cycle phase of interest

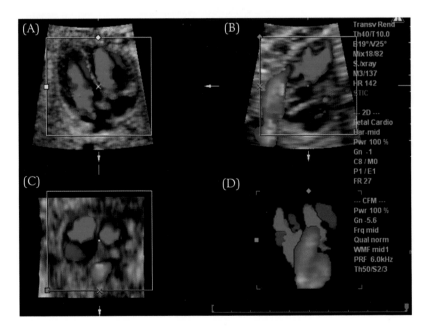

Figure 10.6 Color Doppler spatiotemporal image correlation (STIC) volume of a 27-week fetus displayed in multiplanar and rendering mode. By scrolling through the cine-loop, the different phases of the cardiac cycle can be visualized as diastolic filling of the ventricles, beginning of systole with blood flow streaming in the outflow tracts, and late systole with blood still recognizable in both great vessels. In this view, the cross-crossing of the great vessels can be appreciated in a way not seen before in prenatal diagnosis. Due to presetting of the color persistence the volume in the *d*-plane (D) shows simultaneously late diastole and early systole. Additionally, in the *c*-plane (C) we can appreciate a new anatomic view, the en face view of the atrioventricular valves, with both mitral and tricuspid valves being demonstrated during diastolic flow (red)

by the examiner or by experts at remote sites. Volume datasets can be transmitted via the Internet from remote geographic areas to allow advice or second diagnostic opinions to be obtained from experts in reference centers. Moreover, TELESTIC can be used as a filter in order to relieve the workload in these reference centers. This modality also offers a wide range of possibilities and new applications in the teaching field.[39,40,49]

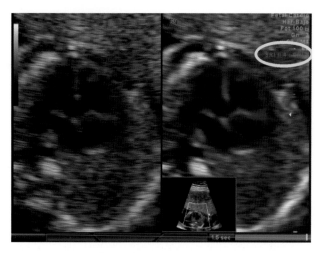

Figure 10.7 Speckle reduction imaging (SRI II) may reduce artifacts, improving image resolution, particularly in difficult scan conditions

Limitations of STIC

There are potential limitations to this technique. Some factors are inherent to conventional sonography, others are specific to 3D technology, some are inherent to color Doppler technology, and a few are related specifically to the STIC method.

Specific limitations of 2D technology

- Resolution limitations typical of 2D imaging.
- Low resolution of the reconstructed planes (*b*- and *c*-planes).
- Low resolution of the image, especially at early gestational ages.

Specific limitations of 3D technology

- During the volume acquisition time, maternal and fetal movements produce artifacts, especially in

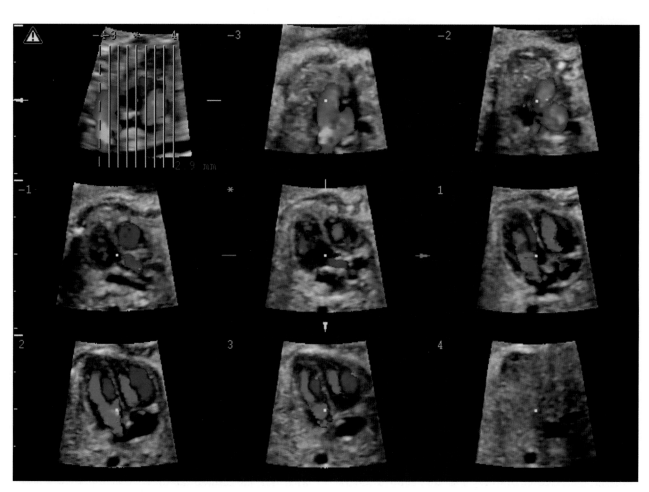

Figure 10.8 Tomographic ultrasound imaging (TUI) in a normal fetal heart at 20 weeks of gestation. TUI allows the diagnosis on one screen of multiple images

the *b*- and *c*-planes. Whenever possible, acquisition must be performed in the absence of maternal and fetal movements.

Specific limitations of color Doppler technology

- Lack of color signal when the region of interest is perpendicular to the insonation (in these cases, it is advisable to modify the angle of insonation).
- On adding color, as in the conventional 2D modality, the resolution is reduced, in comparison with the grayscale image.

Specific limitations of STIC

- Fetal arrhythmias are the main limitation of this technique, since synchronization of the cardiac cycle is not permitted in these cases. When important changes are detected in the fetal heart rate during volume acquisition, calculation of this rate may not be accurate or provide sufficiently useful information due to the appearance of artifacts caused by difficulty in synchronizing the 2D images at the right time within the cycle.
- A learning curve is required to manage this technique, and extra time is needed for post-processing of the image.
- The STIC technology is expensive and only provided by one manufacturer. It is expected that in the near future other companies will provide new software with new possibilities of 3D and 4D acquisition and rendering.

Current applications and new perspectives for STIC

A number of investigators have published their initial experience with this new technology. The current lines of research are focused in the following points.

Clinical application in unselected population and also in populations at risk

Preliminary studies suggest that real-time 3D echocardiography has potential as a screening tool for fetal heart disease, by introducing new screening strategies and new concepts, such as offline echocardiography, screening echocardiography, and tele-echocardiography.[30,48] Some studies of 4D echocardiography using STIC have focused on the acquisition of volume datasets by operators with limited experience in echocardiography and subsequent analysis by an expert.[48]

Systematization of the multiplanar technique

Some studies of 4D echocardiography using STIC have focused on the development of a multiplanar technique to systematically examine the four-chamber view and the outflow tracts.

- Gonçalves et al[45] have described a four-step technique to simultaneously display the right and left ventricular outflow tracts (Figure 10.9). Using the four-chamber view as the starting point, the heart is rotated approximately 45° around the *z*-axis and the reference dot is placed at the center of the interventricular septum. Next, the volume is rotated clockwise around the *y*-axis until the left ventricular outflow tract is visualized. The reference dot is repositioned at the center of the outflow tract, above the aortic valve. A short-axis view of the right ventricular outflow tract is displayed simultaneously in the right upper panel.
- With the same purpose in mind, De Vore et al[50] described a new technique using 3D multiplanar imaging that allows the examiner to identify the outflow tracts within a few minutes of acquiring the 3D volume dataset by rotating the volume dataset around the *x*- and *y*-axes: this is called the spin technique (Figure 10.10). The full length of the main pulmonary artery, ductus arteriosus, aortic arch, and superior vena cava can easily be identified in the normal fetus by rotating the volume dataset along the *x*- and *y*-axes. 3D multiplanar evaluation of the fetal heart allows the examiner to identify the outflow tracts using a simple and reproducible technique that requires only rotation around *x*- and *y*-axes from reference images obtained in a transverse sweep through the fetal chest.

Reproducibility study

Recent studies support the reproducibility of this technique, in terms of intra-observer and inter-observer variability, although these studies are still based on small series. Gonçalves et al,[51] including a series of 20 volume datasets acquired from fetuses with normal cardiac anatomy, concluded that STIC can be used reproducibly to evaluate fetal cardiac outflow tracts by independent examiners.

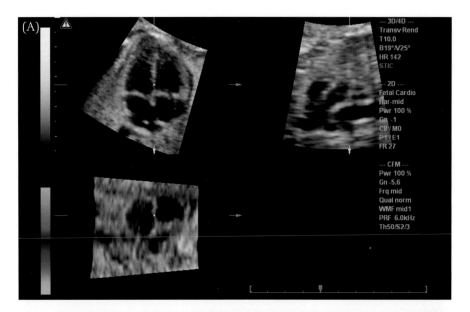

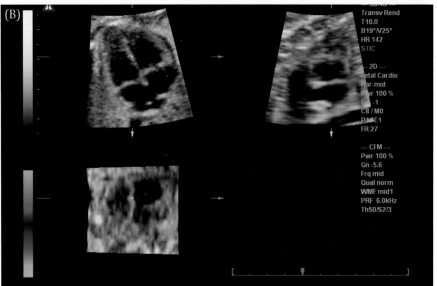

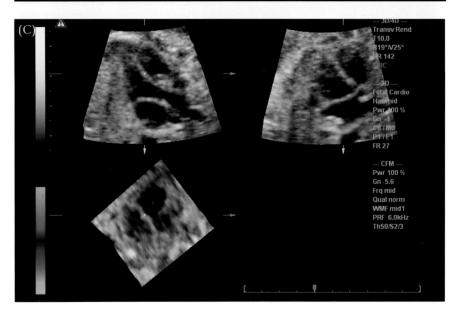

Figure 10.9 Multiplanar technique: four-step technique. With the four-chamber view as starting point (A), the heart is rotated approximately 45° around the *z*-axis and the reference dot is placed at the center of the interventricular septum (B). The volume is rotated clockwise around the *y*-axis until the left ventricular outflow tract is visualized (C). The reference dot is repositioned at the center of the outflow tract, above the aortic valve

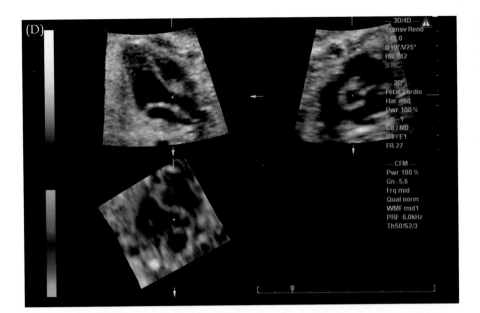

Figure 10.9 A short-axis view of the right ventricular outflow tract is displayed simultaneously in the right upper panel (D)[45]

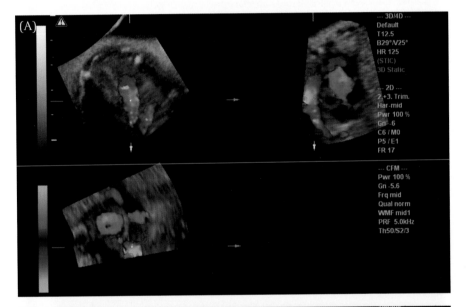

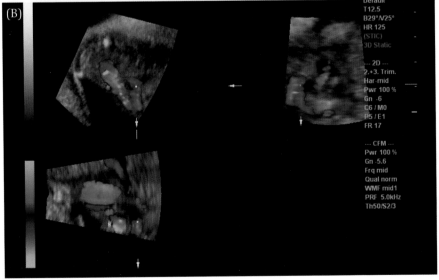

Figure 10.10 Multiplanar technique: spin technique. The full length of the main pulmonary artery and ductus arteriosus (A) and aortic arch (B) can easily be identified in the normal fetus by rotating the volume dataset around the *x*- and *y*-axes[50]

Assessment of diagnosis ability for heart diseases

As already mentioned, with STIC, the multiplanar volume rendering cardiac structures allows accurate documentation of some CHDs that have traditionally been considered difficult to diagnose prenatally with accuracy: these include small ventricular defects,[46] abnormal venous connections[47] and right aortic arch. Additionally, color Doppler STIC has the potential to simplify visualization of the outflow tracts and may improve the diagnosis of some congenital heart abnormalities[42,43] (Figures 10.11–10.14).

Specific applications in the prenatal diagnosis of CHD

4D grayscale and power Doppler STIC can be used to systematically visualize the abnormal relationship of the outflow tracts in fetuses with transposition of the great arteries (TGA)[43,52] (Figure 10.13). The detection rate of TGA by standard obstetric scan evaluation is low, and this disappointing performance has been attributed to technical difficulties in consistently imaging the outflow tracts. 4D sonography may overcome technical limitations related to the skill required to obtain appropriate planes of section.

Estimation of volumes and masses in experimental models

Estimation of ventricular volume and mass is important for baseline and serial evaluation of fetuses with normal and abnormal hearts. Direct measurement of chamber wall volumes and mass can be made without geometric

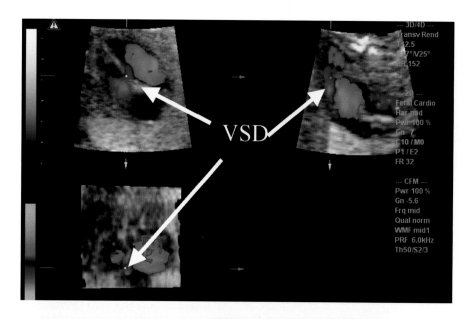

Figure 10.11 One application of the multiplanar mode is demonstrated in this fetus of 22 weeks of gestation with a ventricular septal defect (VSD) showing shunting from the left to the right ventricle (blue color crossing the septum). The arrows point to the dot present in all three planes, which shows the intersection point of these planes. The examiner can place the dot in the region of interest (here in the *a*-plane) and see its position in both of the other planes

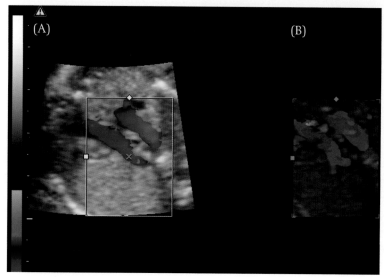

Figure 10.12 A 22-week gestation fetus with a right aortic arch. Two simultaneous images display: (A) the axial plane, the plane of the acquired image obtained during the STIC sweep, corresponding to an axial plane at the level of the upper mediastinum; (B) glass-body rendered image corresponding to the acquisition plane. In both images, we can appreciate the anechoic area representing the trachea surrounded by the ductal arch (on the left side of the trachea) and the aortic arch (on the right side of the trachea)

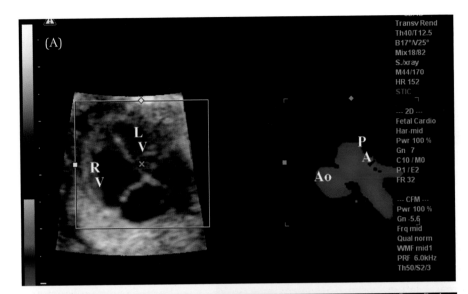

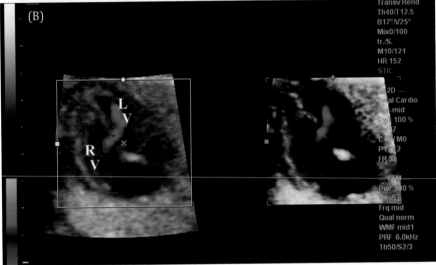

Figure 10.13 A fetus with transposition of the great arteries and ventricular septal defect (VSD) at 22 weeks of gestation. (A) Note the parallel course of both ventricles. The 3D color rendering demonstrates the bifurcation of the pulmonary artery connecting to the left ventricle. (B) Note the additional VSD (red color crossing the septum) in both the 2D four-chamber view and the glass-body rendered image. LV, left ventricle; RV, right ventricle; PA, pulmonary artery; Ao, aorta

assumptions by 3D fetal echocardiography. Recent studies have established the feasibility of fetal ventricular mass measurements with 3D ultrasound technology and have developed normal values from 15 weeks of gestation to term.[53] Non-gated fast 3D fetal echocardiography is an acceptable modality for determination of cardiac chamber wall volume and mass with good accuracy and acceptable inter-observer variability. This method should be especially valuable as an objective serial measurement in clinical fetal studies with structurally or functionally abnormal hearts (Figure 10.14).

Algorithms for the automated acquisition of standard anatomic slices from the stored volume

It is anticipated that algorithms developed to image specific cardiac structures with 3D or 4D volume datasets may eventually be automated using computer software.[54] Despite recent advances in sonography, the acquisition, display, and manipulation of 3D volumes is a technique requiring a substantial 'learning curve'. It is theoretically possible to obtain the volume of a specific organ (e.g. fetal heart) and to allow an automatic program to display from this volume all of the 2D planes that are required for a complete anatomic evaluation of the organ. Abuhamad has termed this new concept 'automatic multiplanar imaging' (AMI). Once a 3D volume of the fetal heart has been obtained from a standardized plane, such as the four-chamber view, AMI will automatically generate all other standardized planes from the acquired volume in an operator-independent manner, improving the reproducibility of AMI-generated sonographic images. Automatic multiplanar imaging allows complete evaluation of anatomically complex organs with a standardized and operator-independent approach.

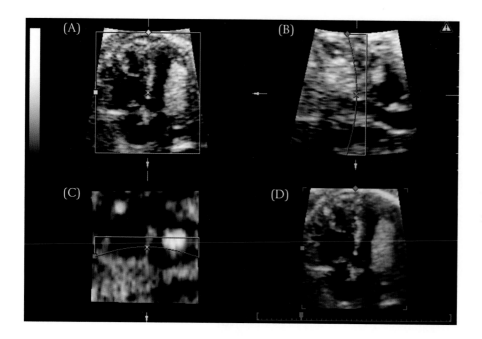

Figure 10.14 A fetus with multiple solid cardiac tumors at 29 weeks of gestation, postnatally diagnosed as tuberous sclerosis. Four simultaneous images display: (A) the axial plane, the plane of the acquired image obtained during the STIC sweep; (B) the orthogonal plane vertical to the plane in (A) (the sagittal plane); (C) the orthogonal plane horizontal to the plane in (A) (coronal plane); (D) gray rendered image

Application of this technology in telemedicine (TELE-STIC)

Preliminary studies suggest that a telemedicine link via the Internet combined with STIC technology (TELE-STIC) is technically feasible.[39,40,49] TELE-STIC allows a second diagnostic opinion to be obtained and also generates a link between different centers, resulting in a new virtual tool for teaching and training.

New diagnostic algorithms

- The minimum projection mode (MPM) is a rendering algorithm available in some 3D and 4D sonography systems that, in one image, allows the visualization of vessels and cystic anatomic structures located in different scanning planes. This algorithm is an alternative rendering modality that facilitates visualization of normal and abnormal vascular connections to the fetal heart, particularly in the three-vessel view.[55] This technique may be useful in prenatal diagnosis of conotruncal abnormalities and in the assessment of the spatial relationships of abnormal vascular connections in the upper mediastinum.
- The inversion-mode algorithm has recently been introduced in fetal imaging as a new tool for 3D rendering of fluid-filled structures.[46,56,57] This novel 3D post-processing algorithm enables any fetal structure with an anechoic content to be converted into an echogenic volume. Numerous fetal disorders have been accurately described using inversion-mode 3D ultrasound including urinary tract anomalies, gastrointestinal obstructions, hydrocephalus, and cysts, and more recently the inversion mode has been employed to display the fetal heart. Using this approach, the beating heart is dynamically transformed into a hyperechogenic 3D structure by signal conversion of the blood flowing within the cardiac structures. Since this technique does not use color or power Doppler sonography as a digital contrast to highlight the blood vessels, it does not have the inherent limitations on image reconstruction related to the angle of insonation, temporal resolution, or the intensity of the Doppler signal. This new rendering modality allows better documentation of some cardiac defects, that have traditionally been difficult to diagnose prenatally (e.g., small ventricular defects[46] and abnormal systemic venous connections[47]), as well as permitting evaluation of complex disorders requiring precise definition of visceral situs, such as heterotaxy syndromes.[56]

FIRST SPANISH STUDY IN STIC TECHNOLOGY

Objective

The objective of this study was to assess the use and performance of the STIC technique in order to perform a basic and extended cardiac fetal evaluation, with online acquisition of the cardiac volume during the morphologic scan by a general sonographer and offline analysis by an expert in fetal cardiology.

Methodology

Cardiac volumes were prospectively stored according to STIC technology[49] during the morphologic ultrasound screening examination, by a general sonographer, in a random selection of obstetric patients attending our unit in the period between December 2004 and February 2005 (Gutenberg Centre, Malaga, Spain). Twenty-eight fetal explorations were included, all of them randomly distributed in our program, depending on the pressure of attendance and the availability of an ultrasound machine equipped with STIC technology. Only fetal explorations considered as normal were included, excluding those cases with cardiac, extracardiac, or chromosomal anomalies. Between one and four volumes were acquired per patient on a grayscale (online acquisition). Afterwards, a second examiner expert in fetal echocardiography assessed the collected volumes in order to make a cardiac basic evaluation and an extended evaluation, in a limited time of 15 minutes per patient (offline analysis).

The acquisition is made from a four-chamber view on grayscale in an automated single sweep in a slow motion, by standardizing the acquisition time in 10 seconds (7.5 to 12.5) and the sweep angle in 25° (20 to 30), depending on the gestational age.

First, only the initial acquisition single plane was examined, followed by a multiplanar study in order to improve the visualization of those structures not identifiable through the initial acquisition plane. The offline analysis included assessment of the situs visceral, cardiac size, cardiac axis, myocardial contractility, symmetry of cavities, cardiac crux, insertion of the atrioventricular valves and their opening, moderator band, foramen ovale, crossing of the great arteries, outflow tracts of both ventricles, and pulmonary and aortic valves. These structures were assessed in the four-chamber view (4CV), the five-chamber view (5CV), the three-vessel view (3VV), and the three-vessel view including the trachea (3VVT). The criteria defining the assessment of the situs visceral were abdominal identification of the position and location of the stomach, abdominal aorta, and inferior vena cava, and identification of the thoracic aorta and cardiac atrial cavities. The criteria defining a basic fetal cardiac study were evaluation of the inflow tract view

(4CV) and evaluation of the outflow tract view (5CV and 3VV or 3VVT) (Figure 10.5). The criteria defining an extended cardiac fetal study were evaluation of the inflow tracts (4CV), evaluation of the outflow tracts (5CV and 3VV or 3VVT), and evaluation of the situs visceral.

We standardized the volume acquisition time to 10 seconds, with a sweep angle of 25°, modifying these variables according to the cardiac size and the conditions in the exploration (fetal movements). The acquisition was achieved from the 4CV – apical (preferable), basal, or lateral, depending on the fetal position – in a sweep covering the initial slice, going under and over it (including the superior abdomen and thorax). Offline analysis was performed by a single investigator using the 4D View Software Version 2.1 (GE Medical Systems, Kretz Ultrasound, Zipf, Austria).

Results

A total of 58 explorations of fetal cardiac volumes in 28 patients were included, with gestational ages ranging between 17 and 35 weeks. The characteristics of the patients and volumes are reported in Table 10.1. The mean visualization scores for the different structures and views are shown in Tables 10.2 and 10.3.

A basic cardiac examination according to set criteria was achieved in 100% of cases, while an extended cardiac examination was achieved in 85% of cases.

Table 10.1 Methodological data: characteristics of patients and volumes

Period of study	December 2004–February 2005
Number of patients	28
Number of analyzed volumes	58
Gestational age (completed weeks)[a]	23 weeks (17–35 weeks)
Acquisition conditions:	
Time[a]	10 seconds (7.5–12.5 seconds)
Angle[a]	25° (20°–30°)
Acquisition plane:	
Apical four-chamber view	68%
Lateral four-chamber view	14%
Basal four-chamber view	18%
Offline analysis (average time)	15 minutes/patient

[a]Average and range

Table 10.2 Visualization rate of cardiac structures: success rate of visualizing different cardiac structures and plans using STIC

Cardiac structures	Visualization rate (%)
Situs visceral	86
Cardiac size	100
Cardiac axis	100
Miocardic contractility	100
Symmetry of cavities	100
Cardiac crux	96
Insertion of atrioventricular valves	93
Opening of atrioventricular valves	100
Moderator band	100
Foramen ovale	100
Crossing of great arteries	100
Left ventricular outflow tract	100
Right ventricular outflow tract	100
Pulmonary valve	100
Aortic valve	100
Four-chamber view	100
Five-chamber view	100
Three-vessel view	100
Three-vessel view including trachea	64
Extended cardiac study[a]	86

[a]The extended cardiac study included evaluation of the inflow tracts, outflow tracts, and situs visceral

Table 10.3 Contribution of the multiplanar study to visualizing different cardiac structures and planes using STIC

	Multiplanar contribution (%)
Four-step technique[a], great arteries	71
IVC-RA[b]	93
SVC-RA[c]	79
Aortic arch (sagittal)	54
Ductal arch (sagittal)	71
Additional contribution[d]	100

[a]A four-step technique to evaluate the outflow tracts from the four-chamber view
[b]Inferior vena cava to right atrium
[c]Superior vena cava to right atrium
[d]Percentage of cases in which the multiplanar examination has contributed to providing additional information

Multiplanar study improved the visualization of those structures not identifiable through the initial acquisition single plane in all cases.

CONCLUSIONS

The detection of CHD is still considered as one of the most problematic areas in the field of prenatal diagno-sis. In spite of being the most frequent and severe congenital malformation in neonates, it is still one of the pathologies least often diagnosed during fetal life. It is also well known that the prognosis of most CHDs, particularly the ductus-dependent anomalies, is significantly better in terms of morbidity and mortality when the anomaly is detected prenatally. These are essential factors motivating interest in improving prenatal detection strategies.

The incorporation of the four-chamber view during the morphologic scan at 20 weeks of gestation, in the so-called 'basic' cardiac scan, has improved the prenatal detection of CHD.[11,12] Recently, inclusion of outflow tract evaluation in the so-called 'extended' cardiac scan has been strongly recommended in order to improve the detection of conotruncal abnormalities.[13,14] Nevertheless, conventional prenatal screening for CHD still involves a time-consuming and highly operator-dependent acquisition of the four-chamber view and outflow tracts. As routine prenatal screening in the general obstetric setting is unsatisfactory, the main objective of this technique is to produce a method able to identify or exclude major CHD in a screening policy. It has recently been demonstrated that STIC acquisition of the fetal heart is feasible with high success rates in visualizing cardiac structures. From our experience and a few published studies,[45,48,49] the anatomy of the fetal heart can be confidentially demonstrated by means of STIC acquisition carried out by an operator unskilled in fetal cardiology. We should point out the high success rate in visualizing the structures and views included in our checklist, suggesting that most of the relevant sonographic data on the fetal heart can be obtained in one STIC volume. By acquiring the entire fetal heart instantaneously as a single volume, STIC may facilitate fetal cardiac screening. The STIC data volume acquired by a non-expert sonographer or general obstetrician can subsequently be used by a fetal echocardiologist for prenatal confirmation of normal heart anatomy or exclusion of major cardiac defects.[48] This could particularly be the case if the dataset volume for analysis is acquired automatically, thus reducing the need for technical skills and expertise from sonographers. Artifacts must also be recognized and minimized, resolution must improve, and substantial training will be necessary prior to widespread clinical use. Real-time 3D examination of the fetal heart with the use of matrix phased-array probes may help to overcome such difficulties in the future.

In summary, the introduction of the STIC technology, overcoming the limitations imposed by cardiac movement on volumetric reconstruction, provides a fast and easy online acquisition of the cardiac volume in the context of a routine ultrasound examination, with the possibility of carrying out a more complete offline analysis of cardiovascular structures. Potential advantages include the possibility of offline analysis in the patient's absence, remote diagnosis, novel scanning planes, and new approaches for medical education. It should be emphasized that there is a high rate of success in volume acquisition and offline analysis, allowing the possibility of an extended cardiac evaluation, in what we have called 'screening offline extended cardiac scan' or 'basic offline echocardiography'. This concept can be introduced as a promising new strategy that can be implemented in the general population in order to improve the prenatal detection rate of congenital heart abnormalities.

REFERENCES

1. Sklansky M. Advances in fetal cardiac imaging. Pediatr Cardiol 2004; 25: 307–21.

2. Campbell S. Isolated major congenital heart disease. Ultrasound Obstet Gynecol 2001; 17: 370–9.

3. Mitchell SC, Korones SB, Berendes HW. Congenital heart disease in 56,109 births. Incidence and natural history. Circulation 1971; 43: 323–32.

4. Allan L, Sharland G, Milburn A, et al. Prospective diagnosis of 1006 consecutive cases of congenital heart disease in the fetus. J Am Coll Cardiol 1994; 23: 1452–8.

5. Garne E, Stoll C, Clementi M, and the Euroscan Group. Evaluation of prenatal diagnosis of congenital heart diseases by ultrasound: experience from 20 European registries. Ultrasound Obstet Gynecol 2001; 17: 386–91.

6. Bonnet D, Coltri A, Butera G, et al. Detection of transposition of the great arteries in fetuses reduces neonatal morbidity and mortality. Circulation 1999; 99: 916–18.

7. Allan LD. Fetal cardiology. Curr Op Obstet Gynecol 1996; 8: 142–7.

8. Gembruch U. Prenatal diagnosis of congenital heart disease. Prenat Diagn 1997; 17: 1283–98.

9. Todros T. Prenatal diagnosis and management of fetal cardiovascular malformations. Curr Opin Obstet Gynecol 2000; 12: 105–9.

10. Levi S, Schaaps JP, De Havay P, Coulon R, Defoort P. End result of routine ultrasound screening for congeni-tal anomalies. The Belgian Multicentric Study 1984–92. Ultrasound Obstet Gynecol 1995; 5: 366–71.

11. Lee W. Performance of the basic fetal cardiac ultrasound examination. J Ultrasound Med 1998; 17: 601–7.

12. Royal College of Obstetricians and Gynaecologists. Ultrasound Screening. London: Royal College of Obstetricians and Gynaecologists, 2000; http://www.rcog.org.uk/mainpages.asp?PageID=439#20week.

13. Carvalho JS, Mavrides E, Shinebourne EA, Campbell S, Thilaganathan B. Improving the effectiveness of routine prenatal screening for major congenital heart defects. Heart 2002; 88: 387–91.

14. Kirk JS, Riggs TW, Comstock CH, et al. Prenatal screening for cardiac anomalies: the value of routine addition of the aortic root to the four-chamber view. Obstet Gynecol 1994; 84: 427–31.

15. Yagel S, Cohen SM, Achiron R. Examination of the fetal heart by five short-axis views: a proposed screening method for comprehensive cardiac evaluation. Ultrasound Obstet Gynecol 2001; 17: 367–9.

16. Yoo SJ, Lee YH, Cho KS, Kim DY. Sequential segmental approach to fetal congenital heart disease. Cardiol Young 1999; 9: 430–44.

17. Chaoui R. The four-chamber view: four reasons why it seems to fail in screening for cardiac abnormalities and suggestions to improve detection rate. Ultrasound Obstet Gynecol 2003; 22: 3–10.

18. Chaoui R. Fetal echocardiography: state of art. Ultrasound Obstet Gynecol 2001; 17: 277–84.

19. Paladini D, Vasallo M, Tartaglione A, Lapadula C, Martinelli P. The role of tissue harmonic imaging in fetal echocardiography. Ultrasound Obstet Gynecol 2004; 23: 159–64.

20. Tutschek B, Zimmermann T, Buck T, Bender HG. Fetal tissue Doppler echocardiography: detection rates of cardiac structures and quantitative assessment of the fetal heart. Ultrasound Obstet Gynecol 2003; 21: 26–32.

21. Paladini D, Lamberti A, Teodoro A, et al. Tissue Doppler imaging of the fetal heart. Ultrasound Obstet Gynecol 2000; 16: 530–5.

22. Sharma S, Parness IA, Kamenir SA, et al. Screening fetal echocardiography by telemedicine: efficacy and clinical acceptance. J Am Soc Echocardiogr 2003; 16: 202–6.

23. Nelson TR, Pretorius DH, Lev-Toaff A, et al. Feasibility of performing a virtual patient examination using three-dimensional ultrasonographic data acquired at remote locations. Ultrasound Med 2001; 20: 941–62.

24. Deng J, Rodeck CH. New fetal cardiac imaging techniques. Prenat Diagn 2004; 30: 1092–103.

25. Sklansky M. New dimensions and directions in fetal cardiology. Curr Opin Pediatr 2003; 15: 463–71.

26. Deng J. Terminology of three-dimensional and four-dimensional ultrasound imaging of the fetal heart and other moving body parts. Ultrasound Obstet Gynecol 2003; 22: 336–44.

27. Chaoui R, Heling KS. New developments in fetal heart scanning: three- and four-dimensional fetal echocardiography. Semin Fetal Neonat Med 2005; 10: 567–77.

28. Sklansky MS, DeVore GR, Wong PC. Real-time 3-Dimensional fetal echocardiography with and instantaneous volume-rendered display: early description and pictorial essay. J Ultrasound Med 2004; 23: 283–9.

29. Slansky MS, Nelson TR, Pretorious DH. Three-dimensional fetal echocardiography: gated versus nongated techniques. J Ultrasound Med 1998; 17: 451–7.

30. Sklansky M, Miller D, DeVore G, et al. Prenatal screening for congenital heart disease using real-time three-dimensional echocardiography and a novel 'sweep volume' acquisition technique. Ultrasound Obstet Gynecol 2005; 25: 435–43.

31. Bega G, Kuhlman K, Lev-Toaff A, Kurtz A, Wapner R. Application of three-dimensional ultrasonography in the evaluation of the fetal heart. J Ultrasound Med 2001; 20: 307–13.

32. Wang PH, Chen GD, Lin LY. Imaging comparison of basic cardiac views between two- and three-dimensional ultrasound in normal fetuses in anterior spine positions. Int J Cardiovasc Imaging 2002; 18: 17–23.

33. Esh-Broder E, Ushakov FB, Imbar T, Yagel S. Application of free-hand three-dimensional echocardiography in the evaluation of fetal cardiac ejection fraction: a preliminary study. Ultrasound Obstet Gynecol 2004; 23: 546–51.

34. Meyer-Wittkopf M, Cole A, Cooper SG, Schmidt S, Sholler GF. Three-dimensional quantitative echocardiographic assessment of ventricular volume in healthy human fetuses and in fetuses with congenital heart disease. J Ultrasound Med 2001; 20: 317–27.

35. Deng J, Yates R, Sullivan ID, et al. Dynamic three-dimensional color Doppler ultrasound of human fetal intracardiac flow. Ultrasound Obstet Gynecol 2002; 20: 131–6.

36. Meyer-Wittkopf M, Cooper S, Vaughan J, Sholler G. Three-dimensional echocardiographic analysis of congenital heart disease in the fetus: comparison with cross-sectional fetal echocardiography. Ultrasound Obstet Gynecol 2001; 17: 485–92.

37. Chaoui R. Three-dimensional ultrasound of the blood flow in the fetal cardiovascular system. In: Kurjak A, ed. Textbook of Perinatal Medicine. New Delhi: Jaypee Brothers Medical Publishers, 2005: 644–53.

38. Jurgens J, Chaoui R. Three-dimensional multiplanar time-motion ultrasound or anatomical M-mode of the fetal heart: a new technique in fetal echocardiography. Ultrasound Obstet Gynecol 2003; 21: 119–23.

39. Michailidis GD, Simpson JM, Karidas C, Economides DL. Detailed three-dimensional fetal echocardiography facilitated by an Internet link. Ultrasound Obstet Gynecol 2001; 18: 325–8.

40. Viñals F, Poblete P, Mandujano L, et al. Prenatal diagnosis of congenital heart diseases using STIC Telemedicine (TELE-STIC) via internet link. Preliminary results of 7 centers. Ultrasound Obstet Gynecol 2005; 26: 412 (Abstr P05.10).

41. Lee W, Kirk JS, Comstock CH, Romero R. Vasa previa: prenatal detection by three-dimensional ultrasonography. Ultrasound Obstet Gynecol 2000; 16: 384–7.

42. Gonçalves LF, Romero R, Espinoza J, et al. Four-dimensional ultrasonography of the fetal heart using Color Doppler STIC. J Ultrasound Med 2004; 23: 473–81.

43. Chaoui R, Hoffmann J, Heling KS. Three-dimensional (3D) and 4D color Doppler fetal echocardiography using spatio-temporal image correlation (STIC). Ultrasound Obstet Gynecol 2004; 23: 535–45.

44. DeVore GR, Falkensammer P, Sklansky MS, Platt LD. Spatio-temporal image correlation (STIC): new technology for evaluation of the fetal heart. Ultrasound Obstet Gynecol 2003; 22: 380–7.

45. Gonçalves LF, Lee W, Chaiworapongsa T, et al. Four-dimensional ultrasonography of the fetal heart with spatiotemporal image correlation. Am J Obstet Gynecol 2003; 189: 1792–802.

46. Ghi T, Cera E, Segata M, et al. Inversion mode spatio-temporal image correlation (STIC) echocardiography in three-dimensional rendering of fetal ventricular septal defects. Ultrasound Obstet Gynecol 2005; 26: 679–86.

47. Espinoza J, Gonçalves LF, Lee W, Mazor M, Romero R. A novel method to improve prenatal diagnosis of abnormal systemic venous connections using three- and four-dimensional ultrasonography and 'inversion mode'. Ultrasound Obstet Gynecol 2005; 25: 428–34.

48. Viñals F, Poblete P, Giuliano A. Spatio-temporal image correlation (STIC): a new tool for the prenatal screening of congenital heart defects. Ultrasound Obstet Gynecol 2003; 22: 388–94.

49. Viñals F, Mandujano L, Vargas G, Giuliano A. Prenatal diagnosis of congenital heart disease using four-dimensional spatio-temporal image correlation (STIC) telemedicine via an Internet link: a pilot study. Ultrasound Obstet Gynecol 2005; 25: 25–31.

50. DeVore GR, Polanco B, Sklansky MS, Platt LD. The 'spin' technique: a new method for examination of the fetal outflow tracts using three-dimensional ultrasound. Ultrasound Obstet Gynecol 2004; 24: 72–82.

51. Gonçalves LF, Espinoza J, Romero R, et al. Four-dimensional fetal echocardiography with spatiotemporal image correlation (STIC): a systematic study of standard cardiac views assessed by different observers. J Matern Fetal Neonatal Med 2005; 17: 323–31.

52. Gonçalves LF, Espinoza J, Romero R, et al. A systematic approach to prenatal diagnosis of transposition of the great arteries using 4–dimensional ultrasonography with STIC. J Ultrasound Med 2004; 23: 1225–31.

53. Bhat AH, Corbett V, Carpenter N, et al. Fetal ventricular mass determination on three-dimensional echocardiography: studies in normal fetuses and validation experiments. Circulation 2004; 110: 1054–60.

54. Abuhamad A. Automated multiplanar imaging. A novel approach to ultrasonography. J Ultrasound Med 2004; 23: 573–6.

55. Espinoza J, Gonçalves LF, Lee W, et al. The use of the minimum projection mode in 4–dimensional examination of the fetal heart wih STIC. J Ultrasound Med 2004; 23: 1337–48.

56. Gonçalves LF, Espinoza J, Lee W, Mazor M, Romero R. Three- and four-dimensional reconstruction of the aortic and ductal arches using inversion mode: a new rendering algorithm for visualization of fluid-filled anatomical structures. Ultrasound Obstet Gynecol 2004; 24: 696–8.

57. Lee W, Gonçalves LF, Espinoza J, Romero R. Inversion mode: a new volume analysis tool for 3-Dimensional ultrasonography. J Ultrasound Med 2005; 24: 201–7.

11 3D sonography in the study of the fetal face

Guillermo Azumendi, Asim Kurjak, and Carmina Comas Gabriel

ULTRASOUND

Ultrasound evaluation of the fetal face is an extremely important part of the structural survey, since a detailed facial examination can provide much information alerting us to the possibility of associated anomalies at other levels of the fetal anatomy. It is well known that some facial and encephalic structures share the same embryologic origin, and for this reason any malformation detected at the facial level must necessitate a corresponding study at encephalic level.[1] We all recognize, with De Meyer et al,[2] that 'The face predicts the brain'.

Under normal conditions, ultrasound examination of the face is easy to perform because of its surrounding fluid. Generally, most sonologists perform a qualitative evaluation of the fetal face using two-dimensional (2D) ultrasound and moving the probe to obtain a proper visualization of the three orthogonal planes:[1]

- the coronal view looking at soft tissues and bones from the surface well into the palate and orbits, and the symmetry of the face
- the transverse view to visualize the mandible, maxilla and palate, tooth buds, and orbits
- the sagittal view for evaluation of the forehead, the nasal bridge, and the mandible.

Usually, with this approach, we do not spend more than one or two minutes, and it lets us carry out at least one detailed and qualitative study revealing the normality of the facial structures.

The conventional 2D ultrasound examination[3] will be sufficient in most cases to rule out the presence of facial abnormalities. Nevertheless, certain additional aspects can turn out to be interesting to assess in some particular cases. In these situations, we can resort to the use of other methods that complement our basic 2D exploration. For instance, we can use the color Doppler ultrasound to evaluate the integrity of the alveolar ridge and palate; and similarly, during respiratory activity, we can visualize the amniotic fluid flow coming through the nostrils. We can also use in some specific cases magnetic resonance imaging (MRI) to better visualize the palate and internal anatomy, and of course, as we will try to explain in this chapter, we can use 3D and 4D sonography to obtain a more precise evaluation of some facial features.

We do not pretend in this chapter to deal in great detail with the conventional sonographic evaluation of the fetal face by 2D sonography – there is already much in the literature[1,3–7] and excellent textbooks[8–22] that describe in a splendid way the use of 2D sonography to rule out facial anomalies in the fetus.

In this chapter, we will review those aspects of the prenatal ultrasound evaluation of the fetal face that can be improved or enriched with the incorporation of 3D sonography beyond its stereotyped image as an instrument or camera to obtain beautiful images for the family album[23] (Figures 11.1 and 11.2).

The use of 3D sonography is becoming an important component of state-of-the-art imaging in obstetrics and gynecology[24] – and nowhere more so than in the study of the fetal face – as highlighted by a panel of physicians and scientists with interest and expertise in 3D ultrasound held in June 2005 by the American Institute of Ultrasound in Medicine (AIUM) to discuss the current diagnostic benefits and technical limitations in obstetrics and gynecology and consider the

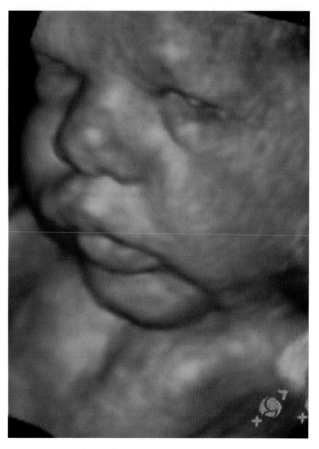

Figure 11.1 Three-dimensional surface rendering of a fetal face at 32 weeks

the same way as real-time ultrasound, transvaginal ultrasound, Doppler ultrasound, color and power-Doppler ultrasound became part of our daily routine in the past, real 4-D ultrasound will stay here. Don´t get left out, because it will constitute the mainstream of ultrasound in the future.'

TECHNICAL CONSIDERATIONS

Technically, in broad outline, the process leading to the achievement of a 3D ultrasound image is made up of two stages. The first is the acquisition of data starting from a 2D image. The second stage is analysis of the acquired information and drawing up of the image, or image display. Current equipment allows us to handle and show this image in many different ways, depending on the aim of our exploration.

DATA ACQUISITION

The data providing the 3D reconstruction are always obtained from a 2D image. The method used to acquire or capture this information differs among different equipment.

utility and role of this type of imaging in clinical practice.[25]

As pointed out by Professor Timor-Tritsch,[26] '4D ultrasound is here to stay. It will never go away, and in

Data acquisition using standard 2D probes

We can resort to systems based on conventional 2D probes. In this case, the movement of the probe during capture can be made by a uniform sweep of the hand

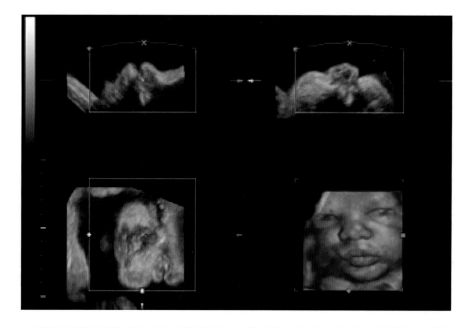

Figure 11.2 Beyond the spectacular beauty of the surface-rendered 3D reconstruction, the multiplanar display will probably provide much more information to aid in diagnosis

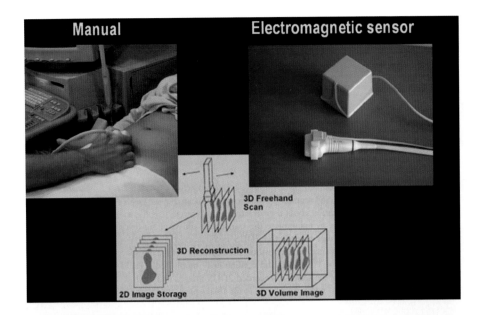

Figure 11.3 The 'freehand' acquisition is made by a conventional 2D probe either moved only by hand or assisted by electromagnetic sensors

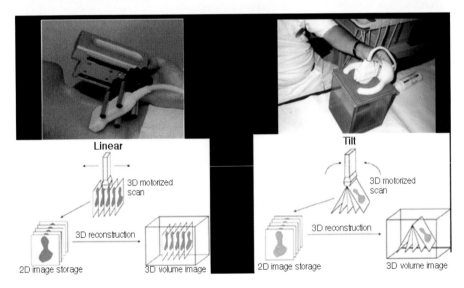

Figure 11.4 Using mechanical devices, a uniform sweep can be made with conventional 2D probe, leading to more reliable images

(the 'freehand' method), either unaided or helped with an electromagnetic sensor connected to the probe that allows the software to identify the movement described by the probe during the acquisition so that the subsequent drawing up is more reliable (Figure 11.3). Both techniques are very operator-dependent, since they depend on the angle of slope of the probe as well as the speed and uniformity of its movement.

In an attempt to improve the uniformity of movement of the probe, mechanical assist devices (Figure 11.4) were introduced some years ago: these were connected to the head of the probe and moved it at a certain speed and direction, allowing a much more standardized capture than the 'freehand' method. However, these devices proved to be uncomfortable for patients and they were consigned to experimental purposes.

The methods acquiring information based on conventional 2D probes had the advantage of low cost and easy implementation with any conventional ultrasound machine. They did not require any investment in new instrumentation, and only the specific software had to be purchased. However, with these systems, at best it is only possible to obtain some superficial reconstructions in a more or less realistic way (Figure 11.5).

For all of these reasons, and although some studies based on this acquisition method still appear in the literature, these systems using conventional 2D probes are effectively obsolete. The clinical application of 3D ultrasound now demands the use of specific probes

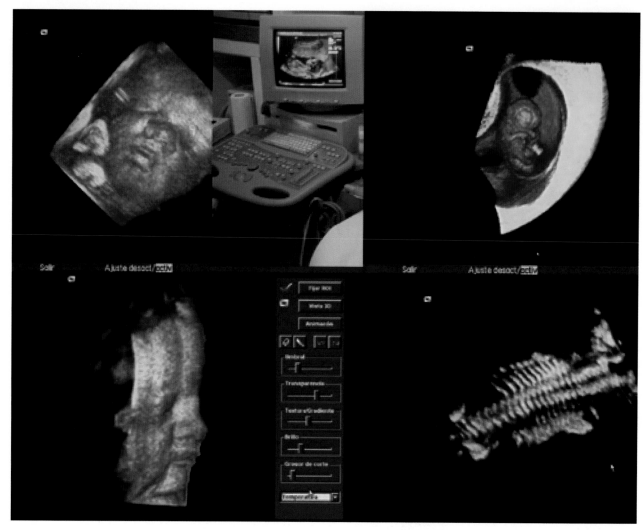

Figure 11.5 Depiction of some surface 3D reconstructions obtained with a 'freehand' acquisition system. No electromagnetic sensors were attached to the probe, which was moved simply by hand. With this method, it was only possible to obtain superficial images, with no measurements or multiplanar navigation through the fetal anatomy

that are dedicated to this kind of sonography and that can produce a precise and reproducible 3D display.

Data acquisition using specific 3D probes

The specific probes for 3D/4D sonography perform a uniform sweep by a motorized mechanism that allows many 2D images to be obtained in a precise layout an exact distance from one another. The set of all these acquired images makes up a 'volume' in which the basic unit is not a pixel as in a 2D image but a voxel, which contains data about its location with respect to three orthogonal planes (Figure 11.6).

It must be noted that in order to achieve a good 3D reconstruction, it is essential that the initially acquired

2D image from which the reconstruction is made be of good quality.[27]

The 3D probe performs a fan-shaped sweep, always in the same direction, and then the information is processed and analyzed in order to obtain the other two planes of the space from the information initially acquired.

In this way, we can visualize on the screen the image in the three orthogonal planes, in the so-called multiplanar display (Figure 11.7). The top left corner is designated as plane A: in this plane, the image appears in the same way as it is usually visualized by conventional 2D ultrasound. It is the plane in which the probe performs the sweep. In the top right and bottom left quadrants, the image developed from that acquisition are displayed, corresponding to the other

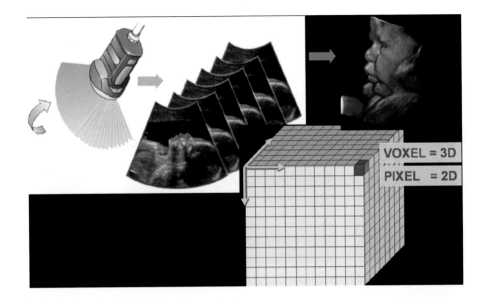

Figure 11.6 Acquisition with specific 3D probes

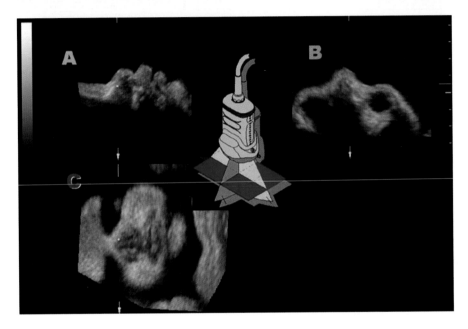

Figure 11.7 Multiplanar display. In the plane *A*, the ultrasound image is seen in the same way as it is usually visualized in conventional 2D examination. In this case, it is depicting the longitudinal view. In the plane *B*, the axial view is displayed. In the plane C, the coronal view is seen: this view is obtained in conventional 2D imaging only with great difficulty. Both *B* and *C* are reconstructed planes, and therefore they show a slight degradation in resolution compared with the acquisition plane *A*

two orthogonal planes. It must be underlined that the C plane (or coronal plane) – also known as the 'bird's-eye view' – is very difficult to achieve by conventional 2D ultrasound: the ability to show this plane is one of the great advantages of 3D sonography. The bottom right quadrant remains for the display of the 3D reconstruction, depending on the modality that is chosen. It must be emphasized that despite the impressive immediate appearance of the 3D view, it is actually the possibility of multiplanar navigation that provides the most valuable information for diagnosis in obstetrics and gynecology.

3D probes are already available for all of the main fields of application, and the latest generation of probes (which are much lighter and easier to use than earlier ones) can also be used for conventional 2D exploration. Thus, it should be possible to perform a 3D acquisition simply with the touch of a key, thus avoiding the risk of losing the opportunity of getting a good 3D image just because the fetus has changed its position.

IMAGE DISPLAY: BASIC SETTINGS AND MODALITIES

To obtain good results, it is necessary to make several basic adjustments not only before acquiring the information but also after having acquired it.

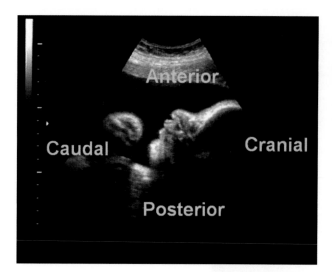

Figure 11.8 2D image orientation before acquisition

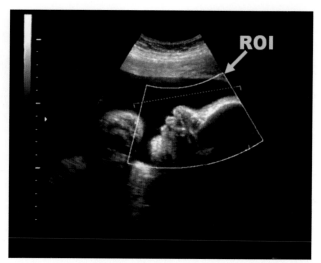

Figure 11.9 Adjusting the region of interest (ROI) box before acquisition

Settings before acquisition

Before proceeding to the acquisition, the 2D image is adjusted, depending on the aim of the exploration and the operator's preferences or favorite presets. Also, the operator will try not to position any structures in front of the intended region of exploration.

It is useful that the operator gets used to directing the 2D image in the longitudinal plane in the same way for each scan: for example, anterior part up, posterior down, cranial on the right, and caudal on the left (Figure 11.8).

The next step is to choose the kind of 3D exploration that is to be performed (static 3D, dynamic 4D, 4D STIC, 4D biopsy, -VCI-A, -VCI-C). The region of interest (ROI) box is then displayed on the screen – this defines the area of the 2D image where the 3D reconstruction will be carried out (Figure 11.9).

It is important to adjust the ROI box properly, taking a number of aspects into account:

- *Size*. Since only part of the 2D image inside the ROI will be reconstructed in 3D, the ROI must be large enough to cover the structures of interest. It should be noted that the larger the ROI, the greater is the time necessary for the equipment to show all of the data, since it must analyze a great deal of information. In the case of 4D imaging, an ROI that is too large will result in a reduction of the number of images per second, and the sensation of imaging in real time will be lost.
- *Orientation*. The sample window is moved to cover the 2D image, with care being taken to ensure that

the dotted green line on the screen remains aligned with the most superficial part of the image that is to be seen in the 3D view. In addition, care should be taken not to position any adjacent structure between the green line and the target of the study.

- An appropriate *sweep angle* must be selected. This parameter is another factor influencing the final size of the acquired volume. If the angle is too large, the volume produced will be too wide and the speed of processing will be reduced.
- Finally, the *quality of acquisition* of the image should be selected. Here again, a compromise must be reached between the quality or resolution of the obtained volume image and the speed of scanning and the number of frames per second that can be visualized in 4D.

Thus, the volume finally acquired will have a size determined by several factors, especially the following:

- the size of the ROI box
- the scanning angle or selected sweep
- the quality or resolution of the image chosen for the acquisition.

The larger these parameters are, the larger will be the volume acquired and the amount of information that the equipment must process, with the consequence that it will have to slow down some of its procedures: it may take longer to capture an image or to display the 3D reconstruction, or the number of sequences per second in the 4D mode may be reduced and the sensation of 'real time' lost.

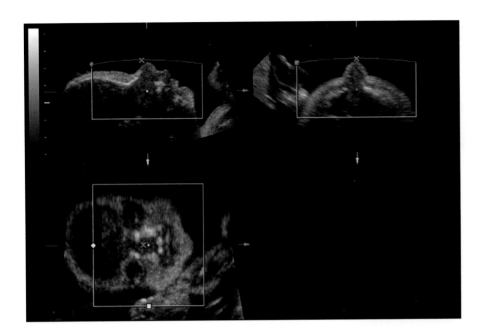

Figure 11.10 Adjusting the rendering box after acquisition

With a little experience and practice, all of these adjustments can become controlled almost automatically by the operator to achieve the desired result.

Settings after acquisition and image display modalities

Multiplanar navigation

After acquiring the information, some adjustments can also be made in the multiplanar mode. The *rendering box* in each of the three orthogonal planes of the screen can be readjusted (Figure 11.10).

It is also possible to *rotate or turn round* (Figure 11.11) the image of any of the three reference planes about the three axes of the space and see the modifications that these changes make in the other two reference images.

Another possibility is to carry out *translations* (Figure 11.12) along the three orthogonal planes in order to visualize each of the multiple slices forming that volume.

With a combination of these transformations, any desired plane through the fetus can be obtained, regardless of fetal position at the time of volume acquisition, although image quality will vary among planes. This technique provides the examiner with a tomographic approach to the fetal anatomy, giving enormous possibilities to the multiplanar navigation mode.

To facilitate orientation in this navigation process, it may be useful to have the central reference dots

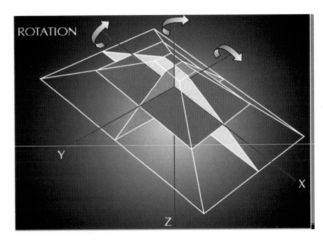

Figure 11.11 Rotation around the three spatial axes

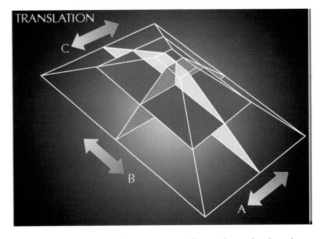

Figure 11.12 Translation or scrolling through the three orthogonal planes

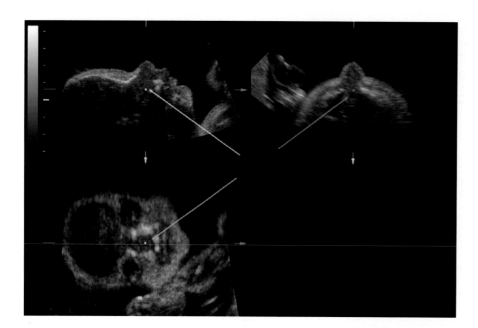

Figure 11.13 Reference color dots are very useful for orientation

displayed in three different colors (Figure 11.13) corresponding exactly to the same point in the space where the three orthogonal planes appearing in the multiplanar display are cut.

In this way, once the information has been acquired, it will remain stored as a volume that can be re-evaluated and navigated through as many times as required, with the settings of the image being altered as necessary to undertake as many measurements as are desired.

This possibility of re-evaluation and navigation offline is undoubtedly one of the great advantages of 3D in comparison with the conventional 2D sonography, where the only chance of re-evaluation lies in recording a video sequence and reviewing it forward and backwards without any possibility of changing the settings of the image or the visualization planes from any point of the space.

The multiplanar view can also be studied simultaneously with rendered images, enabling the planar images to be correlated with 3D rendered images.

3D rendering modes

The volume data may also be processed and reconstructed as 3D rendered images using a variety of rendering algorithms.[28] The terminology used for the rendering parameters has not been standardized and varies among equipment manufacturers. By displaying soft tissue[29] information in the *surface rendering mode* (Figure 11.14A), 3D sonography provides unique and realistic images of the fetal face and body, and this is

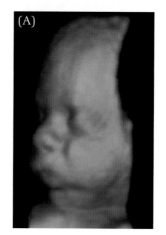 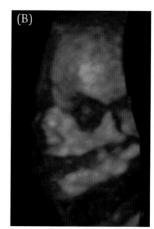

Figure 11.14 Two different renderings of the same face: (A) surface rendering; (B) transparent maximum mode

one of the methods most frequently utilized in the 3D evaluation of the fetal face. This view is achieved by extraction of signals only from the surface of the ROI.

On some occasions, it may be useful to give a transparent appearance to an image for better visualization of some structures, and in that case *transparent mode* can be used, with the possibility of choosing between the *maximum mode* (Figure 11.14B) (which is useful for assessing the skeleton), the *minimum mode* (which is useful for assessing structures with liquid content such as blood vessels and the gallbladder), or the *X-ray mode* (which is useful for enhancing solid lesions in the tissue thickness).

A 3D rendering can be displayed combining two of these modalities in different percentages (surface,

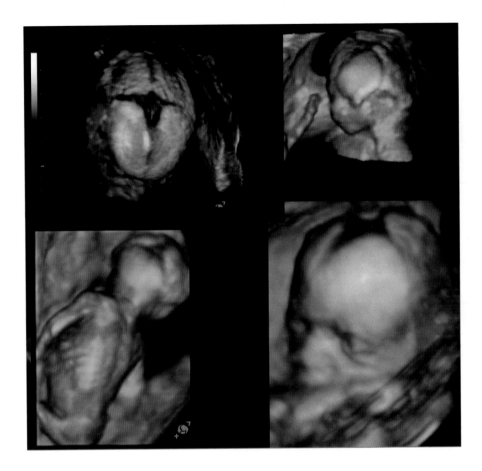

Figure 11.15 Visualization of fontanels and cranial sutures in 3D

maximum mode, minimum mode, or X-ray mode), so that the image highlights features of interest. For instance, it may be desired to visualize in great detail the fontanels and the skull sutures, which are usually very difficult to display on a 2D sonogram as they are curved structures (Figure 11.15).

Electronic scalpels

So-called 'electronic scalpels' can be used to remove unfavorable structures adjacent to the ROI (placenta, umbilical cord, limbs, or uterine wall), allowing free access to the region to be rendered[30] (Figure 11.16).

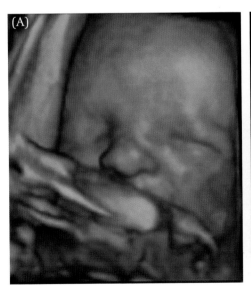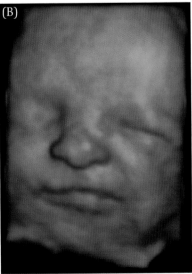

Figure 11.16 (A) Before use of 'electronic scalpels'. (B) After use of 'electronic scalpels' to remove adjacent structures

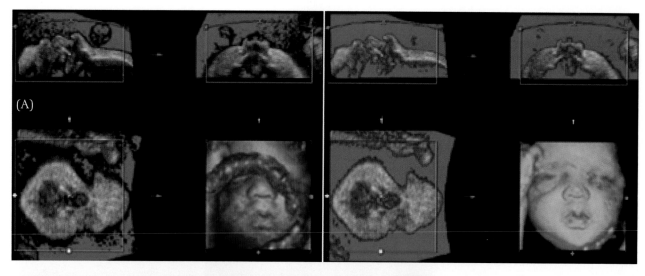

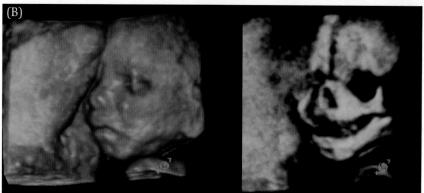

Figure 11.17 By adjusting the threshold level, it is easy to remove adjacent structures such as the umbilical cord (A) or to switch from a surface rendering to a skeleton visualization (B)

Threshold

Another of the settings that can be modified in the 3D reconstruction is the threshold, which can be low or high (Figure 11.17). By adjusting the threshold, it is possible to remove from the 3D reconstruction those echoes whose intensity would be much lower or higher than that of those from the rendered surface.

Transparency

The *transparency* of the reconstruction can also be modified (Figure 11.18) according to the aim of the study.

Volume calculation

The VOCAL mode (<u>v</u>irtual <u>o</u>rgan <u>c</u>omputer aided <u>a</u>na<u>l</u>ysis) is a powerful tool that allows volumetric measurements to be made with great accuracy, which is very helpful in those studies requiring such measurements (Figure 11.19). It offers many possibilities, as well as measurement of the volume contained in the delimited region, it also allows calculation of the area of the surface enclosing that volume. Combined with the Angio 3D mode and application of the Histogram tool, VOCAL allows

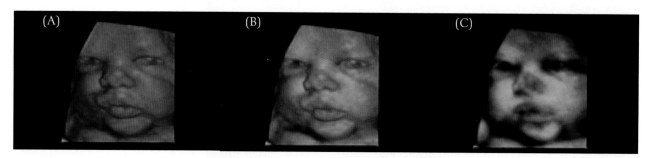

Figure 11.18 (A–C) Different settings of the transparency

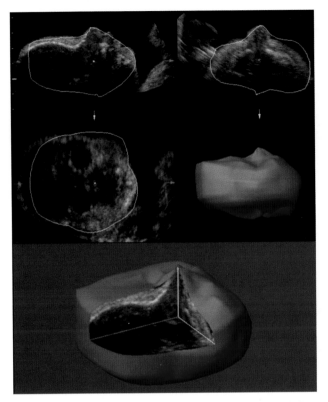

Figure 11.19 Volumentric measurements of fetal face demonstrated using VOCAL mode

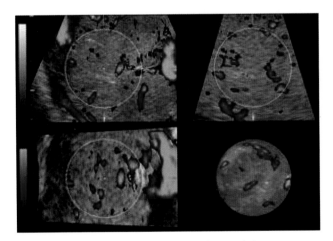

Figure 11.20 Demonstration of placental biopsy using VOCAL mode

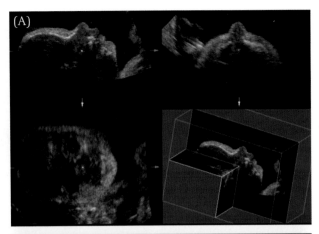

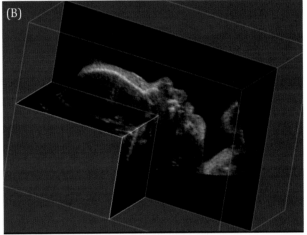

Figure 11.21 (A,B) The 'Niche Mode' allows the viewing of 3 orthogonal planes of fetal face in a stereoscopic view

Niche mode

This is another possibility for 3D display of the information offered by this technology, although, in comparison with the other modalities, it probably has a more limited utility (Figure 11.21).

4D sonography in real time

One of the most exciting developments in 3D visualization is 4D sonography, which has undergone rapid evolution in recent years in terms of progressive improvements in frame rate and image resolution. The latest generation of machines provide a speed of 40 frames/s, allowing visualization almost in real time of fetal movements and an in-depth study of the fascinating world of fetal behaviour (Figure 11.22).[33–38]

It is precisely in the study of the fetal face where 4D sonography may find its most important application, since for the first time it is possible to display in a non-invasive way a wide variety of facial expressions that

study of vascularization in the region under investigation – this had led to the concept of 'vascular biopsy', used by some authors to obtain promising results in the study of the fetus–placental blood circulation[31,32] (Figure 11.20).

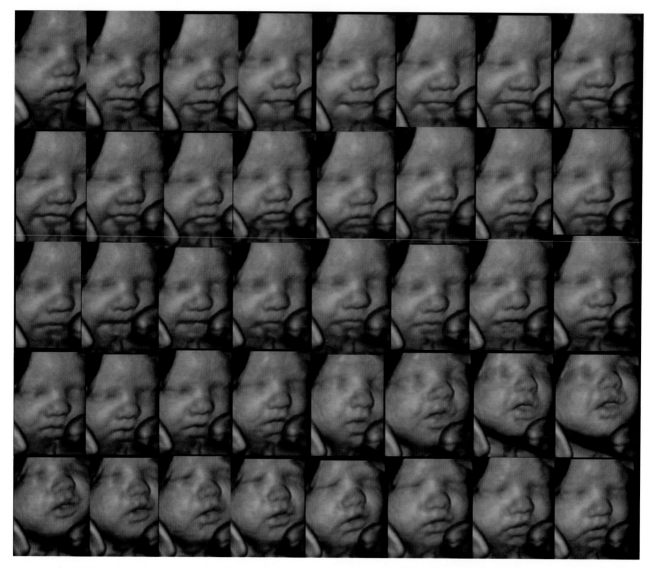

Figure 11.22 In 4D ultrasound, the surface rendering mode provides life-like images almost in real time that are easily comprehended by patients and less-experienced practitioners

could not be shown with conventional 2D sonography. With 4D sonography, it is now feasible to study a full range of facial expressions, including smiling, crying, grimacing, swallowing, sucking, yawning, and eyelid movement[39–41] (Figure 11.23). Nevertheless, as the panel of experts stated in the AIUM Conference on 3D–4D,[25] manufacturers must be encouraged to make 3D ultrasound systems faster and able to display images completely in real time. With no doubt, this goal will be reached in the next few years.

Volume contrast imaging

Volume contrast imaging (VCI) is a 'thick-slice' imaging technique that utilizes 4D probes to acquire a slice of tissue continuously and rapidly in 2D images with enhanced contrast resolution. A special rendering process is performed on the acquired volume data in real-time. The rendering algorithm processes texture, maximum gradient, and transparency parameters. VCI provides more information (from multiple slices) and is of great help in gaining contrast due to an improved signal-to-noise ratio (Figure 11.24).

There are two modes of VCI: VCI-A, where the slice is obtained in the same plane (the *A*-plane) in which the 2D image is being observed, and VCI-C (coronal), which utilizes the same technology but where instead of a longitudinal thick slice, a coronal (C-plane) thick-slice view is presented.

This technique is probably more useful in the study of fetal organs and in gynecologic or breast sonography, although we have employed it for the display of

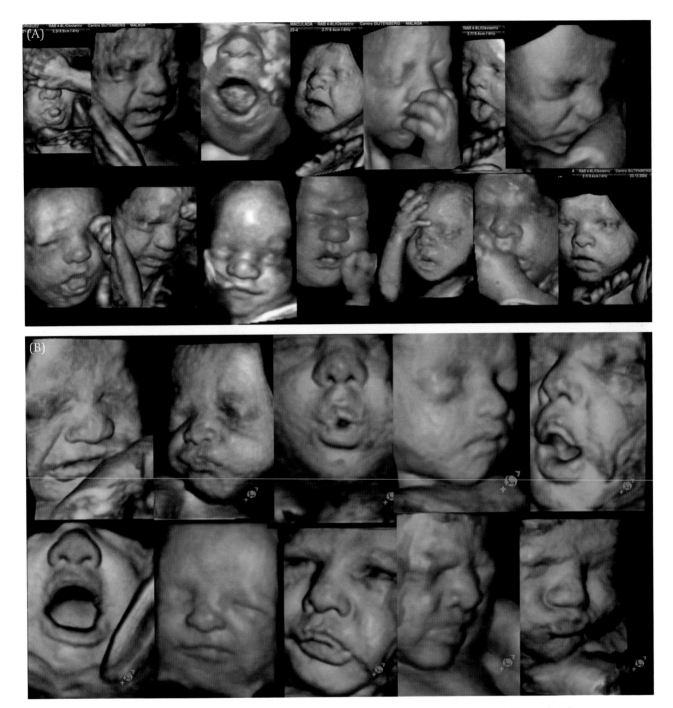

Figure 11.23 (A,B) With 3D and 4D sonography, it is possible to observe the wide range of different facial expressions in a very realistic way not available before with 2D techniques

the corpus callosum in those cases in which it is difficult to obtain a sagittal view of the fetal head, because it is squeezed into the maternal pelvis. In these cases, once we have displayed an axial view of the head similar to that used for measurement of the biparietal diameter, it is very easy to activate the VCI-C mode and place the exploration line over the middle line of the fetal head, achieving immediate visualization of

the corpus callosum in the coronal plane (Figure 11.25).

Multislice view or tomographic ultrasound imaging

These image display modes and algorithms have recently become commercially available. Both, multislice view (Accuvix, Medison, Seoul, Korea) and

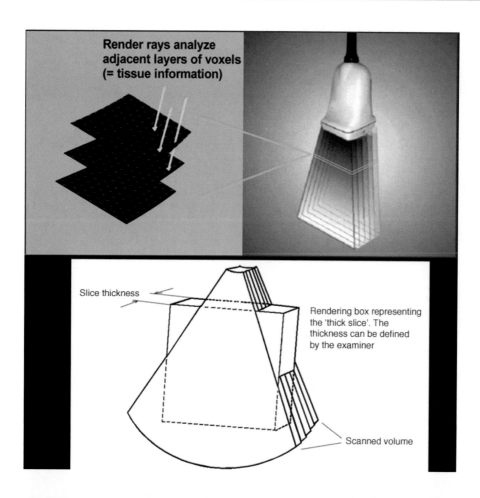

Figure 11.24 Volume contrast imaging (VCI)

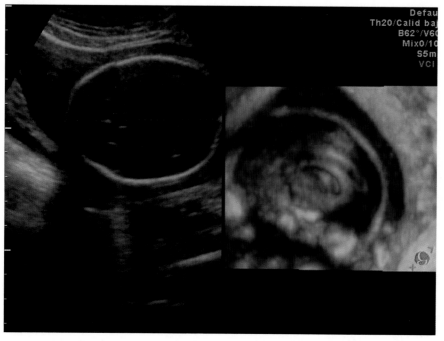

Figure 11.25 With the use of the VCI-C mode in the coronal plane of the head, it is easy to visualize the corpus callosum on a sagittal view

tomographic ultrasound imaging (TUI: Voluson 730, GE Healthcare, Kretztechnik, Zipf, Austria) automatically slice 3D volume datasets and display series of nine or more parallel tomographic images on the screen, similar to the display methods traditionally used in X-ray computed tomography (CT) and MRI.[42]

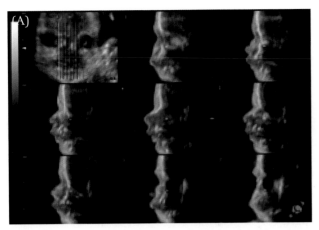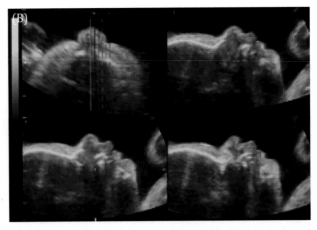

Figure 11.26 Sagittal view of the fetal face using the TUI mode: (A) with 3 mm distance between slices to visualize the central region of the face; (B) with a 2.3 mm distance between slices in a 3-slice display. In this figure and in Figures 11.27–11.29, the upper left image in each set is the reference image, with the vertical lines representing each of the displayed slices

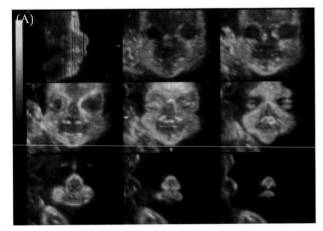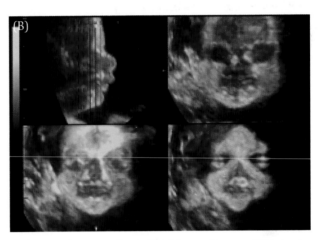

Figure 11.27 TUI display of the facial coronal view: (A) a 2.8 mm distance between slices; (B) 4.2 mm distance. This image display mode allows very nice visualization of several features on the same screen (e.g., orbits, bones, eyelids, nose, and lips)

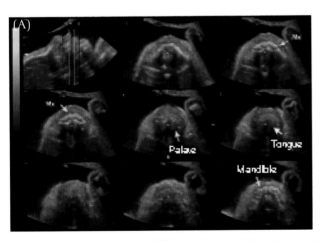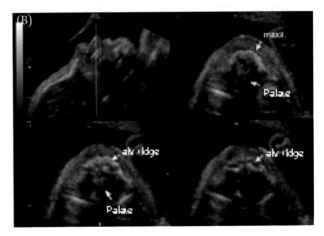

Figure 11.28 TUI display of the axial view of the face at the mouth level. In (A) the distance between slices was 1.9 mm, which was enough to evaluate the integrity of the maxilla (Mx), palate, and mandible. In (B), the distance was 1.7 mm and only three slices were displayed in order to focus attention on the maxilla

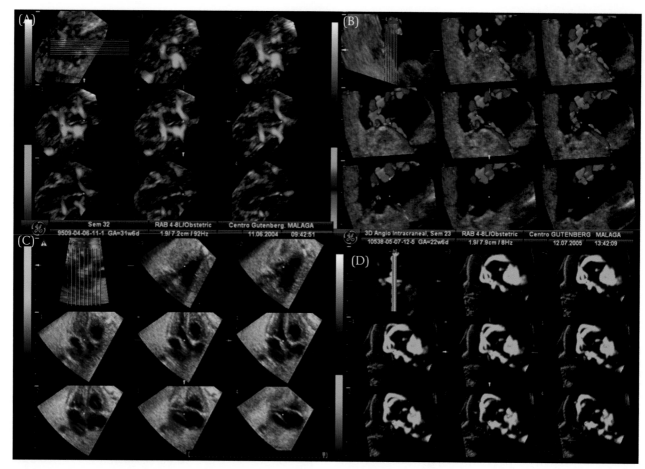

Figure 11.29 The TUI display can be combined with postprocessing techniques, such as C; spatiotemporal image correlation (STIC), B; color Doppler, and A,D; angio 3D

We have some experience with the TUI modality, and we believe that it makes analysis and documentation of dynamic studies easier by providing a simultaneous view of multiple slices of a volume dataset. It provides many management possibilities and simultaneous analysis of 3–20 adjacent slices whose separation can be selected in steps of 0.1 mm. It is even possible to display on the same screen as many as nine of these slices (Figures 11.26–11.28).

In addition, TUI can be combined with other features, including spatiotemporal image correlation (STIC), color Doppler, and angio 3D (Figure 11.29).

These are some of the possibilities offered nowadays by this technology. Every year new tools appear to facilitate and improve the resources available in prenatal sonography. Some of these new techniques have a practical application limited to specific aspects of the sonographic examination, while others have a wide range of applicability. Our approach has been to incorporate them gradually into our daily practice and acquire enough experience to establish their appropriate areas of application.

We shall now list the possible benefits or advantages that can be obtained with the incorporation of 3D and 4D sonography into routine prenatal sonography in general and the study of the fetal face in particular.

CONTRIBUTIONS OR BENEFITS OF 3D SONOGRAPHY IN THE MORPHOLOGIC STUDY OF THE FETAL FACE

In the growing literature on this subject, much data can be found illustrating the several benefits and additional contributions of 3D and 4D sonography in prenatal diagnosis.[43–50]

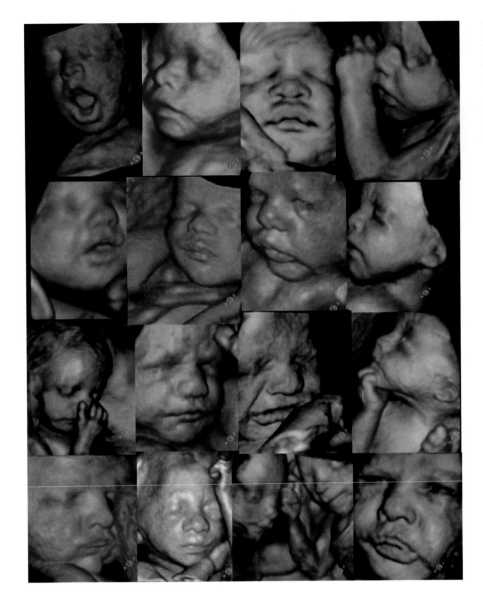

Figure 11.30 Some of the fetal facial images obtained by the authors over the last few years. Even with the earliest commercially available equipment for 4D imaging, some years ago, we obtained very high-quality images, albeit not in all cases. With the great improvements in equipment and experience gained since then, it has now become possible to obtain high-quality images in most examinations

Depiction of fetal anatomy in realistic images

3D sonography offers perspectives that cannot be obtained with 2D techniques and depicts the anatomy in its most appropriate and comprehensive position.[19,51] This standardized display of images helps to provide a better understanding of fetal anatomy both for parents and for less-experienced doctors. Because of its curvature and small anatomic details, the fetal face can be visualized and analyzed only to a limited extent with 2D sonography. The entire face cannot be seen on a single image. 3D sonography provides a spatial reconstruction of the fetal face and simultaneous visualization of all facial structures such as the nose, eyebrows, mouth, and eyelids (Figure 11.30).

Improved identification of anomalies

3D sonography is of great help in the identification of anomalies, since images can be obtained in orientations and planes that are very difficult or impossible with conventional 2D sonography. Several authors have reported improved visualization of the fetal face and neck in pregnancies at high risk for dysmorphic syndromes because of exposure to teratogens (e.g., phenytoin), fetal alcohol syndrome, and chromosomal abnormalities. Cleft lips, micrognathia, malformed ears, and frontal bossing have all been reported to be better displayed and analyzed by 3D sonography.[24,47–49,52–68]

In this context, multiplanar navigation provides invaluable help, allowing re-evaluation of the whole

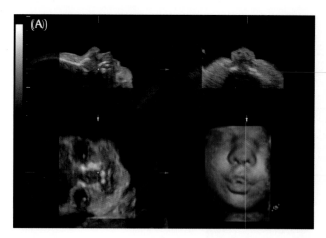 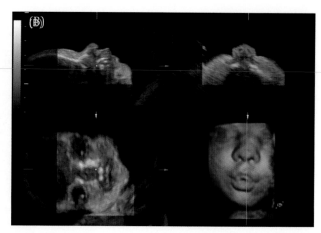

Figure 11.31 These images illustrate how the use of 3D rendering can aid in exact positioning with regard to the midline of the fetal face. Thus, in (A), although the profile in the *A*-plane may seem to be correct, the green reference line superimposed on the rendered image shows that the profile is actually displaced to the left of the face. With the application of an appropriate translation, it is then easy to move the reference line to the middle of the face, ensuring that the profile displayed in the *A*-plane corresponds exactly to the profile in the midsagittal plane (B). This same approach can also be adopted, for example, for correct location of the coronal plane, allowing measurement of ocular diameters and interocular distance to assess the degree of hypo- or hypertelorism

volume, millimeter by millimeter, in the three spatial planes, and navigation through all of the fetal anatomy, visualizing all the facial features from different angles. Some morphogic anomalies are very subtle; consequently, their accurate evaluation must be performed from the most suitable plane, depending on the aim of the assessment. Sometimes, the fetal position or the conditions of the exploration prevent appropriate slices being obtained in the 2D examination. In these cases, with appropriate rotations and translations, it is possible to move through the 3D volume until the target plane is reached.

This possibility offered in general by 3D sonography and particularly by multiplanar navigation has contributed to improving or extending the study of certain morphologic alterations of the fetus in comparison with 2D sonography.

In a recent review of this literature by Gonçalves et al,[69] they found several references reporting diagnostic improvement with the use of 3D sonography.[49,56,59,71–73] Although this advantage is not overwhelming, it certainly extends the initial 2D diagnosis in a number of ways.

One of the most important advantages of 3D sonography is its ability to display a true midsagittal plane of the fetal face[74] (Figure 11.31).

Merz et al[59] analyzed the effect of 3D facial profile reconstruction on 125 fetuses. They found that 30.4% of the profiles were turned 3°–20° from the correct one. Therefore, in only 69.6% of the cases was the true

profile obtained with 2D ultrasound. These findings are of some significance in that it should be borne in mind that when the true middle plane is not identified correctly, anomalies may not be seen or may be overdiagnosed.

In the assessment of anomalies in the midsagittal plane, the important investigations are measurement of the nasofrontal angle, assessment of the ocular biometry and the interorbital distance for the diagnosis of the hyper- or hypotelorism, and assessment of the maxilla and mandible in the diagnosis of micrognathia and retrognathia.[75] Evaluation of the mandible is very important because mandibular anomalies are commonly encountered fetal facial defects[76,77] and are components of more than 100 genetic syndromes,[78] including the Pierre Robin sequence and Treacher–Collins syndrome, and are associated with various chromosomal anomalies such as trisomies 18 and 13, triploidy, and those involving gene deletions or translocations.[78–80]

Fetuses with mandibular anomalies are at risk of acute neonatal respiratory distress syndrome, since the tongue may obstruct the upper airways. There is no strict parallelism between the severity of the anatomic defect and the impairment of respiratory function at birth. Thus, antenatal recognition of even mild cases of mandibular anomalies, is very important, allowing a neonatologist to be present in the delivery room to provide immediate care for the infant and also to prepare everything for ex utero intrapartum treatment (EXIT) if needed.[81]

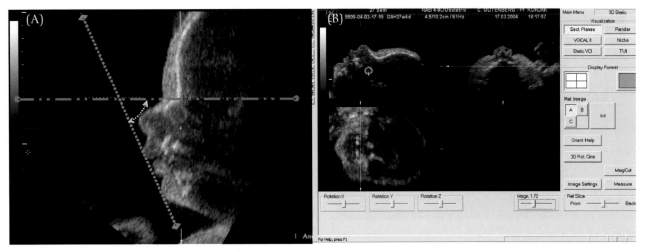

Figure 11.32 (A) Calculating the inferior facial angle, as defined by Rotten et al,[56] on a midsagittal view by crossing of the line orthogonal to the vertical part of the forehead at the level of the synostosis of the nasal bones (reference line in orange), and the line joining the tip of the mentum and the anterior border of the more protruding lip (profile line in green). The cut-off value for the inferior facial angle is 49.2° (mean –2 standard deviations). Any value below this defines retrognathism. (B) This measurement can be made offline by computer-assisted planar navigation through the sagittal plane

Mandibular anomalies are usually diagnosed subjectively by the presence of a prominent upper lip and small chin or a small jaw or posterior displacement of the mandible.[82] Although some attempts have been made to define biometric parameters that would allow an objective distinction between normal and abnormal mandibles,[82,83] they do not differentiate retrognathia (abnormal recession of the chin) from micrognathia (insufficient size of the mandible). In an attempt to apply objective measures to distinguish between these two entities, Rotten et al[77] defined two indices: the inferior facial angle to assess posterior displacement (retrognathia) and the ratio of mandibular width to maxillar width to assess the restriction in size (micrognathia) (Figures 11.32 and 11.33).

Figure 11.34 illustrates the use of the anteroposterior and laterolateral diameters of the mandible for calculation of the jaw index as described by Paladini et al[84] for the diagnosis of micrognathia.

Another possibility offered by multiplanar navigation in the study of the fetal face is scrolling or translation in the coronal plane until the eyelids are

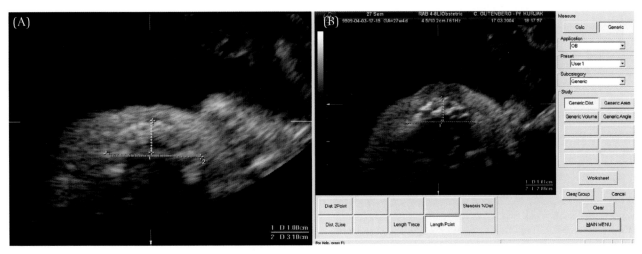

Figure 11.33 Calculation of the mandibular/maxillar width ratio on axial views obtained at the alveolar level as defined by Rotten et al.[77] The mandibular (A) and maxillar (B) widths were measured 10 mm posteriorly to the anterior osteous border (approximately at the level of the canines). The mean value of the mandibular/maxillar width ratio in the 18-28 gestational week interval was 1.017 (SD 0.116). Consequently, a mandibular/maxillar width ratio <0.785 defines micrognathism

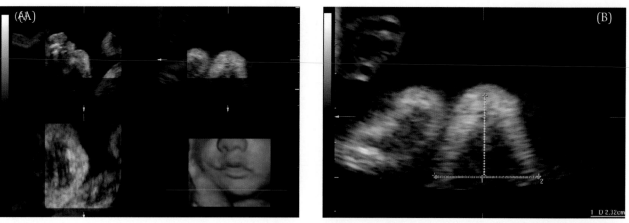

Figure 11.34 Calculation of the jaw index as described by Paladini et al.[84] The fetal mandible is measured in the axial plane at the base of the cranium just caudal to the lower dental arch, where the whole horseshoe mandible is imaged. Anteroposterior and laterolateral diameters are measured as follows: the laterolateral diameter is traced, joining the bases of the two rami; the anteroposterior diameter is measured from the symphysis mentis to the middle of the laterolateral diameter. Care must be taken to obtain the correct plane and to avoid inadvertent partial inclusion of the rami within the calipers. The jaw index is then calculated as anteroposterior mandibular diameter/biparietal diameter × 100

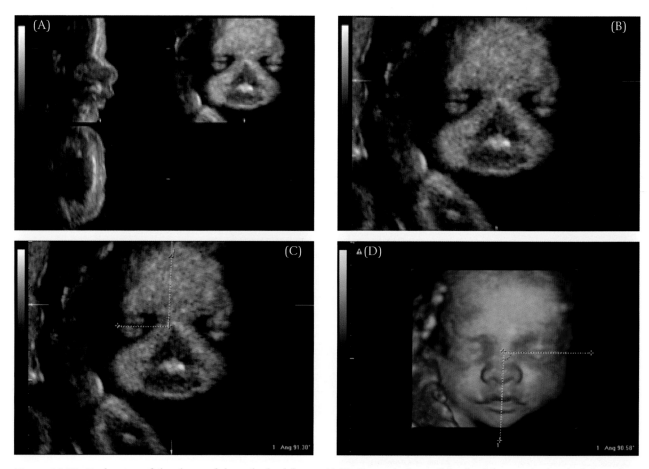

Figure 11.35 Evaluation of the shape of the palpebral fisure. (A,B) Coronal plane of the fetal face at the level of the palpebral fissure. (C,D) Measurement of the angle of slope of the palpebral fissure with respect to the midline of the face: (C) in the coronal plane; (D) in the surface rendering mode (which makes this measurement easier)

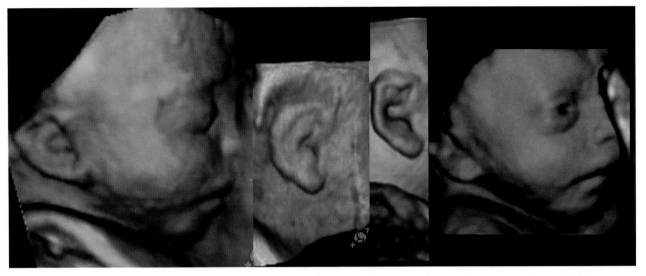

Figure 11.36 Clear visualization of ear morphology by the surface rendering mode. The morphology, location, and orientation of the ear can be checked easily, since the reference points all appear on the same image

reached, in order to evaluate the angle of the palpebral fissure. This is very difficult with 2D sonography, whereas with 3D multiplanar navigation it is simple (Figure 11.35).

It should be emphasized that the measurements and assessments illustrated in Figures 11.31–11.35 were performed on the same volume and took just a matter of seconds, without the patient being present.

It has been shown that 3D sonography can depict in detail the morphology, location, and orientation of the fetal ear.[66] This is important, because anomalous ears may be associated with complex congenital syndromes. 3D surface rendering displays on the same screen all the reference points needed to evaluate the ear position – this cannot be done with 2D sonography because of the curvature of the face (Figure 11.36). As pointed out by Mangione et al,[85] 'Although it is rarely decisive, 3D ultrasound is of interest when it comes to the precise description of craniofacial dysmorphisms and the study of the fetal ears'.

According to Merz et al,[59] 3D sonography is capable of providing a consistent depiction of facial dysmorphology with good accuracy and clarity, particularly in cases with subtle facial abnormalities (Figures 11.37 and 11.38).

Improved assessment of extent and location of fetal anomalies such as cleft lip and palate

Several authors have found 3D sonography useful to identify the location and extent of facial anomalies.[43,44,49,55–57,59–61,63,64,72,86–91]

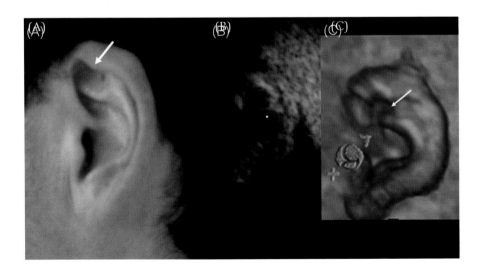

Figure 11.37 Assessment of a subtle auricular dysmorphism with 3D sonography. (A) The ear of the father of the fetus: the previous children had also presented this auricular morphology, and the father wanted his future child to be checked for this feature. (B) The quality of the 2D visualization was sufficient for a broad evaluation of auricular morphology, but the dysmorphism of interest could not be appreciated. (C) It was, hoiwever, clear on a 3D surface rendering

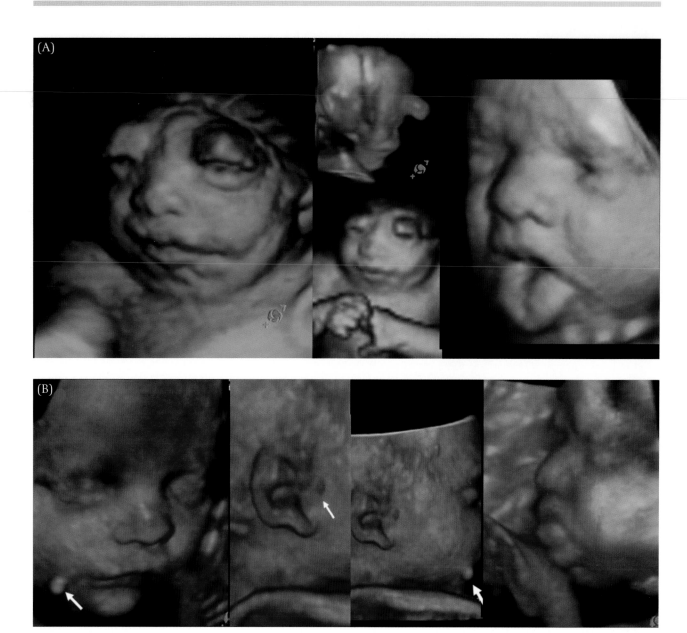

Figure 11.38 It can be seen here how 3D sonography can help to visualize not only severe facial malformations in a realistic way (A), but also subtle dismorphisms such as the small skin tags and the persistent protruding tongue shown in (B) that lead to a diagnosis of macroglossia

Cleft lip and palate is the most common craniofacial malformation; the value of 3D sonography, compared with 2D techniques, for the detection of this anomaly has been studied,[49,55–57,59,64,70,73,92–94] and it has been shown that multiplanar imaging is best used to evaluate the extent of cleaving into the anterior alveolar ridge. Rendered images provide landmarks for the planar images, and are also more easily comprehended and therefore helpful in explaining the abnormality to the family and the consulting surgeon (Figures 11.39 and 11.40). Johnson et al[56] found that 3D sonography has an impact on diagnosis and clinical management, detecting the associated cleft palate much more often than 2D sonography. In 7 of 31 patients, care was affected after the family was shown rendered images of the fetal face.

The TUI display mode can be used for easier analysis and documentation of the defect (Figure 11.41).

Another interesting possibility is to rotate the rendered surface through 180° about the vertical axis

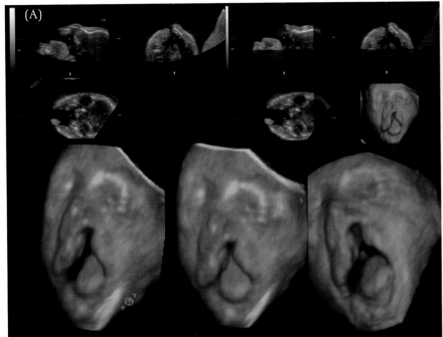

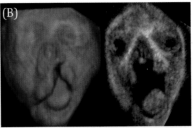

Figure 11.39 Multiplanar navigation in a case of severe unilateral cleft lip and palate. The multiplanar images help to establish the location and extension of the anomaly. The surface rendering mode, is used as being a reference for the multiplanar navigation, also allows one to obtain images that are easy to comprehend, helping parents as well as practitioners to make decisions

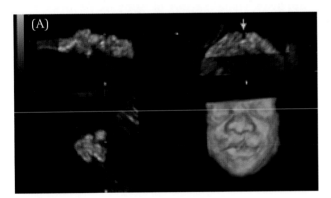

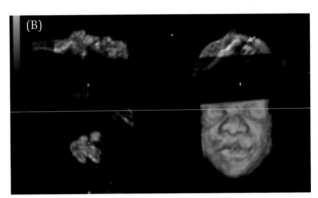

Figure 11.40 (A) Scrolling of the green line through the surface rendering until the location of the upper lip. In the axial plane, a small unilateral cleft lip can be seen (arrow). (B) The green line is moved up to the maxilla; and in the axial plane, a small cleft in the alveolar ridge can be seen (arrow)

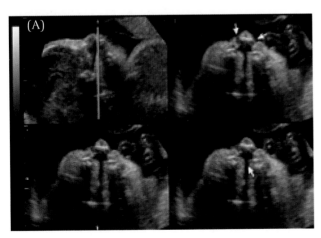

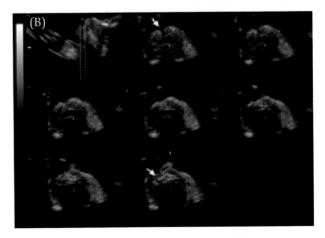

Figure 11.41 (A) TUI display of a bilateral cleft lip and cleft palate (arrows). (B) TUI of this unilateral cleft lip allows easy visualization of the defect and the integrity of the palate on the same screen

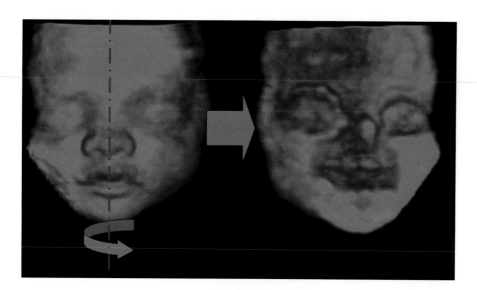

Figure 11.42 It is easy to rotate the rendered image 180° about the vertical axis to obtain the 3D reverse face view

to obtain what has been called by Campbell and co-workers the '3D reverse face view' (Figure 11.42). Campbell and Less[95] obtained interesting results with this approach in the antenatal categorization of facial clefting and in particular clefting of the hard palate. Campbell et al[96] have reported improved categorization of cleft palate using this technique. In our opinion, however, the frequent interposition of structures such as the tongue leads to the appearance of many artifacts, which has an adverse effect on the reproducibility of this technique (Figure 11.43).

Simultaneous visualization of several facial features or anomalies

3D sonography enables the visualization of two or even more anomalies on the same image; using 2D

sonography, at least two different images would be needed[19] (Figure 11.44).

Improved visualization of bony structures

With transparent maximum rendering, the fetal head bones can be visualized very nicely. The threshold level can be modified in order to visualize the facial surface and then the facial bones (Figure 11.45).

Abnormal development of sutures has been associated with dysmorphic syndromes and metabolic disturbances.[97,98] More than 10 years ago, Pretorius and Nelson[99–101] and more recently Faro et al,[102] have shown that 3D sonography offers clearer visualization of cranial structures and bone plates, offering improved understanding of cranial anatomy.[103,104] With 3D, there is improved visualization of 'overlapping' sutures in

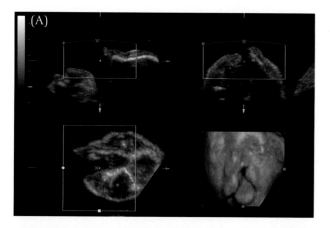

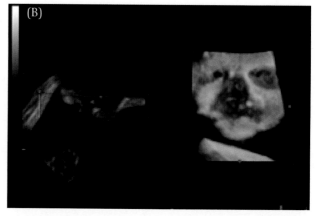

Figure 11.43 (A,B) 3D reverse face view for visualization of a cleft palate. Although Campbell and co-workers[95,96] find this approach quite useful in cases of cleft lip and palate, the frequent interposition of other structures leads to the appearance of artifacts, thus limiting its practical utility

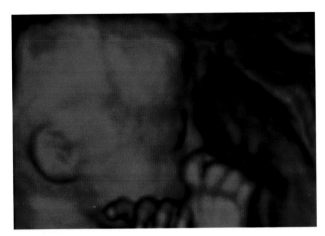

Figure 11.44 One of the benefits of 3D surface rendering is the possibility of simultaneous visualization of several features. In this image, the location and morphology of the ear, one cranial suture, and both hands can be clearly seen together

fetal death and in craniosynostosis or abnormal cranial contours such as cloverleaf skull.[100]

This approach is also very helpful in the evaluation of nasal bones as described by several authors.[105–109]

Offline evaluation and networking

3D sonography offers several options for review of clinical data, which extend beyond those available

with conventional 2D technique.[19] Because the entire volume dataset is saved, physicians and sonographers are able to review the examination findings at a convenient time, even after the patient has been discharged, without loss of information; this has the potential for reducing the duration of the examination and the need for patient callback. The stored data can be reformatted and analyzed in numerous ways. With 3D sonography, numerous arbitrary planes can be shown. Equivocal findings can be scrutinized without pressure of time or any discomfort for the patient, and a second examiner can read and interpret the stored volume independently of the first examiner.[110] Work to date suggests that these postprocessing capabilities make 3D sonography a useful tool in the visualization of normal and abnormal fetal anatomy.[9,29,44,78,87,111–121]

The ability to review volume data and extract diagnostic views also provides new opportunities for 'hands-on' training. Trainees can navigate through saved volume data from cases with abnormalities and test their ability to identify and characterize fetal anomalies.

One of the potential benefits of 3D sonography is the opportunity for networking.[122] This is very important, because interpretation of data from examinations often requires expertise that is usually not available at primary clinical sites. Volumes of data can be copied and stored in digital format, or they can be transferred

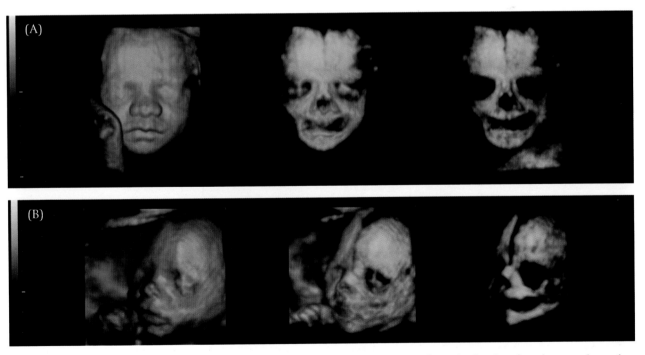

Figure 11.45 (A,B) Simply by modifying the threshold level, it is possible to move from the facial surface down to the underlying skeleton

to the hard disks of workstations through Digital Imaging and Communications in Medicine standard connections. The volume data can be analyzed interactively after the patient has been discharged, facilitating consultation with experts. Volume data can also be compressed and sent over the Internet. This permits clinical data to be obtained at primary care sites and interpreted remotely where sonographic expertise is available.[123]

Volumetric calculation

Another important advantage of 3D sonography is the ability to perform accurate volume measurements.[112–114,116–119,121,124,125]

4D sonography in the assesment of fetal behavior

4D ultrasound has some additional advantages, including the ability to study fetal activity in the surface-rendered mode, and is particularly superior for fast fetal movements.[126]

With 2D sonography, fetal movements such as yawning, swallowing and eyelid movements cannot be displayed simultaneously, while with 4D sonography, simultaneous facial movements can be clearly depicted.[39]

There are several types of jaw movement patterns, such as isolated jaw movement, sucking, and swallowing, which can be observed by 2D sonography.[39,127,128] Observations of facial expressions may be of scientific and diagnostic value, and this approach opens an entirely new field.[129,130] There are many unanswered questions. When do facial expressions start? Which expressions dominate, and at what gestational age do they occur? An important diagnostic aim of the observation of facial expression is prenatal diagnosis of facial paresis. The criterion for the diagnosis is asymmetric facial movement and detection of movements limited to only one side of the face. Unfortunately, during the relaxed phase, it is not possible to evaluate the status of the facial nerve. Therefore, the fetus should be scanned by 4D ultrasound during the active phase.

Since the origin of facial expressions can be external, before a final diagnosis is reached the sonographer should be aware of this pitfall. For example, the force of the fetal hand can alter the facial expression on one side of the face, causing asymmetry. This kind of asymmetry, however, should be differentiated from pathologic features such as unilateral facial paresis.

We believe that the greatest challenges with 4D sonography are in unexplored areas of parental and fetal behavior.[129–134]

2D real-time and 4D sonography are complementary methods used for the evaluation of fetal movements. The quality of each fetal movement can be visualized and evaluated more precisely by 4D

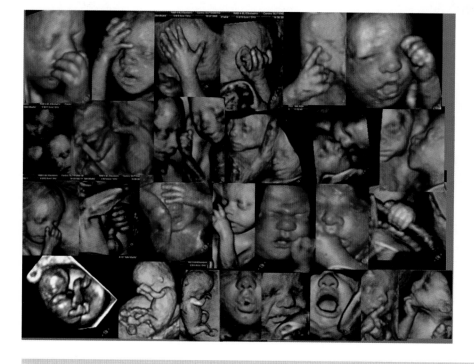

Figure 11.46 3D/4D sonography allows study of fetal behavior from early pregnancy onwards

techniques (Figure 11.46). Our group has been evaluating fetal behavioral patterns in the 3rd trimester between the 30th and 33rd weeks of gestation in 10 pregnancies.[41] The evidence of continuity between fetal and neonatal behavior has been published recently by the Zagreb, Barcelona, and Malaga groups.[37]

Improved maternal–fetal bonding

Several authors have studied the effects of 3D/4D ultrasound on maternal/paternal antenatal attachment.[135,136] Steiner et al[120] have reported that many patients see the 2D image as something abstract whereas on the 3D images they recognize the baby's features (whether or not these are normal), and they can feel more attached to them.

Maier et al[137] looked at the influences of 3D sonography on women with high-risk pregnancy. They offered 3D sonography to 20 high-risk women at 24–32 weeks of pregnancy. After receiving 3D rendered images of their fetuses, 15 of the 20 women thought that 3D sonography had a positive influence on their perception of the fetus. The mothers reported more motivation to endure pregnancy-related difficulties, reduced anxiety, and improved capacity to cope. Pretorius[138] found that this improvement in maternal–fetal bonding can assist mothers in refraining from smoking and other harmful behaviors during pregnancy.

Rustico et al[139] have published a study in which the addition of 4D sonography does not significantly change the perception that women have of their baby nor their antenatal emotional attachment compared with conventional 2D sonography. However, the quality of the 3D acquired images was not taken into account in this study, and we also think the research lacked a valid basis, since a patient can be as satisfied with an isolated 2D examination as a woman undergoing an additional 4D exploration. The appropriate question is whether a patient undergoing a 2D study and then a 4D examination feels different emotions depending on the kind of image. Rustico et al admitted that facial expressions and hand-to-mouth movements were twice as likely to be seen with 4D sonography, although this difference did not reach statistical significance, probably due to the low number of cases analyzed in each group.

In our ultrasound unit we carry out about 11 000 scans every year, performed by nine highly qualified

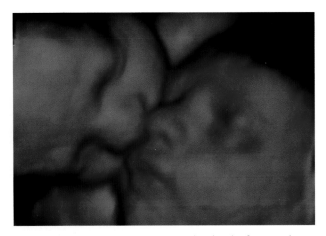

Figure 11.47 In our experience, this kind of image has a clear positive effect in maternal–fetal bonding

practitioners in 2D prenatal sonography and with different levels of expertise in 3D techniques. We started to research this aspect over 2 years ago.[140] We studied the emotional aspects of 302 consecutive 3D examinations performed at our center in 2004 (out of 8500 such examinations carried out in that year). After a 2D ultrasound exploration to detect malformations , a 3D examination between 22 and 34 weeks was performed. After the ultrasound examination, a questionnaire was given to the patient and the relatives attending the examination. Several questions were asked in order to determine the emotional aspects and the level of satisfaction. Among the 302 patients interviewed, 298 (99%) reported beneficial additional aspects with 4D compared with 2D sonography. Of the total number of patients, 210 (69%) pointed out as the principal advantage a stronger feeling of emotion with the 4D image than with the 2D. One hundred and sixty-seven (55%) patients highlighted as the most positive aspect the fact that 4D provided them with an easier interpretation of the images, whereas 136 (45%) patients reported as the most positive characteristic the tightening of the affective bonds with their future child. In summary, in a significant way (99% of our patients), women find positive aspects of undergoing a 4D examination after the 2D one (Figure 11.47). Currently, this study is being extended with several additional parameters, and we are interested in the level of satisfaction with image quality as perceived by the patient in comparison with that perceived by the practitioner or the auxiliary staff in our clinic. We also intend to correlate these data with the level of experience that the doctor has in 3D sonography and the time spent in the acquisition of good images. We have

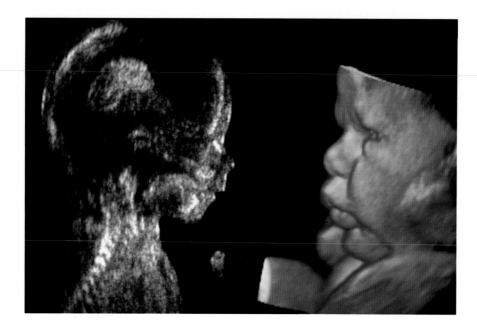

Figure 11.48 These two profiles depicted face to face are among the best achieved in our experience. In the same way, 2D and 3D are often confronted. We strongly believe that they should be used in a complementary way

now collected more than 1000 cases, and in the near future we intend to publish our results, a preliminary analysis of which confirms our earlier finding: the positive assessment made by our patients after the utilization of 3D sonography.

We believe that the positive aspects of 3D/4D sonography in maternal–fetal bonding must not be underestimated, since this represents one of the occasions when we feel closer to our patients from a human point of view. Although medicine does rely to a large extent on statistical data and a scientific basis for its advances, and detractors of 3D sonography can be somewhat critical of the emotional aspects of the 3D image, it is our belief that doctors should transmit humanity as well as science. In this respect, we should sometimes remove our eyes from the screen and glance at our patients' faces to check their emotions when they contemplate these images.

CONCLUSIONS

3D sonography expands our diagnostic abilities in obstetric imaging and provides additional information about the face in ways that are complementary to conventional 2D sonography.[74] It is not only a useful tool in appreciating the severity of a fetal defect, but also provides more convincing evidence of a normal fetus than conventional 2D sonograms in cases with increased risk of a recurrent surface malformation.[89]

This technique does not replace conventional real-time 2D imaging, but rather supplements it (Figure 11.48).[87,141,142] 3D sonography requires an investment of additional time in each case; therefore, it is predominately used (presently in conjunction with 2D sonography) as a problem-solving tool.[123]

As this relatively new technology becomes easier to use and more widely available, recognition of its advantages and clinical utility will likely expand. Numerous investigations have shown the utility of this technique and have defined where and when it is advantageous over conventional 2D sonography.[19,44,89,112–121,143]

Some benefits that may be obtained using 3D sonography are:

- the ability to digitally store and later review an entire volume of ultrasonographic data, even in an automated way[144,145]
- interactive manipulation of volume data to obtain views that are otherwise not obtainable
- correlation of the multiplanar display and rendered images, permitting simultaneous evaluation of cross-sectional views with the rendered image
- display of images in a standardized way, improving understanding of normal and abnormal anatomy
- depiction of fetal anatomy in realistic images, which are more readily comprehended by clinicians and patients
- possible enhancement of maternal–fetal bonding
- improved assessment of the extent and location of fetal anomalies

- accurate volume measurements, which are especially useful for irregular anatomic structures

We agree with Pretorius et al[118] when they affirm that 'although three-dimensional ultrasound will not replace two-dimensional ultrasound, many additional benefits will be identified and its use will continue to grow'.

The specific role and indications for volume sonography are emerging with ongoing clinical studies and there is an urgent need for randomized control studies,[146] but there is little doubt that 3D sonography will have an impact on medical practice.[147,148] It is anticipated that in the future primary clinical sites in remote areas will have access to expert consultation and interpretation offline, promoting high-quality, cost-effective medical care.[123]

4D sonography has an enormous potential in perinatal research and should assist us in better understanding the development of the early embryo and the fetus.

The continuous emergence of new modalities in 3D sonography forces us to a constant update and training leading to a long learning curve. To reduce the length of this curve and for the technique to become widely accepted, work must be done by several groups, including manufacturers, to make the 3D ultrasound systems faster and more user-friendly.[25]

In any case, we consider there are already many reasons to encourage those who have not done it yet to try to gain experience with this technique, and they will surely find numerous possibilities of application in their daily work in prenatal diagnosis.

REFERENCES

1. Hegge FN, Prescott GH, Watson PT. Fetal facial abnormalities identified during obstetric sonography. J Ultrasound Med 1986; 5: 679–84.

2. De Meyer V, Zeman W, Palmer CC. The face predicts the brain: diagnostic significance of medial tacial anomalies for holoprosencephaly (archinencephaly). Pediatrics 1964; 34: 256–8.

3. American Institute of Ultrasound in Medicine. AIUM Practice Guide for the Performance of an Antepartum Obstetric Ultrasound Examination. Laurel, MD: American Institute of Ultrasound in Medicine, 2003. Available at: http://www.aium.org/provider/standards/obstetrical.pdf.

4. Baba K. Obstetrics and gynecology. Nippon Rinsho 2004; 62: 807–14.

5. Benacerraf BR, Frigoletto FO, Bieber FR. The fetal face: ultrasound examination. Radiology 1984; 153: 495–7.

6. Hafner E, Sterniste W, Scholler J, Schuchter K, Philip K. Prenatal diagnosis of facial malformations. Prenat Diagn 1997; 17: 51–8.

7. Pilu G, Reece EA, Romero R, et al. Prenatal diagnosis of craniofacial malformations with ultrasonography. Am J Obstet Gynecol 1986; 155: 45–50.

8. Borruto F, Hansmann M, Wladimiroff JW. Fetal Ultrasonography: The Secret Prenatal Life. Chichester, UK: Wiley, 1982.

9. Chervenak FA, Isaacson G, Campbell S. Ultrasound in Obstetrics and Gynecology. Boston, MA: Little, Brown, 1993.

10. Chervenak FA, Isaacson G, Lorber J. Anomalies of the Fetal Head, Neck, and Spine: Ultrasound Diagnosis and Management. Philadelphia, PA: WB Saunders, 1988.

11. Fleischer AC, Romero R, Manning FA, Jeanty P. The Principles and Practice of Ultrasonography in Obstetrics and Gynecology. Norwalk, CT: Appleton and Lange, 1991.

12. Fleischer AC, Manning FA, Jeanty P, Romero R. Sonography in Obstetrics and Gynecology: Principles and Practice. London: Prentice-Hall, 1996.

13. Fleischer AC, James AE. Diagnostic Sonography. Philadelphia, PA: WB Saunders, 1989.

14. Goldstein SR, Timor-Tritsch IE. Ultrasound in Gynecology. New York: Churchill Livingstone, 1995.

15. Hansmann M, Hackeloeer BJ, Staudach A, Wittmann BK. Ultrasound Diagnosis in Obstetrics and Gynecology. Berlin: Springer-Verlag, 1986.

16. Jeanty P, Romero R. Obstetrical Ultrasound. New York: McGraw-Hill, 1984.

17. Kurjak A, Chervenak FA, eds. Donald School Textbook of Ultrasound in Obstetrics and Gynecology. Boca Raton, FL: Jaypee Brothers Medical Publishers, 2003. New Delhi.

18. Monteagudo A, Timor-Tritsch IE. Fetal face and central nervous system. In Textbook of Fetal Ultrasound. New York: Parthenon, 1999.

19. Nelson TR, Downey DB, Pretorius DH, Fenster A, eds. Three-Dimensional Ultrasound. Philadelphia, PA: Lippincott Williams and Wilkins, 1999: 11–32.

20. Nyberg DA, McGahan JP, Pretorius DH, Pilu G. Diagnostic Imaging of Fetal Anomalies. Philadelphia, PA: Lippincott Williams and Wilkins, 2003.

21. Nyberg DA, Mahony BS, Pretorius D. Diagnostic Ultrasound of Fetal Anomalies: Text and Atlas. Chicago, IL: Year Book, 1990.

22. Romero R, Pilu G, Jeanty P, Ghidini A, Hobbins JC. Prenatal Diagnosis of Congenital Anomalies. Norwalk, CT: Appleton and Lange, 1988.

23. Benacerraf BR. Three-dimensional fetal sonography: use and misuse. J Ultrasound Med 2002; 21: 1063–7.

24. Hata T, Yonehara T, Aoki S, et al. Three-dimensional sonographic visualization of the fetal face. AJR Am J Roentgenol 1998; 170: 481–3.

25. Benacerraf BR, Benson CB, Abuhamad AZ, et al. Three- and 4-dimensional ultrasound in obstetrics and gynecology: Proceedings of the American Institute of Ultrasound in Medicine Consensus Conference. J Ultrasound Med 2005; 24: 1587–97.

26. Timor-Tritsch IE, Platt LD. Three-dimensional ultrasound experience in obstetrics. Curr Opin Obstet Gynecol 2002; 14: 569–75.

27. Nelson TR, Pretorius DH, Riccabona M, Sklansky MS, James G. Sources and impact of artifacts on clinical three-dimensional ultrasound imaging. Ultrasound Obstet Gynecol 2000; 16: 374–83.

28. Riccabona M, Pretorius DH, Nelson TR, Johnson D, Budorick NE. Three-dimensional ultrasound: display modalities in obstetrics. J Clin Ultrasound 1997; 25: 157–67.

29. Matsumoto M, Yanagihara T, Hata T. Three-dimensional qualitative sonographic evaluation of fetal soft tissue. Hum Reprod 2000; 15: 2438–42.

30. Merz E, Miric-Tesanic D, Welter C. Value of the electronic scalpel (cut mode) in the evaluation of the fetal face. Uttrasound Obstet Gynecol 2000; 16: 564–8.

31. Merce LT, Barco MJ, Bau S, Kupesic S, Kurjak A. Assessment of placental vascularization by three-dimensional power doppler 'vascular biopsy' in normal pregnancies. Croat Med J 2005; 46: 765–71.

32. Mercé LT, Barco MJ, Bau S. Reproducibility of the study of placental vascularization by three-dimensional power Doppler. J Perinat Med 2004; 32: 228–33.

33. Andonotopo W, Medic M, Salihagic-Kadic A, et al. The assessment of fetal behavior in early pregnancy: comparison between 2D and 4D sonographic scanning. J Perinat Med 2005; 33: 406–14.

34. Andonotopo W, Stanojevic M, Kurjak A, Azumendi G, Carrera JM. Assessment of fetal behavior and general movements by four-dimensional sonography. Ultrasound Rev Obstet Gynecol 2004; 4: 103–14.

35. Kurjak A, Stanojevic M, Andonotopo W, et al. Fetal behaviour assessed in all three trimesters of normal pregnancy by 4D ultrasonography. Croat Med J 2005; 46: 772–80.

36. Kurjak A, Pooh RK, Carrera JM, et al. Structural and functional early human development assessed by 3D and 4D sonography. Fertil Steril 2005; 84: 1285–99.

37. Kurjak A, Stanojevic M, Andonotopo W, et al. Behavioral pattern continuity from prenatal to postnatal life – a study by four-dimensional (4D) ultrasonography. J Perinat Med 2004; 32: 346–53.

38. Salihagic-Kadic A, Kurjak A, Medic M, Andonotopo W, Azumendi G. New data about embryonic and fetal neurodevelopment and behavior obtained by 3D and 4D sonography. J Perinat Med 2005; 33: 478–90.

39. Kozuma S, Baba K, Okai T, Taketani Y. Dynamic observation of the fetal face by three-dimensional ultrasound. Ultrasound Obstet Gynecol 1999; 13: 283–4.

40. Roodenburg PJ, Vladimiroff IW, van Es A, Prechtl HFR. Classification and quantitative aspect of tetal movements during the second half of normal pregnancy. Early Hum Dev 1991; 25: 19–35.

41. Kurjak A, Azumendi G, Vecek N, et al. Fetal hand movements and facial expression in normal pregnancy studied by four-dimensional sonography. J Perinat Med 2003; 31: 496–508.

42. Leung KY, Ngai CS, Chan BC, et al. Three-dimensional extended imaging: a new display modality for three-dimensional ultrasound examination. Ultrasound Obstet Gynecol 2005; 26: 244–51.

43. Hamper UM, Trapanotto V, Sheth S, DeJong MR, Caskey CI. Three-dimensional US: preliminary clinical experience. Radiology 1994; 191: 397–401.

44. Merz E, Bahlmann F, Weber G. Volume scanning in the evaluation of fetal malformations: a new dimension in prenatal diagnosis. Ultrasound Obstet Gynecol 1995; 5: 222–7.

45. Merz E, Bahlmann F, Weber G, Macchiella D. Three-dimensional ultrasonography in prenatal diagnosis. J Perinat Med 1995; 23: 213–22.

46. Merz E, Miric-Tesanic D. Current status of three-dimensional ultrasonography in prenatal diagnosis. Perinatology 2000; 2: 55–60.

47. Paladini D, Vassallo M, Sglavo G, et al. Cavernous lymphangioma of the face and neck: prenatal diagnosis by three-dimensional ultrasound. Ultrasound Obstet Gynecol 2005; 26: 300–2.

48. Petrikovsky BM, Kaplan GP. Fetal dacryocystocele: comparing 2D and 3D imaging. Pediatr Radiol 2003; 33: 582–3.

49. Pretorius DH, House M, Nelson TR, Hollenbach KA. Evaluation of normal and abnormal lips in fetuses: comparison between three- and two-dimensional sonography. AJR Am J Roentgenol 1995; 165: 1233–7.

50. Wang CJ, Yen CF, Masrani MR, et al. Three-dimensional ultrasonic images of normal fetus. Chang Gung Med J 2001; 24: 476–82.

51. Rotten D, Levaillant JM. Two- and three-dimensional sonographic assessment of the fetal face. 1. A system-

atic analysis of the normal face. Ultrasound Obstet Gynecol 2004; 23: 224–31.

52. Boog G, Le Vaillant C, Winer N, et al. Contribution of tridimensional sonography and magnetic resonance imaging to prenatal diagnosis of Apert syndrome at mid-trimester. Fetal Diagn Ther 1999; 14: 20–3.

53. Candiani F. The latest in ultrasound: three-dimensional imaging. Eur J Radiol 1998; 27: 179–82.

54. Hsu TY, Chang SY, Ou CY, et al. First trimester diagnosis of holoprosencephaly and cyclopia with triploidy by transvaginal three-dimensional ultrasonography. Eur J Obstet Gynecol Reprod Biol 2001; 96: 235–7.

55. Hull AD, Pretorius DH. Fetal face: what we can see using two-dimensional and three-dimensional ultrasound imaging. Semin Roentgenol 1998; 33: 369–74.

56. Johnson DD, Pretorius DH, Budorick NE, et al. Fetal lip and primary palate: three-dimensional versus two-dimensional US. Radiology 2000; 217: 236–9.

57. Lee A, Deutinger J, Bernaschek G. Three dimensional ultrasound: abnormalities of the fetal face in surface and volume rendering mode. Br J Obstet Gynaecol 1995; 102: 302–6.

58. Lin HH, Liang RI, Chang FM, et al. Prenatal diagnosis of otocephaly using two-dimensional and three-dimensional ultrasonography. Ultrasound Obstet Gynecol 1998; 11: 361–3.

59. Merz E, Weber G, Bahlmann F, Miric-Tesanic D. Application of transvaginal and abdominal three-dimensional ultrasound for the detection or exclusion of malformations of the fetal face. Ultrasound Obstet Gynecol 1997; 9: 237–43.

60. Mueller GM, Weiner CP, Yankowitz J. Three-dimensional ultrasound in the evaluation of fetal head and spine anomalies. Obstet Gynecol 1996; 88: 372–8.

61. Nelson TR, Pretorius DH. Three-dimensional ultrasound of fetal surface features. Ultrasound Obstet Gynecol 1992; 2: 166–74.

62. Platt LO, Santulli T Jr, Carlson DE, Greene N, Walla CA. Three-dimensional ultrasonography in obstetrics and gynecology: preliminary experience. Am J Obstet Gynecol 1998; 178: 1199–206.

63. Pretorius DH, Richards RD, Budorick NE, et al. Three-dimensional ultrasound in the evaluation of fetal anomalies. Radiology 1997; 205(P)(Suppl): 245.

64. Pretorius DH, Nelson TR. Fetal face visualization using three-dimensional ultrasonography. J Ultrasound Med 1995; 14: 349–56.

65. Pretorius DH, Nelson TR. Prenatal visualization of cranial sutures and fontanelles with three-dimensional ultrasonography. Ultrasound Obstet Gynecol 1995; 5: 219–21.

66. Shih JC, Shyu MK, Lee CN, et al. Antenatal depiction of the fetal ear with three-dimensional ultrasonography. Obstet Gynecol 1998; 91: 500–5.

67. Sivan E, Chan L, Uerpairojkit B, Chu G, Reece A. Growth of the fetal forehead and normative dimensions developed by three-dimensional ultrasonographic technology. J Ultrasound Med 1997; 16: 401–5.

68. Van Wymersch O, Favre R, Gasser B. Use of three-dimensional ultrasound to establish the prenatal diagnosis of Fryns syndrome. Fetal Diagn Ther 1996; 11: 335–40.

69. Gonçalves LF, Lee W, Espinoza J, Romero R. Three- and 4-dimensional ultrasound in obstetric practice: does it help? J Ultrasound Med 2005; 24: 1599–624.

70. Chen ML, Chang CH, Yu CH, Cheng YC, Chang FM. Prenatal diagnosis of cleft palate by three-dimensional ultrasound. Ultrasound Med Biol 2001; 27: 1017–23.

71. Chmait R, Pretorius D, Jones M, et al. Prenatal evaluation of facial clefts with two-dimensional and adjunctive three-dimensional ultrasonography: a prospective trial. Am J Obstet Gynecol 2002; 187: 946–9.

72. Mittermayer C, Blaicher W, Brugger PC, Bernaschek G, Lee A. Foetal facial clefts: prenatal evaluation of lip and primary palate by 2D and 3D ultrasound. Ultraschall Med 2004; 25: 120–5.

73. Ulm MR, Kratochwil A, Ulm B, et al. Three-dimensional ultrasonographic imaging of fetal tooth buds for characterization of facial clefts. Early Hum Dev 1999; 55: 67–75.

74. Lee W, McNie B, Chaiworapongsa T, et al. Three-dimensional ultrasonographic presentation of micrognathia. J Ultrasound Med 2002; 21: 775–8.

75. Radlanski RJ, Renz H, Klarkowski MC. Prenatal development of the human mandible. 3D reconstructions, morphometry and bone remodelling pattern, sizes 12–117 mm CRL. Anat Embryol (Berl) 2003; 207: 221–32.

76. Tsai MY, Lan KC, Ou CY, et al. Assessment of the facial features and chin development of fetuses with use of serial three-dimensional sonography and the mandibular size monogram in a Chinese population. Am J Obstet Gynecol 2004; 190: 541–6.

77. Rotten D, Levaillant JM, Martinez H, Ducou le Pointe H, Vicaut E. The fetal mandible: a 2D and 3D sonographic approach to the diagnosis of retrognathia and micrognathia. Ultrasound Obstet Gynecol 2002; 19: 122–30.

78. Jones KL. Smith's Recognizable Patterns of Human Malformation, 5th edn. London: WB Saunders, 1997.

79. Nicolaides KH, Salvesen DR, Snijders RJM, Gosden CM. Fetal facial defects: associated malformations and chromosomal abnormalities. Fetal Diagn Ther 1993; 8: 1–9.

80. Turner GM, Twining P. The facial profile in the diagnosis of fetal abnormalities. Clin Radiol 1993; 47: 389–95.

81. Shih JC, Hsu WC, Chou HC, et al. Prenatal three-dimensional ultrasound and magnetic resonance imaging evaluation of a fetal oral tumor in preparation for the ex-utero intrapartum treatment (EXIT) proce-dure. Ultrasound Obstet Gynecol 2005; 25: 76–9; discussion 79.

82. Otto C, Platt LD. The fetal mandible: measurement and objective determination of fetal jaw size. Ultrasound Obstet Gynecol 1991; 1: 12–17.

83. Laitinen SH, Ranta RE. Cephalometric measurements in patients with Pierre Robin syndrome and isolated cleft papate. Scand J Plast Reconstr Hand Surg 1992; 26: 177–83.

84. Paladini D, Morra T, Teodoro A, et al. Objective diagnosis of micrognatia in the fetus: the Jaw Index. Obstet Gynecol 1999; 93: 382–6.

85. Mangione R, Lacombe D, Carles D, et al. Craniofacial dysmorphology and three-dimensional ultrasound: a prospective study on practicability for prenatal diagno-sis. Prenat Diagn 2003; 23: 810–18.

86. Chen CP, Shih JC, Hsu CY, et al. Prenatal three-dimensional/four-dimensional sonographic demonstra-tion of facial dysmorphisms associated with holoprosencephaly. J Clin Ultrasound 2005; 33: 312–8.

87. Devonald KJ, Ellwood DA, Griffiths KA, et al. Volume imaging: three-dimensional appreciation of the fetal head and face. J Ultrasound Med 1995; 14: 919–25.

88. Lai TH, Chang CH, Yu CH, Kuo PL, Chang FM. Prenatal diagnosis of alobar holoprosencephaly by two-dimensional and three-dimensional ultrasound. Prenat Diagn 2000; 20: 400–3.

89. Merz E, Welter C. 2D and 3D ultrasound in the evalu-ation of normal and abnormal fetal anatomy in the second and third trimesters in a level III center. Ultraschall Med 2005; 26: 9–16.

90. Pretorius DH, Johnson DD, Budorick NE, et al. Three-dimensional ultrasound of the fetal lip and palate. Radiology 1997; 205(P)(Suppl): 245.

91. Xu HX, Zhang QP, Lu MD, Xiao XT. Comparison of two-dimensional and three-dimensional sonography in evaluating fetal malformations. J Clin Ultrasound. 2002; 30: 515–25.

92. Lee W, Kirk JS, Shaheen KW, et al. Fetal cleft lip and palate detection by three-dimensional ultrasonography. Ultrasound Obstet Gynecol 2000; 16: 314–20.

93. Rotten D, Levaillant JM. Two- and three-dimensional sonographic assessment of the fetal face. 2. Analysis of cleft lip, alveolus and palate. Ultrasound Obstet Gynecol 2004; 24: 402–11.

94. Tonni G, Centini G, Rosignoli L. Prenatal screening for

fetal face and clefting in a prospective study on low-risk population: Can 3- and 4-dimensional ultrasound enhance visualization and detection rate? Oral Surg Oral Med Oral Pathol Oral Radiol Endod 2005; 100: 420–6.

95. Campbell S, Lees CC. The three-dimensional reverse face (3D RF) view for the diagnosis of cleft palate. Ultrasound Obstet Gynecol 2003; 22: 552–4.

96. Campbell S, Lees C, Moscoso G, Hall P. Ultrasound antenatal diagnosis of cleft palate by a new technique: the 3D 'reverse face' view. Ultrasound Obstet Gynecol 2005; 25: 12–8.

97. Benacerraf BR, Spiro R, Mitchell AG. Using three-dimensional ultrasound to detect craniosynostosis in a fetus with Pfeiffer syndrome. Ultrasound Obstet Gynecol 2000; 16: 391–4.

98. Ginath S, Debby, A, Malinger G. Demonstration of cranial sutures and fontanelles at 15 to 16 weeks of gestation: a comparison between two-dimensional and three-dimensional ultrasonography. Prenat Diagn 2004; 24: 812–15.

99. Pretorius DH, Nelson TR. Prenatal visualization of cranial sutures and fontanelles with three-dimensional ultrasonography. J Ultrasound Med 1994; 13: 871–6.

100. Pretorius DH, Nelson TR. Three-dimensional ultra-sound. J Ultrasound Med 1994; 13: 871–6.

101. Pretorius DH, Nelson TR. Three-dimensional ultra-sound. Ultrasound Obstet Gynecol 1995; 5: 219–21.

102. Faro C, Benoit B, Wegrzyn P, Chaoui R, Nicolaides KH. Three-dimensional sonographic description of the fetal frontal bones and metopic suture. Ultrasound Obstet Gynecol 2005; 26: 618–21.

103. Chaoui R, Levaillant JM, Benoit B, et al. Three-dimen-sional sonographic description of abnormal metopic suture in second- and third-trimester fetuses. Ultrasound Obstet Gynecol 2005; 26: 761–4.

104. Dikkeboom CM, Roelfsema NM, Van Adrichem LN, Wladimiroff JW. The role of three-dimensional ultra-sound in visualizing the fetal cranial sutures and fontanels during the second half of pregnancy. Ultrasound Obstet Gynecol 2004; 24: 412–16.

105. Benoit B, Chaoui R, Three-dimensional ultrasound with maximal mode rendering: a novel technique for the diagnosis of bilateral or unilateral absence or hypoplasia of nasal bones in second-trimester screening for Down syndrome. Ultrasound Obstet Gynecol 2005; 25: 19–24.

106. Gonçalves LF, Espinoza J, Lee W, et al. Phenotypic characteristics of absent and hypoplastic nasal bones in fetuses with Down syndrome: description by 3-Dimensional ultrasonography and dinical significance. J Ultrasound Med 2004; 23: 1619–27.

107. Lee W, DeVore GR, Comstock CH, et al. Nasal bone evaluation in fetuses with Down syndrome during the

second and third trimesters of pregnancy. J Ultrasound Med 2003; 22: 55–60.

108. Peralta CF, Falcon O, Wegrzyn P, Faro C, Nicolaides KH. Assessment of the gap between the fetal nasal bones at 11 to 13 + 6 weeks of gestation by three-dimensional ultrasound. Ultrasound Obstet Gynecol 2005; 25: 464–7.

109. Rembouskos G, Cicero S, Longo D, Vandecruys H, Nicolaides K. Assessment of the fetal nasal bone at 11–14 weeks' gestation by three-dimensional ultrasound. Ultrasound Obstet Gynecol 2004; 23: 232–6.

110. Baba K. Development of 3D ultrasound. In: Kurjak A, Chervenak FA, eds. Donald School Textbook of Ultrasound in Obstetrics and Gynecology. Boca Raton, FL: Jaypee Brothers Medical Publishers (P) Ltd. New Delhi: 2003, 27–42.

111. Bonilla-Musoles F, Machado LE, Osborne NG, et al. Ultrasound diagnosis of facial and cephalic pole malformations: comparative study of different three-dimensional modalities and two-dimensional ultrasound. Ultrasound Q 2000; 16: 97–105.

112. Chang FM, Hsu KF, Ko HC, et al. Three-dimensional ultrasound assessment of fetal liver volume in normal pregnancy: a comparison of reproducibility with two-dimensional ultrasound and a search for a volume constant. Ultrasound Med Biol 1997; 23: 381–9.

113. Hosli IM, Tercanli S, Herman A, Kretschmann M, Holzgreve W. In vitro volume measurement by three-dimensional ultrasound: comparison of two different systems. Ultrasound Obstet Gynecol 1998; 11: 17–22.

114. Hughes SW, D'Arcy TJ, Maxwell DJ, et al. Volume estimation from multiplanar 2D ultrasound images using a remote electromagnetic position and orientation sensor. Ultrasound Med Biol 1996; 22: 561–72.

115. Lee A, Kratochwil A, Deutinger J, Bernaschek G. Three-dimensional ultrasound in diagnosing phocomelia. Ultrasound Obstet Gynecol 1995; 5: 238–40.

116. Merz E. 3-D Ultrasound in Obstetrics and Gynecology. Philadelphia, PA: Lippincott Williams and Wilkins, 1998.

117. Nelson TR, Pretorius DH. 3-dimensional ultrasound volume measurement. Med Phys 1993; 201: 927.

118. Pretorius DH, Borok NN, Coffler MS, Nelson TR. Three-dimensional ultrasound in obstetrics and gynecology. Radiol Clin North Am 2001; 39: 499–521.

119. Riccabona M, Nelson TR, Pretorius DH. Three-dimensional ultrasound: accuracy of distance and volume measurements. Ultrasound Obstet Gynecol 1996; 7: 429–34.

120. Steiner H, Staudach A, Spitzer D, Schaffer H. Three-dimensional ultrasound in obstetrics and gynaecology: technique, possibilities and limitations. Hum Reprod 1994; 9: 1773–8.

121. Steiner H, Gregg AR, Bogner G, et al. First trimester three-dimensional ultrasound volumetry of the gestational sac. Arch Gynecol Obstet 1994; 255: 165–70.

122. Nelson TR, Pretorius DH, Lev-Toaff A, et al. Feasibility of performing a virtual patient examination using three-dimensional ultrasonographic data acquired at a remote location. J Ultrasound Med 2001; 20: 941–52.

123. Bega G, Lev-Toaff A, Kuhlman K, et al. Three dimensional ultrasonographic imaging in obstetrics: present and future. J Ultrasound Med 2001; 20: 391–408.

124. Lee W, Gonçalves L, Espinoza J, Romero R. Inversion mode: a new volume analysis tool for 3-dimensional ultrasonography. J Ultrasound Med 2005; 24: 201–7.

125. Wong J, Gerscovich EO, Cronan MS, Seibert JA. Accuracy and precision of in vitro volumetric measurements by three-dimensional sonography. Invest Radiol 1996; 31: 26–9.

126. Lee A. Four-dimensional ultrasound in prenatal diagnosis; leading edge in imaging technology. Ultrasound Rev Obstet Gynecol 2001; 1: 194–8.

127. Levy DS, Zielinsky P, Aramayo AM, et al. Repeatability of the sonographic assessment of fetal sucking and swallowing movements. Ultrasound Obstet Gynecol 2005; 26: 745–9.

128. Troyano JM, Gomez-Frieiro M, Clavijo M. Fetal kinetics: its quantification by transvaginal Doppler ultrasonography. In: Kurjak A, Arenas JB, eds. Donald School Textbook of Transvaginal Sonography. New Delhi: Jaypee Brothers Medical Publishers, 2005: 84–95.

129. Hata T, Kanenishi K, Akiyama M, Tanaka H, Kimura K. Real-time 3-D sonographic observation of fetal facial expression. J Obstet Gynaecol Res 2005; 31: 337–40.

130. Kurjak A, Stanojevic M, Azumendi G, Carrera JM. The potential of four-dimensional (4D) ultrasonography in the assessment of fetal awareness. J Perinat Med 2005; 33: 46–53.

131. Kuno A, Akiyama M, Yamashiro C, et al. Three-dimensional sonographic assessment of fetal behavior in the early second trimester of pregnancy. J Ultrasound Med 2001; 20: 1271–5.

132. Kurjak A, Vecek N, Kupesic S, Azumendi G, Solak M. Four-dimensional sonography: How much does it improve perinatal practice? In: Carrera JM, Kurjak A, Chervenak FA, eds. Controversies in Perinatal Medicine. London: Parthenon, 2003.

133. Kurjak A, Vecek N, Hafner T, et al. Prenatal diagnosis: What does four-dimensional ultrasound add? J Perinat Med 2002; 30: 57–62.

134. Campbell S. 4D or not 4D: that is the question. Ultrasound Obstet Gynecol 2002; 19: 1–4.

135. Ji EK, Pretorius DH, Newton R, et al. Effects of ultrasound on maternal–fetal bonding: a comparison of two- and three-dimensional imaging. Ultrasound Obstet Gynecol 2005; 25: 473–7.

136. Righetti Pl, Dell' Avanzo M, Grigio M, Nicolini U. Maternal/paternal antenatal attachment and fourth-dimensional ultrasound technique: a preliminary report. Br J Psychol 2005; 96: 129–37.

137. Maier B, Steiner H, Wienerroither H, Staudach A. The psychological impact of three-dimensional fetal imaging on the fetomaternal relationship. In: Baba K, Jurkovic D, eds. Three-dimensional Ultrasound in Obstetrics and Gynecology. New York: Parthenon, 1997: 67–74.

138. Pretorius DH. Maternal Smoking Habit Modification via Fetal Visualization. University of California Tobacco Related Disease Research Program. Annual Report to the California State Legislature, 1996: 76.

139. Rustico MA, Mastromatteo C, Grigio M, et al. Two-dimensional vs. two- plus four-dimensional ultrasound in pregnancy and the effect on maternal emotional status: a randomized study. Ultrasound Obstet Gynecol 2005; 25: 468–72.

140. Azumendi G, Comas C, Romero M. Maternal feelings after 3D and 4D obstetrical examination. Lecture in the 1st Course on Advances in Prenatal Diagnosis, Marbella, Spain, 17 June 2005.

141. Downey DB, Fenster A, Williams JC. Clinical utility of three-dimensional US. Radiographics 2000; 20: 559–71.

142. Dyson RL, Pretorius DH, Budorick NE, et al. Three-dimensional ultrasound in the evaluation of fetal anomalies. Ultrasound Obstet Gynecol 2000; 16: 321–8.

143. Baba K, Okai T, Kozuma S, Taketani Y. Fetal abnormalities: evaluation with real-time-processible three-dimensional US – preliminary report. Radiology 1999; 211: 441–6.

144. Abuhamad AZ. Standardization of 3-dimensional volumes in obstetric sonography: a required step for training and automation. J Ultrasound Med 2005; 24: 397–401.

145. Abuhamad A. Automated multiplanar imaging: a novel approach to ultrasonography. J Ultrasound Med 2004; 23: 573–6.

146. Scharf A, Ghazwiny MF, Steinborn A, Baier P, Sohn C. Evaluation of two-dimensional versus three-dimensional ultrasound in obstetric diagnostics: a prospective study. Fetal Diagn Ther 2001; 16: 333–41.

147. Benacerraf BR, Shipp TD, Bromley B. How sonographic tomography will change the face of obstetric sonography: a pilot study. J Ultrasound Med. 2005 Mar; 24: 371–8.

148. Benacerraf B. The future of ultrasound: viewing the dark side of the moon. Ultrasound Obstet Gynecol 2004; 23: 211–15.

12   CNS: Normal anatomy and malformations

Ritsuko K Pooh, Kyong-Hon Pooh, and Asim Kurjak

INTRODUCTION

Imaging technologies have developed remarkably over recent years and have contributed greatly to the prenatal evaluation of fetal central nervous system (CNS) development and the assessment of CNS abnormalities in utero.

Conventional transabdominal sonography, by which it is possible to observe fetuses through the maternal abdominal wall, uterine wall, and sometimes placenta, has been most widely utilized for antenatal imaging diagnosis. With the transabdominal approach, the whole CNS of a fetus can be demonstrated – for instance, the brain in axial section and the spine in sagittal section. However, the transabdominal approach to the fetal CNS encounters several obstacles, such as the maternal abdominal wall, the placenta, and the fetal cranial bones, and it is difficult to obtain clear and detailed images of fetal CNS structure.

The introduction of high-frequency transvaginal transducers has contributed to establishing the field of 'sonoembryology',[1] and the recent general use of transvaginal sonography in early pregnancy has enabled early diagnosis of major fetal anomalies.[2] In middle and late pregnancy, the fetal CNS is generally evaluated through the maternal abdominal wall. The brain, however, is a three-dimensional (3D) structure, and should be assessed in the three basic cutting planes: the sagittal, coronal, and axial sections (Figure 12.1). Sonographic assessment of the fetal brain in sagittal and coronal sections, requires an approach from the fetal parietal direction. Transvaginal sonography of the fetal brain has opened up a new field in medicine: 'neurosonography'.[3] The transvaginal approach to the

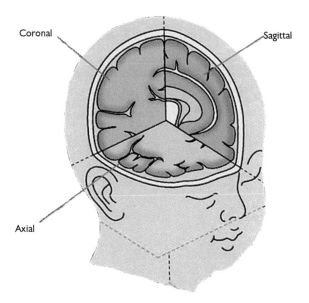

Figure 12.1 The three basic orthogonal cutting planes of the brain. The brain should be understood as a three-dimensional structure. It is important to assess the brain in the three basic planes: the sagittal, coronal, and axial sections

normal fetal brain during the 2nd and 3rd trimesters was introduced at the beginning of 1990s. It was the first practical application of 3D CNS assessment by 2D ultrasound.[4] Transvaginal observation of the fetal brain offers sagittal and coronal views of the brain from the fetal parietal direction[5–8] through the fontanelles and/or the sagittal suture as ultrasound windows. Serial oblique sections[3] via the same ultrasound window reveal the intracranial morphology in detail. This method has contributed to the prenatal assessment of congenital CNS anomalies and acquired brain damage in utero.

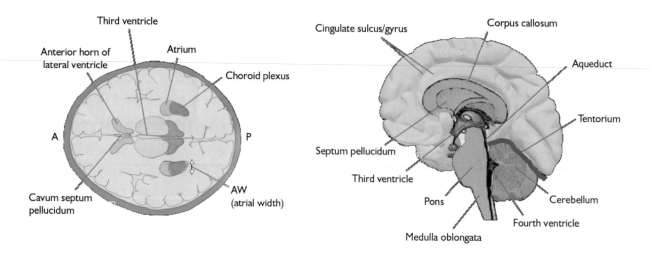

Figure 12.2 Basic anatomy of the fetal brain in axial and sagittal sections

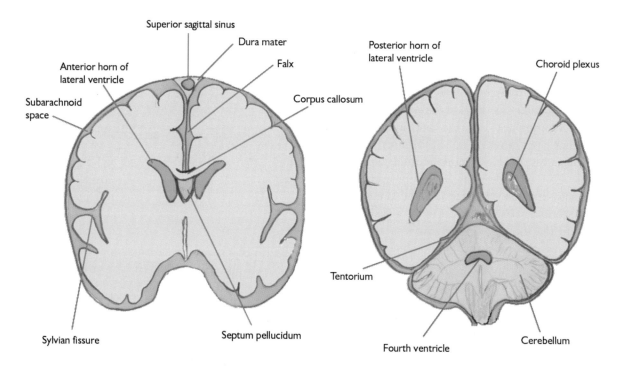

Figure 12.3 Basic anatomy of the fetal brain in coronal section

BASIC ANATOMY OF THE BRAIN

As described above, the brain should be understood as a 3D structure. It is generally believed that the anatomy of the brain is extremely complicated and that there must be lots of terms to remember. However, in order to demonstrate the brain structure and evaluate fetal CNS disorders, it is not necessary to remember all of the detailed structure. Here, essential anatomic structures are selected for neuroimaging and comprehension of fetal CNS diseases. Figure 12.2 shows the basic brain anatomy in axial and sagittal sections and Figure 12.3 the anatomy in anterior coronal and posterior coronal sections.

TRANSVAGINAL 3D SONOGRAPHIC ASSESSMENT OF FETAL CNS

3D sonography is one of the most attractive modalities in the field of fetal ultrasound imaging. There are two scanning methods: freehand scanning and automatic scanning. Automatic scanning with a dedicated 3D transducer uses motor-driven automatic sweeping and is called a 'fan scan'. With this method, a shift and/or change in angle of the transducer is not required during scanning, and the scan duration is only several seconds. After acquisition of the target organ, multiplanar imaging analysis and tomographic imaging analysis are possible. Combination of transvaginal and 3D sonography[9–12] may be of great diagnostic utility in the evaluation of the 3D structure of the fetal CNS. Recent advanced 3D ultrasound equipment may have several useful functions as follows:

- surface anatomic imaging
- bony structural imaging of the calvaria and vertebrae
- multiplanar imaging of the intracranial structure
- tomographic ultrasound imaging of the fetal brain in any cutting section
- thick-slice imaging of intracranial structure
- simultaneous volume contrast imaging of the same section or vertical section of fetal brain structure
- volume calculation of target organs such as the intracranial cavity, ventricles, and choroid plexus, as well as of intracranial lesions
- 3D sono-angiography of the brain circulation (3D power Doppler or 3D color Doppler).

It is well known that 3D sonography can demonstrate surface anatomy. In cases of CNS abnormalities, facial abnormalities and anomalies in the extremities are often also involved. Therefore, reconstructed surface images are helpful. Bony structural imaging of the calvaria (Figure 12.4) and vertebrae (Figures 12.5 and 12.6) are useful in cases of craniosynostosis and spina bifida. The vertebral level of spina bifida may provide important information on postnatal neurologic deficits. In multiplanar imaging of brain structure, it is possible to show not only the sagittal and coronal sections but also the axial section of the brain, which cannot be shown from the parietal direction by conventional 2D transvaginal sonography (Figure 12.7). Transvaginal 3D ultrasound is the principal modality used during the 1st and early 2nd trimesters. In the late 2nd and 3rd trimesters, magnetic resonance imaging (MRI) is occasionally utilized as a prenatal diagnostic tool. During the 2nd trimester, transvaginal 3D sonography may demonstrate more detailed structure of the fetal brain than MRI (Figure 12.8). However, in late pregnancy, MRI can show the whole brain structure, some parts of which transvaginal 3D sonography cannot cover because of a developed calvarium, scan-angle limitation, and acoustic shadowing due to ossifying cranial bone. A comparison of transvaginal 3D sonography and MRI in the assessment of the fetal CNS is given in Table 12.1.

Parallel slicing provides tomographic visualization of internal morphology similar to MRI. Parallel slices were formerly obtained by translating the cutting plane; however, recent developments in technology have allowed the production of tomographic ultrasound images and can show a series of parallel cutting

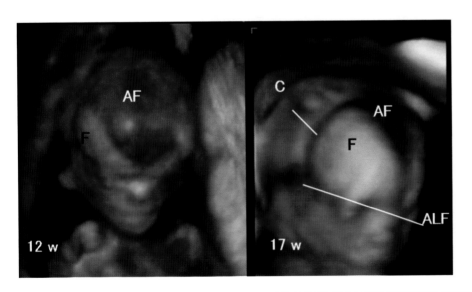

Figure 12.4 Fetal cranial structure at 12 and 17 weeks of gestation. Cranial bone structure develops rapdly in the first half of pregnancy. AF, anterior fontanel; ALF, anterolateral fontanel; F, frontal bone; C, coronal suture; M, metopic suture; S, sagittal suture

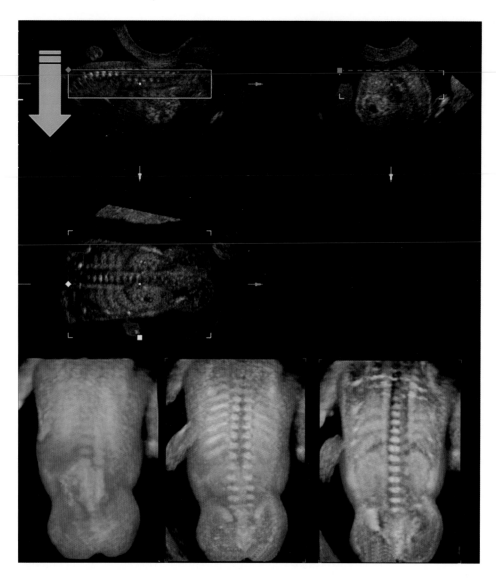

Figure 12.5 Three orthogonal views and 3D reconstructed image of a normal fetus at 16 weeks of gestation. Movement of the region of interest (arrow) provides a 3D reconstruction of the surface level (lower left), neural arch level (lower middle), and vertebral body level (lower right)

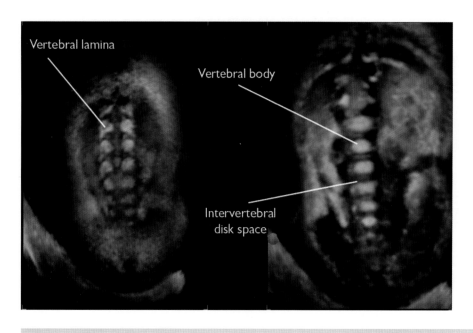

Figure 12.6 Fetal veretebral structure by 3D sonography at 21 weeks of gestation

Vertebral lamina

Vertebral body

Intervertebral disk space

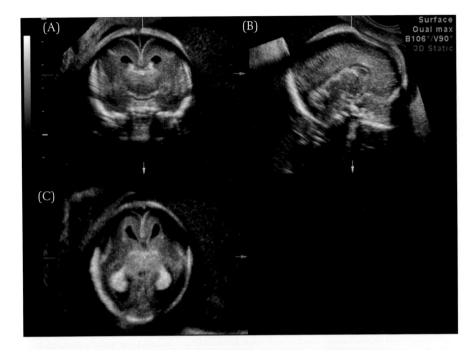

Figure 12.7 3D multiplanar image analysis (normal brain at 18 weeks of gestation). The use of three orthogonal views is helpful in obtaining the orientation of the brain structure. Coronal (A), sagittal (B), and axial (C) images can be visualized on a single screen. Any rotation of the brain image around any (*x,y,z*) axis is possible

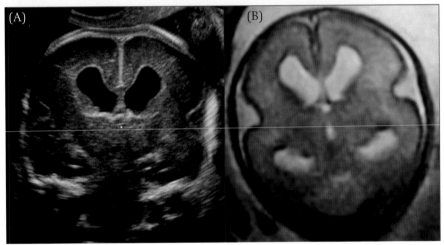

Figure 12.8 Transvaginal sonography and magnetic resonance imaging (MRI). Comparison of an anterior coronal cutting section by transvaginal sonography (A) and MRI (B) in a case of ventriculomegaly. During the 2nd trimester, transvaginal sonography may be superior to MRI in demonstrating the detailed structure of the brain

Table 12.1 3D transvaginal sonography (3D-TVS) and magnetic resonance imaging in the assessment of the fetal CNS

Assessment of fetal CNS	3D-TVS vs MRI
Whole cortical development in late pregnancy	3D-TVS << MRI
Volume calculation, longitudinal study	3D-TVS >> MRI
Intracranial vascular structure	3D-TVS >> MRI
Enlarged ventricles	3D-TVS = MRI
Intracranial cyst	3D-TVS = MRI
Corpus callosum	3D-TVS ≥ MRI
Cerebellum/posterior fossa	3D-TVS ≤ MRI
Brainstem	3D-TVS <<<<<<<< MRI
Abnormal gyration (target study)	3D-TVS = MRI
Calcification	3D-TVS only
Small cystic formation	3D-TVS ≥ MRI
Cysts in cyst	3D-TVS >>> MRI

slices on a single screen as well as MRI does. As shown in Figure 12.9, images obtained by tomographic ultrasound imaging (TUI) are quite similar to pictures from MRI. The superiority of TUI over MRI lies in the possibility with the former to change slice width, rotate images, magnify images, and rotate images in any direction. These functions are extremely useful for detailed CNS assessment and also for consultation with neurosurgeons and neurologists. Thick-slice imaging of intracranial structures (Figure 12.10) and simultaneous volume contrast imaging (VCI) of the same plane or the vertical plane of a conventional 2D image (Figure 12.11) are often convenient to observe gyral formation and inside lateral ventricles.[13] The premature brain image obtained using VCI (shown in Figure 12.12) clearly demonstrates the CNS anatomic structure.

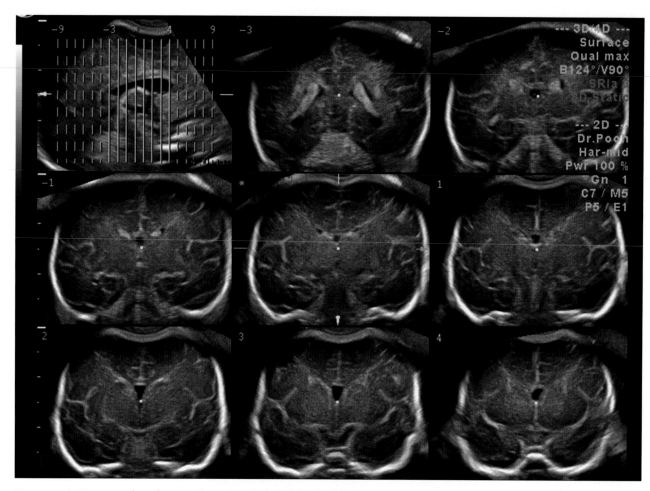

Figure 12.9 Tomographic ultrasound imaging (TUI) of the fetal brain. Normal brain in coronal section at 31 weeks of gestation. Intracranial structures, including gyral formation, are clearly demonstrated

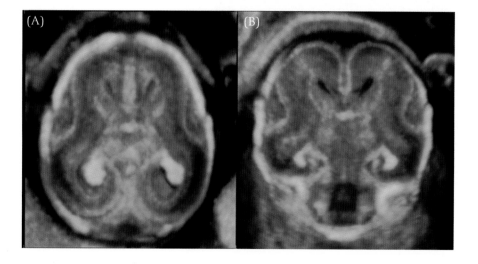

Figure 12.10 3D thick slices of the brain (20 weeks of gestation). Axial thick slice (A) and coronal thick slice (B) of the premature brain. With these slices, imaging of the anatomy of cortical structure and inside ventricles can be comprehensive

Volume-extracted imaging and volume calculation of the fetal brain in early pregnancy was reported in the 1990s.[14,15] In our institute, the Voluson 730 Expert (GE Medical Systems, Milwaukee, USA) with transvaginal 3D transducer and 3D View or 4D View software (Kretztechnik AG, Zipf, Austria) has been used for volume extraction and volume estimation of brain structure.[16–18] On three orthogonal images, the target

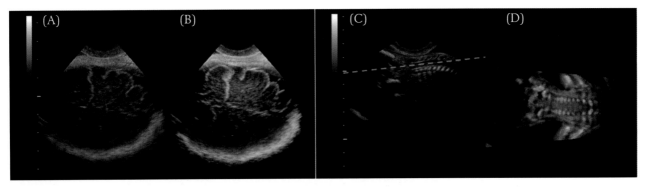

Figure 12.11 3D volume contrast imaging (VCI) of the brain and spine. (A,B) Cerebral gyri and sulci at 33 weeks of gestation: (A) normal 2D sonogram; (B) simultaneous VCI. Gyral formation was demonstrated by VCI. (C,D) Cerebrospinal view at 18 weeks of gestation: (C) normal 2D sonogram; (D) simultaneous view of rectangular VCI

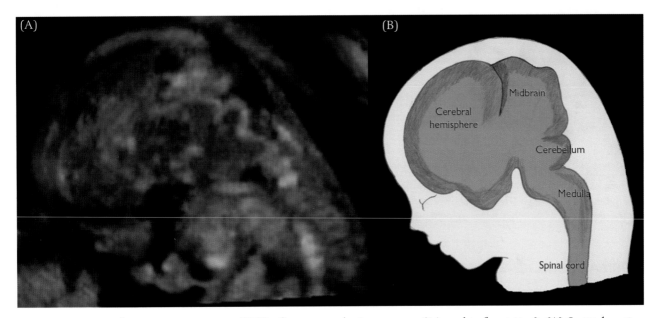

Figure 12.12 3D volume contrast imaging (VCI) of premature brain structure (14 weeks of gestation). (A) Sagittal section of the premature brain by VCI. (B) Brain structure at this gestational age. The detailed structures of the midbrain, cerebellum, and medulla can be detected on the ultrasound image

organ can be traced automatically or manually with rotation of volume imaging data. After tracing, the volume-extracted image is shown and volume calculation data are exhibited (Figure 12.13). 3D fetal brain volume measurements show good intra- and inter-observer reliability,[19,20] and could be used to estimate gestational age.[19] Volume analysis by 3D sonography provides exceedingly informative imaging data. Volume analysis of the structure of interest provides an intelligible complete evaluation of brain structure, and longitudinal and objective assessment of enlarged ventricles and intracranial lesions. Any intracranial organ can be chosen as a target for volumetry, no matter how distorted its shape and appearance may be.

The brain circulation as demonstrated by transvaginal 2D power Doppler was first reported in 1996.[21] Thereafter, fetal brain vascularity was successfully assessed by transvaginal 3D power Doppler.[17,22] With the use of advanced techniques of directional power Doppler, 3D angiostructural imaging has become increasingly sophisticated (Figures 12.14 and 12.15).

Fetal neuroimaging with advanced 3D technology is easy, non-invasive, and reproducible. It produces not only comprehensible images but also objective imaging data. Easy storage and extraction of the raw volume dataset enables easy offline analysis and consultation with neurologists and neurosurgeons.

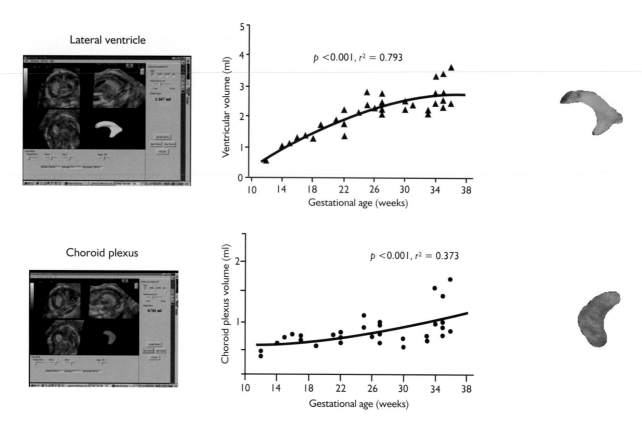

Figure 12.13 3D volume extraction and volumetric analysis of lateral ventricle and choroid plexus. On three orthogonal sections, the target organ can be traced automatically or manually with rotation of volume imaging data. After tracing, the volume-extracted image (right) is shown and the volume calculation data are exhibited. The graphs show nomograms of ventricular volume and choroid plexus volume during pregnancy

NORMAL FETAL CNS IMAGING

The three primary brain vesicles of the forebrain (prosencephalon), midbrain (mesencephalon), and hindbrain (rhombencephalon) are formed in the early embryonic period. At 7 and 8 weeks of gestation, these three primary brain vesicles are demonstrated in the midsagittal plane (Figure 12.16). The forebrain partly divides into the two secondary brain vesicles of the telencephalon and diencephalon, and the hindbrain partly divides into the metencephalon and myelencephalon. The five secondary brain vesicles are consequently formed. The telencephalon forms derivatives of the cerebral hemisphere and lateral ventricles.[23] At 9 weeks of gestation, these secondary vesicles are detected by sonography (Figure 12.17). Thereafter, the premature brain vesicles develop rapidly during the first half of pregnancy. The choroid plexuses develop in the roof of the third ventricle, in the medial walls of the lateral ventricles, and in the roof of the fourth ventricle.[23] The choroid plexuses secrete ventricular fluid, which becomes cerebrospinal fluid

(CSF). The choroid plexuses are highly echogenic structures, detectable from the 9th week of gestation and conspicuous during the 1st trimester (Figures 12.18 and 12.19). From the beginning of the 2nd trimester, the choroid plexus of the lateral ventricle gradually shifts backward (Figures 12.20 and 12.21). As the cerebral cortex develops, the commissures connect corresponding areas of the cerebral hemispheres with one another. The largest cerebral commissure is the corpus callosum, connecting neocortical areas. The corpus callosum initially lies in the lamina terminalis, but fibers are added to it as the cortex enlarges; as a result, it gradually extends beyond the lamina terminalis. The rest of the lamina terminalis lies between the corpus callosum and the fornix. It becomes stretched to form the thin septum pellucidum, a thin plate of brain tissue. The corpus callosum extends over the roof of the diencephalon.[23] The corpus callosum (Figure 12.22) is detectable by ultrasound from around 16 weeks of gestation in some cases and at 18 weeks in most cases. On neuroimaging in the 3rd trimester, gyral formation is a main change

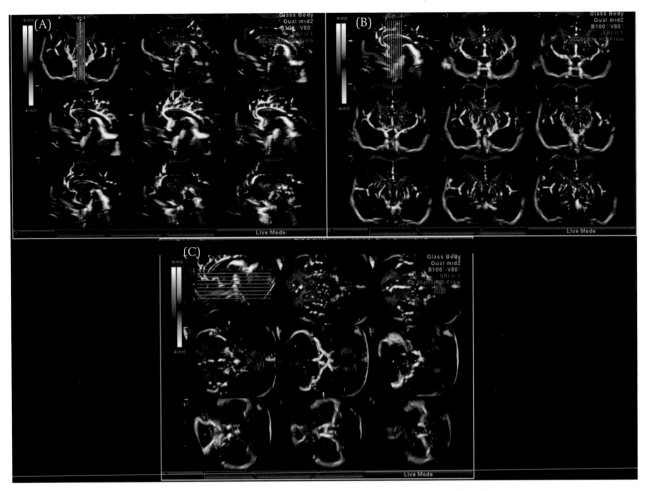

Figure 12.14 Tomographic ultrasound imaging of normal cerebral circulation at 31 weeks of gestation. Tomographic directional power Doppler imaging of sagittal (A), coronal (B), and axial (C) sections. Anterior cerebral arteries and their branches are seen in the sagittal plane, middle cerebral arteries and their branches in the coronal plane, and the circle of Willis in the axial plane

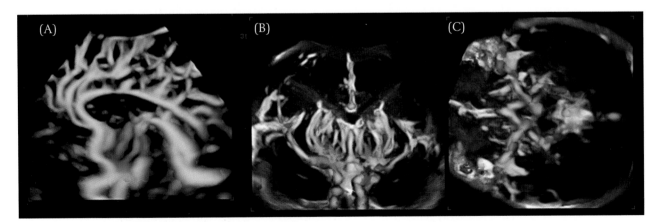

Figure 12.15 Tomographic ultrasound imaging of normal cerebral circulation at 31 weeks of gestation. 3D sonoangiography by directional power Doppler: sagittal (A), coronal (B), and axial (C) views. Anterior cerebral arteries and their branches are seen in the sagittal plane, middle cerebral arteries and their branches in the coronal plane, and the circle of Willis in the axial plane. These images can be rotated in any directions, and the 3D angiostructure is comprehensible

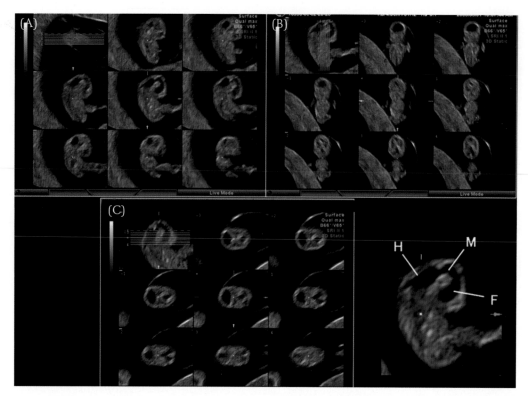

Figure 12.16 Normal brain at 8 weeks of gestation. Tomographic ultrasound imaging of sagittal (A), coronal (B), and axial (C) sections. The premature ventricular system is demonstrated. The three primary brain vesicles of forebrain (F), midbrain (M), and hindbrain (H) are well demonstrated

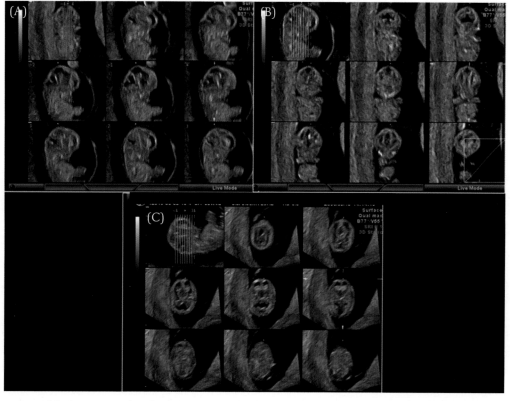

Figure 12.17 Normal brain at 9 weeks of gestation. Tomographic ultrasound imaging of sagittal (A), coronal (B), and axial (C) sections. The premature ventricular system is demonstrated. In the coronal and axial sections, the already-divided bilateral hemispheres can be visualized

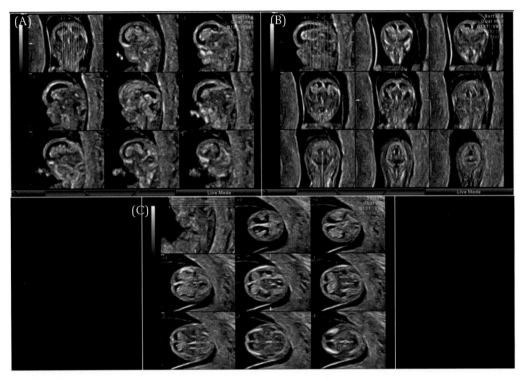

Figure 12.18 Normal brain at 10 weeks and 6 days of gestation. Tomographic ultrasound imaging of sagittal (A), coronal (B), and axial (C) sections. Rapid development of the cerebral and ventricular system is seen compared with Figure 12.17. Bilateral echogenic structure indicates the choroid plexus of lateral ventricles

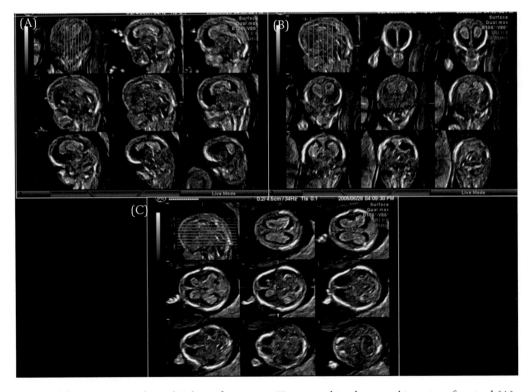

Figure 12.19 Normal brain at 12 weeks and 5 days of gestation. Tomographic ultrasound imaging of sagittal (A), coronal (B), and axial (C) sections. The rate of occupation of the cerebral hemispheres becomes larger compared with Figure 12.18. The bilateral echogenic structure is the choroid plexus of the lateral ventricles

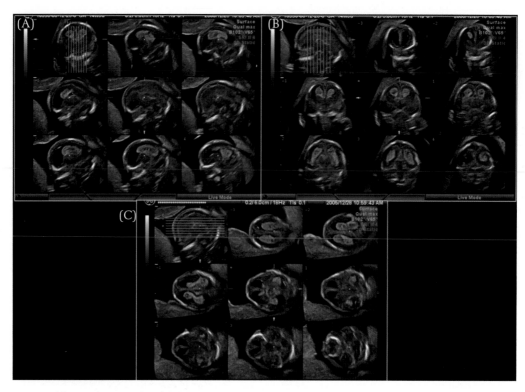

Figure 12.20 Normal brain at 14 weeks and 6 days of gestation. Tomographic ultrasound imaging of sagittal (A), coronal (B), and axial (C) sections. The rate of occupation of the cerebral hemisphere is still large

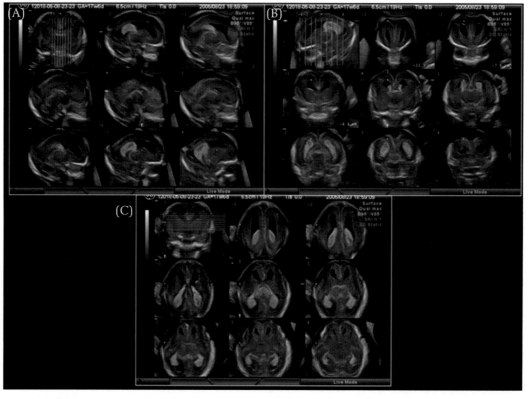

Figure 12.21 Normal brain at 17 weeks of gestation. Tomographic ultrasound imaging of sagittal (A), coronal (B), and axial (C) sections. The choroid plexus (echogenic part) shifts to the posterior half of the lateral ventricles

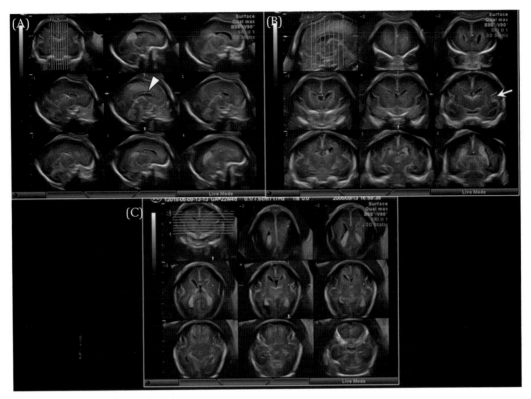

Figure 12.22 Normal brain at 22 weeks of gestation. Tomographic ultrasound imaging of sagittal (A), coronal (B), and axial (C) sections. The normal ventricular shape is seen. Lateral ventricular asymmetry is often observed in normal fetuses. The corpus callosum (arrowhead) can be clearly observed from 18 weeks of gestation. The Sylvian fissure (arrow) is still dull

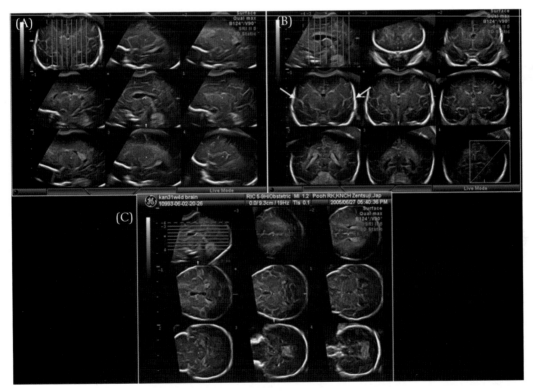

Figure 12.23 Normal brain at 31 weeks of gestation. Tomographic ultrasound imaging of sagittal (A), coronal (B), and axial (C) sections. Formation of sulci and gyri is clearly observed from around 30 weeks of gestation. The Sylvian fissure (arrows) is formed as the lateral sulcus

in brain development (Figure 12.23). Initially, the surfaces of the hemispheres are smooth; however, as growth proceeds, sulci (grooves or furrows) and gyri (convolutions or elevations) develop. The sulci and gyri permit a considerable increase in the surface area of the cerebral cortex without requiring an extensive increase in cranial size. As each cerebral hemisphere grows, the cortex covering the external surface of the corpus striatum grows relatively slowly and is soon overgrown. This buried cortex, hidden from view in the depths of the lateral sulcus (fissure) of the cerebral hemisphere, is the insula.[23]

HYDROCEPHALUS AND VENTRICULOMEGALY IN UTERO

'Hydrocephalus' and 'ventriculomegaly' are both terms used to describe dilatation of the lateral ventricles. However, they should be distinguished: hydrocephalus signifies dilated lateral ventricles resulting from an increased amount of CSF inside the ventricles and increased intracranial pressure, while ventriculomegaly is a dilatation of the lateral ventricles without increased intracranial pressure, due to cerebral hypoplasia or a CNS anomaly such as agenesis of the corpus callosum.[8,24] Of course, ventriculomegaly can sometimes change into a hydrocephalic state. In sonographic imaging, those two intracranial conditions can be differentiated by visualization of the subarachnoid space and the appearance of the choroid plexus. In the normal condition, the subarachnoid space, visualized around both cerebral hemispheres, is well preserved during pregnancy. The choroid plexus is a soft tissue and is easily affected by external pressure. An obliterated subarachnoid space and a dangling choroid plexus are observed in the case of hydrocephalus. In contrast, the subarachnoid space

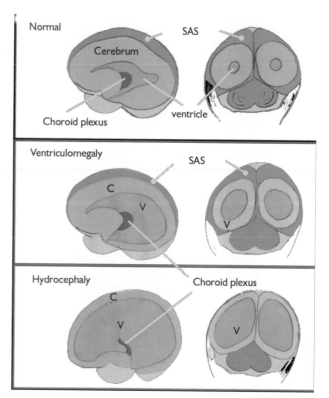

Figure 12.24 Schematic illustration of ventriculomegaly and hydrocephalus. In the case of ventriculomegaly without increased intracranial pressure, the appearance of the subarachnoid space (SAS) and choroid plexus appearance is well preserved, while in the case of hydrocephalus with increased intracranial pressure, a dangling choroid plexus and gradual disappearance of the SAS can be seen

and choroid plexus are well preserved in the case of ventriculomegaly (Figure 12.24). It is difficult to evaluate the subarachnoid space in the axial plane because it is observed on the parietal side of the hemispheres (Figure 12.25). Therefore, the transabdominal approach may not differentiate accurately between hydrocephalus with increased intracranial pressure and ventriculomegaly without pressure. It has

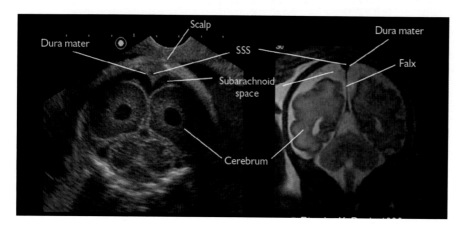

Figure 12.25 Normal structure outside of the cerebral hemispheres. Outside of the hemispheres, the subarachnoid space can normally be observed. Outside of the subarachnoid space, the dura mater, cranial bone, and scalp cover the brain. SSS, superior sagittal sinus

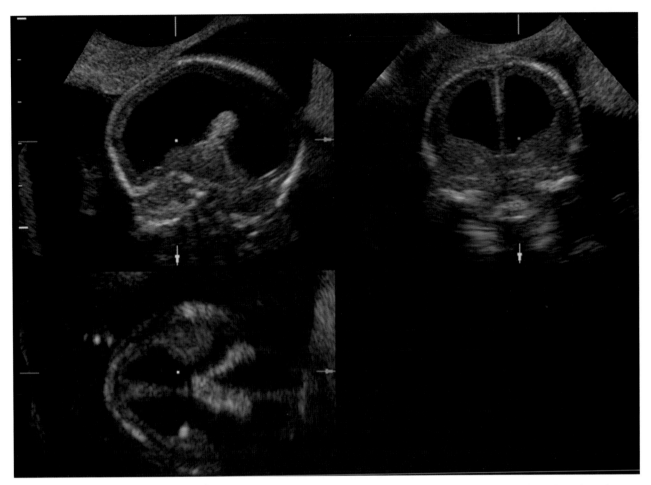

Figure 12.26 Hydrocephalus due to myelomeningocele and spina bifida at 17 weeks of gestation. The subarachnoid space has disappeared and the choroid plexus is dangling

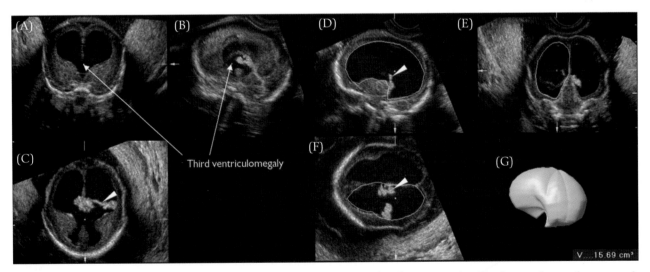

Figure 12.27 Hydrocephalus due to aqueductal obstruction at 19 weeks of gestation. (A–C) Three orthogonal views with anterior coronal (A) and median sagittal (B) and axial (C) slices. Bilateral ventriculomegaly and third ventriculomegaly can be seen. The lack of enlargement of the fourth ventricle indicates obstruction of the aqueduct. (D–F) Three orthogonal views with parasagittal (D) and posterior coronal (E) and axial (F) slices. The subarachnoid space is already obliterated, and a dangling choroid plexus (arrowheads) is seen. (G) Extracted 3D ventricular image from the VOCAL mode. In this case, the ventricle was ten times the size of a normal 19-week ventricle

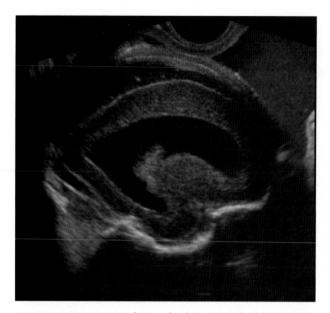

Figure 12.28 Ventriculomegaly due to cerebral hypoplasia at 29 weeks of gestation. There is an enlarged ventricle, but the subarachnoid space is well preserved and no dangling choroid plexus can be seen. These findings indicate the absence of an increase in intracranial pressure (ICP). This condition should be differentiated from hydrocephalus with increased ICP

been suggested that evaluation of enlarged ventricles should be made in the parasagittal and coronal views by a transvaginal approach to the fetal brain or by 3D multidimensional analysis. Transvaginal images are shown of hydrocephalus in Figures 12.26 and 12.27 and of ventriculomegaly in Figures 12.28 and 12.29. In some cases of hydrocephalus, the septum pellucidum is destroyed and the ventricles are fused to each other (Figure 12.30). This condition should be differentiated from the lobar type of holoprosencephaly. Intracranial venous blood flow may be related to increased intracranial pressure. In normal fetuses, the blood flow waveforms of dural sinuses, such as the superior sagittal sinus, the vein of Galen, and the straight sinus have a pulsatile pattern.[25] However, in cases with progressive hydrocephalus, normal pulsation disappears and the blood flow waveforms have a flat pattern.[25] In the case of progressive hydrocephalus, there may be seven stages of progression: (1) increased fluid collection in the lateral ventricles; (2) incresed intracranial pressure; (3) dangling choroid plexus; (4) disappearance of the subarachnoid space; (5) excessive extension of the dura and superior sagittal sinus; (6) disappearance of venous pulsation; and finally (7) an enlarged skull. In general, both hydrocephalus and ventriculomegaly are still evaluated by

measurement of the biparietal diameter (BPD) and atrial width (AW) in transabdominal axial section. As a screening examination, the measurement of AW is useful with a cut-off value of 10 mm,[26,27] although isolated mild ventriculomegaly with an AW of 10–12 mm may be a normal variant.[28] As described above, however, hydrocephalus and ventriculomegaly should be differentiated from each other, and the hydrocephalic state should be assessed from the changing appearance of intracranial structure. To evaluate enlarged ventricles, examiners should carefully observe the following structures and specific causes of hydrocephalus;

- choroid plexus – dangling or not
- subarachnoid space – obliterated or not
- ventricles – symmetry or asymmetry
- visibility of the third ventricle
- pulsation of the dural sinuses
- ventricular size (3D volume calculation, if possible)
- other abnormalities.

Genetic hydrocephalus is rare, but important when counseling couples regarding subsequent pregnancy. X-linked hydrocephalus (HSAS, hydrocephalus due to stenosis of the aqueduct of Sylvius), MASA (mental retardation–aphasia–shuffling gait–adducted thumbs) syndrome, X-linked complicated spastic paraparesis (SP1), and X-linked corpus callosum agenesis (ACC) are all due to mutations in the *L1* gene.[29] This gene is located near the telomere on the long arm of the X chromosome at Xq28. It has therefore been suggested that this clinical syndrome be referred to by the acronym CRASH (corpus callosum hypoplasia, retardation, adducted thumbs, spastic paraplegia, and hydrocephalus).[29] It has been reported that mutations that produce truncations in the extracellular domain of the L1 protein are more likely to produce severe hydrocephalus, grave mental retardation, or early death than point mutations in the extracellular domain or mutations affecting only the cytoplasmic domain of the protein.[30] For the families, prenatal CNS diagnosis of male infants is important. A morphology-based approach becomes feasible between postmenstrual weeks 15 and 20. Prior to this gestational age, the diagnosis should rely on molecular biological tests.[31]

Borderline ventriculomegaly is defined as a width of the atrium of the lateral cerebral ventricles of 10–15 mm. The majority of fetuses with prenatally detected isolated mild ventriculomegaly are developmentally normal.[32]

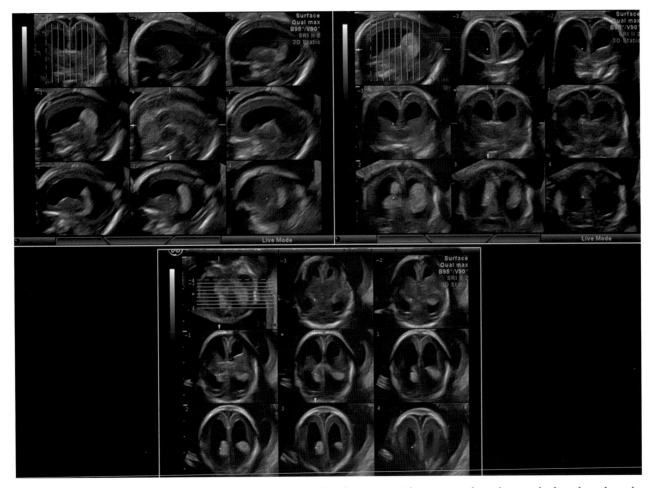

Figure 12.29 Ventriculomegaly of unknown cause at 17 weeks of gestation. There is an enlarged ventricle, but the subarachnoid space is well preserved and no dangling choroid plexus can be seen. In this case, spontaneous resolution of ventriculomegaly occurred during the next few weeks

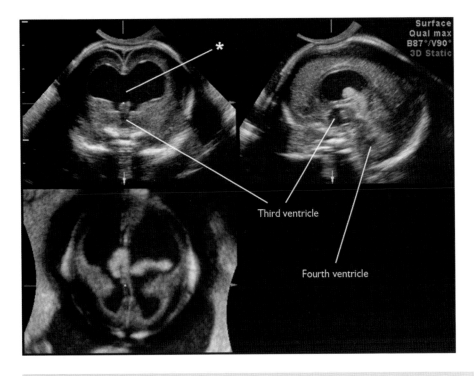

Figure 12.30 Hydrocephalus at 21 weeks of gestation. The subarachnoid space has disappeared and the choroid plexus is dangling. The septum pellucidum is destroyed and the ventricles are fused to each other (*)

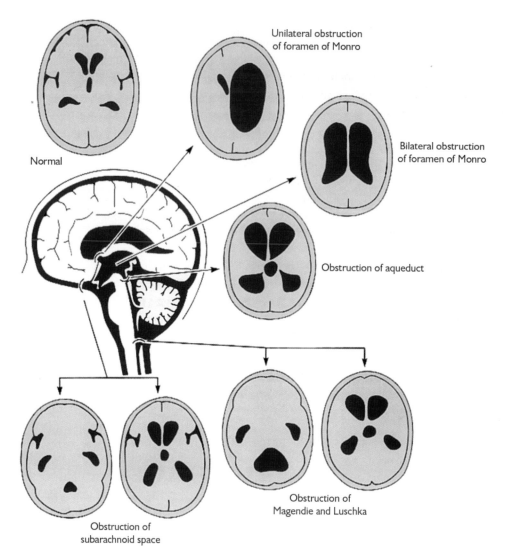

Unilateral obstruction
of foramen of Monro

Bilateral obstruction
of foramen of Monro

Obstruction of aqueduct

Normal

Obstruction of
Magendie and Luschka

Obstruction of
subarachnoid space

Figure 12.31 Types of hydrocephalus due to various sites of obstruction of cerebrospinal fluid flow (from: Handbook on Hydrocephalus for Patients. Research Committee on Intractable Hydrocephalus, Japanese Ministry of Health and Welfare, ©1993, with permission, and by courtesy of the Chairman of the Committee, Professor K Mori)

Pilu et al[33] reviewed 234 cases of borderline ventriculomegaly, with an abnormal outcome in 22.8%, and concluded that borderline ventriculomegaly carries an increased risk of cerebral maldevelopment, delayed neurologic development, and possibly chromosomal aberrations.

The term 'hydrocephalus' does not identify a specific disease, but is a generic term meaning a serial pathologic condition due to abnormal circulation of CSF. Treatment of hydrocephalus should be selected according to age of onset and symptoms. Congenital hydrocephalus is classified into three categories by causes that disturb the CSF circulation pathway: simple hydrocephalus, dysgenetic hydrocephalus, and secondary hydrocephalus.[24]

- Simple hydrocephalus: this is caused by a developmental abnormality localized within the CSF circulation pathway and includes aqueductal stenosis, atresia of the foramen of Monro, and maldevelopment of arachnoid granulation. Types of hydrocephalus due to various obstructive sites of CSF flow are shown in Figure 12.31.
- Dysgenetic hydrocephalus: this results from a cerebral developmental disorder in the early stages of development, and includes hydranencephaly, holoprosencephaly, porencephaly, schizencephaly, Dandy–Walker malformation, dysraphism, and Chiari malformation.
- Secondary hydrocephalus: this is a generic term indicating hydrocephalus caused by an intracranial

pathologic condition, such as a brain tumor, intracranial infection, or intracranial hemorrhage.

The treatment of hydrocephalus includes the use of a miniature reservoir,[34,35] shunt procedures, and neuro-endoscopy. Ventriculoperitoneal shunting is the most popular procedure. The effectiveness of a shunt procedure for congenital hydrocephalus was proven early on. However, there are various complications of shunting, such as shunt infection, obstruction of the shunt tube, overdrainage, underdrainage, and slit-ventricle syndrome. To reduce those complications, various types of shunt devices, such as antisiphon devices and pressure-programmable valve shunt devices, have been developed. Third ventriculostomy by neuroendoscopy has recently been performed in children with obstructive hydrocephalus, and the number of shunt-independent cases has been increased. It is controversial, however, whether infants younger than one year have a higher risk of treatment failure after neuroendoscopic procedures than older children. Some workers have concluded that neuroendoscopy is an effective alternative for the treatment of hydrocephalus in cases under the age of one.[36] However, third ventriculostomy still does not seem to be effective in neonates because of the prematurity of absorption ability in neonates and small infants.

CONGENITAL CNS ANOMALIES

During the fetal period, the embryonic premature CNS structures develop rapidly into mature structures with formation of gyri. With this rapid development, various developmental disorders and/or insults result in various phenotypes of fetal CNS abnormalities. To understand fetal CNS diseases, a basic knowledge of the development of the nervous system is essential. The developmental stages and their major disorders are described in Table 12.2.

Cranium bifidum

Prevalence. Anencephaly; 0.29/1000 births;[37] overall neural tube defect (NTD): 0.58–1.17/1000 births.[38–40] There have been many reported remarkable reductions in the prevalence of NTDs after the use of folic acid supplementation and fortification,[37–40] although some have reported no decline in the anencephaly rate.[41]

Definition. As with spina bifida, cranium bifidum is classified into four types of encephaloschisis (including anencephaly and exencephaly): meningocele, encephalomeningocele, encephalocystocele, and cranium bifidum occultum. Encephalocele occurs in the occipital region in 70–80% of cases. Acrania, exencephaly, and anencephaly are not independent anomalies. It is considered that dysraphia (absent cranial vault, acrania) occurs in the very early stages, and disintegration of the exposed brain (exencephaly) during the fetal period results in anencephaly.[42]

Etiology. Multifactorial inheritance; single mutant genes; specific teratogens (valproic acid); maternal

Table 12.2 Developmental stages and major disorders

Developmental stage	Disorders
Primary neurulation (3–4 weeks of gestation)	Spina bifida aperta Cranium bifidum
Caudal neural tube formation (secondary neurulation, from 4 weeks of gestation)	Occult dysraphic states
Procencephalic development (2–3 months of gestation)	Holoprosencephaly Agenesis of the corpus callosum Agenesis of the septum pellucidum Septo-optic dysplasia
Neuronal proliferation (3–4 months of gestation)	Micrencephaly Macrencephaly
Neuronal migration (3–5 months of gestation)	Schizencephaly Lissencephaly Pachygyria Polymicrogyria
Organization (5 months of gestation–postnatal years)	Idiopathic mental retardation
Myelination (Birth–postnatal years)	Cerebral white matter hypoplasia

diabetes; environmental factors; predominant in females.

Pathogenesis. Failure of anterior neural tube closure or a restricted disorder of neurulation.

Associated anomalies. Open spina bifida (inien-cephaly); Chiari type III malformation; bilateral renal cystic dysplasia and postaxial polydactyly with occipital cephalocele (Meckel–Gruber syndrome); hydrocephalus; polyhydramnios.

Prenatal diagnosis. Acrania (Figure 12.32); anencephaly (Figure 12.33); early detection of inien-cephaly (Figure 12.34).

Differential diagnosis. Amniotic band syndrome (ABS). In cases of ABS, cranial destruction occurs secondarily to an amniotic band, and a similar appearance is observed. However, ABS has a completely different pathogenesis from acrania/excencephaly.

Prognosis. Anencephaly is a uniformly lethal anomaly. In other types of cranium bifidum, various neurologic deficits may occur, depending on types and degrees.

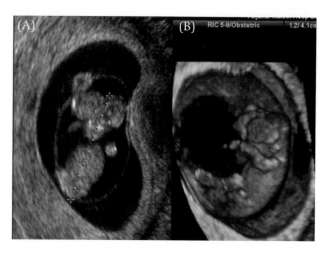

Figure 12.32 Acrania at 10 weeks of gestation. (A) Coronal image. Note the normal appearance of the amniotic membrane, which indicates that this is not amniotic band syndrome. (B) 3D sonography of the same fetus

Recurrence risk. There used to be a high recurrence risk of 5–13%; however, this has recently declined because of the use of folic acid supplementation and fortification.

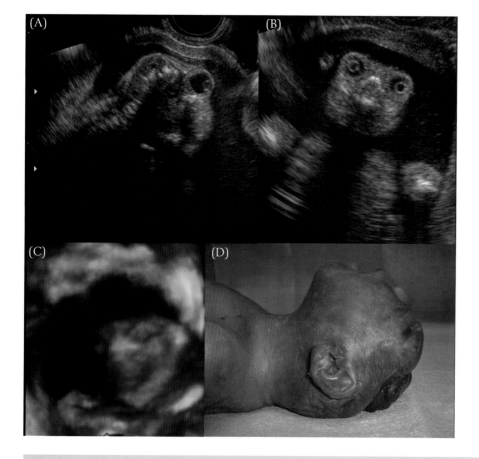

Figure 12.33 Anencephaly in middle gestation (the same case as in Figure 12.32). (A) Sagittal image at 23 weeks of gestation. (B) Coronal image. (C) 3D image. (D) External appearance of stillborn fetus at 25 weeks of gestation. It is clear that there is exencephalic brain tissue scattered in the amniotic space compared with this case at 10 weeks

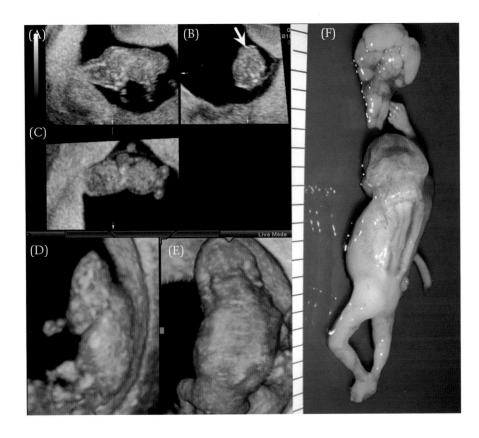

Figure 12.34 3D sonographic detection of a fetus with iniencephaly and acrania at 10 weeks of gestation. (A–C) Three orthogonal views of the fetus. Spina bifida (arrow) was demonstrated in the coronal section. (D,E) 3D images show the fetal lateral and dorsal views. (F) Appearance of aborted fetus at the end of 11 weeks of gestation. The brain and part of the spinal cord were detached at delivery

Obstetric management. Termination of pregnancy can be offered in cases with anencephaly.

Neurosurgical management. For other cases of cranium bifidum, surgery aims at transposition of cerebral tissue into the intracranial cavity. Ventriculoperitoneal shunt can be used for hydrocephalus.

Spina bifida

Prevalence. 0.22/1000 births.[37] As mentioned above, the use of folic acid supplements has reduced the prevalence of NTDs.[37–41]

Definition. Spina bifida aperta – the manifest form of spina bifida – is classified into four types: meningocele, myelomeningocele, myelocystocele, and myeloschisis. Spina bifida occuluta is a generic term for spinal diseases covered with normal skin tissue, and does not include spinal diseases that cannot be diagnosed by external appearance. Cutaneous abnormalities near the spinal lesion are found: skin bulge (subcutaneous lipoma), dimple, hair tuft, pigmentation, skin appendage, and hemangioma. In cases with thickened film terminale, dermal sinus, or diastematomyelia

(split cord malformation), there is abnormal tethering and fixation of the spinal cord.

Etiology. Multifactorial inheritance; single mutant genes; autosomal recessive; chromosomal abnormalities (trisomies 18 and 13); specific teratogens (valproic acid); maternal diabetes; environmental factors; predominant in females.

Pathogenesis.
- Spina bifida aperta: impairment of neural tube closure
- Spina bifida occuluta: caudal neural tube malformation due to canalization and retrogressive differentiation.

Associated anomalies. Chiari type II malformation; hydrocephalus; scoliosis (above L2); kyphosis (Figures 12.35 and 12.36); polyhydramnios; additional non-CNS anomalies.

Prenatal diagnosis. See Figures 12.35–12.38.

Differential diagnosis. Sacrococcygeal teratoma.

Prognosis. Disturbance of motor, sensory, and sphincter functions, depending on lesion levels. Below S1:

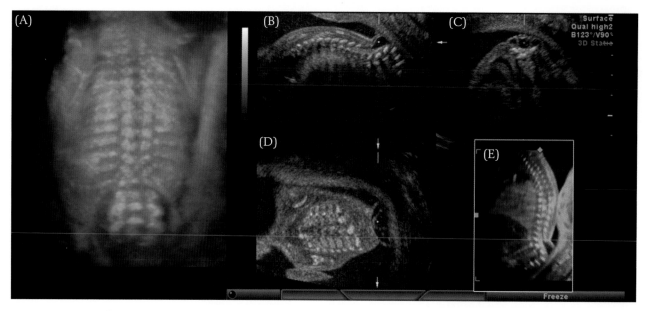

Figure 12.35 Myelomeningocele with severe kyphosis at 20 weeks of gestation. (A) 3D surface reconstruction shows the large myelomeningocele from T12. (B–D) Three orthogonal views of vertebral structure and myelomeningocele with severe kyphosis. (E) 3D thick slice of vertebral structure

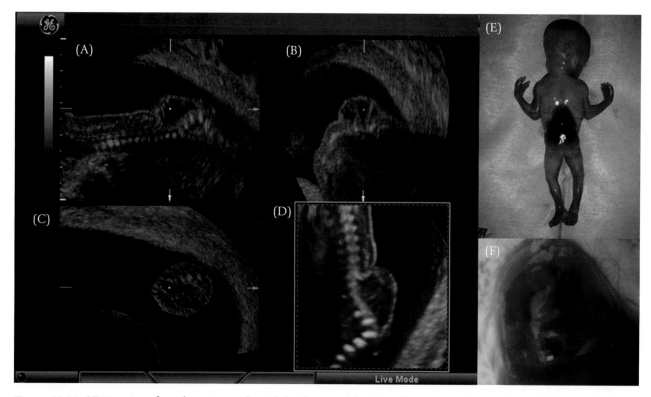

Figure 12.36 3D imaging of myelomeningocele with kyphosis at 16 weeks of gestation. (A–D) Three orthogonal views and surface reconstruction. (A) Sagittal image: the spinal cord protrudes completely into the sac surface from the spinal canal, and severe kyphosis can be seen. (B) Axial view. (C) Coronal view of myelomeningocele. (D) Sagittal vertebral bony structure by 3D thick slice. (E) Aborted fetus at 17 weeks. (F) Tortuous structure of spinal cord

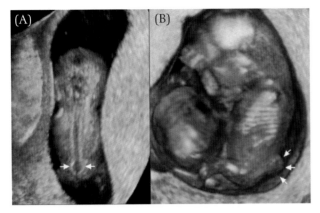

Figure 12.37 Myelomeningocele in the 1st trimester. (A) The 3D dorsal view at 9 weeks of gestation clearly demonstrates a neural tube defect at the lower lumbar and sacral level (arrows). (B) The same fetus at 12 weeks of gestation. Arrows indicate the lumbosacral myelomeningocele

unable to walk unaided; above L2: wheelchair dependent; variable at intermediate level.

Recurrence risk. Decreased; almost no recurrence rate[43] with the use of folic acid supplementation and fortification.

Obstetric management. In cases of spina bifida aperta, especially with skin defects, cesarean section is preferable to protect the spinal cord and nerves and prevent infection.

Neurosurgical management.
- Spina bifida aperta. In cases with defects of normal skin tissue, immediate closure of spina bifida after birth reduces spinal infection. Spinal cord reconstruction is the most important aim of operation. Placement of a miniature Ommaya reservoir and a subsequent ventriculoperitoneal shunt is required for hydrocephalus. For symptomatic Chiari malformation, posterior fossa decompressive craniectomy and/or tonsillectomy is performed.
- Spina bifida occuluta. The aim of surgical treatment is decompression of the spinal cord and cutting off tethering to the cord.

Chiari malformation

Prevalence. This depends on the prevalence of spina bifida (Chiari type II malformation). With the recent

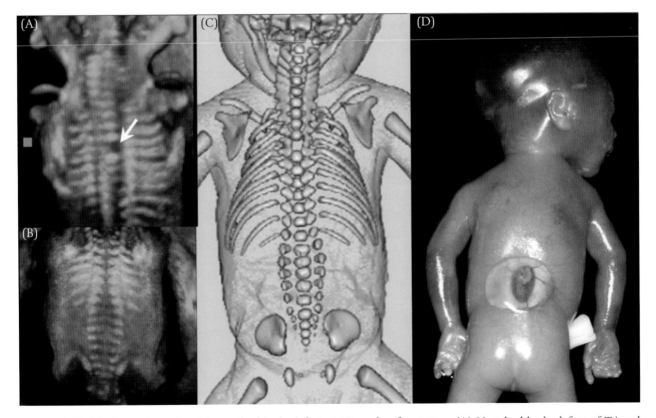

Figure 12.38 Myelomeningocele with vertebral body defect at 17 weeks of gestation. (A) Vertebral body defect of T4 and T5 (arrow). (B) Spina bifida from T11 level. (C) 3D-CT image of aborted fetus at 20 weeks of gestation. The L4 and L5 vertebral body defect and spina bifida are well demonstrated. (D) Myelomeningocele of aborted fetus

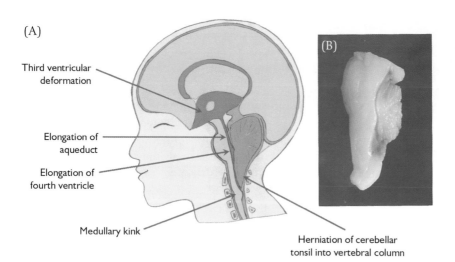

(A)

Third ventricular deformation

Elongation of aqueduct

Elongation of fourth ventricle

Medullary kink

(B)

Herniation of cerebellar tonsil into vertebral column

Figure 12.39 Schematic illustration and macroscopic finding of Chiari type II malformation. (A) Chiari type II malformation is characterized by inferior displacement of the lower cerebellum through the foramen magnum with obliteration of the cisterna magna, inferior displacement of the medulla into the spinal canal, and elongation of the fourth ventricle and aqueduct. (B) Macroscopic view of the elongated aqueduct, fourth ventricle, and cerebellum from a specimen of an aborted fetus at 21 weeks of gestation

remarkable reduction in prevalence of NTDs after using folic acid supplementation and fortification, the prevalence has declined. Other types are rare.

Definition. Chiari classified anomalies with cerebellar herniation in the spinal canal into three types by the content of the herniated tissue: in type I, it contains a lip of cerebellum; in type II, part of the cerebellum, the fourth ventricle, the medulla oblongata, and the pons; and in type III, a large herniation of the posterior fossa. Type IV with just cerebellar hypogenesis was added later. However, this classification occasionally leads to confusion in neuroimaging diagnosis. Therefore, at present, the following classification is advocated.

- *Type I:* herniation of only the cerebellar tonsil, not associated with myelomeningocele
- *Type II* (Figure 12.39): herniation of the cerebellar tonsil and brainstem; medullary kink, tentorial dysplasia, associated with myelomeningocele
- *Type III:* associated with cephalocele or craniocervical meningocele, in which the cerebellum and brainstem are herniated
- *Type IV:* associated with marked cerebellar hypogenesis and shrinkage of the posterior fossa.

Synonyms. Arnold–Chiari malformation.

Etiology. This depends on the type.

Pathogenesis. Chiari malformation occurs as a result of (1) inferior displacement of the medulla and the fourth ventricle into the upper cervical canal; (2) elongation and thinning of the upper medulla and lower pons and persistence of the embryonic flexure of these structures; (3) inferior displacement of the lower cerebellum through the foramen magnum into the upper cervical region; (4) a variety of bony defects of the foramen magnum, occiput, and upper cervical vertebrae.[44]

Associated anomalies. Hydrocephalus caused by obstruction of fourth ventricular outflow or associated aqueductal stenosis. Myelomeningocele or myeloschisis (type II); cephalocele or craniocervical meningocele (type III); cerebellar hypogenesis (type IV); syringomyelia (type I).

Prenatal diagnosis. Prenatal sonographic diagnosis by features: lemon sign, indicating deformity of the frontal bone; banana sign, indicating abnormal shape of cerebellum without the cisterna magna (Figure 12.40); medullary kink; small clivus–supraocciput angle.[45] The lemon and banana signs provide circumstantial evidence for Chiari malformation. Sonographic detection of the Chiari malformation itself is occasionally possible (Figure 12.41).

Differential diagnosis. Craniosynostosis.

Prognosis. Nearly every case of myelomeningocele is accompanied by morphologic Chiari II malformation. Many cases with Chiari II are asymptomatic. However, clinical features due to Chiari malformation, such as feeding disturbances, laryngeal stridor, and apneic episode, are found in approximately 9–30% of cases. In cases with these clinical features, the prognosis is often poor.

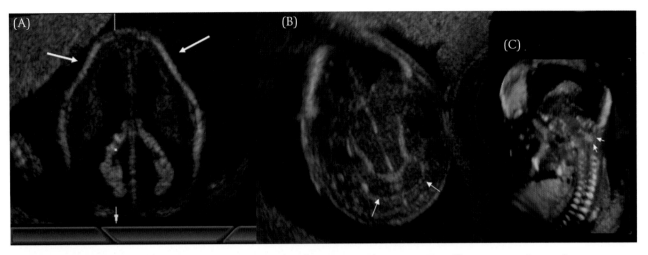

Figure 12.40 Chiari type II malformation at 16 weeks of gestation. Chiari type II malformation is observed in most cases with myelomeningocele and myeloschisis. (A) Typical lemon sign (arrows). (B) Typical banana sign (arrows). (C) 3D reconstruction of interval image of Chiari type II malformation (arrows)

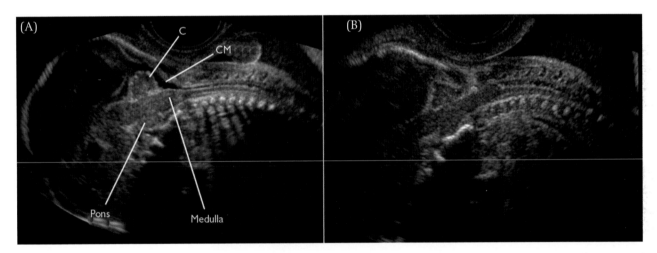

Figure 12.41 Ultrasound imaging of Chiari II malformation at 20 weeks of gestation. (A) Normal sagittal section of cerebrospinal region. The brainstem (pons and medulla) and cerebellum (C) are well demonstrated. The cisterna magna (CM) is well preserved. (B) The same cutting section of Chiari II malformation. Herniation of the cerebellum and medulla into the spinal cord is demonstrated. The posterior fossa, including the cisterna magna, is compressed

Recurrence risk. This depends on the types of Chiari malformation. It has decreased with the decline in NTD recurrence rate following the use of folic acid supplementation and fortification.

Neurosurgical management. Neurosurgical decompression of the foramen magnum (FMD) for any types of Chiari malformation. Syringo-subarachnoid shunt for Chiari type I.

Holoprosencephaly

Incidence. 1/15 000–20 000 live births; however, the initial incidence may be more than 60-fold greater in aborted human embryos.[46,47]

Classification.[44] Holoprosencephalies are classified into three varieties:

- *Alobar type*: A single-sphered cerebral structure with a single common ventricle, posterior large cyst of third ventricle (dorsal sac), absence of olfactory bulbs and tracts and a single optic nerve
- *Semilobar type*: with formation of a posterior portion of the interhemispheric fissure
- *Lobar type*: with formation of the interhemispheric fissure anteriorly and posteriorly, but not

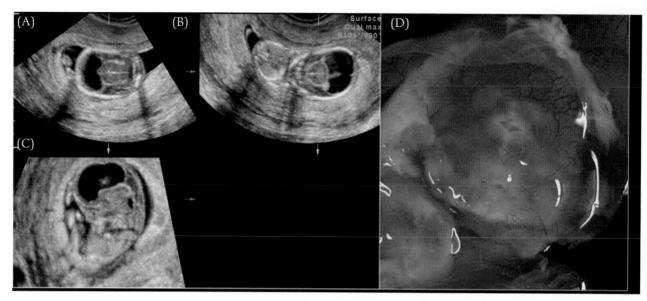

Figure 12.42 Alobar holoprocencephaly in the 1st trimester. (A–C) Three orthogonal views demonstrating holoprocencephaly at 13 weeks of gestation. The crown–rump length was compatible with 10 weeks of gestation. (D) Face of the aborted fetus, with cyclopia, arrhinia, and small mouth

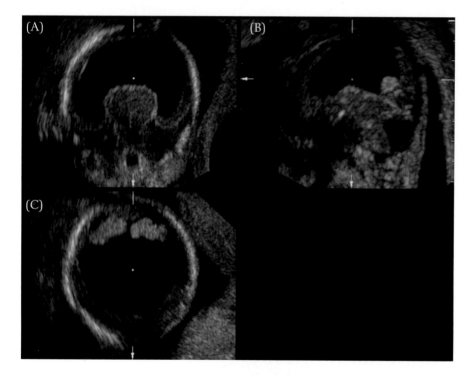

Figure 12.43 Alobar holoprosencephaly at 15 weeks of gestation. (A–C) Three orthogonal images of intracranial structure showing a complete single ventricle within a single-sphered cerebral structure

in the midhemispheric region; fusion of the fornices is seen.[48]

Etiology. 75% of cases of holoprosencephaly have normal karyotype, but chromosomes 2, 3, 7, 13, 18, and 21 have been implicated in holoprosencephaly.[44] In particular, trisomy 13 has most commonly been observed. Autosomal dominant transmission is rare.

Pathogenesis. Failure of cleavage of the prosencephalon and diencephalon during the early 1st trimester (5–6 weeks) results in holoprosencephaly.

Associated anomalies. Facial abnormalities such as cyclopia, ethmocephaly, cebocephaly, flat nose, and cleft lip and palate are invariably associated with horoprosencephaly. Extracerebral abnormalities are

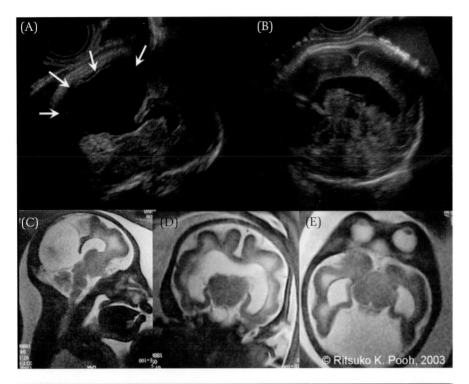

Figure 12.44 Semilobar holoprosencephaly at 33 weeks of gestation. (A) Dorsal sac (arrows) in median section. (B) Fused ventricle. (C–E) Fetal magnetic resonance images: sagittal (C), coronal (D), and axial (E) sections. The blind end of the nasal cavity and hypotelorism are seen in (C) and (E), respectively

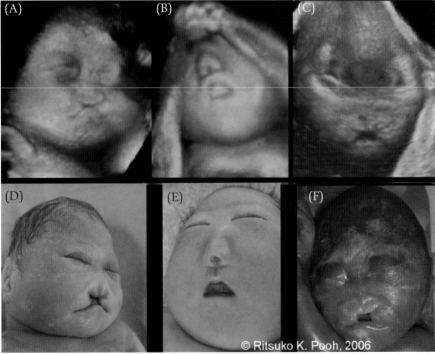

Figure 12.45 Facial abnormalities in cases of holoprosencephaly. (A–C) Prenatal 3D facial images. (D–F) Respective postpartum facial appearances. (A/D) Alobar holoprosencephaly (image in (A) is at 20 weeks of gestation). (B/E, C/F) Semilobar type (images in (B,C) are in late pregnancy). Hypotelorism and exophthalmos are common. The cases in (A/D) and (B/E) had cleft lip and palate and obstruction of the nasal cavity. The case in (C/F) had a single, obstructed nasal cavity

also invariably associated, such as renal cysts/dysplasia, omphalocele, cardiac disease, and/or myelomeningocele.

Prenatal diagnosis. Alobar holoprosencephaly in the 1st trimester and at 15 weeks of gestation is shown in Figures 12.42 and 12.43, respectively, and the semilobar type in late pregnancy is shown in Figure 12.44.

Figure 12.45 shows the facial appearance in cases of holoprosencephaly.

Differential diagnosis. Hydrocephalus; hydranencephaly.

Prognosis. Extremely poor in alobar holoprosencephaly; uncertain in the lobar type; variable but poor in the semilobar type.

Recurrence risk. 6%;[49] but much lower in sporadic or trisomy cases, and much higher in genetic cases.

Management. Chromosomal evaluation is offered.

Agenesis of the corpus callosum

Prevalence Uncertain, but 3–7/1000 in the general population is estimated.

Definition. Absence of the corpus callosum, which may be subclassified into (complete) agenesis, partial agenesis, or hypogenesis of the corpus callosum:

- complete agenesis: complete absence of the corpus callosum
- partial agenesis (hypogenesis): absence of splenium or posterior portion to various degrees.

Etiology. Chromosomal aberration in 20% of affected cases, such as trisomies 8, 13, or 18. Autosomal dominant, autosomal recessive, X-linked recessive, part of Mendelian syndromes such as Walker–Warburg syndrome, and X-linked dominant such as Aicardi syndrome.

Pathogenesis. Uncertain, but callosal formation may be associated with a migration disorder.

Associated anomalies. Colpocephaly (ventriculomegaly with disproportionate enlargement of trigones, occipital horns and temporal horns, not hydrocephalus); superior elongation of the third ventricle; interhemispheric cyst; lipoma of the corpus callosum.

Prenatal diagnosis. Median sonographic images of complete agenesis and hypogenesis of the corpus callosum are shown in Figure 12.46 and fetal MRI in Figure 12.47. Abnormal brain vessels in a case of agenesis of the corpus callosum are demonstrated in Figure 12.48.

Diagnosis. As the corpus callosum is depicted only after 17–18 weeks of gestation by ultrasound, it is impossible to diagnose agenesis prior to this age.[50]

Prognosis. This is variable, depending on associated anomalies. Most cases with isolated agenesis of the corpus callosum without other abnormalities are asymptomatic and prognosis is good. Complete agenesis has a worse prognosis than partial agenesis.[51] Epilepsy, intellectual impairment, or psychiatric disorder[52] may occur later on.

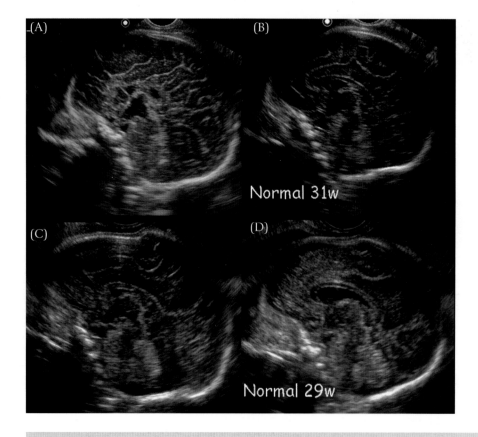

Figure 12.46 Complete agenesis (A) and hypogenesis (C) of the corpus callosum. All images are transvaginal median (midsagittal) images. (B) and (D) are normal images of the corpus callosum at the same gestational age as (A) and (C), respectively

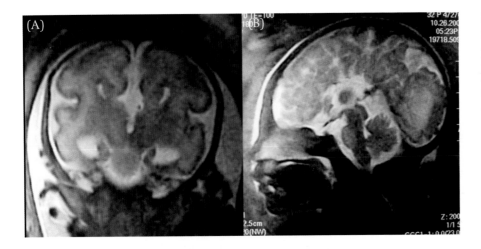

Figure 12.47 Fetal magnetic resonance images of complete agenesis of the corpus callosum at 33 weeks of gestation. (A) Anterior coronal section; (B) median section. No communicating bridge is seen. Note the bull's horn-like appearance of the anterior horns of the lateral ventricle in (A)

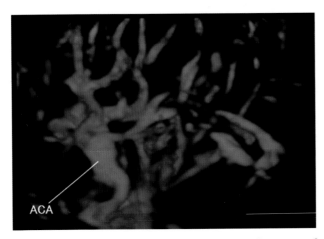

Figure 12.48 Abnormal brain vessels in a case of agenesis of the corpus callosum at 36 weeks of gestation. Intracranial angiostructure by 3D power Doppler. A normal pericallosal artery does not exist and radial formation of the branches of the anterior cerebral arteries (ACA) can be seen

Recurrence risk. This depends on the etiology: chromosomal 1%; autosomal recessive 25%; X-linked recessive male 50%.

Management. Standard obstetric care. Chromosomal evaluation is offered. In cases with interhemispheric cyst, postnatal fenestration or shunt procedure may be performed.

Absent septum pellucidum and septo-optic dysplasia

Incidence. Unknown, but rare.

Definition.
- Absent septum pellucidum: absence of the septum pellucidum with or without associated anomalies.

The septum pellucidum can be destroyed by concomitant hydrocephalus or by contiguous ischemic lesions such as porencephaly. An isolated absent septum pellucidum[53] can exist, but is rare.
- Septo-optic dysplasia: absence of the septum pellucidum and unilateral or bilateral hypoplasia of the optic nerve.

Synonyms. de Morsier syndrome (septo-optic dysplasia).

Etiology. Maternal drug use (multidrug, valproic acid,[54] cocaine[55]); autosomal recessive; *HESX1* homeobox gene mutation.[56]

Pathogenesis. It may occur as part of a vascular disruption sequence, with other prosencephalic or neuronal migration disorders.

Associated anomalies. Schizencephaly; gyral abnormalities; heterotopias; hypotelorism; ventriculomegaly; communicating lateral ventricles; bilateral cleft lip and palate; hypopituitarism.

Differential diagnosis. Dysgenesis of the corpus callosum; lobar holoprosencephaly.

Prognosis. This depends on associated anomalies. There is a variable degree of mental deficit and multiple endocrine dysfunction. In cases with isolated absence of septum pellucidum, prognosis may be good.

Recurrence risk. Unknown.

Management. Confirmation of diagnosis after birth is important for genetic counseling. Endocrine dysfunction should be sought and corrected. A shunt procedure can be employed in cases with progressive ventriculomegaly.

Lissencephaly

Incidence. Unknown, but rare.

Definition. It is characterized by a lack of gyral development and is divided into two types:

- *Lissencephaly type I*: a smooth surface of the brain. The cerebral wall is similar to that of an approximately 12-week-old fetus:[57]
  - isolated lissencephaly
  - Miller–Dieker syndrome, with additional craniofacial abnormalities, cardiac anomalies, genital anomalies, sacral dimple, creases, and/or clinodactyly
- *Lissencephaly type II*: cobblestone appearance:
  - Walker–Warburg syndrome, with macrocephaly, congenital muscular dystrophy, cerebellar malformation, and retinal malformation
  - Fukuyama congenital muscular dystrophy, with microcephaly and congenital muscular dystrophy.

Synonyms. Agyria; pachygyria; Walker–Warburg syndrome was known as HARD±E syndrome (<u>h</u>ydrocephalus, <u>a</u>gyria, retinal <u>d</u>ysplasia, with or without <u>e</u>ncephalocele).

Etiology. Isolated lissencephaly is linked to chromosomes 17p13.3 and Xq24–q24. Miller–Dieker syndrome is also linked to chromosome 17p13.3. Walker–Warburg syndrome has an autosomal recessive inheritance. Fukuyama congenital muscular dystrophy is linked to chromosome 9q31 and fukutin.[58]

Pathogenesis. Defective neuronal migration, with four, rather than six, layers in the cortex.

Associated anomalies. Polyhydramnios; less fetal movement; colpocephaly; agenesis of the corpus callosum; Dandy–Walker malformation. In Miller–Dieker syndrome: micrognathia; flat nose; high forehead; low-set ears; cardiac anomalies; genital anomalies are often observed in males.

Prenatal diagnosis. A few reports of prenatal diagnosis of lissencephaly have been published.[59–61] Without previous history of an affected child, diagnosis probably cannot be reliably made until 26–28 weeks of gestation.[42]

Prognosis. Type I: hypotonia; paucity of movements; feeding disturbance; seizures – the prognosis is poor, and death occurs. Type II: severe seizures; mental disorders; severe muscle disease with hypotonia – death in the first year is common.

Recurrence risk. This depends on the etiology.

Management. Karyotyping is recommended to detect the chromosomal defect.

Schizencephaly

Incidence. Rare.

Definition. This disorder is characterized by congenital clefts in the cerebral mantle, lined by pia-ependyma, with communication between the subarachnoid space laterally and the ventricular system medially. 63% of cases are unilateral and 37% bilateral. The frontal region is involved in 44% and the frontoparietal region in 30%.[57]

Etiology. Uncertain. In a familial case, a point mutation was found in the homeobox gene *EMX2*.[62,63] Cytomegalovirus infection has also been reported in some cases.[64]

Pathogenesis. Neuronal migration disorder.

Associated anomalies. Ventriculomegaly; microcephaly; polymicrogyria; gray matter heterotopias; dysgenesis of the corpus callosum; absence of the septum pellucidum; optic nerve hypoplasia.

Differential diagnosis. Porencephaly; arachnoid cyst or other intracranial cystic masses. MRI is useful in diagnosis of schizencephaly.[65]

Prognosis. This is variable, with affected infants generally suffering from mental retardation, seizures, developmental delay, and motor disturbances.

Recurrence risk. Unknown.

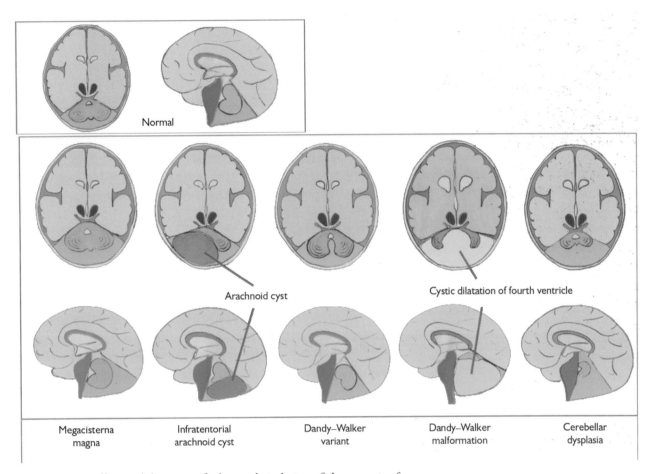

Normal

Arachnoid cyst

Cystic dilatation of fourth ventricle

| Megacisterna magna | Infratentorial arachnoid cyst | Dandy–Walker variant | Dandy–Walker malformation | Cerebellar dysplasia |

Figure 12.49 Differential diagnosis of a hypoechoic lesion of the posterior fossa

Management. Ventriculoperitoneal shunt for progressive hydrocephalus.

Dandy–Walker malformation, Dandy–Walker variant, and megacisterna magna

Incidence. Dandy–Walker malformation has an estimated prevalence of about 1/30 000 births, and is found in 4–12% of all cases of infantile hydrocephalus.[66] The incidences of Dandy–Walker variant and megacisterna magna are unknown.

Definition. At present, the term Dandy–Walker complex[67] is used to indicate a spectrum of anomalies of the posterior fossa that are classified by axial CT scans as listed below. Dandy–Walker malformation, Dandy–Walker variant, and megacisterna magna seem to represent a continuum of developmental anomalies of the posterior fossa.[67] Figure 12.49 shows the differential diagnosis of a hypoechoic lesion of the posterior fossa.

- *(Classic) Dandy–Walker malformation:* cystic dilatation of the fourth ventricle; enlarged posterior fossa; elevated tentorium; complete or partial agenesis of the cerebellar vermis
- *Dandy–Walker variant:* variable hypoplasia of the cerebellar vermis, with or without enlargement of the posterior fossa
- *Megacisterna magna:* enlarged cisterna magna, with integrity of both cerebellar vermis and the fourth ventricle.

Etiology. Mendelian disorders such as Warburg syndrome; chromosomal aberrations such as 45,X and partial monosomy/trisomy; viral infections; diabetes.

Pathogenesis. During development of the fourth ventricular roof, a delay or total failure of the foramen of Magendie to open occurs, allowing a build-up of cerebrospinal fluid (CSF) and development of a cystic dilatation of the fourth ventricle. Despite the subsequent opening of the foramina of Luschka (usually patent in Dandy–Walker malformation), cystic

245

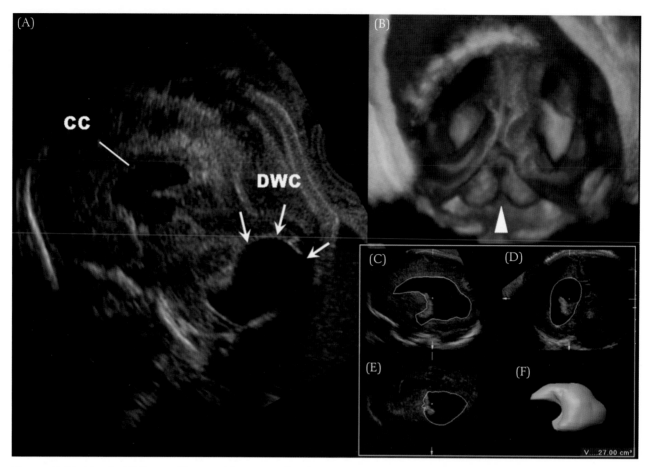

Figure 12.50 Dandy–Walker malformation at 28 weeks of gestation. (A) Median section of the brain: the corpus callosum (CC) is normally demonstrated and a Dandy–Walker cyst (DWC, arrows) is seen in the posterior fossa. (B) 3D view in the posterior coronal section: hypoplastic vermis of the cerebellum (arrowhead) is seen. Three orthogonal views (C–E) and an extracted ventricular appearance (F) demonstrate moderate ventriculomegaly in this case

dilatation of the fourth ventricle persists and CSF flow is impaired.

Anomalies associated with Dandy–Walker malformation. Hydrocephalus; other midline anomalies such as agenesis of the corpus callosum, holoprosencephaly, and occipital encephalocele; extracranial abnormalities such as congenital heart diseases, neural tube defects, and cleft lip/palate. The frequency of additional anomalies ranges between 50% and 70%.

Prenatal diagnosis. For Dandy–Walker malformation, see Figures 12.50 and 12.51. For Dandy–Walker variant, see Figure 12.52. To observe the agenesis of the cerebellar vermis, the axial section is preferable. To observe the elevated tentorium, the sagittal section is preferable.

Differential diagnosis. Infratentorial arachnoid cyst; other intracranial cystic tumors; hydrocephalus; cerebellar dysplasia.

Prognosis. There is progressive hydrocephalus – not observed in neonates but often progressive during the first month. For cases diagnosed in utero or in the neonatal period, the outcome is generally unfavorable: nearly 40% die, and 75% of survivors exhibit cognitive deficits. Prognosis of Dandy–Walker variant is good. The clinical significance of megacisterna magna is uncertain.

Recurrence risk. This depends on the etiology: generally 1–5% (Dandy–Walker malformation).

Management. Cyst–peritoneal shunt or cyst–ventriculoperitoneal shunt.

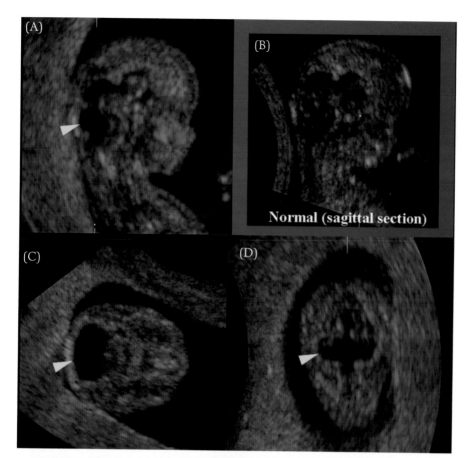

Figure 12.51 (A,C,D) Early stage of Dandy–Walker malformation or variant at 11 weeks of gestation. Abnormal dilatation of the posterior fossa (arrowheads). (B) Sagittal image at the same gestational age in a normal case. Amniocentesis revealed trisomy 9 mosaicism, and the fetus died in utero at 19 weeks

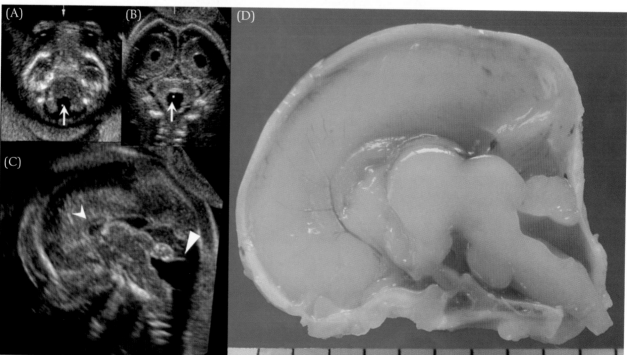

Figure 12.52 Dandy–Walker variant at 20 weeks of gestation. (A,B) 2D axial and 2D posterior coronal 3D thick slices of oblique coronal and axial sections. Hypoplasia of the vermis (arrows) is demonstrated, and no marked ventriculomegaly can be seen. (C) Median section. Partial agenesis of the corpus callosum (arrowhead), floated cerebellum, and cystic formation of the posterior fossa (triangular arrowhead) can be seen. (D) Median section of a specimen of an aborted fetus at 21 weeks of gestation. This case had other complicated anomalies, and the karyotype was partial trisomy of chromosome 10

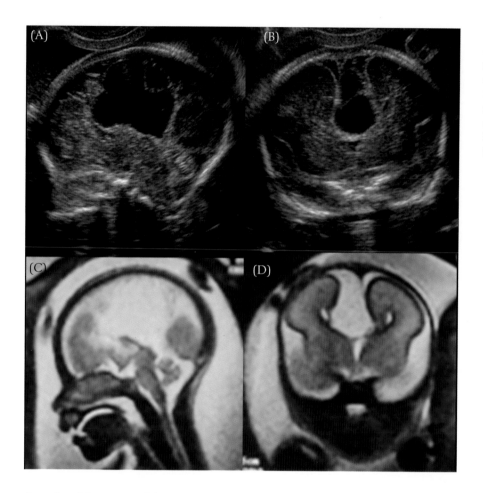

Figure 12.53 Sonographic (A,B) and magnetic resonance (C,D) images of an interhemispheric cyst at 24 weeks of gestation. (A,C) Median sections; (B,D) anterior coronal sections. There is a cystic lesion between the hemispheres. An intracystic cyst is visible on the sonograms (A,B)

Arachnoid cyst and interhemispheric cyst

Prevalence. 1% of intracranial masses in newborns.

Definition. This is a congenital or acquired cyst, lined by arachnoid membranes, and filled with a fluid collection that is of the same character as the CSF. The cysts are mostly single, but two or more can occasionally be observed. The location of arachnoid cysts is variable: approximately 50% of cysts arise from the Sylvian fissure (middle fossa); 20% from the posterior fossa; and 10–20% each from the convexity, suprasellar, interhemisphere, and quadrigeminal cistern. Interhemispheric cysts are often associated with agenesis or hypogenesis of the corpus callosum.

Etiology. Unknown.

Pathogenesis. Congenital arachnoid cysts are formed by maldevelopment of the arachnoid membrane. CSF accumulation in the subarachnoid space or intra-arachnoid layers from a choroid plexus-like tissue within the cyst wall leads to a progressive distension of the lesion.

Associated anomalies. Unilateral or bilateral hydrocephalus; macrocrania.

Prenatal diagnosis. See Figure 12.53. Detection in the first trimester has been reported.[68]

Differential diagnosis. Porencephaly; schizencephaly; third ventriculomegaly; intracranial cystic-type tumor; vein of Galen aneurysm; Dandy–Walker malformation; large cisterna magna; external hydrocephalus.

Prognosis. This is generally good. Postnatally, many are asymptomatic and remain quiescent for years, although others expand and cause neurologic symptoms by compressing adjacent brain, ventriculomegaly, and/or expanding the overlying skull.

Recurrence risk. Unknown.

Obstetric management. Arachnoid cysts may increase or decrease in size. Therefore, expectant management of antenatally diagnosed cases is suggested.[69] In cases with accompanying hydrocephalus, the mode and timing of delivery may be modified.

Postnatal management. In cases with symptoms or with prospects of neurologic symptoms, treatment should be considered. Operative methods include:

- cyst fenestration by craniotomy
- cyst fenestration by neuroendoscopy
- cyst–peritoneal shunt.

Craniotomy, shunting, or neuroendoscopic methods are still controversial.[70,71]

CRANIOSYNOSTOSIS

Incidence. Unknown.

Definition. This is premature closure of cranial sutures, affecting one or more of these. Simple sagittal synostosis is most common. The various cranial shapes depend on the affected suture(s):

- sagittal suture — scaphocephaly or dolichocephaly
- bilateral coronal suture — brachycephaly
- unilateral coronal suture — anterior plagiocephaly
- metopic suture — trigonocephaly
- lambdoid suture — acrocephaly
- unilateral lambdoid suture — posterior plagiocephaly
- coronal/lambdoid/metopic or squamous/sagittal suture — cloverleaf skull
- total cranial sutures — oxycephaly.

Syndromes.
- *Crouzon syndrome:* acrocephaly; synostosis of coronal, sagittal, and lambdoid sutures; with ocular proptosis, maxillary hypoplasia
- *Apert syndrome:* brachycephaly; irregular synostosis, especially coronal suture; with midfacial hypoplasia, syndactyly, broad distal phalanx of thumb and big toe
- *Pfeiffer syndrome:* brachycephaly; synostosis of coronal and/or sagittal sutures; with hypertelorism, broad thumbs and toes, partial syndactyly
- *Antley–Bixler syndrome:* brachycephaly; multiple synostosis; especially of coronal suture; with maxillary hypoplasia, radiohymeral synostosis, choanal atresia, arthrogryposis.

Etiology. Crouzon syndrome is autosomal dominant, variable; Apert syndrome is autosomal dominant, usually a new mutation; Pfeiffer syndrome is autosomal dominant; Antley–Bixler syndrome is autosomal recessive. Five autosomal dominant craniosynostosis syndromes (Apert, Crouzon, Pfeiffer, Jackson–Weiss, and Crouzon with acanthosis nigricans) result from mutations in *FGFR* (fibroblast growth factor receptor) genes.[72]

Pathogenesis.[73] (1) Cranial vault bones with decreased growth potential. (2) Asymmetric bone deposition at perimeter sutures. (3) Sutures adjacent to the prematurely fused suture compensate in growth more than those sutures that are not contiguous with the closed suture. (4) Enhanced symmetric bone deposition occurs along both sides of a non-perimeter suture continuing a prematurely closed suture.

Associated anomalies. Hypertelorism; syndactyly; polydactyly; exophthalmos.

Prenatal diagnosis. Figure 12.54 shows facial abnormality in a case of Pfeiffer syndrome. The intracranial structure with an abnormal shape of the ventricles is demonstrated in Figure 12.55. Abnormal craniofacial appearance can be detected by 2D/3D ultrasound.[74,75]

Prognosis. This varies: in some of the trigonocephaly and syndromic types, the prognosis is poor.

Recurrence risk. This depends on the etiology.

Management. The aim of cranioplasty is improvement of intracranial pressure and cosmetic change.

Vein of Galen aneurysm

Incidence. Rare.

Definition. These are direct arteriovenous fistulas between choroidal and/or quadrigeminal arteries and an overlying single median venous sac.

Synonyms. Vein of Galen malformation.

Etiology. Unknown.

Pathogenesis. The venous sac most probably represents persistence of the embryonic median

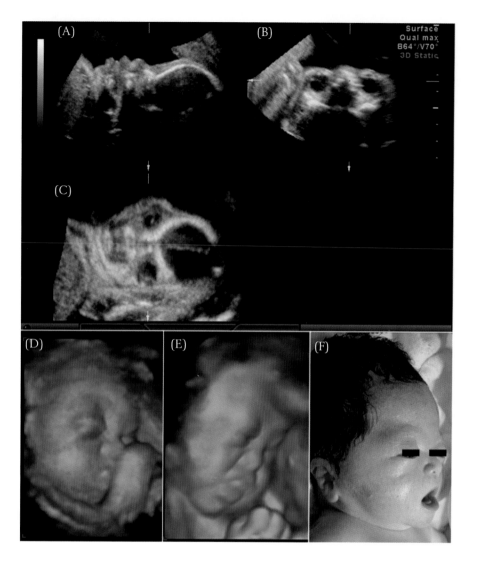

Figure 12.54 Facial abnormality in a case of craniosynostosis. (A–C) Three orthogonal views of the fetal face at 26 weeks of gestation. Hypertelorism, proptosis, and a flat face are demonstrated. (D,E) 3D surface images of the fetal face. (F) The baby's face at birth. Pfeiffer syndrome was strongly suspected

prosencephalic vein of Markowski, not the vein of Galen per se.[76]

Associated anomalies. Cardiomegaly; high cardiac output; secondary hydrocephalus; macrocrania; cerebral ischemia (intracranial steal phenomenon); subarachnoid/cerebral/intraventricular hemorrhages.

Prenatal diagnosis. 2D and 3D color/power Doppler detection is possible.

Differential diagnosis. Arachnoid cyst; porencephalic cyst; intracranial teratoma. Color/power Doppler is helpful for differential diagnosis.

Prognosis. According to earlier reviews, outcome did not differ between treated and untreated groups, and over 80% of cases died.[77] However, recent advances in treatment have improved outcome, such that 60–100% survive and over 60% have a good neurologic outcome.[78,79]

Recurrence risk. Unknown.

Management. Evaluation of the fetal high-output cardiac state is necessary for proper obstetric management. Percutaneous embolization by microcoils is the current main postnatal treatment and has markedly improved outcome.

Choroid plexus cysts

Incidence. 0.61–2.89% of all fetuses scanned.[80–86]

Definition. These are cysts with fluid collection within the choroid plexus; these may be unilateral or bilateral. They are depicted in the 2nd trimester and usually resolve by the 24th week of gestation.

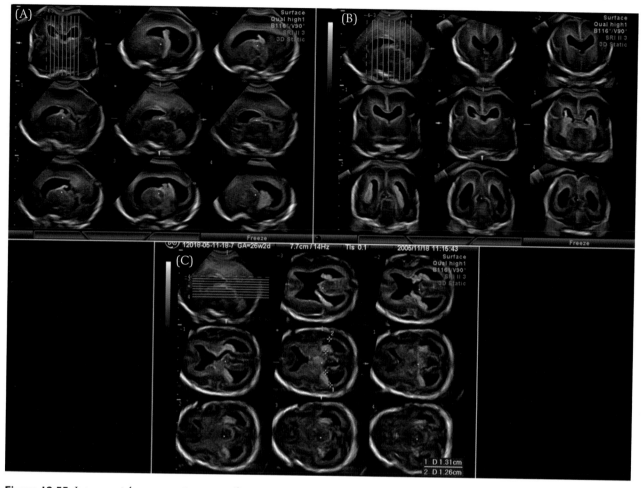

Figure 12.55 Intracranial structure in a case of craniosynostosis. Tomographic ultrasound imaging of sagittal (A), coronal (B), and axial (C) sections. Fusion of enlarged ventricles and abnormal shape of the ventricles due to craniosynostosis can be seen

Etiology. This is a normal variant.

Pathogenesis. The choroid plexus is located within the ventricular system and produces CSF. Within the choroidal villi, choroid plexus cysts exist, surrounded by the loose stroma of the choroid plexus.[83] Choroid plexus cysts probably result from entrapment of CSF within tangled villi of the fetal ventricular system.[87]

Associated anomalies. In cases of trisomy 18, associated anomalies include growth retardation, congenital heart diseases such as ventricular septal defect and double-outlet right ventricle, overlapping fingers, facial anomalies, cerebellar dysplasia, and others.

Prenatal diagnosis. Figure 12.56 shows prenatal sonograms of choroid plexus cysts in cases of trisomy 18 and normal karyotype. It is impossible to distin-

guish normal from abnormal karyotypes just by the location and appearance of choroid plexus cysts. Detection of additional anomalies is important for differential diagnosis.

Differential diagnosis. Intraventricular hemorrhage.

Prognosis. Choroid plexus cysts per se are usually asymptomatic and benign, but rarely may be symptomatic and disturb CSF flow.[88,89] Isolated choroid plexus cysts may be a normal variation.

Recurrence risk. Unknown.

Management. An isolated choroid plexus cyst is an indication to perform a detailed and accurate examination of other markers of aneuploidy. If the choroid plexus cyst is an isolated finding, there is no reason to perform amniocentesis.[84]

251

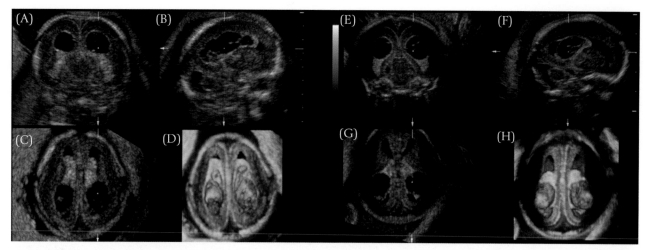

Figure 12.56 Choroid plexus cysts in cases of trisomy 18 and normal karyotype. (A–D) Three orthogonal views (A–C) and inside 3D view (D) of a choroid plexus cyst in a case of trisomy 18 at 17 weeks of gestation. Various additional anomalies were detected. Three orthogonal views (E–G) and inside 3D view (H) of a choroid plexus cyst in a case with normal karyotype at 16 weeks of gestation. No additional abnormalities were detected and the postnatal course was normal. It is impossible to distinguish normal from abnormal karyotypes just by the location and appearance of a choroid plexus cyst. Detection of additional anomalies is important for differential diagnosis

ACQUIRED BRAIN ABNORMALITIES IN UTERO

In terms of encephalopathy or cerebral palsy, the timing of brain insult – antepartum, intrapartum, or postpartum – is a controversial issue, involving medical, social, legal, and ethical aspects.[24] Although brain insults may be related to antepartum events in a substantial number of term infants with hypoxic–ischemic encephalopathy, the timing of the insult cannot always be determined. It is difficult to obtain antepartum evidence of brain injury predictive of cerebral palsy. Fetal heart rate monitoring cannot reveal the presence of encephalopathy, and neuroimaging by ultrasound and MRI is the most reliable modality for disclosure of silent encephalopathy. In many cases with cerebral palsy with acquired brain insults especially, term-delivered infants with reactive fetal heart rate tracing and good Apgar score at delivery are not suspected to have encephalopathy and are often overlooked for months or years. Recent imaging technology has revealed brain insults in utero.

Brain tumors

Incidence. Extremely rare.

Definition. Tumors located in the intracranial cavity.

Histologic types. Brain tumors are devided into *teratomas*, which are the most commonly reported, and non-teratomatous tumors. The latter include *neuroepithelial tumors*, such as medulloblastoma, astrocytoma, choroid plexus papilloma, choroid plexus carcinoma, ependymoma, and ependymoblastoma, *mesenchymal tumors*, such as craniopharyngioma, sarcoma, fibroma, hemangioblastoma, hemangioma, and meningoma, and *others*, such as lipoma of the corpus callosum and subependymal giant-cell astrocytoma associated with tuberous sclerosis (often accompanied by cardiac rhabdomyoma).[90,91]

Location of tumor. There is a supratentorial predominance among neonatal tumors as a whole, but an infratentorial predominance in medulloblastoma. Choroid plexus papilloma is located within the lateral ventricles.

Associated abnormalities. Macrocrania or local skull swelling; epignathus; secondary hydrocephalus; intracranial hemorrhage; intraventricular hemorrhage; polyhydroamnios; heart failure due to high cardiac output;[92] hydrops.

Diagnosis. Intracranial masses with solid, cystic, or mixed pattern with or without visualization of hypervascularity are seen on sonography and fetal MRI. Brain tumors should be considered in cases with unexplained intracranial hemorrhage.

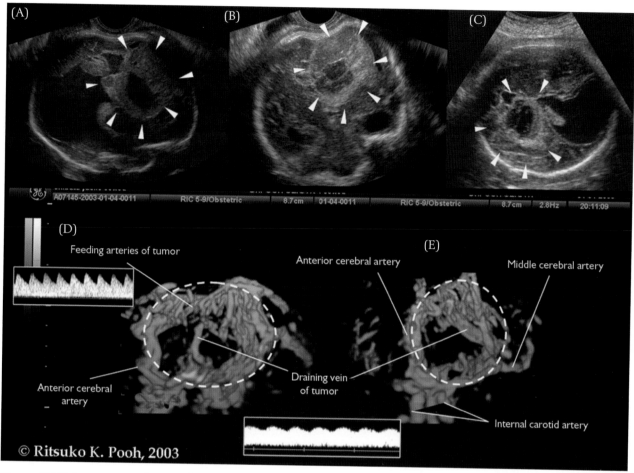

Figure 12.57 Sonograms and tumoral vascular visualization by 3D power Doppler in a fetus with an intracranial tumor with interventricular hemorrhage (35 weeks and 5 days of gestation). (A–C) Sagittal, coronal, and axial images. There is a huge tumor (arrowheads) with hemorrhage within the tumor in the frontoparietal lobe, complicated with unilateral hydrocephalus with intraventricular hemorrhage. (D) Oblique sagittal view from the fetal left side. (E) Oblique coronal view from the fetal front side. The tumor is fed by numerous feeding arteries from the anterior cerebral artery. The feeder arteries have a low-resistance flow waveform. One large vein draining blood from the tumor is visible. The draining vein has a pulsatile flow

Prenatal diagnosis. Prenatal diagnosis of an intracranial tumor and its vascularization by 3D power Doppler is shown in Figure 12.57.

Differential diagnosis. Arachnoid cyst; vein of Galen aneurysm; porencephaly; schizencephaly; periventricular leukomalacia; subdural hemorrhage.

Prognosis. Fetal demise – stillbirth may occur. Prognosis in neonates is generally poor, but depends on the timing of diagnosis and the histologic type of the tumor. Choroid plexus papilloma has a minimal mortality rate and a high likelihood of neonatal outcome. The mortality rate of teratomas is over 90%; that of medulloblastoma over 80%. Other tumors have various prognoses.

Recurrence risk. Unknown.

Management. Cesarean section may be considered. Neurosurgical tumor resection, including subtotal hemispherectomy by craniotomy, and chemotherapy are possible treatments for neonatal tumors. Radiotherapy is usually not indicated in neonates.

Subependymal pseudocysts

Prevalence. 2.6–5% of all neonates; 1% of premature newborns; unknown in fetuses.

Definition. Cystic formation, located in the caudothalamic groove or in the caudate nucleus, lateral to the wall of the anterior horns of the lateral ventricles.

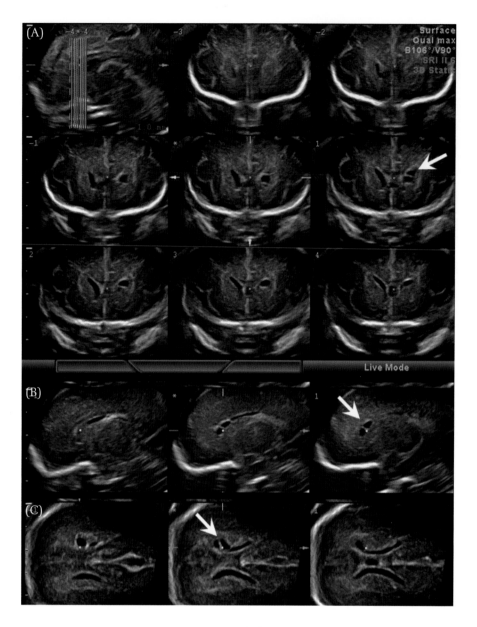

Figure 12.58 Subependymal cysts. (A) Coronal tomographic ultrasound images of unilateral subependymal cysts. Two clear cysts are demonstrated (arrow). (B) Sagittal tomographic images. (C) Axial tomographic images

Synonyms. Periventricular pseudocysts.[93,94]

Etiology. Infection (cytomegalovirus or rubella); subependymal hemorrhage; metabolic diseases; chromosomal deletions (del (q6) or del (p4)); cocaine exposure; and others.

Pathogenesis. The cystic cavity is lined by a pseudo-capsule consisting of aggregates of germinal cells and glial tissue, but no epithelium can be found. The origin of pseudocysts is uncertain – they may be due to cystic matrix regression or germinolysis.

Associated anomalies. Congenital infection (e.g., cytomegalovirus); congenital heart diseases; associated CNS abnormalities.

Prenatal diagnosis. Figure 12.58 shows tomographic ultrasound imaging of subependymal cysts.

Differential diagnosis. Periventricular leukomalacia.

Prognosis. This is good in cases with isolated subependymal pseudocysts. In cases with accompanying abnormalities (e.g., cardiac disease, cytomegalovirus infection, or other intracranial abnormalities), or cases with atypical pseudocysts, the prognosis may be poor.[93–95]

Recurrence risk. Unknown.

Management. In many cases, cysts regress several months after birth. Obstetric/neonatal care is normal.

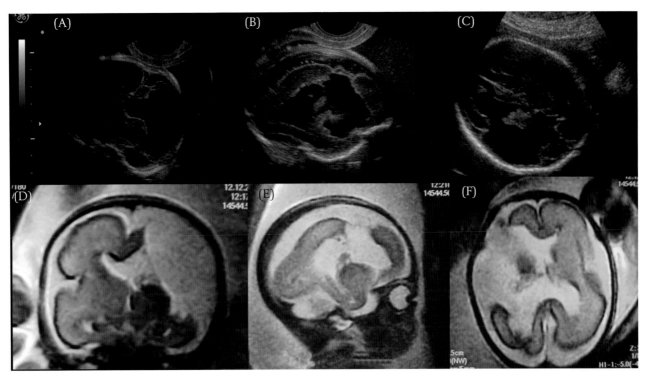

Figure 12.59 Fetal sonographic and magnetic resonance images of porencephaly at 25 weeks of gestation. (A) Transvaginal coronal sonogram showing a defect in the parietolateral part of the unilateral cerebrum. This case also has an absent septum pellucidum. (B) Parasagittal sonogram: the porencephalic part is fused with the unilateral ventricle, and the echogenicity of the inside of the ventricular wall indicates intraventricular hemorrhage. (C) Transabdominal axial sonogram. (D–F) Fetal magnetic resonance images on the same day: coronal (D), parasagittal (E), and axial (F) sections from the left side

Porencephaly

Incidence. Unknown.

Definition Fluid-filled spaces replace normal brain parenchyma, and may or may not communicate with the lateral ventricles or subarachnoid space.

Synonyms. Porencephalic cyst.

Etiology. Ischemic episode; trauma;[96] demise of one twin; intercerebral hemorrhage; infection.

Pathogenesis. This occurs when the immature cerebrum has a propensity to dissolution and cavitation (due to a high water content, myelinated fiber bundles, or a deficient astroglial response). The timing of ischemic injury (maybe as early as the 2nd trimester) is closely related to porencephaly and hydranencephaly.[97]

Associated anomalies. Intercerebral hemorrhage; interventricular hemorrhage; hydrocephalus.

Prenatal diagnosis. Figure 12.59 shows porencephaly after intracerebral hemorrhage at 25 weeks of gestation. Some cases have been reported in utero.[98,99]

Differential diagnosis. Schizencephaly; arachnoid cyst; intracranial cystic tumor; other cysts. A porencephalic cyst never causes a mass effect, which is observed with arachnoid cysts and other cystic mass lesions. This condition is an acquired brain insult and should be differentiated from schizencephaly of migration disorder.

Prognosis. This is variable, depending on the timing and size of the lesion. Seizures, neurologic deficits, and cerebral palsy often occur.[100]

Recurrence risk. Unknown.

Management. A ventriculoperitoneal shunt should be applied if hydrocephalus progresses.

Hydranencephaly

Incidence. 1–2.5/10 000 births.

Definition. Absence of the cerebral hemispheres and a sac-like structure containing CSF surrounding the brainstem and basal ganglia.

Etiology. Ischemic episode; trauma; demise of one twin; intercerebral hemorrhage; infection. There are several theories, but bilateral occlusion of the supra-clinoid segment of the internal carotid arteries[101] or of the middle cerebral arteries is one cause of subtotal defects of the cerebral hemisphere.

Pathogenesis. It may occur when the immature cerebrum has a propensity to dissolution and cavitation (due to a high water content, myelinated fiber bundles, or a deficient astroglial response). The timing of ischemic injury (may be as early as the 2nd trimester) is closely related to porencephaly and hydranencephaly.

Prenatal diagnosis. Hydranencephaly from 11 weeks of gestation has been reported.[102]

Differential diagnosis. Massive hydrocephalus; alobar holoprosencephaly; porencephaly.

Prognosis. Extremely poor.

Recurrence risk. Unknown.

Management. There is no active treatment. A shunt procedure may be used for progressive increase in the size of the infant's head.

Intracranial hemorrhage

Incidence. Unknown, but rare in utero.

Definition. Hemorrhage, with bleeding inside of the cranium. Intracranial hemorrhage includes subdural hemorrhage, primary subarachnoid hemorrhage, intracerebellar hemorrhage, intraventricular hemorrhage, and intraparenchymal hemorrhage other than cerebellar.[103]

Etiology. Trauma; alloimmune and idiopathic thrombocytopenia; von Willebrand disease; specific medications (warfarin) or illicit drug (cocaine) abuse; seizures; fetal conditions, including congenital factor X and factor V deficiencies; intracranial tumors; twin–twin transfusion; demise of a co-twin; vascular diseases; fetomaternal hemorrhage; extracorporeal membrane oxygenation (ECMO).[104]

Associated anomalies. Hydrocephalus; hydranencephaly; porencephaly; microcephaly.

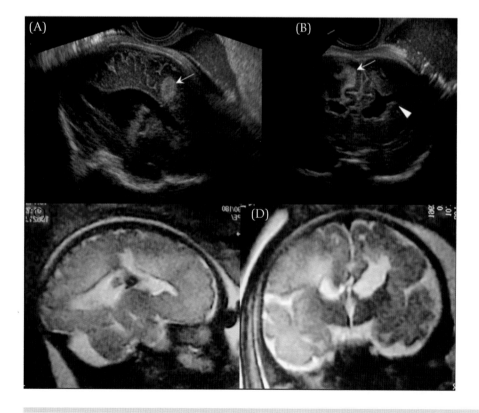

Figure 12.60 Sonographic and magnetic resonance images in a fetus with cerebral hemorrhage and mild ventriculomegaly at 35 weeks of gestation. Parasagittal (A) and anterior coronal (B) sonograms of the brain. The arrows indicate intracerebral hemorrhage. The arrowhead shows a porencephalic part fused with the lateral ventricle. (C,D) Magnetic resonance images showing the same cutting sections as (A) and (B), respectively

Prenatal diagnosis. Figure 12.60 shows multiple intracerebral hemorrhage at 35 weeks.

Differential diagnosis. Intracranial tumor.

Prognosis. This is poor in premature infants, with apnea, seizures, and other neurologic symptoms.

Recurrence risk. This depends on the etiology.

Management. A ventriculoperitoneal shunt may be used if hydrocephalus progresses.

Fetal periventricular leukomalacia (PVL)

Incidence. 25–75% of premature infants at autopsy are complicated with periventricular white matter injury. However, clinically, the incidence may be much lower: 5–10% of infants of <1500 g birthweight. PVL is very rare in at-term infants.

Definition. Multifocal areas of necrosis are found deep in the cortical white matter; they are often symmetrical and occur adjacent to the lateral ventricles. PVL represents a major precursor to neurologic and intellectual impairment, and cerebral palsy in later life.

Etiology. Birth trauma; asphyxia and respiratory failure; cardiopulmonary defects; premature birth/low birthweight; associated immature cerebrovascular development and lack of appropriate autoregulation of cerebral blood flow in response to hypoxic–ischemic insults.[105]

Pathogenesis. Distinctive, consisting primarily of both focal periventricular necrosis and more diffuse cerebral white matter injury. The two most common sites are at the level of the cerebral white matter near the trigone of the lateral ventricles and around the foramen of Monro. Volpe[97] describes three factors closely related to PVL: (1) periventricular vascular anatomic and physiologic factors; (2) cerebral ischemia; (3) intrinsic vulnerability of cerebral white matter of premature newborn.

Differential diagnosis. Subarachnoid (periventricular) pseudocysts; porencephaly; other intracranial cystic formation.

Prognosis. Neurologic features of PVL in the neonatal period are lower limb weakness and (as features of long-term sequelae) spastic diplegia, intellectual deficits, and visual deficits.[97]

Recurrence risk. Unknown.

Management. Early rehabilitation.

REFERENCES

1. Timor-Tritsch IE, Peisner DB, Raju S. Sonoembryology: an organ-oriented approach using a high-frequency vaginal probe. J Clin Ultrasound 1990; 18: 286–98.

2. Pooh RK. B-mode and Doppler studies of the abnormal fetus in the first trimester. In: Chervenak FA, Kurjak A, eds. Fetal Medicine. Carnforth, UK: Parthenon, 1999: 46–51.

3. Timor-Tritsch IE, Monteagudo A. Transvaginal fetal neurosonography: standardization of the planes and sections by anatomic landmarks. Ultrasound Obstet Gynecol 1996; 8: 42–7.

4. Monteagudo A, Reuss ML, Timor-Tritsch IE. Imaging the fetal brain in the second and third trimesters using transvaginal sonography. Obstet Gynecol 1991; 77: 27–32.

5. Monteagudo A, Timor-Tritsch IE, Moomjy M. In utero detection of ventriculomegaly during the second and third trimesters by transvaginal sonography. Ultrasound Obstet Gynecol 1994; 4: 193–8.

6. Monteagudo A, Timor-Tritsch IE. Development of fetal gyri, sulci and fissures: a transvaginal sonographic study. Ultrasound Obstet Gynecol 1997; 9: 222–8.

7. Pooh RK, Nakagawa Y, Nagamachi N, et al. Transvaginal sonography of the fetal brain: detection of abnormal morphology and circulation. Croat Med J 1998; 39: 147–57.

8. Pooh RK, Maeda K, Pooh KH, Kurjak A. Sonographic assessment of the fetal brain morphology. Prenat Neonat Med 1999; 4: 18–38.

9. Pooh RK. Three-dimensional ultrasound of the fetal brain. In: Kurjak A, Kupesik S, eds. Clinical Application of 3D Ultrasonography. Carnforth, UK: Parthenon, 2000: 176–80.

10. Pooh RK, Pooh KH, Nakagawa Y, Nishida S, Ohno Y. Clinical application of three-dimensional ultrasound in fetal brain assessment. Croat Med J 2000; 41: 245–51.

11. Timor-Tritsch IE, Monteagudo A, Mayberry P. Three-dimensional ultrasound evaluation of the fetal brain: the three horn view. Ultrasound Obstet Gynecol 2000; 16: 302–6.

12. Monteagudo A, Timor-Tritsch IE, Mayberry P. Three-dimensional transvaginal neurosonography of the fetal

brain: 'navigating' in the volume scan. Ultrasound Obstet Gynecol 2000; 16: 307–13.

13. Pooh RK, Pooh KH. Fetal neuroimaging with new technology. Ultrasound Rev Obstet Gynecol 2002; 2: 178–81.

14. Blaas HG, Eik-Nes SH, Kiserud T, et al. Three-dimensional imaging of the brain cavities in human embryos. Ultrasound Obstet Gynecol 1995; 5: 228–32.

15. Blaas HG, Eik-Nes SH, Berg S, Torp H. In-vivo three-dimensional ultrasound reconstructions of embryos and early fetuses. Lancet 1998; 352: 1182–6.

16. Pooh RK. Fetal brain assessment by three-dimensional ultrasound. In: Kurjak A, Kupesic S, eds. Clinical Application of 3D Sonography. Carnforth, UK: Parthenon, 2000: 171–9.

17. Pooh RK, Pooh KH. Transvaginal 3D and Doppler ultrasonography of the fetal brain. Semin Perinatol 2001; 25: 38–43.

18. Pooh RK, Pooh KH. The assessment of fetal brain morphology and circulation by transvaginal 3D sonography and power Doppler. J Perinat Med 2002; 30: 48–56.

19. Endres LK, Cohen L. Reliability and validity of three-dimensional fetal brain volumes. J Ultrasound Med 2001; 20: 1265–9.

20. Roelfsema NM, Hop WC, Boito SM, Wladimiroff JW. Three-dimensional sonographic measurement of normal fetal brain volume during the second half of pregnancy. Am J Obstet Gynecol 2004; 190: 275–80.

21. Pooh RK, Aono T. Transvaginal power Doppler angiography of the fetal brain. Ultrasound Obstet Gynecol 1996; 8: 417–21.

22. Pooh RK. Two-dimensional and three-dimensional Doppler angiography in fetal brain circulation. In: Kurjak A, ed. 3D Power Doppler in Obstetrics and Gynecology. Carnforth, UK: Parthenon, 1999: 105–11.

23. Moore KL, Persaud TVN. The Developing Human. Clinically Oriented Embryology, 7th edn. Pennsylvania, PA: Saunders, 2003.

24. Pooh RK, Maeda K, Pooh KH. An Atlas of Fetal Central Nervous System Disease. Diagnosis and Management. London: Parthenon/CRC Press, 2003.

25. Pooh RK, Pooh KH, Nakagawa Y, et al. Transvaginal Doppler assessment of fetal intracranial venous flow. Obstet Gynecol 1999; 93: 697–701.

26. Alagappan R, Browning PD, Laorr A, McGahan JP. Distal lateral ventricular atrium: reevaluation of normal range. Radiology 1994; 193: 405–8.

27. Almog B, Gamzu R, Achiron R, et al. Fetal lateral ventricular width: What should be its upper limit? A prospective cohort study and reanalysis of the current and previous data. J Ultrasound Med 2003; 22: 39–43.

28. Signorelli M, Tiberti A, Valseriati D, et al. Width of the fetal lateral ventricular atrium between 10 and 12 mm: a simple variation of the norm? Ultrasound Obstet Gynecol 2004; 23: 14–18.

29. Fransen E, Lemmon V, Van Camp G, et al. CRASH syndrome: clinical spectrum of corpus callosum hypoplasia, retardation, adducted thumbs, spastic paraparesis and hydrocephalus due to mutations in one single gene, L1. Eur J Hum Genet 1995; 3: 273–84.

30. Yamasaki M, Thompson P, Lemmon V. CRASH syndrome: mutations in L1CAM correlate with severity of the disease. Neuropediatrics 1997; 28: 175–8.

31. Timor-Tritsch IE, Monteagudo A, Haratz-Rubinstein N, Levine RU. Transvaginal sonographic detection of adducted thumbs, hydrocephalus, and agenesis of the corpus callosum at 22 postmenstrual weeks: the MASA spectrum or L1 spectrum. A case report and review of the literature. Prenat Diagn 1996; 16: 543–8.

32. Patel MD, Filly AL, Hersh DR, Goldstein RB. Isolated mild fetal cerebral ventriculomegaly: clinical course and outcome. Radiology 1994; 192: 759–64.

33. Pilu G, Falco P, Gabrielli S, et al. The clinical significance of fetal isolated cerebral borderline ventriculomegaly: report of 31 cases and review of the literature. Ultrasound Obstet Gynecol 1999; 14: 320–6.

34. Wakayama A, Morimoto K, Kitajima H, et al. Extremely low birth-weight infant with hydrocephalus; management of hydrocephalus using a miniature Ommaya's reservoir. No Shinkei Geka 1991; 19: 795–800.

35. Morimoto K, Hayakawa T, Yoshimine T, Wakayama A, Kuroda R. Two-step procedure for early neonatal surgery of fetal hydrocephalus. Neurol Med Chir 1993; 33: 158–65.

36. Fritsch MJ, Mehdorn M. Endoscopic intraventricular surgery for treatment of hydrocephalus and loculated CSF space in children less than one year of age. Pediatr Neurosurg 2002; 36: 183–8.

37. Martinez de Villarreal L, Perez JZ, Vazquez PA, et al. Decline of neural tube defects cases after a folic acid campaign in Nuevo Leon, Mexico. Teratology 2002; 66: 249–56.

38. Ray JG, Meier C, Vermeulen MJ, et al. Association of neural tube defects and folic acid food fortification in Canada. Lancet 2002; 360: 2047–8.

39. Persad VL, Van den Hof MC, Dube JM, Zimmer P. Incidence of open neural tube defects in Nova Scotia after folic acid fortification. CMAJ 2002; 167: 241–5.

40. Mathews TJ, Honein MA, Erickson JD. Spina bifida and anencephaly prevalence – United States, 1991–2001. MMWR Recomm Rep 2002; 51: 9–11.

41. Green NS. Folic acid supplementation and prevention of birth defects. J Nutr 2002; 132: 2356S-60S.

42. Monteagudo A, Timor-Tritsch IE. Fetal neurosonography of congenital brain anomalies. In: Timor-Tritsch IE, Monteagudo A, Cohen HL, eds. Ultrasonography of the Prenatal and Neonatal Brain, 2nd edn. New York: McGraw-Hill, 2001: 151–258.

43. Stevenson RE, Allen WP, Pai GS, et al. Decline in prevalence of neural tube defects in a high-risk region of the United States. Pediatrics 2000; 106: 677–83.

44. Volpe JJ. Neural tube formation and prosencephalic development. In: Neurology of the Newborn, 4th edn. Philadelphia, PA: WB Saunders, 2001, 3–44.

45. D'Addario V, Pinto V, Del Bianco A, et al. The clivus–supraocciput angle: a useful measurement to evaluate the shape and size of the fetal posterior fossa and to diagnose Chiari II malformation. Ultrasound Obstet Gynecol 2001; 18: 146–9.

46. Matsunaga E, Shiota K. Holoprosencephaly in human embryos: epidemiologic studies of 150 cases. Teratology 1977; 16: 261–72.

47. Cohen MM Jr. Perspectives on holoprosencephaly. I. Epidemiology, genetics and syndromology. Teratology 1989; 40: 211–35.

48. Pilu G, Ambrosetto P, Sandri F, et al. Intraventricular fused fornices: a specific sign of fetal lobar holoprosencephaly. Ultrasound Obstet Gynecol 1994; 34: 259–62.

49. Cohen MM. An update on the holoprosencephalic disorders. J Pediatr 1982; 101: 865–9.

50. Pilu G, Porelo A, Falco P, Visentin A. Median anomalies of the brain. In: Timor-Tritsch IE, Monteagudo A, Cohen HL, eds. Ultrasonography of the Prenatal and Neonatal Brain, 2nd edn. New York: McGraw-Hill, 2001: 259–76.

51. Goodyear PW, Bannister CM, Russell S, Rimmer S. Outcome in prenatally diagnosed fetal agenesis of the corpus callosum. Fetal Diagn Ther 2001; 16: 139–45.

52. Taylor M, David AS. Agenesis of the corpus callosum: a United Kingdom series of 56 cases. J Neurol Neurosurg Psychiatry 1998; 64: 131–4.

53. Schmidt-Riese U, Zieger M. Ultrasound diagnosis of isolated aplasia of the septum pellucidum. Ultraschall Med 1994; 15: 286–92.

54. McMahon CL, Braddock SR. Septo-optic dysplasia as a manifestation of valproic acid embryopathy. Teratology 2001; 64: 83–6.

55. Dominguez R, Aguirre Vila-Coro A, Slopis JM, Bohan TP. Brain and ocular abnormalities in infants with in utero exposure to cocaine and other street drugs. Am J Dis Child 1991; 145: 688–95.

56. Dattani MT, Martinez-Barbera JP, Thomas PQ, et al. Mutations in the homeobox gene HESX1/Hesx1 associated with septo-optic dysplasia in human and mouse. Nat Genet 1998; 19: 125–33.

57. Volpe JJ. Neuronal proliferation, migration, organization and myelination. In: Neurology of the Newborn, 4th edn. Philadelphia, PA: WB Saunders, 2001: 45–99.

58. Kobayashi K, Nakahori Y, Miyake M, et al. An ancient retrotransposal insertion causes Fukuyama-type congenital muscular dystrophy. Nature 1998; 394: 388–92.

59. McGahan JP, Grix A, Gerscovich EO. Prenatal diagnosis of lissencephaly: Miller–Dieker syndrome. J Clin Ultrasound 1994; 22: 560–3.

60. Greco P, Resta M, Vimercati A, et al. Antenatal diagnosis of isolated lissencephaly by ultrasound and magnetic resonance imaging. Ultrasound Obstet Gynecol 1998; 12: 276–9.

61. Kojima K, Suzuki Y, Seki K, et al. Prenatal diagnosis of lissencephaly (type II) by ultrasound and fast magnetic resonance imaging. Fetal Diagn Ther 2002; 17: 34–6.

62. Granata T, Farina L, Faiella A, et al. Familial schizencephaly associated with EMX2 mutation. Neurology 1997; 48: 1403–6.

63. Brunelli S, Faiella A, Capra V, et al. Germline mutations in the homeobox gene EMX2 in patients with severe schizencephaly. Nat Genet 1996; 12: 94–6.

64. Iannetti P, Nigro G, Spalice A, Faiella A, Boncinelli E. Cytomegalovirus infection and schizencephaly: case reports. Ann Neurol 1998; 43: 123–7.

65. Denis D, Maugey-Laulom B, Carles D, et al. Prenatal diagnosis of schizencephaly by fetal magnetic resonance imaging. Fetal Diagn Ther 2001; 16: 354–9.

66. Osenbach RK, Menezes AH. Diagnosis and management of the Dandy–Walker malformation: 30 years of experience. Pediatr Neurosurg 1991; 18: 179–85.

67. Barkovich AJ, Kjos BO, Normal D, et al. Revised classification of the posterior fossa cysts and cystlike malformations based on the results of multiplanar MR imaging. AJNR Am J Neuroradiol 1989; 10: 977–88.

68. Bretelle F, Senat MV, Bernard JP, Hillion Y, Ville Y. First-trimester diagnosis of fetal arachnoid cyst: prenatal implication. Ultrasound Obstet Gynecol 2002; 20: 400–2.

69. Elbers SE, Furness ME. Resolution of presumed arachnoid cyst in utero. Ultrasound Obstet Gynecol 1999; 14: 353–5.

70. Ciricillo SF, Cogen PH, Harsh GR, et al. Intracranial arachnoid cysts in children. A comparison of the effects of fenestration and shunting. J Neurosurg 1991; 74: 230–5.

71. Nakamura Y, Mizukawa K, Yamamoto K, Nagashima T. Endoscopic treatment for a huge neonatal prepontine-suprasellar arachnoid cyst: a case report. Pediatr Neurosurg 2001; 35: 220–4.

72. Hollway GE, Suthers GK, Haan EA, et al. Mutation

detection in *FGFR2* craniosynostosis syndromes. Hum Genet 1997; 99: 251–5.

73. Delashaw JB, Persing JA, Broaddus WC, Jane JA. Cranial vault growth in craniosynostosis. J Neurosurg 1989; 70: 159–65.

74. Benacerraf BR, Spiro R, Mitchell AG. Using three-dimensional ultrasound to detect craniosynostosis in a fetus with Pfeiffer syndrome. Ultrasound Obstet Gynecol 2000; 16: 391–4.

75. Pooh RK, Nakagawa Y, Pooh KH, Nakagawa Y, Nagamachi N. Fetal craniofacial structure and intracranial morphology in a case of Apert syndrome. Ultrasound Obstet Gynecol 1999; 13: 274–80.

76. Raybaud CA, Strother CM, Hald JK. Aneurysms of the vein of Galen: embryonic considerations and anatomical features relating to the pathogenesis of the malformation. Neuroradiology 1989; 31: 109–28.

77. Hoffman HJ, Chuang S, Hendrick EB, Humphreys RP. Aneurysms of the vein of Galen. Experience at The Hospital for Sick Children, Toronto. J Neurosurg 1982; 57: 316–22.

78. Campi A, Rodesch G, Scotti G, Lasjaunias P. Aneurysmal malformation of the vein of Galen in three patients: clinical and radiological follow-up. Neuroradiology 1998; 40: 816–21.

79. Friedman DM, Verma R, Madrid M, Wisoff JH, Berenstein A. Recent improvement in outcome using transcatheter embolization techniques for neonatal aneurysmal malformations of the vein of Galen. Pediatrics 1993; 91: 583–6.

80. Kupferminc MJ, Tamura RK, Sabbagha RE, et al. Isolated choroid plexus cyst(s): an indication for amniocentesis. Am J Obstet Gynecol 1994; 171: 1068–71.

81. Reinsch R. Choroid plexus cysts – association with trisomy: prospective review of 16,059 patients. Am J Obstet Gynecol 1997; 176: 1381–3.

82. Snijders RJ, Shawa L, Nicolaides KH. Fetal choroid plexus cysts and trisomy 18: assessment of risk based on ultrasound findings and maternal age. Prenat Diagn 1994; 14: 1119–27.

83. Nadel AS, Bromley BS, Frigoletto FD Jr, Estroff JA, Benacerraf BR. Isolated choroid plexus cysts in the second-trimester fetus: Is amniocentesis really indicated? Radiology 1992; 185: 545–8.

84. Coco C, Jeanty P. Karyotyping of fetuses with isolated choroid plexus cysts is not justified in an unselected population. J Ultrasound Med 2004; 23: 899–906.

85. Morcos CL, Platt LD, Carlson DE, et al. The isolated choroid plexus cyst. Obstet Gynecol 1998; 92: 232–6.

86. Geary M, Patel S, Lamont R. Isolated choroid plexus cysts and association with fetal aneuploidy in an unselected population. Ultrasound Obstet Gynecol 1997; 10: 171–3.

87. Kennedy KA, Carey JC. Choroid plexus cysts: significance and current management practices. Semin Ultrasound CT MR 1993; 14: 23–30.

88. Lam AH, Villanueva AC. Symptomatic third ventricular choroid plexus cysts. Pediatr Radiol 1992; 22: 413–16.

89. Parizek J, Jakubec J, Hobza V, et al. Choroid plexus cyst of the left lateral ventricle with intermittent blockage of the foramen of Monro, and initial invagination into the III ventricle in a child. Childs Nerv Syst 1998; 14: 700–8.

90. Wakai S, Arai T, Nagai M. Congenital brain tumors. Surg Neurol 1984; 21: 597–609.

91. Volpe JJ. Brain tumors and vein of Galen malformation. Neurology of the Newborn, 4th edn. Philadelphia, PA: WB Saunders, 2001: 841–56.

92. Sherer DM, Abramowicz JS, Eggers PC, et al. Prenatal ultrasonographic diagnosis of intracranial teratoma and massive craniomegaly with associated high-output cardiac failure. Am J Obstet Gynecol 1993; 168: 97–9.

93. Lu JH, Emons D, Kowalewski S. Connatal periventricular pseudocysts in the neonate. Pediatr Radiol 1992; 22: 55–8.

94. Malinger G, Lev D, Ben Sira L, et al. Congenital periventricular pseudocysts: prenatal sonographic appearance and clinical implications. Ultrasound Obstet Gynecol 2002; 20: 447–51.

95. Bats AS, Molho M, Senat MV, et al. Subependymal pseudocysts in the fetal brain: prenatal diagnosis of two cases and review of the literature. Ultrasound Obstet Gynecol 2002; 20: 502–5.

96. Eller KM, Kuller JA. Porencephaly secondary to fetal trauma during amniocentesis. Obstet Gynecol 1995; 85: 865–7.

97. Volpe JJ. Hypoxic–ischemic encephalopathy: neuropathology and pathogenesis. In: Neurology of the Newborn, 4th edn. Philadelphia, PA: WB Saunders, 2001: 296–330.

98. Meizner I, Elchalal U. Prenatal sonographic diagnosis of anterior fossa porencephaly. J Clin Ultrasound 1996; 24: 96–9.

99. de Laveaucoupet J, Audibert F, Guis F, et al. Fetal magnetic resonance imaging (MRI) of ischemic brain injury. Prenat Diagn 2001; 21: 729–36.

100. Scher MS, Belfar H, Martin J, Painter MJ. Destructive brain lesions of presumed fetal onset: antepartum causes of cerebral palsy. Pediatrics 1991; 88: 898–906.

101. Stevenson DA, Hart BL, Clericuzio CL. Hydranencephaly in an infant with vascular malformations. Am J Med Genet 2001; 104: 295–8.

102. Lam YH, Tang MH. Serial sonographic features of a fetus with hydranencephaly from 11 weeks to term. Ultrasound Obstet Gynecol 2000; 16: 77–9.

103. Sherer DM, Anyaegbunam A, Onyeije C. Antepartum fetal intracranial hemorrhage, predisposing factors and prenatal sonography: a review. Am J Perinatol 1998; 15: 431–41.

104. Hardart GE, Fackler JC. Predictors of intracranial hemorrhage during neonatal extracorporeal membrane oxygenation. J Pediatr 1999; 134: 156–9.

105. Rezaie P, Dean A. Periventricular leukomalacia, inflammation and white matter lesions within the developing nervous system. Neuropathology 2002; 22: 106–32.

13 Fetal thorax by 3D sonography

Ashok Khurana and Vishal Mittal

INTRODUCTION

Congenital malformations of the fetal thorax are being diagnosed in the antenatal period with an increasing frequency, and the clinical outcomes in these fetuses seem to be quite different from conventional concepts and general belief. There is an emerging consensus that follow-up data on these fetuses in the first year of life indicates a far better outcome than previously believed.[1] Concurrent with this awareness, practitioners of fetal medicine have been witness to revolutions in neonatal anesthesia, neonatal surgical technique, and novel methods of in utero surgery. These factors, combined with a pressing social and legal need for informed parental counseling, have placed new responsibilities on the shoulders of the sonologist

involved in the care of these pregnancies. Advances in transducer technology and computer software are changing the way in which ultrasound scans are performed today, and three-dimensional (3D) and real-time three-dimensional (4D) technology is being used extensively to gain and display anatomic and hemodynamic information. This chapter reviews the application of these newer techniques in enhancing the data that can be obtained by sonography.

DATA ACQUISTION AND DISPLAY: GENERAL CONSIDERATIONS

3D sonography first became popular because of its ability to display the fetal face in a surface rendering

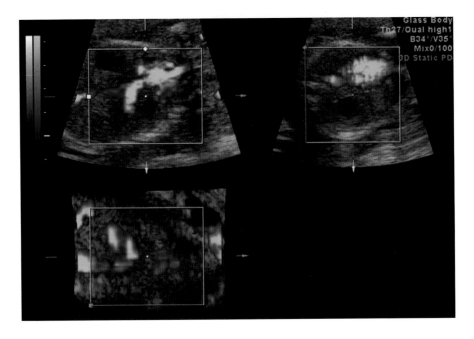

Figure 13.1 3D multiplanar display of a lung cyst. 3D acquisition of data permits any abnormality in the acquired volume of interest to be displayed in one desired plane and two corresponding planes perpendicular to the desired plane. These data permit excellent evaluation of organ relationships, lesion localization, and a display of vascularity

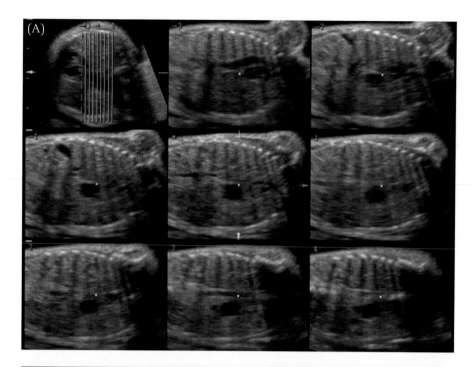

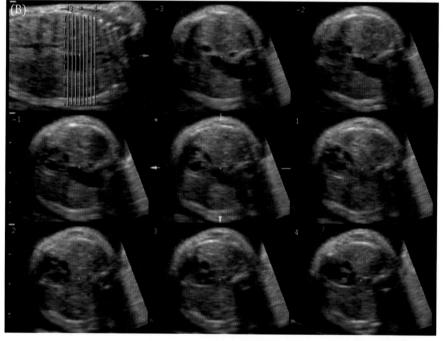

Figure 13.2 Tomographic ultrasound imaging is an extension of 3D and 4D acquisition of 4D data displayed in serial sections in any desired planes. This method not only shows a lesion in a format that is familiar to physicians and surgeons because it is akin to CT and MRI formats, but also permits a unique evaluation of normal anatomy, disordered anatomy, and the ability to appreciate a lesion in the depth of its own anatomy. (A–C) show a congenital diaphragmatic hernia of the entire stomach into the thorax on the left side and also demonstrate the absence of cardiac and mediastinal displacement, the absence of pleural effusions, good lung field extent, and a normal rib structure. This is made possible by a short and simple volume acquisition over the field of interest. Storage of such volume data, apart from excellent anatomic display, gives an opportunity for simple electronic storage of data with easy access to recall for review and retrospective analysis, for transmission to colleagues over a long distance by appropriate internet or telephone lines, and for teaching purposes

mode. Currently available equipment has gone a long way beyond this, and permits the automatic acquisition of volume datasets that can then be processed for display in various modes. Volume acquisition can be done using a static 3D method or a 4D real-time method. Power Doppler flow information from the entire volume of tissue being imaged can be acquired at the same time. Once the data have been acquired, they can be analyzed, processed, and displayed using various software capabilities that facilitate obtaining optimal information. The specific advantage of a 3D/4D dataset is that cross-sectional views can be obtained in any plane, at any orientation, in any direction, and at any depth. It is possible to scroll through the entire volume using buttons, keys, and track balls on the control panel. The display can be made in various ways: in a single plane, of a multiplanar type with a simultaneous view of three orthogonal planes, a tomographic multislice type akin to X-ray computed tomography (CT) and magnetic resonance imaging

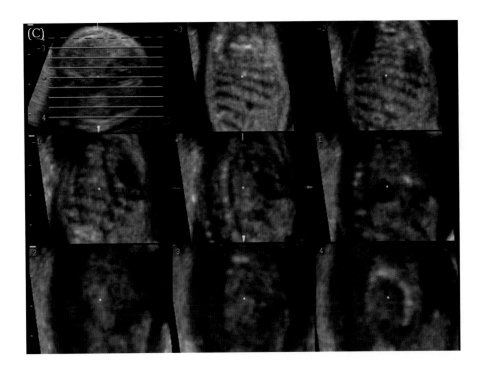

Figure 13.2 *Continued*

(MRI), or a rendering of the data in various modes. These rendering modes include surface, minimum, inversion, and glassbody modes. In a multiplanar display, three planes are displayed perpendicular to each other (Figure 13.1). Since any such three planes intersect at a point, it is possible to navigate through the volume by moving the point. Tomographic multi-slice display is a newer volume technique that displays cross-sections parallel to each other, at any selected slice thickness in any selected plane orientation. After acquiring a volume, instead of scrolling through the volume, a series of slices can be displayed in any selected dataset orientation (Figures 13.2–13.4). Information can be displayed as a grayscale for structure, in color for vascular morphology or as a combination of grayscale structure and color vascular morphology information (Figures 13.5 and 13.6). Volume contrast imaging is another new 4D technique that can enhance the information obtained. All of these modes are discussed in the following sections.

VOLUME DISPLAY WITH TRANSPARENT MINIMUM MODE

Choosing this mode renders anechoic structures such as cysts, fluid collections, and blood vessels black or dark in a surrounding of more echogenic tissue. This results in highlighting of fluid areas and greatly enhances the delineation of organ relationships (Figure 13.7). The technique is useful in the evaluation of mediastinal cysts and cystic spaces in congenital cystic cystadenomatoid malformations, and in delineating the extent of pleural effusions.

VOLUME DISPLAY WITH SURFACE RENDERING MODE

Thoracic wall masses such as lymphangiomas and hemangiomas can be dramatically displayed by this mode, and the technique enhances the appreciation of extent of the lesion by the parents and the surgical team (Figure 13.8).

VOLUME DISPLAY WITH INVERSION MODE

This mode commences with the minimum mode, but then reverses the color of the lesion of interest as in a positive–negative photographic manner (Figure 13.9). Anechoic structures end up being seen as echogenic solids, and the mode also obscures information on surrounding tissue. Any fluid-filled structure is highlighted appropriately. This mode can be used to ascertain the relationships of larger vessels in the thorax to abnormalities in the region of interest without using power Doppler. The latter has the drawback of slower acquisition, and hence the chance

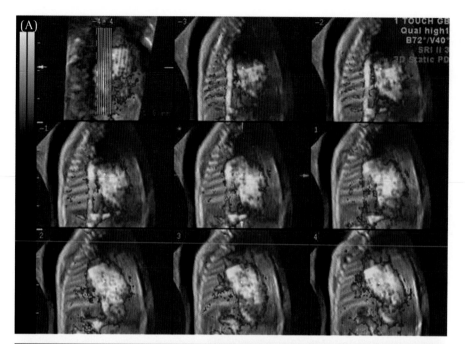

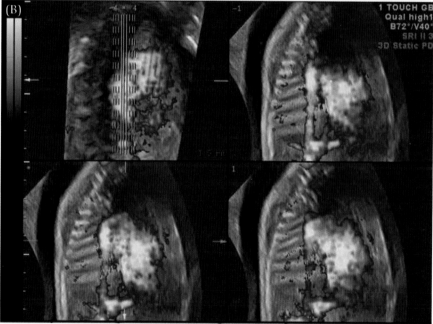

Figure 13.3 Sepia-toned tomographic ultrasound imaging display with simultaneous power Doppler information. Since data are acquired over an entire volume, it can be displayed to variably demonstrate structural anatomy in relation to vascular anatomy. It also offers immense possibilities of visualizing tissue planes anywhere in the data, at any distance from each other, and at variable slice thicknesses

of cardiac activity-induced motion artifact. Volume display with inversion also overcomes other specific disadvantages of Doppler such as angle of insonation and temporal resolution. It may not work well, however, for lesions of poor tissue contrast.

VOLUME DISPLAY WITH SKELETAL MODE

Choosing this mode displays the spine, ribs, sternum, clavicles, and mandible to advantage (Figure 13.10),

thereby enabling the identification and characterization of skeletal dysplasia.[2] This is useful in classifying short-rib polydactyly syndromes, asphyxiating thoracic dystrophy, and thanatophoric dwarfism.

VOLUME DISPLAY WITH GLASSBODY MODE

This mode acquires color or power Doppler along with grayscale, and permits simultaneous display of

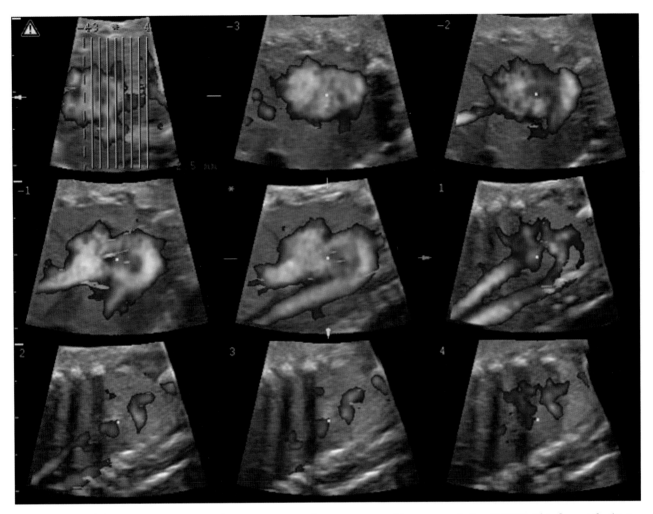

Figure 13.4 Still from a 4D power Doppler acquisition with spatiotemporal image correlation (STIC). This format facilitates excellent delineation of structural anatomy, vascular maps, and anatomic–vascular relationships. This figure shows a lung lesion supplied by vascular channels from the descending aorta

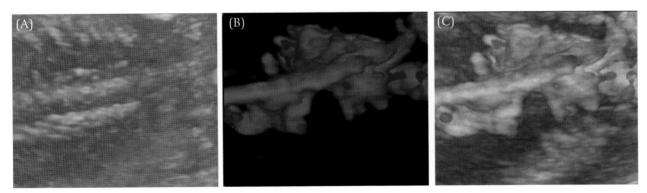

Figure 13.5 Volume data can be displayed as a grayscale (A) for anatomic structure, in power Doppler mode (B) for vascular delineation, and as a combination of grayscale and power Doppler information (C)

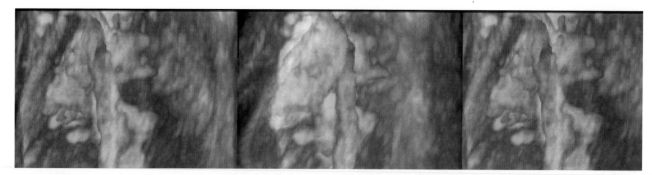

Figure 13.6 3D acquisition of grayscale and power Doppler data permits a glassbody reconstruction of the area of interest. When processed in the rotation/cine mode, this offers not only a display of disordered structure but also a unique perspective for the evaluation of disease processes. These stills from a 3D rotation cine reconstruction reveal a lesion with no vascular supply. The differential diagnosis includes a bronchogenic cyst or a mediastinal cyst

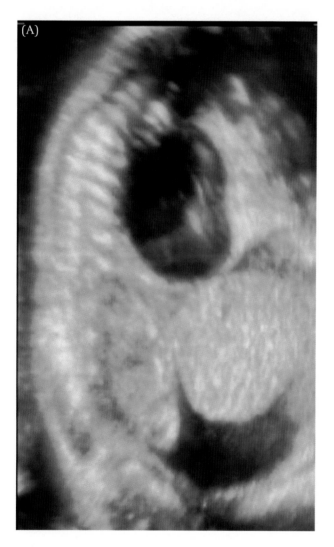

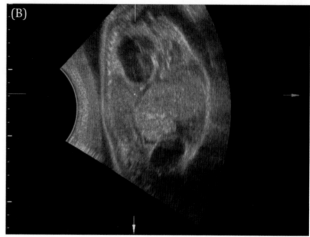

Figure 13.7 Any acquired 3D or 4D volume data can be evaluated in various software settings referred to as modes. The transparent minimum mode highlights fluid areas and enhances the delineation of organs in the region of interest. The transparent minimum mode shown here displays a neurenteric cyst in relation to displaced pulmonary vasculature, compressed lung parenchyma, cardiac displacement, and abnormal vertebrae

matoid malformations, which are supplied by the pulmonary artery, and sequestrations, which have a systemic supply (Figure 13.11).

VOLUME CONTRAST IMAGING

Volume contrast imaging (VCI) enhances contrast between tissues. It consists of a 5–20 mm thick slice-shaped volume image projected on a 2D screen. Due to a very small elevation sweep angle, the render box has a large surface but relatively small thickness, thus increasing contrast resolution. The speckle pattern of

structure and vascular morphology. This is invaluable in vascular delineation[3] and in identifying the vascular supply of lung lesions. The latter is particularly useful in differentiating between congenital cystic cystadeno-

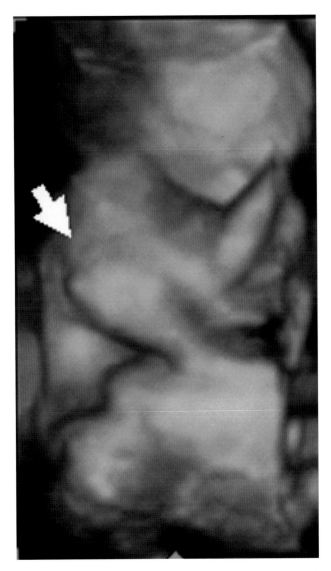

Figure 13.8 To appreciate superficial thoracic lesions such as those in the wall, appropriate mode settings can reveal skeletal and soft tissue abnormalities. This still from a 4D surface rendering mode reveals a large mass in the axilla preventing the fetal arm from resting against the anterior abdominal wall. This was an axillary lymphangioma

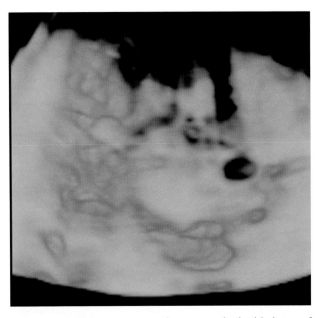

Figure 13.9 The inversion mode permits the highlighting of relationships of fluid-filled structures and larger thoracic vessels. This mixed congenital cystic adenomatoid malformation shows displacement of pulmonary arterial vasculature, several large cysts, and one large branch of the pulmonary artery showing up as a black void

the image is smoothed by filling up the gaps with tissue information from the adjacent layers.[4] The technique enhances the contrast between fetal lung and diaphragm, fetal lung and mediastinum, lesions within the lungs, herniated viscera into the thorax, the thymus, and pericardial solid lesions (Figure 13.12). Information about lung maturity as provided by this technique still needs adequate laboratory and clinical re-evaluation.[5]

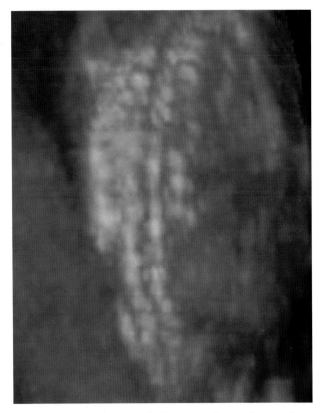

Figure 13.10 Skeletal mode displays enhance the visualization of fetal bones. This still from a 3D rotation cine clip reveals short ribs, thereby offering support to a diagnosis of a pulmonary hypoplasia secondary to a short-rib syndrome

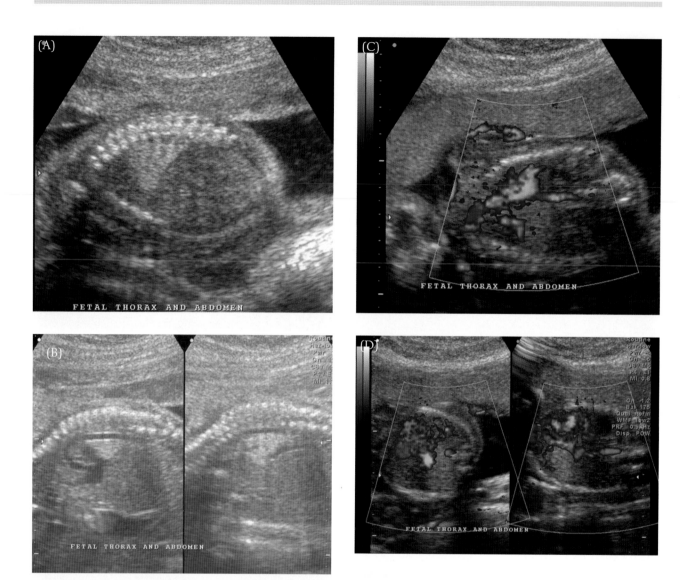

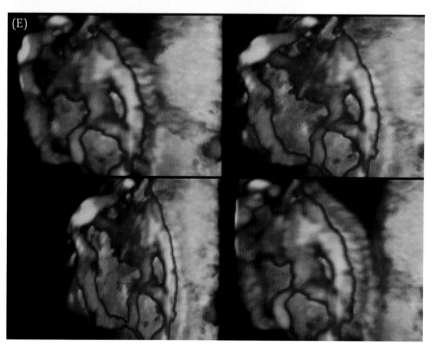

Figure 13.11 Glassbody rendering of volume data offers a unique view into the vascular anatomy of lung lesions. (A,B) These show a triangular echogenic lesion in the left lung base. (C,D) These 2D power Doppler frames do not adequately reveal the origin of the vasculature of this lesion, which exhibits the echogenicity, location, and configuration of a bronchopulmonary sequestration. A grayscale and power Doppler rotation cine display throws up a surprise. (E) These stills from a rotation cine reconstruction reveal that the lesion has no supply from the aorta and is fed by pulmonary arterial branches and drained by enlarged pulmonary veins leading to the left atrium. This was the primary pointer to the diagnosis of a congenital cystic adenomatoid malformation

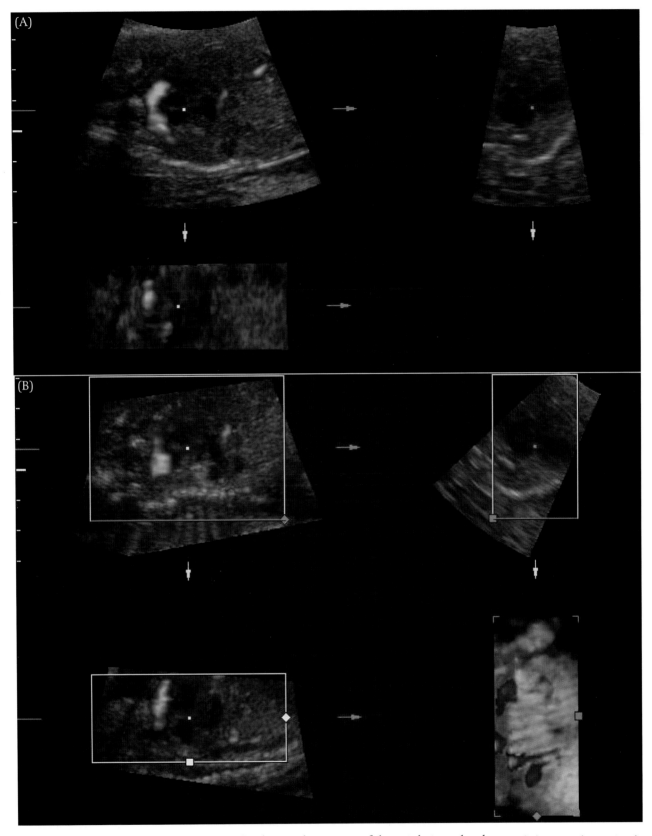

Figure 13.12 Volume contrast imaging (VCI) enhances the contrast of thoracic lesions, thereby permitting superior anatomic detail and more accurate organ relationships. (A) A multiplanar power Doppler display in the routine multiplanar mode gives only the slightest hint of a pericardial lesion. (B) A VCI rendering, however, convincingly demonstrates an avascular echogenic pericardial lesion. This was a pericardial teratoma

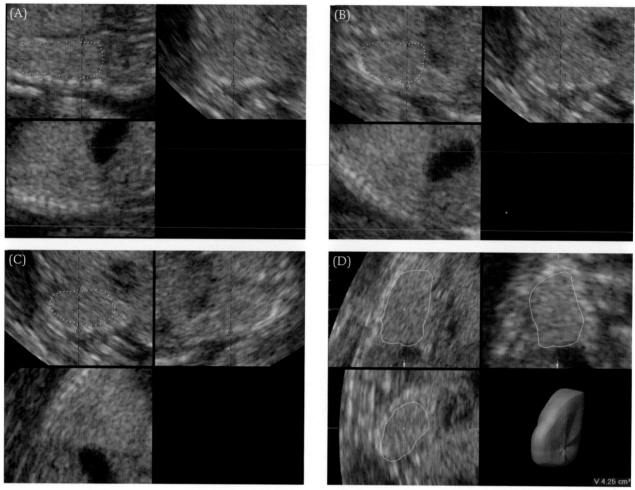

Figure 13.13 Virtual organ computer-aided analysis (VOCAL) is software that permits accurate volume calculations. (A–C) These demonstrate serial planes in which the lung is outlined, and when the entire thickness of the lung has been scrolled through, the software automatically calculates the volume and shows an organ display (D). 3D calculations such as this are accurate to a degree of ±5% compared with 2D formulae, which can be off by as much as ±15%

LUNG VOLUMES

Adequate lung development is central to fetal viability.[6,7] Hypoplastic lungs show a low ratio of lung to body weight and demonstrate a reduced number of alveoli on histopathological examination.[8] The pathogenesis of pulmonary hypoplasia is consequent to either inadequate thoracic space for growth, inadequate breathing movements of whatever cause, inadequate fluid within the lung, or suboptimal quantities of amniotic fluid.[9] It is therefore seen in a variety of conditions, including prolonged severe oligoamnios,[10–13] skeletal dysplasias with a small bony thorax, sizable thoracic masses, consequent to neuromuscular dysfunction (as in the Pena Shokeir syndrome), trisomies, and conditions with decreased pulmonary

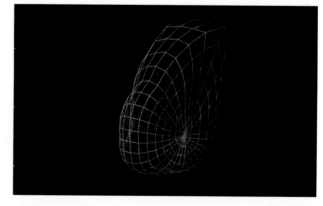

Figure 13.14 Several methods of displaying the VOCAL volume dataset improve the appreciation of volume information by the viewer. This shows a lung volume displayed as a blue wire mesh. This is permitted by automatically working software at the press of a button

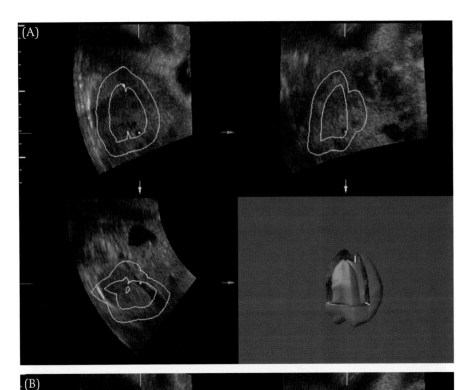

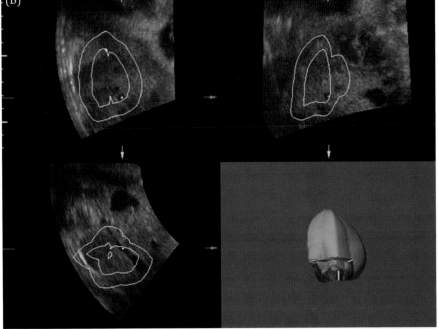

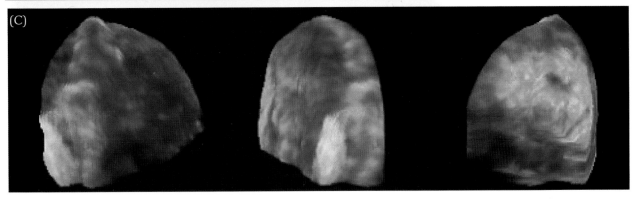

Figure 13.15 VOCAL datasets contain complete grayscale and power Doppler information on the region of interest. (A,B) The entire volume can be scrolled through in any plane. The entire organ can be displayed in any perspective using control panel buttons. (C) Video stills showing a fetal lung with normal volume and configuration

perfusion.[14] Lung hypoplasia is rarely primary and rarely unilateral.[15,16]

D'Arcy et al[17] were among the first to describe the estimation of lung volume. Following this pioneering attempt, several methods at 3D evaluation of fetal lung volume have been described.[18,19] These were based on subtracting fetal heart volumes from fetal thoracic volumes. This was followed by an attempt to estimate lung volumes by successively outlining the lung contour in parallel slices.[20] Rotational measurement of volume has become possible through the introduction of virtual organ computer-aided analysis (VOCAL).[21] Fetal lung volumes are easy to obtain using VOCAL (Figures 13.13–13.15). The accuracy and precision of prenatal 3D ultrasound in estimating fetal lung volume using VOCAL by comparing it with postmortem volume measurements has been extensively evaluated.[22] In this study, fetal lung volume was measured during 3D ultrasound examination using a rotational multiplanar technique in eight cases of congenital diaphragmatic hernia (CDH) (six left- and two right-sided) and in 25 controls without pulmonary malformation, immediately before termination of pregnancy. Prenatal 3D sonographic estimates of fetal lung volume were compared with postmortem measurement of fetal lung volume achieved by water displacement. The intraclass correlation coefficient of fetal lung volume estimated by 3D ultrasound and measured at postmortem examination was 0.95 in CDH cases and 0.99 in controls. Based on Bland–Altman analysis, the bias, precision and limits of agreement were, respectively, 0.35 cm^3, 1.46 cm^3, and between –2.51 and +3.21 cm^3 in cases with CDH and 0.08 cm^3, 2.80 cm^3, and between –5.41 and +5.57 cm^3 in controls. The mean relative error of 3D ultrasound fetal lung volume measurement was –7.19% (from –42.70% to +18.11%) in CDH cases and –0.72% (from –30.25% to +19.22%) in controls, while the mean absolute error of 3D ultrasound fetal lung volume measurement was 1.40 cm^3 (range 0.71–2.52 cm^3) and 2.12 cm^3 (range 0.05–4.98 cm^3), respectively. The accuracy of 3D ultrasound for measuring fetal lung volumes was 84.86% (range 57.30–99.48%) in cases with CDH and 91.38% (range 69.75–99.45%) in controls. The mean intra-observer variability for lung volume estimated by 3D ultrasound was 0.28 cm^3 in controls and 0.17 cm^3 in CDH cases. Fetal 3D ultrasound can estimate accurately fetal lung volume using VOCAL, even in fetuses with very small lungs, such as cases with isolated CDH.

2D and 3D methods of measuring fetal pulmonary volume have been formulated and compared along with establishing nomograms of fetal pulmonary volume according to gestational age for the accurate diagnosis of pulmonary hypoplasia.[23] In this study, three methods of measuring fetal pulmonary volume in 39 normal fetuses were compared: 2D ultrasound measurement assuming that the lung is a geometric pyramid, 3D ultrasound using the VOCAL rotational method, and the conventional multiplanar 3D mode. Linear regression was used to construct an equation for 3D volume calculation from 2D measurements (the re-evaluated pulmonary volume equation: RPVE). Lung volume measurements were recorded from 622 singleton fetuses in order to construct nomograms. There was no statistically significant difference between the lung volume values obtained using the two 3D modes. However, in comparison with the 2D measurements, the volumes obtained were larger (mean difference 11.99, $p < 0.1 \times 10^{-6}$). The relationship between the 2D and 3D volumes was determined using a statistical linear regression method:

$$\text{RPVE (ml)} = 4.24 + (1.53 \times 2\text{DGPV})$$

where the 2D geometric pulmonary volume is given by:

$$2\text{DGPV} = [\text{surface area right lung base (cm}^2)$$
$$+ \text{ surface area left lung base (cm}^2)]$$
$$\times \frac{1}{3} \times \text{height of right lung (cm)}$$

Two nomograms were constructed: one for use with 2D and one for use with 3D technology. The study reasonably concluded that pulmonary volume assessment can be used in clinical situations where fetal prognosis depends on lung volume and its growth potential. It is easy to perform, particularly when repeat measurements are required in the evaluation of lung growth.

3D estimation of fetal lung volumes correlates well with postmortem measurements in fetuses with CDH. In this study by Ruano et al,[24] two fetuses with CDH were studied, in whom the fetal lung volumes were estimated by 3D ultrasound and the results were compared with the postmortem lung volume measurements. Both examiners (sonographer and pathologist) were blinded to each other's results. The first case was a right CDH diagnosed at 20 weeks of gestation. The second case was a left CDH diagnosed at 22 weeks of gestation. Both pregnancies were terminated upon request of the parents. 3D ultrasound estimation of fetal lung volume was performed 1 day before termination of pregnancy using the technique of rotation of the three perpendicular planes. The left and right lung volumes estimated by 3D ultrasound were 3.88 and 1.87 cm^3, respectively, in the first case and 0 and 5.52 cm^3, respectively, in the second. On postmortem examination, the left and right lung volumes were 3.0 and 2.2 cm^3, respectively, in the first case, and 1.1 and 5.6 cm^3, respectively, in the second.

The agreement of 3D sonography and magnetic resonance imaging (MRI) in estimating fetal lung volume in cases with isolated congenital diaphragmatic hernia has been studied.[25] In this study, fetal lung volume was measured in 11 cases of congenital diaphragmatic hernia (10 left and 1 right) by 3D sonography and MRI. These examinations were performed during the same week. The operators were blinded to each other's results. Intraclass correlation was used to evaluate the agreement between 3D sonography and MRI estimates of the ipsilateral, contralateral, and total fetal lung volume. A Bland–Altman graph was plotted to detect possible discordant observations. The global intraclass correlation coefficient between MRI and 3D sonographic measurement of fetal lung volume was 0.94 (95% confidence interval (CI) 0.78–0.98), with no outliers being observed on the Bland–Altman plot, thereby demonstrating a good agreement between 3D sonography and MRI for fetal lung volume estimation in cases with CDH.

OVERVIEW OF CONGENITAL THORACIC ABNORMALITIES

Not all lung masses can be delineated in the 18–20 week anomalies scan, although embryologically they do exist.[26,27] Depending on their size and growth, they result in unilateral or bilateral hypoplasia of the lungs. Prognosis depends on the size of the lesion, heart and mediastinal displacements, presence of hydrops, associated structural anomalies, underlying chromosomal abnormalities, and the bearing of associated polyhydramnios on preterm premature rupture of membranes and prematurity.[28–30]

Common chest masses include CDH and congenital cystic adenomatoid malformations (CCAMs). Other lung masses include bronchogenic cysts, neurenteric cysts, congenital lobar emphysema (CLE),

bronchial atresia, pulmonary gigantism, bronchopulmonary sequestration (BPS), and mediastinal masses. The mediastinal lesions include teratomas,[31] thymomas,[32] goiter, cardiac lesions such as rhabdomyoma, myxoma and fibroma,[33–35] esophageal duplication cysts,[36] enteric cysts[36] and neurenteric cysts,[37–39] and thoracic neuroblastoma. Mediastinal lesions are rare but important in the perspective of a differential diagnosis of a mass adjacent to the mediastinum but arising from the adjacent lung or from the abdomen. Since the pathologic panorama is so vast and the prognosis so variable, it is imperative to obtain as much information as possible on imaging studies. The role of newer ultrasound techniques in giving additional clinically useful information is detailed below.

CONGENITAL DIAPHRAGMATIC HERNIA

CDH has an incidence of 1–4.5/10 000 live births.[40] CDH is more common on the left side, but is not infrequently right-sided or bilateral. The diaphragm forms between the 6th to 14th weeks of pregnancy by fusion of the septum transversum, pleuroperitoneal membranes, mesentery of the esophagus, and the body wall. Failure of fusion, especially of the pleuroperitoneal membranes, results in a herniation of abdominal contents into the thorax when the gut returns to the abdomen. The disorder is progressive, and the organs that herniate include the stomach, liver, spleen, small bowel, and colon. Left-sided CDH usually involves the stomach. Right-sided CDH usually involves herniation of the liver. Over four of five fetuses die in the neonatal period – usually because of pulmonary hypoplasia and pulmonary hypertension. It is important, therefore, that both lungs in these fetuses should be evaluated for their volume using VOCAL (Figure 13.16). 2D sonographic signs[41] include a low abdominal perimeter, failure to visualize the fetal stomach in the fetal abdomen, visualization of the herniated viscera in the thorax, cardiomediastinal shift, pleural effusions, and hydrops. There may also be failure to delineate the diaphragm in its entire extent. This can be overcome by using the 4D VCI option. Right-sided hernias are difficult to identify because of isoechoic lung, and these should be evaluated by color Doppler to confirm the portal vein location in the thorax. 3D and 4D glassbody rendering is extremely useful for delineating the liver and the portal vein in the thorax (Figure

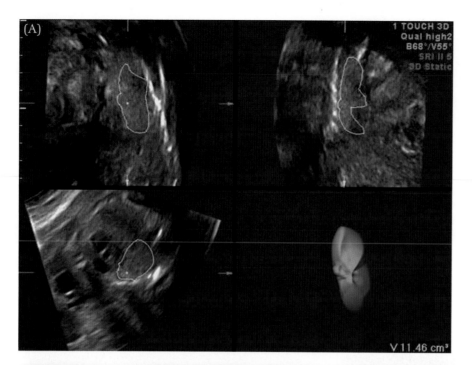

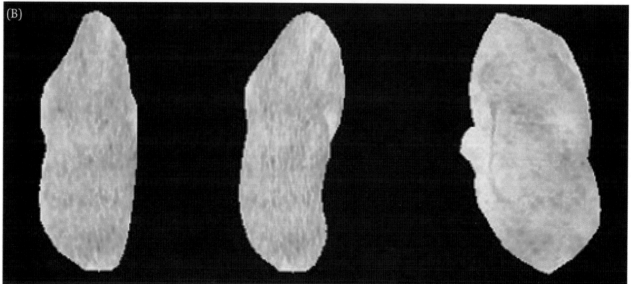

Figure 13.16 VOCAL lung volume calculation in a patient with a congenital diaphragmatic hernia. The VOCAL display (A) and stills from a VOCAL rotation cine sequence (B) show a largely normal extent and configuration of the left lung. Such information greatly enhances the verdict of a reasonably good prognosis in this fetus

13.17). Although identification of the liver is not critical for a diagnosis of CDH, it has a major bearing on the prognosis.[42,43] This is so because, after surgical repair, the ductus venosus and umbilical vein often become kinked or compromised, thereby contributing to morbidity and often mortality. The presence of the left lobe of the liver in a left-sided hernia has a bearing on poor prognosis (Figure 13.18) as the vascularity becomes kinked after a repair. This pattern of herniation is excellently displayed using the glass body rendering mode. Occasionally, a gallbladder may be seen in the CDH, and this would be more convincing using the minimum transparent mode. Bilateral hernias may be difficult to detect because of the absence of cardiomediastinal shift, and here again the VCI mode is useful for delineation (Figure 13.19). Ascites within a herniation may be mistaken for a pleural effusion.

Not all fetuses with a CDH have a poor prognosis.[44–47] Prognosis depends on gestational age at diagnosis (particularly if this is 24 weeks or earlier), large size, dilated stomach, presence of the liver (even its left lobe in left-sided lesions), small contralateral lung, bilateral herniation, and the presence of associated anomalies. Because of the higher incidence of CDH in certain syndromes, a 4D surface rendering of the fetal

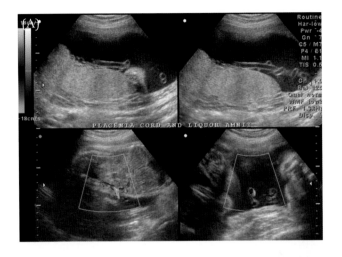

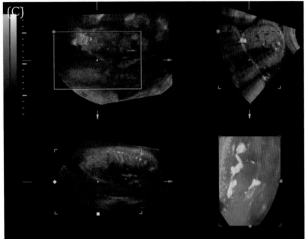

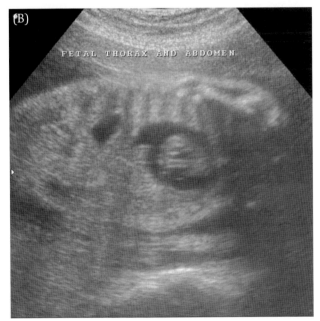

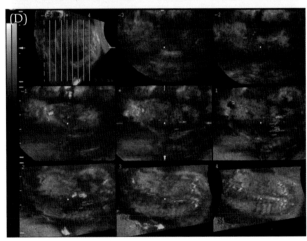

Figure 13.17 This fetus with a Bochdalek hernia and with a single umbilical artery (A) and abnormal appearance of the thorax (B) shows an abnormal extent of the portal vein (C) into the thorax. This information, obtained by 3D power Doppler and also demonstrated by tomographic ultrasound imaging (D), enhances the diagnosis of the liver into the fetal thorax

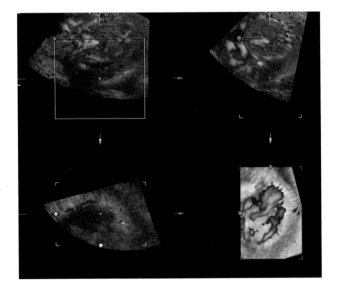

Figure 13.18 3D power Doppler renderings greatly increase the appreciation of disordered anatomy and vascularity. These images of a fetus with a left-sided herniation of the stomach into the thorax additionally reveal the vascularity of the left lobe of the liver to be located in the thorax. This indicates an additional herniation of the liver into the left hemithorax. This has a tremendous bearing on the outcome of this fetus. This is so because when the liver is returned into the abdomen by the pediatric surgical team, this vascularity often becomes kinked and results in a significant hepatic infarction

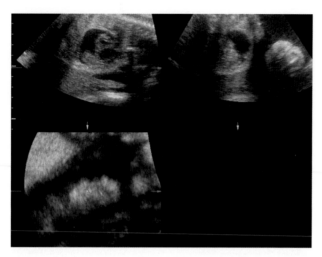

Figure 13.19 Volume contrast imaging of this diaphragmatic hernia confirms the suspicion of bilateral diaphragmatic discontinuity, a right-sided herniation of the liver into the thorax, loculated ascites along the cardiac border, and a herniation of the fetal stomach into the left side of the fetal thorax

face and a cardiac survey merit special attention. These syndromes include trisomy 18, Fryn syndrome, lethal pterygium, Beckwith–Wiedemann and Cornelia de Lange, Apert, and Goldenhar syndromes.[48,49]

Fetal therapy has found a reasonable place in the treatment of CDH.[50] The aim of surgery is to prevent lung hypoplasia. Although fetal therapy initially involved reduction of the hernia by open repair in utero, current practice involves clipping of the trachea. In follow-up evaluation, the lung volume can be estimated using the VOCAL option.

Currently, videofetoscopic techniques are under evaluation. Tracheal occlusion results in increased lung volume and accelerated lung maturity similar to the pathophysiology seen in laryngeal and tracheal atresia.[51]

CONGENITAL CYSTIC ADENOMATOID MALFORMATIONS

CCAMs occur consequent to failure of induction of mesenchyme by bronchiolar epithelium. Lack of normal cellular development is considered to be consequent to focal bronchial atresia. The lesion is hamartomatous and characterized by focal abnormal proliferation of bronchiolar-like air spaces and absence of alveoli.[52] It is usually unilateral. Some may be associated with sequestration in the same lung. Diagnosis depends on the demonstration of a mass in the thorax.[53] This may be macrocystic (cysts

2–10 mm), microcystic (cysts 0.3–0.5 mm), or mixed.[26,27] These may cause a cardiomediastinal shift, ipsilateral and contralateral lung compression, pulmonary hypoplasia and hydrops. The lesion may regress spontaneously.[54] It is therefore important that an accurate estimation of the volume be made for future comparison. Since the accuracy of VOCAL estimations is considerably higher than that of any 2D methods, it is logical to use this 3D method. Prognosis depends on associated pulmonary hypoplasia, pulmonary hypertension, hydrops, associated anomalies, polyhydramnios, and prematurity. 3D lung volume estimations are accurate and useful in formulating a prognosis. Microcystic lesions are more likely to cause pulmonary hypoplasia and hydrops. The arterial supply is via a pulmonary artery and drainage into a pulmonary vein. 3D glassbody rendering and 3D and 4D power Doppler tomographic ultrasound imaging offer a unique mapping of the vascularity of CCAMs, particularly in demonstrating the origin of the arterial supply and confirming it to have a pulmonary arterial source and not an aortic or systemic artery source (Figures 13.20 and 13.21). The arterial supply delineation is also useful in surgical treatment planning. Treatment of the lesion consists of expectant management, monitoring for hydrops, or premature/term delivery followed by lobectomy if necessary.[28] Referral to a tertiary care center is important because emergency thoracic surgery is often needed. Recurrence is rare in later pregnancies. Since Klinefelter syndrome and trisomy 18 are known for an association with CCAMs, it is appropriate to obtain a karyotype when the condition is diagnosed.

In utero aspiration of a larger cyst, thoraco-amniotic shunting of a larger cyst, and in utero resections have been attempted, and are methods of gaining time to achieve viability. In utero resection has been tried only in fetuses with the poorest prognosis, since the procedure itself carries a high morbidity and mortality.

BRONCHOPULMONARY SEQUESTRATION

Also known as pulmonary sequestration and accessory lung, BPS is a congenital malformation consisting of lung parenchyma that is separated from normal lung. It receives arterial supply of systemic origin and does not communicate with the normal tracheobronchial tree. Sequestrations arise from a supernumerary anomalous outpouching of the foregut. If they arise prior to closure of the pleura, they have no separate

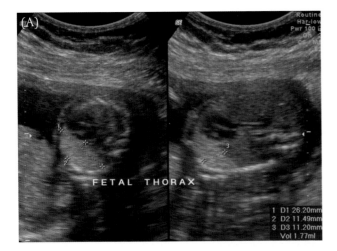

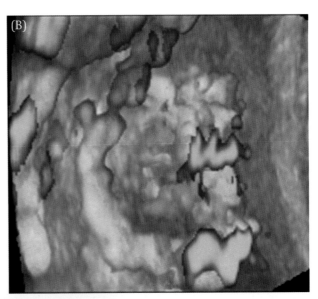

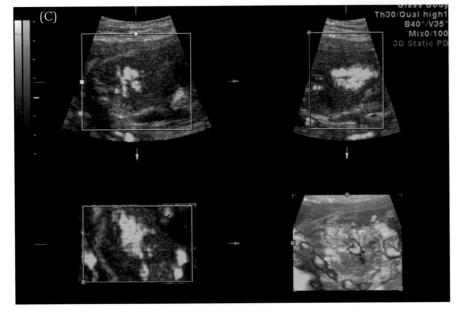

Figure 13.20 This fetal thorax reveals a triangular opacity in the lung (A), which shows extensive pulmonary arterial vascularization (B), confirming that this is a congenital cystic adenomatoid malformation (CCAM), and not a congenital lobar emphysema. Multiplanar views (C) reveal a normal aorta, thereby confirming that this is not a sequestration. The lesion shows occasional vascular twigs rising from the pulmonary artery. This minimal vascularity and the CCAM resolved completely shortly before birth

pleural envelope and are called intralobar sequestrations. If they originate after closure of the pleura, they are called extralobar sequestrations and have their own pleura. Intralobar sequestrations drain into pulmonary veins, while extralobar sequestrations usually drain into a systemic vein, usually the azygos, hemiazygos, or inferior vena cava. Extralobar sequestrations may be thoracic or extrathoracic, and may even communicate with the esophagus.[55] They are occasionally associated with other thoracic and foregut anomalies such as CDH, CCAMs, bronchogenic cysts, and neurenteric cysts. A wide variety of extrapulmonary anomalies, including congenital heart disease, renal anomalies, and hydrocephalus, have been reported to coexist with sequestrations. Many sequestrations show extensive subpleural lymphatics, which account for ipsilateral pleural effusions. Typical sonographic appearances[56] include a lobar or triangular echogenic lesion in the lung base, usually left basal. Color and power Doppler studies reveal a systemic arterial supply.[57] The arterial supply and venous drainage are more accurately and more convincingly demonstrated using a combination of glassbody rendering (Figures 13.22 and 13.23) and 4D power Doppler tomographic ultrasound imaging. There is a variable mediastinal shift and hydrops. Several sequestrations have regressed spontaneously.[58] No specific features indicate which sequestrations are likely to resolve. Persistent sequestrations may stabilize or may need postnatal surgical resection.

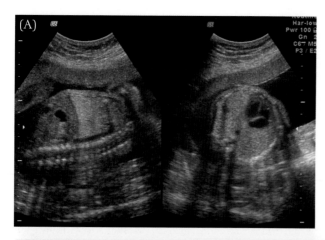

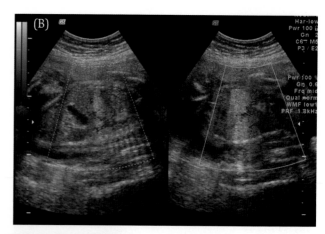

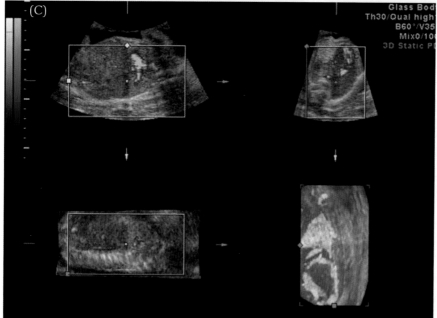

Figure 13.21 This large echogenic lesion seen on 2D ultrasound (A) reveals doubtful vascularity on 2D studies (B). The multiplanar display and 3D glass-body rendering (C) reveals a doubtful pulmonary artery supply to this. Stills from a rotation cine 3D and power Doppler rendering (D) reveal a subtle but definite pulmonary arterial supply strongly suggesting a diagnosis of a microcystic CCAM

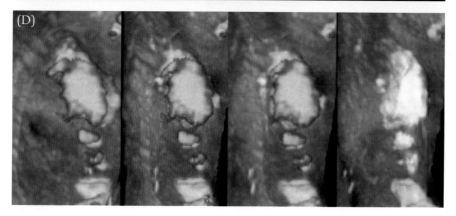

BRONCHOGENIC CYSTS

These arise as a consequence of abnormal foregut budding, and show variable echogenicity and variable progress. They may be mediastinal or peripheral, and often show associated foregut malformations and hemivertebrae. The usual manifestation is an echogenic lesion representing fluid-filled lung beyond the stenosis. The left upper lobe is the most frequent site. Occasionally, they are multiple. These lesions are

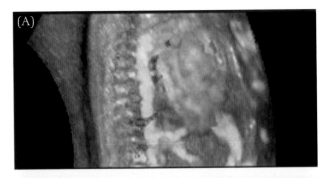

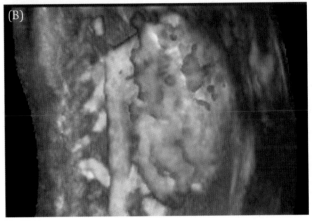

Figure 13.22 (A,B) Glassbody renderings of a bronchopulmonary sequestration reveal an exclusive supply from the pulmonary artery and drainage to a pulmonary vein. These videos reveal hypertrophied vessels arising from the aortic arch and coursing into the lesion

uniquely avascular and complete absence of either a pulmonary arterial or a systemic arterial supply or venous drainage is demonstrated. They are usually innocuous and do not require specific obstetric management. Their importance lies in being among the differential diagnoses of a fetal lung mass.[53]

LARYNGEAL AND TRACHEAL ATRESIA

These are rare congenital anomalies that are associated with demise soon after birth, unless treated antenatally. These arise consequent to subglottic laryngeal atresia, tracheal stenosis, or atresia, or tracheal webs or cysts, and are also known as congenital high airways obstruction (CHAOS). Embryologically, persistent fusion of the sixth branchial arches is apparently involved. Pathologically, failure of efflux of fluid from the fetal lung results in exaggerated lung development. Ultrasound features[59,60] include symmetric enlargement of both lungs, with anterior displacement of the heart. The lungs are homogeneously echogenic, textu-

rally often similar to autosomal recessive infantile polycystic kidneys, since the underlying lesion consists of numerous fluid-filled spaces. In situations where the altered echogenicity is borderline and the subjective evaluation of lung size is doubtful, the enlargement of the lungs can be objectively assessed by a VOCAL estimation. The diaphragm is flat or inverted and cutaneous edema is common, as is hydrops. Polyhydramnios is seen consequent to esophageal compression. The distal trachea and bronchii may be identified as tubular bulging fluid-laden structures in the mediastinum. Over half of the fetuses with this abnormality have renal agenesis, facial anomalies, and central nervous system malformations. To salvage a fetus with this anomaly, it is necessary to establish a functional airway before the fetus is removed from placental support.[61]

CONGENITAL LOBAR EMPHYSEMA

Although this condition has clinical manifestations in the pediatric age group, it can be seen in the fetus as a solid lung mass akin to a microcystic CCAM or an extralobar sequestration. It is usually located in the upper lobe, unlike an extralobar sequestration. There is one case report of a spontaneous regression after indomethacin treatment.[62]

PLEURAL EFFUSION

Unlike a small amount of pericardial fluid, which may be physiologic, a fetal pleural fluid collection is always abnormal.

Primary pleural effusions are accumulations of pleural fluid, which may be idiopathic or consequent to thoracic duct malformations.[63] They are unilateral, or, if bilateral, then markedly asymmetric. Mediastinal shifts are common, and there are no associated findings except hydrops, which is ominous. Pulmonary hypoplasia is common in large chronic effusions. The condition may resolve spontaneously, and does very well after thoracocentesis or thoracoamniotic shunting.[64,65]

Secondary pleural effusions are consequent to other fetal anomalies, and are often the earliest sign of immune or non-immune hydrops fetalis (NIHF).[66] The causes therefore include anemia, infection, cardiac anomalies, anomalies with large arteriovenous shunts, chromosomal abnormalities, skeletal

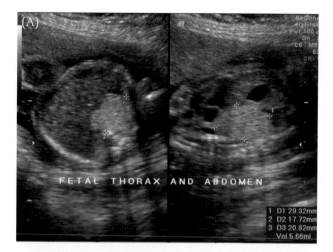

Figure 13.23 This fetus shows an echogenic subdiaphragmatic mass (A). This shows an arterial supply from the abdominal aorta, as seen in these glassbody renderings (B,C), confirming it to be an extralobar sequestration. Stills from a 3D rotation cine (D) reconfirm vascularization from the aorta

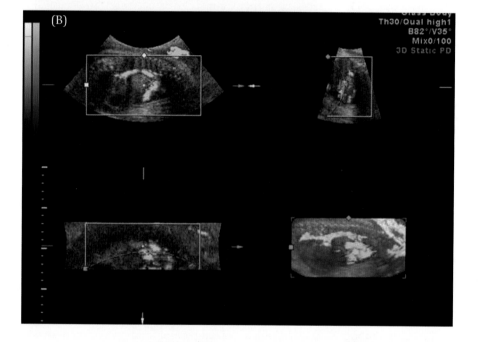

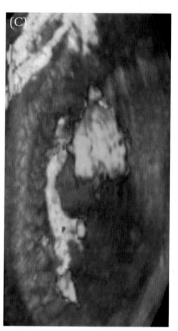

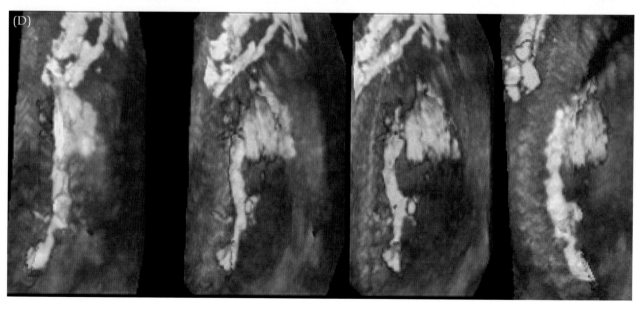

dysplasias, and thoracic malformations. Secondary effusions are usually bilateral, and are often associated with early onset of other signs of hydrops. Prior to instituting any treatment procedure, it is wise to exclude an abnormal fetal karyotype and assess fetal anemia. It is also useful to objectively quantify the effusion for serial comparison. For this, 3D calculations are superior to conventional ellipse formulae.

CONCLUSION

The sensitivity and specificity of prenatal diagnosis of thoracic malformation have improved due to technological advances and innovations.[67] 3D and 4D techniques have been central to this revolution, and should be used liberally to enhance the availability of relevant information to the practicing specialist of fetal medicine.

REFERENCES

1. Pumberger W, Hormann M, Deutinger J, et al. Longitudinal observation of antenatally detected congenital lung malformations (CLM): natural history, clinical outcome and long-term follow-up. Eur J Cardiothorac Surg 2003; 24: 703–11.

2. Ruano R. Recent advanes in sonographic imaging of fetal thoracic structures. Exp Rev Med Devices 2005; 2: 217–22.

3. Chaoui R, Heling KS. New development in fetal heart scanning: three- and four-dimensional fetal echocardiography. Semin Fetal Neonat Med 2005; 10: 567–77.

4. Ruano R, Benachi A, Aubry MC, Dumez Y, Dommergues M. Volume contrast imaging: a new approach to identify fetal thorax structures. J Ultrasound Med 2004; 23: 403–8.

5. Kwittken J, Reiner L. Congenital cystic adenomatoid malformation of the lung. Pediatrics 1962; 30: 759–63.

6. Kilbride HW, Yeast J, Thibeault DW. Defining limits of survival: Lethal pulmonary hypoplasia after midtrimester premature rupture of membranes. Am J Obstet Gynecol 1996; 175: 651–81.

7. Vergani P, Ghidini A, Locatelli A, et al. Risk factors for pulmonary hypoplasia in second trimester premature rupture of membranes. Am J Obstet Gynecol 1994; 170: 3159–64.

8. Askenazi SS, Perlman M. Pulmonary hypoplasia: lung weight and radial alveolar count as criteria of diagnosis. Arch Dis Child 1979; 54: 614–18.

9. Rizzo G. Use ultrasound to predict preterm delivery: do not lose the opportunity (Editorial). Ultrasound Obstet Gynecol 1996; 8: 289–92.

10. McNamara MF, McCurdy CM, Reed KL, et al. The relation between pulmonary hypoplasia and amniotic fluid volume: lessons learned from discordant urinary tract anomalies in monoamniotic twins. Obstet Gynecol 1995; 85: 867–9.

11. Nicolini U, Fisk NM, Rodeck CH, et al. Low amniotic pressure in oligohydramnios – Is this the cause of pulmonary hypoplasia? Am J Obstet Gynecol 1989; 161: 1098–101.

12. Alcorn D, Adamson TM, Lambert TF, et al. Morphological effects of chronic tracheal ligation and drainage in the fetal lamb lung. J Anat 1977; 123: 649–60.

13. Hislop A, Hey E, Reid L. The lungs in congenital bilateral renal agenesis and dysplasia. Arch Dis Child 1979; 54: 32–8.

14. Mitchell JM, Roberts AB, Lee A. Doppler waveforms from the pulmonary arterial system in normal fetuses and those with pulmonary hypoplasia. Ultrasound Obstet Gynecol 1998; 11: 167–72.

15. Bromley B, Benacerraf BR. Unilateral lung hypoplasia: report of three cases. J Ultrasound Med 1997; 16: 599–601.

16. Yancey MK, Richards DS. Antenatal sonographic findings associated with unilateral pulmonary agenesis. Obstet Gynecol 1993; 81: 847–9.

17. D'Arcy TJ, Huges SW, Chiu WS, et al. Estimation of fetal lung volume using enhanced 3-dimensional ultrasound: a new method and first result. Br J Obstet Gynaecol 1996; 103: 1015–20.

18. Lee A, Kratochwil A, Stumpflen I, Deutinger J, Bernaschek G. Fetal lung volume determination by three-dimensional ultrasonography. Am J Obstet Gynecol 1996; 175: 588–92.

19. Laudy JA, Janssen MM, Struyk PC, Stijnen T, Wladimiroff JW. Three-dimensional ultrasonography of normal fetal lung volume: a preliminary study. Ultrasound Obstet Gynecol 1998; 11: 13–16.

20. Phis UG, Rempen A. Fetal lung volumetry by three-dimensional ultrasound. Ultrasound Obstet Gynecol 1998; 11: 6–12.

21. Raine-Fenning NJ, Clewes JS, Kendall NR, et al. The interobserver reliability and validity of volume calculation from three-dimensional ultrasound datasets in the in vitro setting. Ultrasound Obstet Gynecol 2003; 21: 283–91.

22. Ruano R, Benachi A, Joubin L, et al. Three-dimensional ultrasonographic assessment of fetal lung volume as prognostic factor in isolated congenital diaphragmatic hernia. Br J Obstet Gynaecol 2004; 111: 423–9.

23. Moeglin D, Talmant C, Duyme M, Lopez AC; CFEF.

Fetal lung volumetry using two- and three-dimensional ultrasound. Ultrasound Obstet Gynecol 2005; 25: 119–27.

24. Ruano R, Benachi A, Martinovic J, et al. Can three-dimensioanl ultrasound be used for the assessment of the fetal lung volume in cases of congenital diaphragmatic hernia? Fetal Diagn Ther 2004; 19: 87–91.

25. Ruano R, Joubin L, Sonigo P, et al. Fetal lung volume estimated by 3-dimensional ultrasonography and magnetic resonance imaging in cases with isolated congenital diaphragmatic hernia. J Ultrasound Med 2004; 23: 353–8.

26. Adzick NS, Harrison MR, Crombleholme TM, et al. Fetal lung lesions: management and outcome. Am J Obstet Gynecol 1998; 179: 884–9.

27. Bromley B, Parad R, Estroff JA, et al. Fetal lung masses: prenatal course and outcome. J Ultrasound Med 1995; 14: 927–36; quiz, 1378.

28. Thorpe-Beeston JG, Nicolaides KH. Cystic adenomatoid malformation of the lung: prenatal diagnosis and outcome. Prenat Diagn 1994; 14: 677–88.

29. Rice HE, Estes JM, Hedrick MH, et al. Congenital cystic adenomatoid malformation. A sheep model of fetal hydrops. J Pediatr Surg 1994; 29: 692–6.

30. Dommergues M, Louis-Sylvestre C, Mandelbrot L, et al. Congenital adenomatoid malformation of the lung: When is active fetal therapy indicated? Am J Obstet Gynecol 1997; 177: 953–8.

31. Todros T, Gaglioti P, Presbitero P. Management of a fetus with intrapericardial teratoma diagnosed in utero. J Ultrasound Med 1991; 10: 287–90.

32. de Miguel Campos E, Casanova A, Urbano J, et al. Congenital thymic cyst: prenatal sonographic and postnatal magnetic resonance findings. J Ultrasound Med 1997; 16: 365–7.

33. Gushiken BJ, Callen PW, Silverman NH. Prenatal diagnosis of tuberous sclerosis in monozygotic twins with cardiac masses. J Ultrasound Med 1999; 18: 165–8.

34. Green KW, Bors-Koefoed R, Pollack P, et al. Antepartum diagnosis and management of multiple fetal cardiac tumors. J Ultrasound Med 1991; 10: 697–9.

35. Schmaltz AA, Apitz J. Primary heart tumors in infancy and childhood. Report of four cases and review of literature. Cardiology 1981; 67: 12–22.

36. Reed JC, Sobonya RE. Morphologic analysis of foregut cysts in the thorax. AJR Am J Roentgenol 1974; 120: 851–60.

37. Fernandes ET, Custer MD, Burton EM, et al. Neurenteric cyst: surgery and diagnostic imaging. J Pediatr Surg 1991; 26: 108–10.

38. Maculay KE, Winter TC III, Shields LE. Neurenteric cyst shown by prenatal sonography. AJR Am J Roentgenol 1997; 169: 563–5.

39. Wilkinson CC, Albanese CT, Jennings RW, et al. Fetal neurenteric cyst causing hydrops: Case report and review of the literature. Prenat Diagn 1999; 19: 118–21.

40. Katz Al, Wiswell TE, Baumgart S. Contemporary controversies in the management of congenital diaphragmatic hernia. Clin Perinatol 1998; 25: 219–21.

41. Guibaud L, Filiatrault D, Garel L, et al. Fetal congenital diaphragmatic hernia: accuracy of sonography in the diagnosis and prediction of the outcome after birth. AJR Am J Roentgenol 1996; 166: 1195–202.

42. Albanese CT, Lopoo J, Goldstein RB, et al. Fetal liver position and perinatal outcome for congenital diaphragmatic hernia. Prenat Diagn 1998; 18: 1138–42.

43. Bootstaylor BS, Filly RA, Harrison MR, et al. Prenatal sonographic predictors of liver herniation in congenital diaphragmatic hernia. J Ultrasound Med 1995; 14: 515–20.

44. Dommergues M, Louis-Sylvestre C, Mandelbrot L, et al. Congenital diaphragmatic hernia: Can prenatal ultrasonography predict outcome? Am J Obstet Gynecol 1996; 174: 1377–81.

45. Geary MP, Chitty LS, Morrison JJ, et al. Prenatal outcome and prognostic factors in prenatally diagnosed congenital diaphragmatic hernia. Ultrasound Obstet Gynecol 1998; 12: 107–11.

46. Sharland GK, Lockhart SM, Heward AJ, et al. Prognosis in fetal diaphragmatic hernia. Am J Obstet Gynecol 1992; 166: 9–13.

47. Losty PD, Vanamo K, Rintala RJ, et al. Congenital diaphragmatic hernia – Does the size of the defect influence the incidence of associated malformations? J Pediatr Surg 1998; 33: 507–10.

48. Sheffield JS, Twickler DM, Timmons C, et al. Fryns syndrome: prenatal diagnosis and pathologic correlation. J Ultrasound Med 1998; 17: 585–9.

49. Harrison MR, Adzick NS, Estes JM, et al. A prospective study of the outcome for fetuses with diaphragmatic hernia. JAMA 1994; 271: 382–4.

50. Geary M. Management of congenital diaphragmatic hernia diagnosed prenatally: an update. Prenat Diagn 1998; 18: 1155–8.

51. Silver MM, Thurston WA, Patrick JE. Perinatal pulmonary hyperplasia due to laryngeal atresia. Hum Pathol 1988; 19: 110–13.

52. Moerman P, Fryns JP, Vandenberghe K, et al. Pathogenesis of congenital cystic adenomatoid malformation of the lung. Histopathology 1992; 21: 315–21.

53. Mayden KL, Tortora M, Chervenak FA, et al. The antenatal sonographic detection of lung masses. Am J Obstet Gynecol 1984; 148: 349–51.

54. Budorick NE, Pretorius DH, Leopold GR, et al. Spontaneous improvement of intrathoracic masses diagnosed in utero. J Ultrasound Med 1992; 11: 653–62.

55. Gerle RD, Jaretzki AD, Ashley CA, et al. Congenital bronchopulmonary–foregut malformation. Pulmonary sequestration communicating with the gastrointestinal tract. N Engl J Med 1968; 278: 1413–19.

56. Lopoo JB, Albanese CT, Goldstein RB, et al. Fetal pulmonary sequestration: a favorable cystic lung lesion. Obstet Gynecol 1999; 94: 567–71.

57. Hernanz-Schulman M, Stein SM, Neblett WW, et al. Pulmonary sequestration: diagnosis with color Doppler sonography and a new theory of associated hydrothorax. Radiology 1991; 180: 817–21.

58. Langer B, Donato L, Riethmuller C, et al. Spontaneous regression of fetal pulmonary sequestration. Ultrasound Obstet Gynecol 1995; 6: 33–9.

59. Scott JN, Trevenen CL, Wiseman DA, et al. Tracheal atresia: ultrasonographic and pathologic correlation. J Ultrasound Med 1999; 18: 375–7.

60. Choong KK, Trudinger B, Chow C, et al. Fetal laryngeal obstruction: Sonographic detection. Ultrasound Obstet Gynecol 1992; 2: 357–9.

61. DeCou JM, Jones DC, Jacobs HD, et al. Successful ex utero intrapartum treatment (EXIT) procedure for congenital high airway obstruction syndrome (CHAOS) owing to laryngeal atresia. J Pediatric Surg 1998; 33: 1563–5.

62. Richards DS, Langham MR Jr, Mahaffey SM. The prenatal ultrasonograhic diagnosis of cloacal exstrophy. J Ultrasound Med 1992; 11: 507–10.

63. Longaker MT, Laberge JM, Dansereau J, et al. Primary fetal hydrothorax: natural history and management. J Pediatr Surg 1989; 24: 573–6.

64. Benacerraff BR, Frigoletto FD Jr. Mid-trimester fetal thoracentesis. J Clin Ultrasound 1985; 13: 202–4.

65. Wilkins Haug LE, Doubilet P. Successful thoracoamniotic shunting and review of the literature in unilateral pleural effusion with hydrops. J Ultrasound Med 1997; 16: 153–60.

66. Weber AM, Philipson EH. Fetal pleural effusion: a review and meta-analysis for prognostic indicators. Obstet Gynecol 1992; 79: 281–6.

67. Achiron R, Zalel Y, Lipitz S, et al. Fetal lung dysplasia: clinical outcome based on a new classification system. Ultrasound Obstet Gynecol 2004; 24: 127–33.

14 Gastrointestinal tract and internal abdominal wall

Fernando Bonilla-Musoles and Luiz Eduardo Machado

INTRODUCTION

Malformations of the gastrointestinal tract and abdominal wall are infrequent. Their global incidence is estimated to be below 3–6 cases in every 1000 newborns, although it is probably higher, since many of them are part of very severe polymalformative syndromes, with a high incidence of intrauterine death even in the early stages of pregnancy. Some 10% of cases of polyhidramnios are associated with upper digestive atresia, and another 10% with lower digestive atresia.[1,2]

Colon atresia is responsible for 5–10% of all intestinal atresias. Anal atresia is the most frequent type, with an incidence of around 1 in every 5000 live births. Many other intestinal fetal disorders have been described by ultrasound, including small-intestine or anorectal atresia, Hirschprung's disease, megacolon with anourethral atresia, and distended and descended colon, which is associated with Johansson–Blizzard syndrome.

In the past, the approach to diagnosis was based on radiologic procedures, especially the injection of contrast in the amniotic fluid so that the fetus would swallow it and fill the digestive system with contrast. Nowadays, however, these procedures have been replaced by sonography, using which most of these defects can be diagnosed.

Care should be taken to differentiate physiologic findings (swallowing, gastrointestinal fluid formation, peristaltic, meconium accumulation, and urine production) from pathologic occurrences. It is also important to diagnose possible malformations in other organs and systems that can be related to these defects and therefore have a bearing on neonatal prognosis.

These well-known anomalies can be diagnosed using two-dimensional sonography, many of them even in the 1st trimester, but the advent of 3D and 4D techniques has led to a remarkable advance in better definitions of these defects, with many reports already being available.[1,2]

EMBRYOLOGY

During the 6th week of gestation, the endodermal lining epithelium of the primitive gut proliferates and obliterates the lumen. In the following 2 weeks, it vacuolizes and undergoes recanalization.

Stenosis or colon duplication results from incomplete recanalization that produces an intestinal obstruction. Rotation or abnormal fixation of the gut loops results in a variety of malformations, including compression or intestinal volvulus.

BASIS FOR DIAGNOSIS

A complete gastrointestinal tract examination must include:

- visualization of the stomach, starting at week 9, in the upper-left quadrant of the abdomen
- visualization of the small and large intestines, starting at the 16th week, checking the appearance of peristalsis (in the 16th week) and the progressive maturation of the loops with their austras and meconium accumulation
- visualization of the gallbladder and liver and their blood supply
- checking the integrity of the anterior abdominal wall

- checking the integrity of the diaphragm
- checking the umbilical cord insertion
- differentiating possible anomalies from those occurring in other organs, especially kidney, suprarenal, bladder, ovarian anomalies.

The observation of abnormal images of these structures will allow diagnosis of the most common abdominal wall or/and gastrointestinal tract defects.

CLASSIFICATION OF ABDOMINAL DEFFECTS

Abdominal defects may be classified as follows (see also Figure 14.1).

- esophageal atresia
- situs inversus
- ascites and anasarca
- diaphragmatic defects
- abdominal wall defects:
  - omphalocele
  - gastroschisis
  - Cantrell pentalogy
  - exstrophy: bladder; cloaca
  - ectopia cordis
  - limb–body wall complex
  - body stalk complex
- intestinal atresia:
  - duodenal
  - intestinal
  - cloacal
- Miscellaneous:
  - umbilical cord herniation
  - liver calcifications
  - meconium peritonitis.

The sensitivity of 2D sonography for these malformations is estimated to be 46–86%.[3]

ESOPHAGEAL ATRESIA

This is a sporadic anomaly the incidence of which is estimated to be 2–12 cases in every 10 000 live births and that is associated in 90% of cases with a trachea–esophageal (TE) fistula. Both conditions result from failure in the division of the anterior primitive gut, in the formation of the trachea in front and the esophagus behind, which normally takes place between weeks 3 and 5, and is completed in week 8.

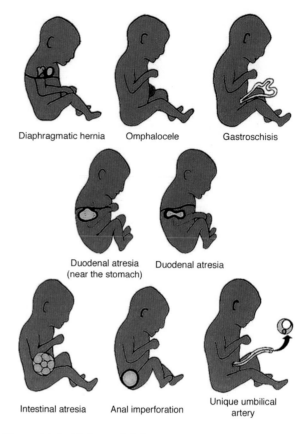

Figure 14.1 Abdominal defects

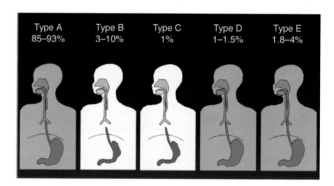

Figure 14.2 Esophageal atresia–fistula

Esophageal atresia is classified as follows (Figure 14.2):[4]

- Type A esophageal atresia without TE fistula
- Type B proximal esophageal atresia with proximal TE fistula
- Type C proximal esophageal atresia with distal TE fistula
- Type D proximal esophageal atresia with both proximal and distal TE fistulas
- Type E TE fistula without esophageal atresia.

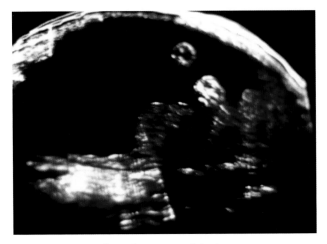

Figure 14.3 Esophageal atresia: polyhydramnios

The most common is the third type 3 (80%), followed by the first type (8%).

This condition is associated in 3–4% of cases with chromosomal anomalies.

The initial diagnosis can be made following the observation of a polyhydramnion, and in successive sonographic examinations, a gastric chamber cannot be seen (Figure 14.3). Also, very occasionally, a distended esophagus can be seen above the atresia, with regurgitation of amniotic fluid after the fetus has swallowed it – however, these are exceptional findings. Failure of visualization of the gastric chamber is not very valuable, however:

- the gastric chamber produces gastric juices that allow its visualization;
- when there is a fistula associated with the chamber, this is also filled up.

Therefore, a prenatal diagnosis can be securely established in less than 10% of cases.

Up to 50–70% of cases affected by this condition are also associated with cardiovascular (29%) and gastrointestinal (28%) malformations, such as intestinal malrotation, anorectal atresia, and duodenal and annular pancreas. This anomaly is also part of the VATER syndrome: vertebral or interventricular septal defects, anal atresia, tracheoesophageal fistula, esophageal atresia, radial dysplasia and renal anomalies, and single-artery umbilical cord.

The prognosis, with or without a TE fistula, will depend on the associated malformations. Consequently, a morphologic study and karyotyping of the amniotic fluid must always be performed after reaching a prenatal diagnosis of an esophageal atresia based on ultrasound.

SITUS INVERSUS

In this condition, the thoracic and abdominal organs are on the opposite sides from usual (situs inversus totalis). A partial variant is known in which only the thoracic organs are abnormally located on the other side (situs inversus partialis). The incidence is estimated to be 1–2 cases in every 10 000 live births. Rarely, the thoracic organs are normally placed, while the abdominal organs are in the reverse position.

Situs inversus partialis is classified as asplenic (both on the right side) or polysplenic (both on the left side). The association between the heart and the spleen, both of which develop in the 6th week of gestation suggests that an unknown factor might exist and might act before or during the formation of these organs. In the asplenic variant, there is no spleen, both lungs are trilobulated, and the liver is centered and symmetric. There is intestinal malrotation and the stomach can be on either side or even in the center. In the polysplenic variant, there are generally two spleens and a variable number of other, smaller, spleens; the liver and stomach can be on the left or right side, and a bilateral superior vena cava can be seen.

The initial diagnosis can be made sonographically when reversed abdominal organs and heart anomalies are observed (Figure 14.4).

The anomalies most frequently associated with situs inversus are complex heart malformations, which

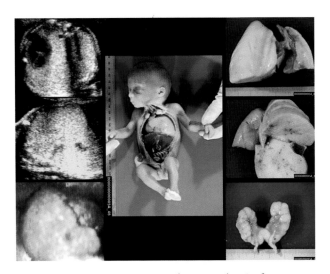

Figure 14.4 Situs inversus totalis in week 24 of gestation. There is dextrocardia and intestinal malrotation, polycystic kidney, left pulmonary hypoplasia, and a cystic adenoma in the right lung. On the left-hand side of the figure can be seen the heart and liver in 2D and 3D at the right side lung, liver and kidneys

are present in 90% of the asplenic variant and 70% of the polysplenic variant. Genitourinary tract malformations and neural tube defects also occur frequently in situs inversus partialis, although they are rarely associated with situs inversus totalis.

The prognosis is very poor, since 90% of newborns affected by this condition die from the associated malformations.

ASCITES AND ANASARCA

Ascites or hydrops fetalis occurs in 1 case in every 1500–4000 newborns. It is a relatively frequent finding, always secondary to severe obstetric problems. Ascites is an accumulation of fluid in the abdominal cavity. Anasarca is generalized edema with accumulation of fluid in the subcutaneous connective tissue all throughout the body. It is generally an advanced stage of ascites, and is sometimes associated with pleural and pericardial effusion (Figures 14.5–14.7).

There are many causes of this fluid retention: immunologic causes (of which Rhesus sensitization is the most common), infections, and metabolic disorders (e.g., diabetes, anemia, and hypoproteinemia), as well as numerous anomalies and malformations.

On sonographic examination, hydrops fetalis is characterized by abdominal distension with a very thin wall and a variable increase in intraperitoneal fluid. There are reduced echoes from intestinal masses, since these are compressed by the fluid and are usually displaced against the vertebral column or towards one of the sides; gut loops are also compressed, but are sometimes partially visible floating in the ascitic fluid (Figure 14.6). The presence of ascites fluid facilitates the identification of abdominal organs, which are also better defined (Figure 14.7).

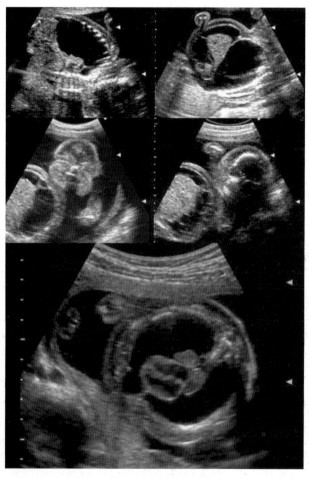

Figure 14.5 Generalized fetal edema, ascites, and anasarca. The edema can be observed underneath the skin. The ascites can be found in the central images. The anasarca with pleural effusion can be seen in the top and bottom images

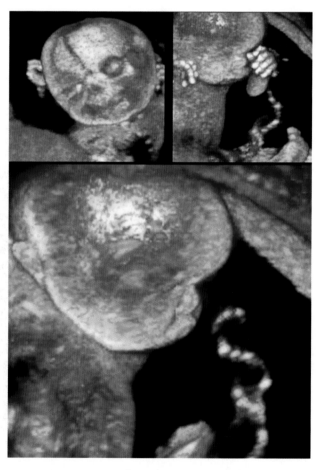

Figure 14.6 3D image from the same case as in Figure 14.5. The transparency produced by the edema underneath the skin is the reason for such fetuses being called 'glass babies'

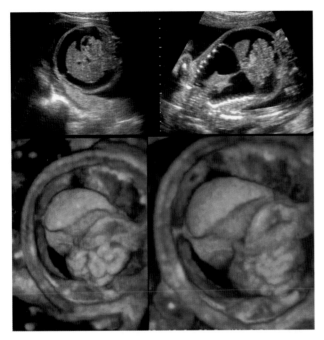

Figure 14.7 2D and 3D sonograms of ascites. The 3D images show the hepatic ligamentum teres and the gut loops immersed in the ascites fluid

When the edema surrounds and extends throughout the whole fetal body, it is called anasarca, generalized hydrops fetalis, or Ballantyne syndrome.

The presence of hydrops indicates a serious danger to the fetus, which is probably in a very compromised situation, most likely terminal (Table 14.1). In 50–70% of cases there is a coexisting polyhydramnios, which is usually very accentuated.

It is essential to determine as precisely as possible the cause of the ascites, in order to start any treatment and to determine the prognosis.

Hydrops fetalis can appear as an isolated occurrence or can be associated with other findings such as hydrothorax, pericarditis, hernia, hepatosplenomegaly, or an increase in the thickness and hyperechogenicity of the placenta.

Ascites or fetal isolated anasarca is generally associated with anomalies of the abdominal lymphatic system. Sonographically guided paracentesis will show the typical lymphocytosis. If the hydrops fetalis is

Table 14.1 Causes of fetal ascites

- Diseases in the mother
- Abnormalities in the placenta
- Fetal diseases or anomalies
- Umbilical cord anomalies

associated with heart beat disorders, supraventricular tachycardia or a cardiopathy must be suspected.

If the hydrops fetalis is associated with other anomalies such as hydrothorax, pericarditis, hernia, hepatosplenomegaly, or an increase in the thickness, hyperechogenicity, or irregularity of the placenta, it could be a non-immune hydrops fetalis. In these cases, there could be a multiple etiology. The obstetrician must consider several causes, such as anomalies/malformations, cardiac, urinary, pulmonary, or polymalformative syndromes, chromosomal syndromes, fetal infections, or other metabolic or hematologic diseases that can affect the fetus.

The finding of hydrops fetalis implies the need for a systematic examination of the fetus and the placenta; a color Doppler and an echocardiographic evaluation should also be performed in order to determine the cardiac and hemodynamic situation of the fetus. Maternal screening should also be performed to rule out any metabolic pathology or infections.

It is important to obtain fetal blood and ascites fluid from the fetus so that fetal anemia, chromosomopathies, hypoproteinemias, bacterial or viral infections, and thalassemia can be ruled out.

Finally, regardless of how much effort is made to reach a diagnosis, in 30% of cases hydrops fetalis will still be considered idiopathic.

DIAPHRAGMATIC DEFECTS

Diaphragmatic defects appear between the 9th and 10th weeks of gestation, and are due to a failure of the closure of the peritoneal pleura that allows the entrance or the herniation of abdominal organs, especially of gut loops inside the thoracic cavity. It is estimated to have an incidence of 1 in every 3000–5000 live births, although the real incidence is doubtless higher, since many of these fetuses die in utero.

The prognosis is very poor, since the origin of these malformations occurs very early on, the defects are substantial, there are other associated malformations, and they can produce pulmonary hypoplasia.

The etiology of these malformations is unknown, although their origin could be sporadic or familial. Some cases have been related to the use of drugs, including anticonvulsants, quinine, and thalidomide.

Pathogenesis can occur by a double mechanism:

- a delay in diaphragmatic fusion
- a primary defect in the development of the diaphragm.

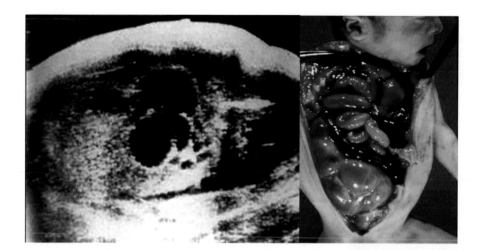

Figure 14.8 Bochdalek hernia

Classification depends on location:

- diaphragmatic hernias: Bochdalek and Morgagni
- septum transversum defects – consist of a defect of the central tendon
- hiatus hernia – occurs through a congenitally large esophageal orifice
- eventration of the diaphragm
- agenesis of the diaphragm.

Bochdalek hernias (Figure 14.8) are the most common type of diaphragmatic defect. They are caused by a posterolateral defect that can be located on either the left side (80%) or the right (15%), or even on both sides (5%). Stomach, spleen, and colon are the most frequently herniated organs. Herniations of the pancreas and liver are less frequent. When the defect is on the right side, herniation of the liver and gallbladder occurs. A peritoneal sac is present in only 10% of cases.

Morgagni hernias are produced by a parasternal defect located on the anterior portion of the diaphragm between the costal and sternum origins of the muscle. They are relatively infrequent (1–2% of all hernias), and even though they can be bilateral, they generally affect the right side. The foramen is usually small, and it can only contain the liver, although sometimes the stomach and the small and large intestines can herniate. If only the liver herniates, it is almost impossible to diagnose this malformation sonographically, since the appearance of the liver and lungs on ultrasound is almost identical. A peritoneal sac is always present.

Hiatus hernias (Figures 14.9 and 14.10), similar to those that occur in adults, are simple defects of the area close to the juncture of the esophagus through

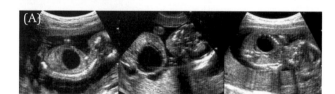

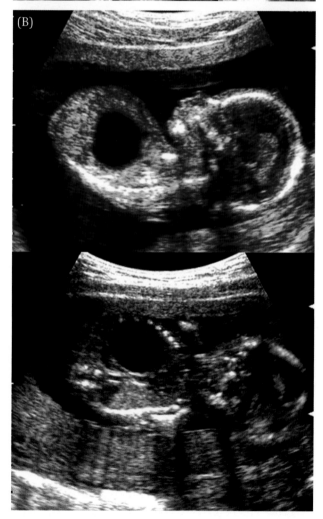

Figure 14.9 (A,B) Hiatus hernias

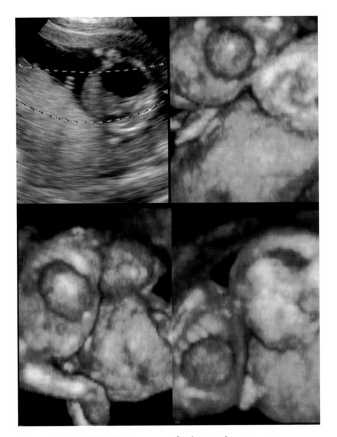

Figure 14.10 3D/4D images of a hiatus hernia

which the gastric cavity can penetrate into the thoracic cavity. A hiatus hernia generally appears as a single cyst.

Eventration involves displacement of the abdominal contents towards the thoracic cavity, due to the development of a weak diaphragm, reduced practically to a simple and thin aponeurotic layer that has no muscle fibers. It comprises 5% of all diaphragmatic defects, and most frequently affects the right side.

Diagnosis of a diaphragmatic defect may be established following the observation of several organs, especially stomach or loops, and also the heart, which is usually displaced towards the right side. If peristaltic movements of the loops are detected, a differential diagnosis can be made with those thoracic pathologies that present similar cystic images, such as pulmonary adenomatosis and bronchogenic and mediastinic cysts.

During the sonographic examination, the absence of a gastric cavity in the abdomen must always be sought – this is usually accompanied by polyhydramnion and a decrease in fetal abdominal circumference.

These defects are commonly associated with anomalies and defects of the central nervous system (25–75%), cardiac anomalies, omphalocele, cleft lip, and chromosomal malformations (trisomies 21, 18, and 13).

DUODENAL ATRESIA

This sporadic condition, caused by atresia or stenosis, has an incidence of 1 in every 10 000 newborns. Familial inheritance has been suggested by an autosomal recessive pattern.

At week 5 of gestation, the lumen of the duodenum is obliterated by proliferation of the epithelium. The path of the lumen is usually restored by week 11, and failure of vacuolization may lead to stenosis or atresia.

A number of causes have been postulated:

- vascular: a vascular accident or interruption of the lumen by a diaphragm or membrane may cause ischemia of a segment of bowel
- drugs: exposure to thalidomide between the 4th and 6th weeks may cause atresia, during a critical time for development
- an annular pancreas is an associated finding (20%); and whereas some believe that this is another feature of an abnormal development, others think that abnormal development of the pancreas may be the cause of the obstruction.

Prenatal diagnosis is based on demonstration of the characteristic 'double-bubble' appearance of the dilated stomach and proximal duodenum, commonly associated with polyhydramnion (Figure 14.11). However, obstruction due to a central web may result in only a 'single bubble' representing the fluid-filled stomach.

Approximately 50% of fetuses have associated malformations, such as skeletal defects (vertebral and rib anomalies, sacral agenesis, radial abnormalities, or talipes), gastrointestinal abnormalities (esophageal atresia, tracheoesophageal fistula, intestinal malrotation, Meckel's diverticulum, or anorectal atresia), cardiovascular malformations (endocardial cushion defects or ventricular septal defects), and renal defects.

Chromosomal anomalies have been observed quite commonly (trisomy 21 in 29% of cases).

The overall mortality rate is high (36%); this is mainly due to the associated abnormalities. Prenatal diagnosis may reduce the morbidity associated with diagnostic delay.

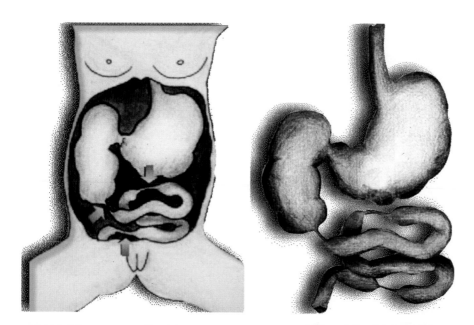

Figure 14.11 'Double bubble': duodenal atresia proximal to the stomach

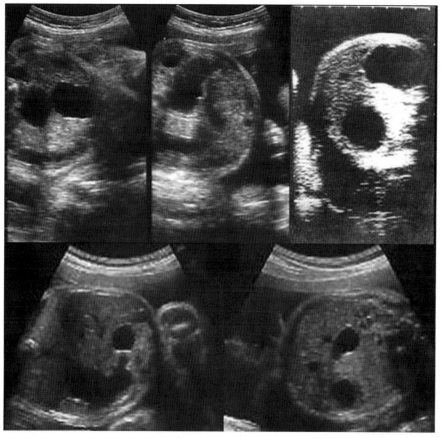

BOWEL OBSTRUCTION

Small-bowel atresia and stenosis occur in 2–3 of every 10 000 newborns. They are sporadic, although familial cases have been described, particularly with the type IV variety. The most common sites of atresia are the distal ileum (36%), proximal jejunum (31%), distal jejunum (20%), and proximal ileum (13%). Intestinal obstruction at any level may lead to proximal bowel dilation and on rare occasions even to perforation. Intestinal atresia is more common than stenosis, and is usually multiple. There are four types of small-bowel atresia:

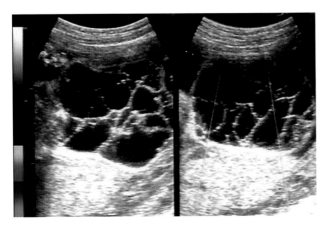

Figure 14.12 Ileal atresia, characterized by multiple cystic intestinal dilatations

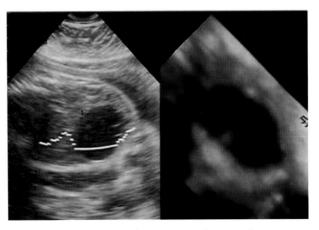

Figure 14.13 Anorectal atresia, with imperforate anus. These pictures have to be differentiated from ovarian cysts, distended urinary bladder, and kidney cysts

- *type I:* mucosal diaphragm (20%)
- *type II:* blind ends of intestine joined by a fibrous band (32%)
- *type III:* blind ends of intestine not connected by a fibrous band (48%)
- *type IV:* absence of a large portion of the small bowel, with a typical apple peel configuration of the small bowel along the mesenteric artery.

Small-bowel atresia is thought to result from vascular accidents, although volvulus or intussusception may lead to vascular impairment at a later stage. Type IV atresia is probably due to occlusion of a branch of the superior mesenteric artery.

Sonographic diagnosis is based on the observation of jejunal and ileal obstructions as multiple fluid-filled loops of bowel (Figure 14.12). The abdomen may be significantly distended, and active peristalsis may be observed.

If bowel perforation occurs, transient ascites, meconium peritonitis, and meconium pseudo cysts may ensue.

Another presentation of small-bowel obstruction is hyperechogenicity in the fetal abdomen. Polyhydramnion is usually also observed, and occurs more frequently with proximal obstructions. Similar bowel appearances and polyhydramnion may be found in fetuses with Hirschsprung's disease and megacystic–microcolon–intestinal hypoperistalsis syndrome. Occasionally, calcified intraluminal meconium in the fetal pelvis is seen, which suggests a diagnosis of anorectal atresia.

Prognosis is related to gestational age at delivery, the presence of associated anomalies, and the site of obstruction.

ANORECTAL ATRESIA

Anorectal atresia, with an incidence of 2 in every 10 000 live births, results from abnormal division of the cloaca during the 9th week of gestation.

Sonographically, it is characterized by a cystic tumor, frequently with irregular contour and a gray ultrasound content (Figure 14.13).

Additional abnormalities are found in 44% of cases, including malrotation, imperforate anus (Figure 14.13), meconium peritonitis and ileus, omphalocele or gastroschisis (20%), and cardiovascular, other gastrointestinal, and chromosomal anomalies (7%).

REFERENCES

1. Bonilla-Musoles F, Machado L, Osborne N, eds. Three-Dimensional Ultrasound for the New Millenium. Text and Atlas. Madrid, Spain: Aloka, 2000.

2. Bonilla-Musoles F. Defectus de la Pared Abdominal Visión con ecografía tridimensional (3D). In: Bonilla-Musoles F, Machado L, eds. 3D–4D Ultrasound in Obstetrics. Madrid, Spain: Panamericana, 2005: 289–304.

3. D'Addario, De Salvia V. Fetal malformations: the central nervous and gastrointestinal systems. In: Kurjak A, ed. Text Book of Perinatal Medicine. London: Parthenon, 1998: 299–324.

4. Thorpe-Beeston JG, Nicolaides KH. The fetal abdomen. In: Chervenak F, Isaacson GC, Campbell S, eds. Ultrasound in Obstetrics and Gynecology. Boston, MA: Little, Brown, 1993: 953–65.

15　The fetus with an abdominal wall defect

Abdallah Adra, Fernando Bonilla-Musoles, and Asim Kurjak

Abdominal wall defects represent a heterogeneous group of fetal malformations ranging from the most common types, namely gastroschisis and omphalocele, to very rare and complex types such as pentalogy of Cantrell and limb–body wall complex. With the more widespread use of biochemical serum screening (α-fetoprotein, AFP) during pregnancy and advances in sonography, prenatal diagnosis of these defects is becoming very common. Visualization of a normal cord insertion and an adjacent anterior abdominal wall excludes the majority of ventral wall defects (Figure 15.1). Prognosis varies markedly, depending on the type of defect, associated anomalies, and certain characteristics that vary with the specific defect. For example, while the prognosis for gastroschisis is generally good, depending mostly on condition of the eviscerated bowel at birth, the prognosis for omphalocele is less optimistic and depends on the presence or absence of concurrent structural and/or chromosomal malformations and the extent of organ evisceration. The role of prenatal sonography is not only to establish the correct diagnosis, which is usually easy, but also to provide an accurate evaluation of the prognostic variables mentioned above to allow expectant parents to make an informed decision regarding pregnancy options, after proper counseling. Similarly it can help the obstetrician to determine the place, time, and perhaps route of delivery, and aid the pediatric surgeon in explaining to the couple the potential complications after neonatal surgical repair and delineate the outcome for them as accurately as possible.

The two most common types of ventral wall defects – gastroschisis and omphalocele – will be discussed first in this chapter. The role of sonography in making

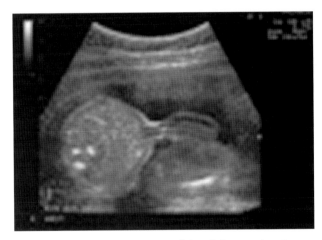

Figure 15.1　Transverse view of the abdomen showing an intact abdominal wall with a normal umbilical cord insertion into the fetus

the initial diagnosis and its importance in fetal surveillance and pregnancy management will be heavily emphasized. Sonographic findings of diagnostic or prognostic value will be discussed in detail. The value of three-dimensional (3D) sonography in confirming the diagnosis, and allowing both physicians and expectant parents to better visualize the malformation through reconstructed images and hence make genetic counseling more comprehensive, will be delineated for each specific defect, and the available literature will be summarized and cited.

GASTROSCHISIS

Gastroschisis is a periumbilical abdominal wall defect, nearly always located to the right of the umbilical insertion. This defect causes various segments of the bowel, from stomach to colon, to herniate into the amniotic fluid. In rare instances, other organs, such as the liver, spleen, urinary bladder, and gonads, may eviscerate.

The incidence of gastroschisis is approximately 1.36 per 10 000 births. This varies considerably with maternal age, being higher in teenage pregnancies.[1] There has been a general trend of increasing incidence reported during the last decade, probably due to improved antenatal sonographic diagnosis and the widespread use of biochemical maternal serum (MS) AFP screening during pregnancy.

The etiology of gastroschisis is uncertain, but it has been generally thought to be related to a vascular accident during early fetal development. Possible mechanisms that have been suggested involve (i) interruption of the omphalomesenteric artery, with infarction and necrosis of the base of the cord and herniation of the gut through this infarcted area;[2] (ii) abnormal involution of the right umbilical vein, resulting in a paraumbilical defect through which the small bowel prolapses at approximately 37 days of life;[3] and (iii) an abnormality in the development of the somites responsible for the integrity of the anterior abdominal wall.

Gastroschisis has been associated with substance abuse, with an increased incidence being reported among cocaine, marijuana, amfetamine, and alcohol users.[4,5]

The defect is more common in smokers.[6] In addition, various medications have been implicated in being associated with an increased risk, including cyclooxygenase (COX) inhibitors (aspirin and ibuprofen) and decongestants (pseudoephedrine) – drugs known to be vasoactive – suggesting a vascular origin for the pathogenesis of gastroschisis.[7,8]

Finally, the existence of familial cases may indicate a genetic factor.[9] Although gastroschisis has generally been considered a sporadic event, there have been reports of isolated gastroschisis in successive siblings,[10] with a 4.3% sibling recurrence rate in a population-based study,[9] and couples should be offered screening in future pregnancies with MSAFP and prenatal sonography for detection or reassurance.

Diagnosis

The majority of fetuses with gastroschisis are diagnosed before 20 weeks, with the widespread use of biochemical MSAFP screening and the routine

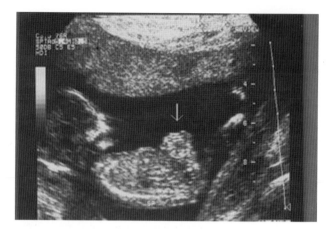

Figure 15.2 Gastroschisis at 17 weeks. Exteriorized bowel appears as a cauliflower lesion (arrow) surfacing on the anterior abdominal wall of the fetus

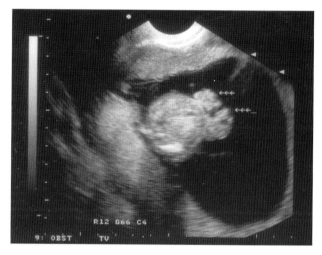

Figure 15.3 Gastroschisis at 19 weeks. Transverse axial view of the fetal abdomen showing eviscerated bowel (arrows) floating in the amniotic fluid

ultrasound examination at 18–20 weeks of gestation. Gastroschisis is detectable on prenatal sonographic examination, with demonstration of a variable amount of bowel protruding through a defect and floating in the amniotic fluid (Figures 15.2 and 15.3). Although earlier studies showed false-positive and false-negative diagnoses of abdominal wall defects, these pitfalls have been avoided by using optimal scanning techniques and color Doppler sonography.[11]

In fact, the detection of gastroschisis in a non-selected population at the National Center for Fetal Medicine in Norway, where MSAFP screening is not available, has recently been reported to be 100% at a mean gestational age of 19 + 2 weeks, with an accuracy of diagnosis of 100%.[12]

On the other hand, in a large study evaluating prenatal sonographic diagnosis of fetal abdominal wall defects by 19 European registries, with a total of 690 123 monitored pregnancies, the overall prenatal detection rate for gastroschisis was 83% and the mean gestational age at diagnosis was 20 ± 7.0 weeks; detection rates varied between registries from 18% to 100%.[13]

In addition, a more recent study looking at the frequency with which severe structural congenital malformations are detected prenatally in Europe and at the gestational age at detection reported an 89% prenatal detection rate of gastroschisis cases, with 79% diagnosed prior to 24 weeks of gestation and a median gestational age at diagnosis of 17 weeks.[14]

Role of prenatal sonography

Prenatal sonography can provide significant information with regard to the prognosis of a fetus with gastroschisis, allowing the expectant mother to make an informed decision concerning pregnancy options, including termination, especially in the case of a large defect with significant organ evisceration and/or the presence of associated malformations.

Perinatal care can be coordinated with the neonatologist and the pediatric surgeon, and decisions can be made regarding mode, time, and place of delivery. In this respect, initial diagnosis in the 3rd trimester can allow for maternal transport to a perinatal center that is able to handle the malformation in the neonatal period and the use of corticosteroids to enhance fetal lung maturation, in the case of elective preterm delivery based on antenatal testing of fetal well-being.

Serial ultrasound examinations allow the following:

- Exclusion of associated malformations and chromosomal aberrations (although these are rare with gastroschisis[15]) that may not have been detected during the initial examination when the defect was discovered.
- Assessment of the degree of organ evisceration as the pregnancy evolves, as cases have been described with herniation of various organs after identification of only loops of small bowel floating in the amniotic fluid on initial examination.[16]
- Assessment of fetal growth interval since it is well known that fetuses with gastroschisis are at an increased risk of intrauterine growth restriction (IUGR).[17,18]

- Assessment of amniotic fluid volume, since both polyhydramnios and oligohydramnios have been noted in association with gastroschisis – the former has been described as being significantly associated with severe bowel complications[19] (and a potential indicator of high bowel obstruction, atresia, and poor neonatal outcome), while the latter has been described as a cause of the increased incidence of fetal distress and intrauterine demise seen in gastroschisis-affected fetuses due to umbilical cord accidents.[20]
- Evaluation of the condition of the bowel – both intraabdominal and herniated – since this sometimes correlates with immediate postnatal outcome and since complications that may dictate immediate delivery have been described, such as acute bowel perforation[21] and vanishing gastroschisis with short-bowel syndrome.[22]
- The use of Doppler and biophysical profile to monitor fetal well-being, since fetuses with gastroschisis are known to be at an increased risk of intrauterine demise.[23]

Prenatal sonography can be used to investigate the value of fetal therapy in gastroschisis – specifically the role of serial exchange amnioinfusion in improving neonatal outcome by reducing the bowel injuries seen in affected fetuses due to the severe perivisceritis and chronic inflammatory process (chemical peritonitis) induced by prolonged exposure of bowel to fetal urine and the gastrointestinal wastes present in amniotic fluid.[24]

Associated anomalies

Extra-intestinal abnormalities are usually rare with gastroschisis. In a study assessing the current accuracy of routine prenatal ultrasound examination in the detection of abdominal wall defects in different regions of Europe, Barisic et al[13] noted that in only 14% of fetuses with gastroschisis were there other defects. As far as chromosomal aberrations are concerned, a fetus with gastroschisis and no associated anomalies carries the normal age-related background risk of a chromosomal abnormality.[25] However, there were two cases of trisomy (one Down syndrome with isolated gastroschisis and one trisomy 13 with multiple malformations) in the series of low-risk pregnancies described by Barisic et al.[13] The decision to perform invasive fetal karyotyping in the case of an

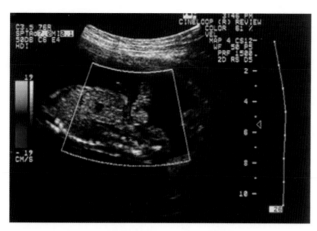

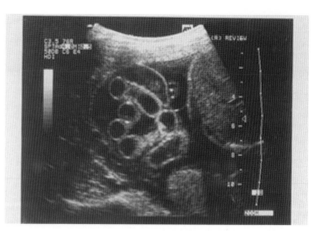

Figure 15.4 Longitudinal scan with color Doppler showing a normal cord insertion with bowel herniating through a small para-umbilical defect

Figure 15.5 Gastroschisis. Scan at 26 weeks demonstrating relatively normal appearing loops of herniated small bowel

isolated gastroschisis should be an informed choice by the mother after she has been counseled about the risks and the value of the information obtained through the test. Cardiovascular malformations have been reported in up to 15% of fetuses with gastroschisis, stressing the importance of performing fetal echocardiography in these cases.[26]

Bowel-related abnormalities remain the most common and most clinically significant complications related to gastroschisis; they include atresia, malrotation, volvulus, and microcolon.[27,28] Intestinal atresia or stenosis may result either from compression of mesenteric vessels by the relatively small defect or from torsion of the eviscerated bowel.[29,30]

Sonographic evaluation of eviscerated organs

Sonographic diagnosis of gastroschisis relies on the demonstration of a full-thickness anterior abdominal wall defect, usually to the right of a normal umbilical cord insertion (Figure 15.4), and herniation of loops of small bowel floating in the amniotic fluid (Figure 15.5). Small bowel is always eviscerated, but progressive evisceration of various segments of the gastrointestinal tract, from stomach to large bowel, has been reported. Other structures that may eviscerate include the liver and spleen, fallopian tubes, ovaries, testicles, and urinary bladder.[16,27,31] Ikhena et al[31] reported a case of gastroschisis associated with bladder evisceration and complicated by rapidly progressive unilateral hydronephrosis, necessitating early cesarean delivery at 34 weeks of gestation with successful primary

closure. This case, among others, highlights the need for continuing sonographic surveillance of fetuses with gastroschisis to identify further associated complications that may influence mode, timing, and place of delivery, as well as neonatal care.

Sonographic evaluation of eviscerated bowel

Many studies have tried to answer the question whether sonography of the fetal bowel can accurately predict postnatal outcome and to produce agreement on certain guidelines regarding mode and (more importantly) timing of delivery, based on sonographic evaluation of eviscerated bowel.[32–39] Langer et al[32] noted that a bowel diameter of at least 18 mm was associated with a significantly longer time to oral feeding and with a significantly greater need for bowel resection, and they concluded that prenatal sonography may be useful in selecting appropriate fetuses for preterm delivery. Pryde et al[33] concurred that fetal bowel dilatation of more than 17 mm appears to be associated with increased short- and long-term infant morbidity, but they questioned whether this finding warrants obstetric intervention in the preterm gastroschisis-affected pregnancy. Adra et al[34] observed that fetuses with prenatally dilated bowel had significantly more bowel edema at birth, longer operative time, and a higher rate of postoperative complications (Figure 15.6). In contrast, Alsulyman et al[35] concluded, based on a 7-year retrospective study involving 21 cases of gastroschisis, that using a cut-off of maximal bowel diameter of 17 mm or more is not

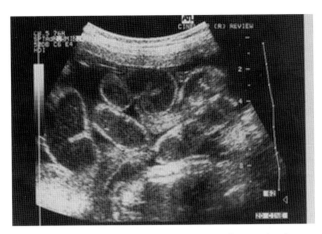

Figure 15.6 Gastroschisis. Scan at 32 weeks – with advancing gestation and prolonged exposure to amniotic fluid, small bowel loops become dilated with thickened wall

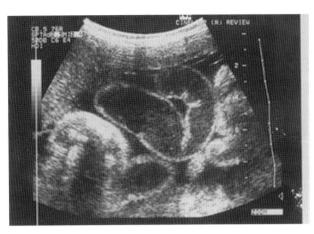

Figure 15.7 Gastroschisis. Scan at 34 weeks demonstrating marked eviscerated small bowel dilatation. This infant had resection of an atretic segment causing proximal intestinal obstruction

an appropriate indication for preterm delivery in the absence of other evidence of fetal compromise. In addition, a more recent study from Australia has evaluated the usefulness of various sonographic parameters to predict neonatal outcome of gastroschisis.[19] Among the parameters assessed – gestation at first diagnosis, maximum bowel diameter, maximum bowel wall thickness, presence of other anomalies, evidence of growth restriction, and polyhydramnios – the authors concluded that polyhydramnios was the only one that was strongly predictive of severe bowel complications in the neonatal period. Finally, infants with gastroschisis with a prenatally dilated stomach had a higher incidence of volvulus and neonatal death, a significantly delayed time to full oral feeding, and a longer hospitalization, when compared with infants with a non-dilated stomach prenatally.[36] Based on the available literature regarding the sonographic appearance of fetal bowel in gastroschisis and its correlation with neonatal outcome and prognosis, one can conclude the following:

- Abnormally dilated bowel segments visualized on prenatal sonography usually correlate with a high rate of neonatal bowel complications, a more difficult surgical repair with a longer operative time, a greater need for intestinal resection, a longer time to full oral feeding and a longer hospital stay.[32,34,36]
- There is no clinically meaningful cut-off point for maximal bowel dilatation that has been shown to be an indicator for preterm delivery to improve neonatal outcome.[37,38] In other words, there are no conclusive data to support the hypothesis that

sonographic evaluation of the fetal bowel, in the setting of isolated gastroschisis, can be useful in identifying the at-risk fetus that might benefit from early delivery.

- Polyhydramnios, when present, is strongly predictive of severe bowel complications in the neonatal period, and should suggest the possibility of bowel obstruction or atresia (Figure 15.7).[19,39,40]

The role of Doppler velocimetry

Fetuses with gastroschisis are known to be at an increased risk of intrauterine demise.[41] There is no apparent explanation for this increase in the risk of fetal death in utero. Robinson et al[42] reported on two cases of notching in the umbilical artery Doppler waveform in pregnancies with gastroschisis, presenting strong evidence that the notching was due to external compression of the umbilical artery by the herniated fetal stomach. Similarly, Kalache et al[43] emphasized the importance of diastolic notching in the umbilical artery during the antepartum surveillance of fetuses with gastroschisis, and questioned whether unexplained intrauterine demise of fetuses with gastroschisis in the 3rd trimester can be caused by umbilical cord compression due to acute extra-abdominal bowel dilatation. These case reports may shed some light on the cause of unexplained fetal demise in gastroschisis cases.[42,43]

On the other hand, after conducting a prospective longitudinal study on 17 fetuses with gastroschisis, Abuhamad et al[44] concluded that Doppler velocimetry of the superior mesenteric artery and its branches is not predictive of neonatal outcome.

Fetal therapy in gastroschisis

The majority of cases of gastroschisis undergo postnatal surgical repair with good results and excellent survival, especially with isolated cases, with minimal long-term morbidity. Nevertheless, some newborns end up losing variable segments of their small intestine, due to damaged, ischemic, and matted bowel at birth.

The benefits of in utero therapy in gastroschisis, namely exchange amnioinfusion, need to be proven before fetal therapy becomes the standard of care for this congenital malformation. Most of the work relating to this mode of in utero therapy has come from the same group in the Hôpital Robert Debre in Paris. Earlier studies of prognostic factors for gastroschisis revealed that fetuses with both severe perivisceritis and meconium-stained amniotic fluid were born earlier than fetuses with mild perivisceritis and normal amniotic fluid.[45]

In 1999, Luton et al[46] conducted a case–control trial to study the effect of amnioinfusion on the outcome of prenatally diagnosed gastroschisis. Ten fetuses with gastroschisis underwent amnioinfusion and were matched to controls according to characteristics of the defect, fetal growth, and amniotic fluid volume. Transabdominal exchange amnioinfusion with saline was performed at a mean gestational age of 32.3 ± 3.2 weeks, with a mean volume infused of 500 ± 239 ml. Amniotic fluid was assayed for specific inflammatory cytokines and ferritin levels. Amnioinfusion had a favorable impact on outcome, mainly on the duration of curarization, delay before full oral feeding, and overall length of hospitalization, although the latter two variables did not reach statistical significance; there was no difference in gestational age at delivery. In addition, amniotic fluid levels of both interleukin-6 and ferritin were significantly lower in amnioinfused fetuses compared with controls, suggesting a milder inflammatory reaction involving the eviscerated bowel.

In addition, Sapin et al[47] reported on the benefits of serial amnioinfusion to avoid fetal demise and intestinal damage in two fetuses with gastroschisis and severe oligohydramnios, where exteriorized bowel was normal at birth and primary closure could be performed with favorable outcome.

In a more recent study, Burc et al[48] measured amniotic fluid inflammatory concentrations of proteins, ferritin, and digestive compounds before each amnioexchange performed in fetuses with gastroschisis, and showed a positive correlation between digestive compounds and ferritin on the one hand and all digestive compounds and total proteins at the final amnioexchange on the other. Finally, studies conducted in animal models of gastroschisis have demonstrated intestinal damage caused by meconium, as evidenced by serosal thickening, fibrin deposition, and various degrees of bowel peel coverage and adherence.[49,50]

In conclusion, the amnioexchange procedure, where the amniotic fluid is changed regularly in the 3rd trimester, involves a new therapeutic approach, aiming at reducing bowel dysfunction in fetuses with gastroschisis. Preliminary data look promising, since amnioinfused fetuses appear to have lesser degrees of perivisceritis at birth, probably due to a lower degree of inflammatory reaction involving the exteriorized bowel, as evidenced by significantly lower levels of inflammatory mediators in the amniotic fluid at the final amnioexchange procedure when compared with initial levels before the first procedure.[48] However, until a randomized controlled trial of exchange amnioinfusion in fetuses with gastroschisis confirms the benefits of this procedure on the degree of bowel dysfunction and neonatal outcome, amnioexchange should be offered only to patients in the context of experimental or research protocols.

Value of 3D sonography

In the evaluation of abdominal wall defects, 3D sonography can play a particularly important role. Although the diagnosis of gastroschisis is often made easily with 2D sonography, expectant parents can often understand 3D ultrasound images of the defect more readily than 2D images (Figure 15.8). In addition, there is improved recognition of the anomaly by less experienced physicians. In a study by Bonilla-Musoles et al[51] comparing 2D versus 3D sonographic diagnosis of abdominal wall defects, 3D sonography in orthogonal planes with surface rendering established a definitive diagnosis of gastroschisis at 14 weeks of gestation. The improved comprehension of fetal anatomy by families after 3D sonographic imaging of the defect (Figure 15.9) allows for more efficient counseling and postnatal therapeutic planning.[51]

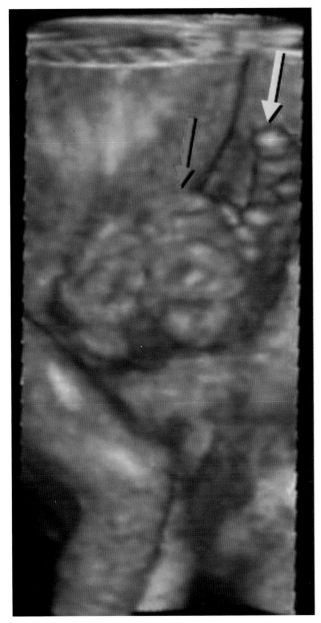

Figure 15.8 3D gastroschisis. The 3D picture shows the intestines (red arrow), floating in the amniotic fluid. The yellow arrow shows the umbilical cord

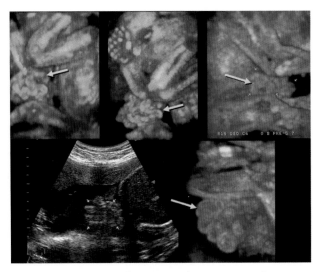

Figure 15.9 Gastroschisis 2D and 3D images. The arrows show the intestines floating in amniotic fluid

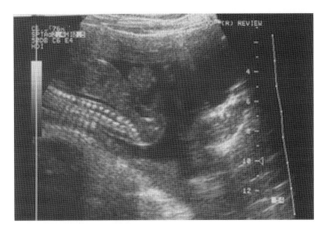

Figure 15.10 Gastroschisis. Sonogram of a fetus at 18 weeks' gestation with elevated MSAFP. Eviscerated bowel appears as a well-delineated rounded mass resting on the surface of the anterior abdominal wall

The diagnosis of gastroschisis by conventional 2D sonography is mostly made after demonstration of a cauliflower-shaped mass on the anterior aspect of the abdominal wall, which usually represents loops of bowel floating freely in the amniotic fluid (Figure 15.10). The actual defect in the abdominal wall is not easily visualized and the relation of the defect to the umbilical cord insertion is not always ascertained with 2D sonography. In this respect, 3D sonography, along with color Doppler, can help to visualize the paraum-bilical defect (usually to the right of a normal cord insertion), and sometimes to assess its size and the degree of organ evisceration. Most importantly, it can help expectant parents to see the malformation better (Figure 15.11), and hence have a clearer understanding of information and counseling regarding pregnancy options (including the potential need for fetal therapy in selected cases), prognosis, and what to expect after birth.

In addition, 3D sonography should be considered a complementary modality in the evaluation of gastroschisis to exclude coexisting malformations that are not readily seen with 2D sonography but may influence prognosis and hence parents' decisions

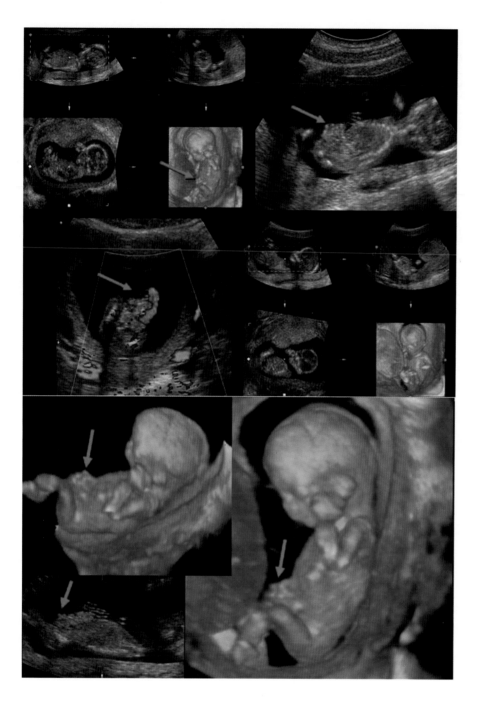

Figure 15.11 Gastroschisis in week 18. 2D color Doppler and 3D. Red arrows are depicting the abdominal defect with intestines emerging through a small hole

regarding pregnancy options. In a study by Brantberg et al,[12] the rate of associated anomalies (excluding intestinal anomalies) in a series of gastroschisis cases prospectively evaluated from a national center in fetal medicine was 6.3%. There were two cases of arthrogryposis of the amyoplasia type – limb anomalies usually due to vascular compromise, and not easily seen on 2D sonography. 3D sonography would probably allow families to appreciate the significance of these limb malformations involving severe muscular atrophy, which are present in 3–5% of fetuses with

gastroschisis, and which are usually associated with a poor prognosis.[52]

Finally, no information is yet available regarding the value of 3D sonography in the evaluation of the eviscerated organs and whether it will be superior to and more accurate than conventional 2D sonography, nor has it been established whether 3D sonography could be of use in evaluating the condition of the exteriorized bowel and its correlation with short-term neonatal outcome. However, 3D sonography will probably be helpful in assessing bowel thickening and

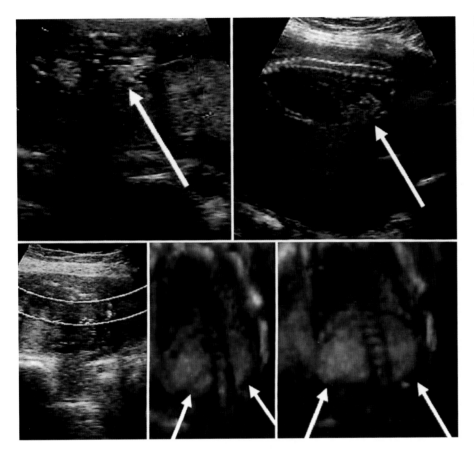

Figure 15.12 Diffuse meconium peritonitis. The arrows show dense, round hyperechogenic intraabdominal masses which correspond to meconium and microcalcifications in the meconium

dilatation, as well as fibrin deposits on the surface, and more importantly acute bowel complications in utero such as perforation or meconium peritonitis (Figure 15.12), which may dictate immediate delivery.

Pregnancy management and postnatal repair

As mentioned earlier, the diagnosis of gastroschisis is easily detected by ultrasound, with the majority of cases being diagnosed prior to 24 weeks, with the widespread using of serum AFP screening and advances in real-time sonography. What then is next?

The expectant parents receive in-depth counseling and pregnancy options are discussed (preferably with the involvement of a pediatric surgeon), chromosomal analysis is sometimes obtained through amniocentesis, and the pregnancy is usually allowed to continue, especially with an isolated defect.

Relevant aspects of perinatal care then include the following:

- Surveillance of the fetus should be carried out with serial sonographic examinations to evaluate fetal growth and well-being and the status of eviscerated bowel – variables that may influence the timing and mode of delivery.

- While some suggest a planned preterm delivery in fetuses with gastroschisis to avoid bowel complications and dysfunction that may result from prolonged exposure to intestinal wastes and meconium,[53] most authorities recommend delivery at term,[54] unless non-reassuring antenatal testing occurs[55] or acute bowel perforation is detected in utero.[21] If fetal therapy in the form of amnioexchange proves to be beneficial in decreasing the incidence of bowel dysfunction,[24] then the issue of elective preterm delivery in gastroschisis will be further contested.

- There is no consensus on the mode of delivery in fetuses with gastroschisis. The conclusions from most studies are limited by their retrospective nature and small sample size.[56–59] While some studies have shown a trend towards a better perinatal outcome with a less difficult repair and a shorter time to enteral feedings with elective cesarean delivery,[56] others (including by our group) have refuted this.[34,57–59] Although the rate

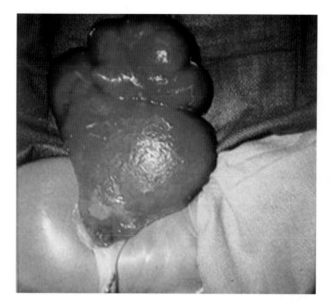

Figure 15.13 Gastroschisis. A surgical photograph shows markedly dilated bowel with thickened serosal layer due to multiple sites of atresia, requiring secondary closure. Note the normal cord insertion with a small para-median abdominal wall defect (courtesy of D. Buckner, MD, Jackson Children's Hospital, Miami, Florida)

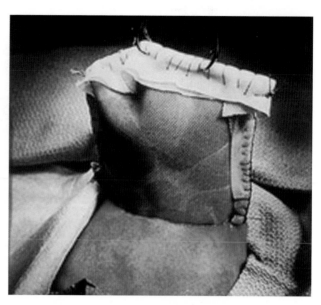

Figure 15.14 A silo bag keeps the bowel (seen in Figure 15.13) sterile and protected allowing periodic inspection of the bowel with gradual replacement of bowel segments into the abdominal cavity

of cesarean delivery is usually high, even in women who are given a trial of labor (high incidence of IUGR with non-reassuring fetal heart rate tracings[55]), the controversy regarding the optimal route of delivery in gastroschisis-affected pregnancies will continue, with little scientific evidence being available.[60,61] A randomized controlled trial may resolve this issue, but it seems that it would be difficult to recruit patients to this kind of trial.

- Irrespective of the route of delivery, the bowel should be handled with great care at birth and kept moist and warm. Delivery should take place in a tertiary care center where pediatric surgical expertise in the repair of gastroschisis is available, since the neonatal outcome after surgical repair of out-born, when compared with in-born babies, has been shown to be worse – mainly due to complications, namely respiratory distress, sepsis, and meconium aspiration.[62,63]

- Prompt repair with primary abdominal wall closure is preferred when the bowel can be returned to the abdomen without difficulty due to visceroabdominal disproportion and without causing bowel compromise. When primary repair is not possible, a silo placement is necessary to protect eviscerated bowel from trauma and infection, and a staged repair is then carried out, with

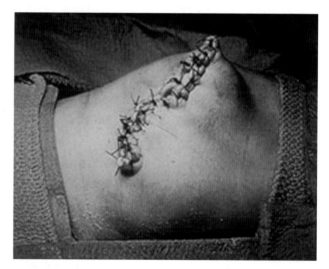

Figure 15.15 Final repair – the defect was successfully closed by 18 days of age. The infant suffered from short-bowel syndrome 6 months after birth

longer time to full oral feeding and a longer hospital stay[64,65] (Figures 15.13–15.15). Infants with gastroschisis will invariably experience various degrees of bowel dysfunction, but there is minimal long-term morbidity, except for short-bowel syndrome that may develop following intestinal resection at birth due to ischemia or atresia (Figure 15.16).[22,66]

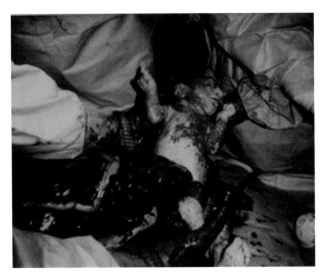

Figure 15.16 Gross appearance at birth of ischemic bowel in gastroschisis

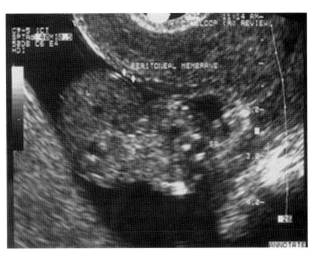

Figure 15.17 Omphalocele. Transverse scan of the fetal abdomen at 15 weeks shows an omphalocele sac containing liver (L), stomach (S), and bowel (B)

OMPHALOCELE

Omphalocele is a central abdominal wall defect characterized by herniation of the bowel, liver, and other organs into the intact umbilical cord. At birth, the eviscerated organs are usually covered by a membrane (unless this has ruptured in utero) that is actually composed of two layers: the peritoneum and amnion (Figure 15.17). The total prevalence rate was reported to be 1 in 4000 births, based on a survey of 3 million births from 21 regional registries in Europe during the period 1980–90.[67] The omphalocele defect is caused by an abnormality that occurred early in embryogenesis during the process of body infolding at 3–4 weeks of gestation. While cephalic folding defects result in a ventral wall defect situated cranially to the umbilicus, as seen in pentalogy of Cantrell (see below), lateral folding defects result in the 'classic' omphalocele with a midabdominal or central defect, while caudal folding defects result in a low or hypogastric omphalocele, as seen in bladder or cloacal extrophy.

Omphaloceles are associated with structural malformations (up to 74% in a study of 265 858 consecutive births from the registry of congenital malformations of Strasbourg), and chromosomal aberrations are seen in 30% of fetuses.[1] Specific syndromes have also been reported in 10% of cases of omphalocele.[13]

Although no known teratogens are associated with omphalocele, several factors have been reported in association with the defect. Preconception use of multivitamins has been shown to decrease the risk of omphalocele,[68] while assisted reproductive technology and consanguinity have been reported in epidemiologic studies to increase the risk.[1,69]

The inheritance of omphalocele is usually sporadic, with a recurrence risk of less than 1%.[70] Familial cases of non-syndromal omphalocele are rare.[71]

The prognosis for omphalocele depends greatly on whether or not there are associated structural or chromosomal abnormalities. Prematurity and mortality rates are increased compared with controls.[72] Surgical repair after birth can be immediate, delayed, or staged, depending on the size of the lesion.

Diagnosis

An omphalocele is often diagnosed during routine prenatal sonographic examination or following the evaluation of elevated MSAFP. MSAFP has been reported to be positive in 42% of omphaloceles.[73] Both gastroschisis and omphalocele are associated with elevated MSAFP. The median value for MSAFP is 9.42 multiples of the median (MOM) in gastroschisis and 4.18 MOM in omphalocele.[74]

The sensitivity of antenatal ultrasound examination in detecting omphalocele was 75% in a European study evaluating the effectiveness of routine prenatal sonographic screening in detecting gastroschisis and omphalocele, with the mean gestational age at the first detection being 18 ± 6.0 weeks.[13]

The value of prenatal sonography in the evaluation and management of the fetus with omphalocele lies in the following:

- It can establish the correct diagnosis during the initial evaluation and can exclude associated malformations or specific syndromes, both chromosomal and non-chromosomal. Expectant parents can then be counseled about the neonatal outcome, and the prognosis can be delineated for them so that they can make an informed decision after discussing pregnancy options.

- Because a high proportion of omphaloceles are associated with concurrent malformations, syndromes, or chromosomal aberrations that may have been missed on the initial evaluation, a repeat detailed examination by an experienced sonographer should become a standard procedure.

- If pregnancy continues, serial sonographic examinations every 2–4 weeks are indicated to assess the size of the defect, the organs herniated (especially the liver), amniotic fluid, fetal growth interval, fetal well-being, and the rare possibility of in utero rupture of the covering membrane – variables that may influence the timing and mode of delivery.

Initial diagnosis and evaluation

The vast majority of fetuses with omphalocele can be identified with prenatal 2D sonography using the five American Institute of Ultrasound Medicine/American College of Radiologists (AIUM/ACR) recommended views: abdominal circumference, stomach, renal area, bladder, and cord insertion.[75] However, a recent study looking at the frequency with which severe structural congenital malformations are detected prenatally in Europe found that the prenatal detection rate of omphalocele was 77%.[14]

The accuracy of prenatal sonographic diagnosis of omphalocele can be improved markedly by assessing the following key features to decrease the rates of false-positive and false-negative diagnoses:

- The central location of the defect at the base of the umbilical cord (rather than to the right of the insertion) is a primary and diagnostic feature of omphalocele. It is important to look for an acute angle between the fetal abdomen and the origin of the sac on a transverse plane; this reduces the chance of the finding being artifactual (pseudo-omphalocele) secondary to an oblique imaging plane or excessive transducer pressure. In addition, color Doppler interrogation of the umbilical cord can help locate the exact site of the

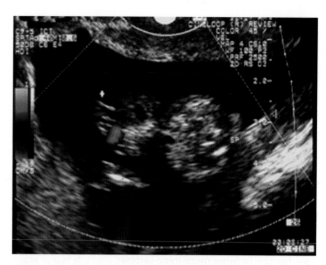

Figure 15.18 Omphalocele. Color Doppler demonstrating the umbilical cord inserting into the caudal-apical portion of the herniated sac

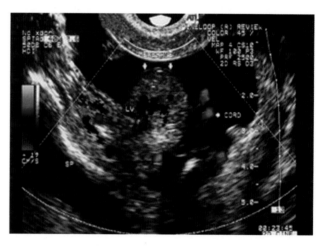

Figure 15.19 Omphalocele. Color Doppler showing cord insertion into the defect with the intrahepatic (LV) umbilical vein coursing through the defect. Note the surrounding membrane (arrows)

defect (Figure 15.18), and demonstration of the intrahepatic umbilical vein coursing through the defect is also evidence of the central location of the lesion (Figure 15.19).

- The presence of a limiting membrane is another essential feature of omphalocele (Figure 15.20). The abdominal contents are enclosed, rounded, and not free-floating in the amniotic fluid like in gastroschisis. It is not always easy to visualize the membrane unless it is outlined by ascites.

- Evaluation of the contents and size of the omphalocele sac is also a key procedure, not only

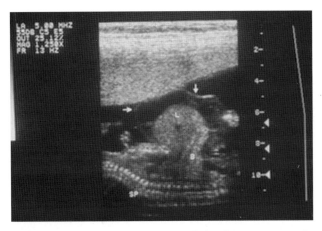

Figure 15.20 Longitudinal scan of the fetus at 20 weeks showing the limiting membrane (arrows), which is a characteristic feature of an omphalocele

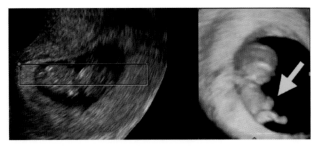

Figure 15.21 Omphalocele in 11th week. The fetal abdomen shows an irregular herniation and bigger than 7 mm

from a diagnostic point of view, but also because of its prognostic value. It is known that omphaloceles containing liver have a lower rate of abnormal karyotype than omphaloceles containing only bowel.[76,77] Similarly, it is generally accepted in the pediatric and surgical literature that large omphaloceles are associated with a poor prognosis because a high incidence of respiratory failure and the increased probability of the need for multiple surgical postnatal interventions.[78,79]

- Finally, it is important to remember that if the defect is detected early (Figure 15.21), prior to 12 weeks, caution should be exercised before diagnosing prior to completion of the physiologic herniation (Figure 15.22). Similarly, a recent study by Blazer et al[80] of fetal omphaloceles diagnosed by endovaginal sonography at 12–16 weeks of gestation reported that in 50% of fetuses with isolated small omphaloceles associated with a normal karyotype, the omphalocele disappeared at 20–24 weeks of gestation and no defect was seen at delivery.

Value of 3D sonography

Diagnosis of omphalocele is usually easy by 2D sonography during a routine fetal examination, and an early diagnosis is possible. Although 3D sonography may not be essential for prenatal diagnosis, it can be of considerable value for the following reasons:

- It does help to identify the omphalocele more clearly and completely, allowing expectant parents to see the malformation better, hence facilitating parental counseling and making the consultation more comprehensive (Figure 15.23).
- The rate of associated anomalies with omphalocele is extremely high even when the karyotype is normal, reaching 89% as reported in a recent case series.[81] Some of these associated structural anomalies are better characterized by 3D sonography, including facial, vertebral, and hand/feet malformations, allowing more accurate diagnosis of non-chromosomal syndromes and thus helping in parental counseling regarding prognosis and outcome.
- Cysts or pseudocysts of the umbilical cord have been reported to be associated with both trisomy 18 and omphalocele.[82,83] A recent study reported an abnormal karyotype in 85% of fetuses with

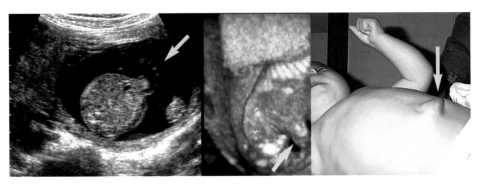

Figure 15.22 Physiological umbilical cord herniation. 2D/3D and the newborn (arrows). This finding, a dilatation of the umbilical cord implantation, is nowadays considered physiologic

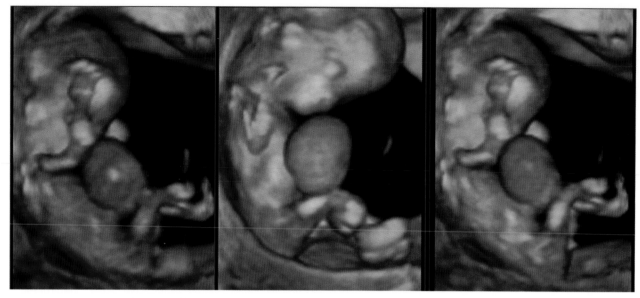

Figure 15.23   3D visualization of omphalocele at 12 weeks of gestation. Pregnancy was allowed to progress till term

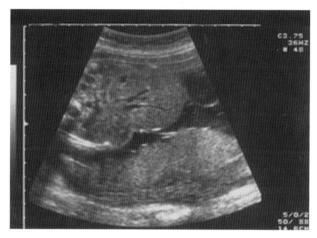

Figure 15.24   Transverse scan of the fetal abdomen at 20 weeks showing a moderate-sized omphalocele with extra-corporeal liver. Genetic amniocentesis revealed a normal karyotype

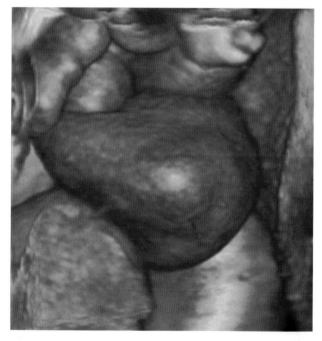

Figure 15.25   The same case as in Figure 15.23 at 30 weeks gestation shown by 3D sonography

omphalocele when an umbilical cord cyst was present.[81] 3S sonography may help to provide better evaluation of the umbilical cord to diagnose a cyst, which, if present, dramatically increases the risk of fetal aneuploidy.

- 3D sonography may also provide more accurate evaluation of the contents of the omphalocele sac (Figures 15.24 and 15.25). In this respect, confirming the presence of an extracorporeal liver by 3D sonography may influence perinatal care regarding mode of delivery, since dystocia and potential liver damage may occur with vaginal birth.[58,61] Similarly, 3D sonography may be helpful in the diagnosis of a ruptured omphalocele sac in utero (Figure 15.26) in order to differentiate it from gastroschisis, which carries a different prognosis and outcome.

Diagnosis of omphalocele using 3D sonography has been described.[51,84,85] Anandakumar et al[84] reported

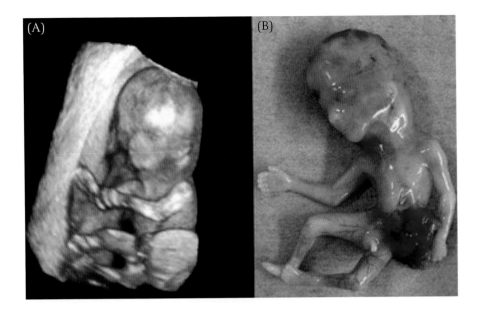

Figure 15.26 Omphalocele detected by 3D sonography in the first trimester. During interruption of pregnancy the omphalocele sac has been ruptured (courtesy of Dr. Ritsuko K. Pooh, CRIFM Clinical Research Institute of Fetal Medicine Pooh Maternity Clinic, Kagawa, Japan)

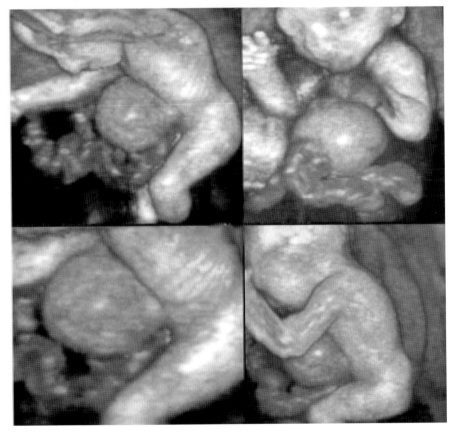

Figure 15.27 3D of an omphalocele. These figures show a case of omphalocele with a very small abdominal opening

the 3D sonographic diagnosis of omphalocele at 12 weeks of gestation using a transvaginal probe in a 35-year-old woman being evaluated because of an abnormal nuchal translucency. Surface rendering was applied to view the omphalocele clearly, and the image was rotated and tilted at various angles to help with explanation and counseling for expectant parents. Similarly, Chuang et al[85] showed how 3D

transabdominal sonographic visualization of a fetal omphalocele at 14 weeks of gestation allowed the parents to comprehend the lesion easily and to make an informed decision after genetic counseling. In addition, Bonilla-Musoles et al[51] emphasized the valuable additional role of 3D sonography in the 2nd trimester for the evaluation of fetuses with abdominal wall defects (Figures 15.27 and 15.28), including

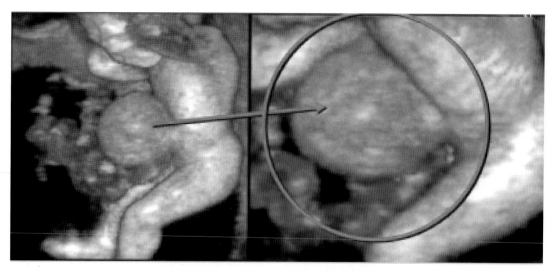

Figure 15.28 Detail of the omphalocele of Figure 15.27 using the zoom

detection of associated subtle malformations not easily detected on 2D imaging and diagnosis of recognizable syndromes such as pentalogy of Cantrell and prune-belly syndrome. The authors, however, noted that 2D was superior to 3D sonography for detection of the contents of omphaloceles.[51]

Management and surgical repair

Once the prenatal diagnosis of omphalocele has been confirmed by conventional 2D sonography (and perhaps has been evaluated further and shown to the parents with 3D sonography), chromosome analysis should be performed, since the risk of trisomies in fetuses with omphalocele is 340 times higher than in those without omphalocele.[86] In an ultrasound screening study involving 15 726 viable singleton pregnancies at 11–14 weeks of gestation, the frequency of trisomy 18, trisomy 13, or triploidy in fetuses with omphalocele was 61%.[87] In addition, because of an increased risk of both congenital and perinatal cardiac abnormalities in fetuses with omphalocele, especially persistent pulmonary hypertension of the newborn, parents should be counseled about the importance of performing echocardiography both prenatally and postnatally in these cases.[26] If the karyotype is normal with no associated serious malformations, and the pregnancy is allowed to continue, close clinical surveillance and serial sonographic evaluation are necessary to monitor for preterm birth and fetal growth and well-being, since prematurity, growth restriction, and perinatal mortality rates are high.[72,88,89] Because the risk of bowel

complications with omphalocele is low, since the bowel is usually protected and not free-floating in the amniotic cavity, most patients are expected to deliver at term unless non-reassuring antenatal testing dictates earlier delivery. With regard to the route of delivery, this continues to be controversial in fetuses identified with an omphalocele.[60,61] In an old study of 112 infants with abdominal wall defects where obstetric management took place without knowledge of the anomaly, vaginal delivery did not appear to adversely affect outcome, although visceral injury from the delivery procedure was suggested in one case.[90] More recent studies have shown that cesarean delivery is not associated with increased primary closure rates, decreased neonatal morbidity and mortality, or significantly increased incidence of visceral trauma.[91,92] Although no conclusive data are currently available showing that cesarean delivery is beneficial for fetuses with small omphaloceles,[60,93] it appears that elective cesarean delivery may be recommended for fetuses with giant omphaloceles (>5 cm), where there is a high risk of sac disruption and trauma to the abdominal viscera.[61,79]

Following delivery, postnatal evaluation is important to exclude genetic syndromes and associated anomalies that may not have been diagnosed in utero. Preoperative stabilization of the newborn is necessary to secure good oxygenation, and sterile wrapping of the omphalocele is required to prevent infection and minimize fluid losses (Figure 15.29), before attempting primary fascial closure, which has been the traditional approach to omphalocele. However, in the case of a giant omphalocele (Figure 15.30) with a narrow abdominal ring and an extracorporeal liver, extra care

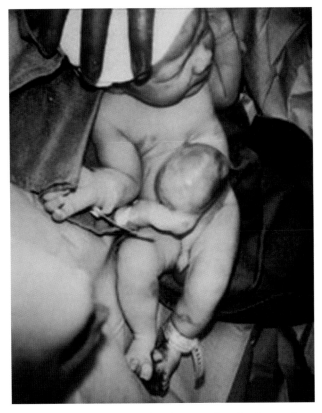

Figure 15.29 Omphalocele. Photograph at birth correlates with prenatal findings seen in Figure 15.19. Note the thick umbilical cord covered inserting into the base of the defect

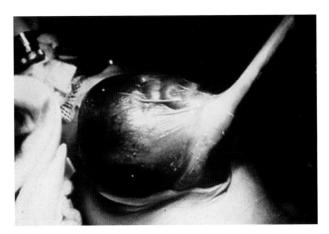

Figure 15.30 Photograph at surgery of a giant omphalocele. Note the large abdominal wall defect and the contents of the omphalocele sac with bowel loops showing through the transparent surrounding membrane. This defect required staged closure

should be taken to avoid overmobilization of the liver, which may injure the hepatic vessels and result in a high risk of liver infarction.[79] Similarly, primary closure of large omphaloceles with increased intra-

abdominal pressure may not be possible, and staged closure with gradual reduction of the viscera into the abdomen over a few days using a silastic pouch is recommended to avoid bowel necrosis and hepatic dysfunction.[94] In a recent case series from the National Center for Fetal Medicine in Norway of 90 fetuses with an omphalocele followed from the time of prenatal diagnosis to birth and into the postnatal period, the rate of primary closure was 60%, with an overall survival rate of 21%.[81]

PENTALOGY OF CANTRELL

Pentalogy of Cantrell is an association of distal sternal cleft, supraumbilical omphalocele, diaphragmatic hernia, defect of the apical pericardium, and congenital intracardiac defects. There was a uniformly fatal outcome in a series of 10 cases diagnosed prenatally, with 2 found to have trisomy 18.[95] Prenatal diagnosis has been reported using both conventional and 3D sonography, and it seems that the complexity of the intracardiac anomaly is the best predictor of neonatal mortality.[96] A recent case report noted the association of the pentalogy with craniorachischisis and alerted sonographers to the fact that open cranial and spinal defects can coexist with this already complex malformation.[97] Again, the value of 3D sonography lies in better visualization of the malformation by experienced sonographers (Figure 15.31), allowing more comprehensive counseling of expectant parents so that they can make an informed decision regarding pregnancy continuation or interruption if the diagnosis is made prior to viability.

ECTOPIA CORDIS

Ectopia cordis is defined as an anomaly in which the fetal heart lies outside the thoracic cavity (Figure 15.32). This condition is very rare, with an incidence of less than 1 in 100 000. Its etiology remains obscure, with a suggestion of mechanical teratogenesis following rupture of the chorion or yolk sac during early embryogenesis, which might interfere with cardiac descent.[98] Associated anomalies seen in a series of eight fetuses diagnosed with ectopia cordis in the 2nd trimester included omphalocele, cardiovascular malformations, and craniofacial and limb defects.[99] The prognosis is generally poor, even in exceptional survivors who have undergone neonatal repair.[100,101] Prenatal diagnosis of

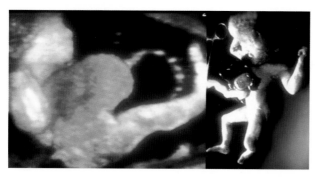

Figure 15.31 Cantrell pentalogy. This fetus shows an abdominal and thoracic herniation with the heart inside of the tumor

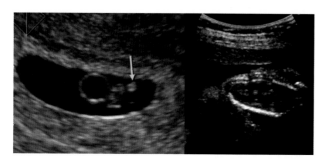

Figure 15.32 Ectopia cordis. On the left side a 9th week pregnancy 2D transvaginal ultrasound. Showing (arrow) the heart beating in the amniotic fluid. On the right side a second trimester ultrasound of the same case showing the heart in the amniotic fluid

ectopia cordis has been reported in the 1st trimester at 11 and 12 weeks, using both transabdominal and transvaginal 2D sonography, coupled with the use of color Doppler.[102,103] Liang et al[104] reported the earliest prenatal diagnosis of ectopia cordis, at 10 weeks of gestation, with 3D sonography clearly showing in a reconstructed image of the fetus a solid mass protruding from the ventral wall, which was confirmed by histopathologic examination at autopsy demonstrating a thoracoabdominal ectopia cordis. The authors emphasized that 3D reconstructed images provided a complete view of the anomaly prenatally, although this was not essential to establish the diagnosis.

LIMB–BODY WALL COMPLEX

Limb–body wall complex (LBWC) is generally characterized by the presence of at least two of the following three abnormalities: (i) meningomyelocele and/or caudal regression; (ii) thoraco- and/or abdominoschisis; and (iii) limb defects.[105] The condition is uniformly

lethal – hence, early and accurate prenatal diagnosis is essential. Prenatal diagnosis has been reported in the 1st trimester as early as 10 weeks with both conventional[106,107] and 3D sonography.[108,109] Chen et al,[108] after suspecting the diagnosis from 2D sonography at 17 weeks of gestation in a 24-year-old primigravida being evaluated for an elevated MSAFP level of 11.45 MOM, demonstrated the anatomic features with a complete view using 3D sonography. Sonographic findings included abdominoschisis, displacement of the heart, sheets of amnion attached broadly to the fetus and the placenta, limb defects, scoliosis, and absence of a normal umbilical cord. 3D sonography enhanced the visualization of the complex malformation in utero, and color power angiography helped the reconstruction of the aberrant umbilical vasculature around the connecting stalk. Similarly, Liu et al[109] emphasized the value of 3D sonography in the survey of LBWC since it can detect almost all of the defects simultaneously, making the diagnosis much more precise than with conventional 2D sonography. In addition, the use of the surface-rendering mode of 3D sonography in illustrating LBWC assisted markedly in genetic counseling and helped the expectant parents comprehend the malformation much better than 2D sonography could do.

REFERENCES

1. Stoll C, Alembik Y, Dott B, et al. Risk factors in congenital abdominal wall defects (omphalocele and gastroschisis): a study in a series of 265,858 consecutive births. Ann Genet 2001; 44: 201–8.

2. Hoyme HE, Higginbottom MC, Jones KL. The vascular pathogenesis of gastroschisis: intrauterine interruption of the omphalomesenteric artery. J Pediatr 1981; 98: 228–31.

3. deVries PA. The pathogenesis of gastroschisis and omphalocele. J Pediatr Surg 1980; 15: 245–51.

4. Torfs CP, Velie EM, Oechsli FW, et al. A population-based study of gastroschisis: demographic, pregnancy, and lifestyle risk factors. Teratology 1994; 50: 44–53.

5. Morrison JJ, Chitty LS, Peebles D, et al. Recreational drugs and fetal gastroschisis: maternal hair analysis in the peri-conceptional period and during pregnancy. Br J Obstet Gynaecol 2005; 112: 1022–5.

6. Haddow JE, Palomaki GE, Holman MS. Young maternal age and smoking during pregnancy as risk factors for gastroschisis. Teratology 1993; 47: 397–403.

7. Martinez-Frias ML, Rodriguez-Pinilla E, Prieto L. Prenatal exposure to salicylates and gastroschisis: a case-control study. Teratology 1997; 56: 241–3.

8. Torfs CP, Katz EA, Bateson TF, et al. Maternal medications and environmental exposures as risk factors for gastroschisis. Teratology 1996; 54: 84–92.

9. Torfs CP, Curry CJR. Familial cases of gastroschisis in a population-based registry. Am J Med Genet 1993; 45: 465–7.

10. Snelling CM, Davies GA. Isolated gastroschisis in successive siblings: a case report and review of the literature. J Obstet Gynaecol Can 2004; 26: 591–3.

11. Lindfors KK, McGahan JP, Walter JP. AJR Am J Roentgenol 1986; 147: 797–800.

12. Brantberg A, Blaas HG, Salvesen KA, et al. Surveillance and outcome of fetuses with gastroschisis. Ultrasound Obstet Gynecol 2004; 23: 4–13.

13. Barisic I, Clementi M, Hausler M, et al. Evaluation of prenatal ultrasound diagnosis of fetal abdominal wall defects by 19 European registries. Ultrasound Obstet Gynecol 2000; 18: 309–16.

14. Garne E, Loane M, Dolk H, et al. Prenatal diagnosis of severe structural congenital malformations in Europe. Ultrasound Obstet Gynecol 2005; 25: 6–11.

15. Nicolaides KH, Snijders RJM, Cheng HH, et al. Fetal gastrointestinal and abdominal wall defects: associated malformations and chromosomal abnormalities. Fetal Diagn Ther 1992; 7: 102–15.

16. Pinzon M, Barr RG. Extracorporeal liver and spleen in gastroschisis. AJR Am J Roentgenol 1995; 164: 1025.

17. Blakelock RT, Upadhyay V, Pease PW, et al. Are babies with gastroschisis small for gestational age? Pediatr Surg Int 1997; 12: 580–2.

18. Raynor BD, Richards D. Growth retardation in fetuses with gastroschisis. J Ultrasound Med 1997; 16: 13–16.

19. Japaraj RP, Hockey R, Chan FY. Gastroschisis: can prenatal sonography predict neonatal outcome? Ultrasound Obstet Gynecol 2003; 21: 329–33.

20. Adair CD, Rosnes J, Frye AH, et al. The role of antepartum surveillance in the management of gastroschisis. Int J Gynaecol Obstet 1996; 52: 141–4.

21. Haberman S, Burgess T, Klass L, et al. Acute bowel perforation in a fetus with gastroschisis. Ultrasound Obstet Gynecol 2000; 15: 542–4.

22. Barsoom MJ, Prabulos A, Rodis JF, et al. Vanishing gastroschisis and short-bowel syndrome. Obstet Gynecol 2000; 96: 818–19.

23. Crawford RAF, Ryan G, Wright VM, et al. The importance of serial biophysical assessment of fetal well-being in gastroschisis. Br J Obstet Gynaecol 1992; 99: 899–902.

24. Luton D, Guibourdenche J, Vuillard E, et al. Prenatal management of gastroschisis: the place of the amnioexchange procedure. Clin Perinatol 2003; 30: 551–72.

25. Salvensen KA. Fetal abdominal wall defects – easy to diagnose – and then what? Ultrasound Obstet Gynecol 2001; 18: 301–4.

26. Gibbin C, Touch S, Broth RE, et al. Abdominal wall defects and congenital heart disease. Ultrasound Obstet Gynecol 2003; 21: 334–7.

27. Novotny A, Klein RJ, Boeckman CR. Gastroschisis: an 18–year review. J Pediatr Surg 1993; 28: 650–2.

28. Saxena AK, Hulskamp G, Schleef J, et al. Gastroschisis: a 15–year, single-center experience. Pediatr Surg Int 2002; 18: 420–4.

29. Luck SR, Sherman J, Raffensperger JG, et al. Gastroschisis in 106 consecutive newborn infants. Surgery 1985; 98: 677–83.

30. Mabogunje OOA, Mahour GH. Omphalocele and gastroschisis: trends in survival across two decades. Am J Surg 1984; 148: 679–86.

31. Ikhena SE, de Chazal RC, Konje JC. Gastroschisis associated with bladder evisceration complicated by hydronephrosis presenting antenatally. Ultrasound Obstet Gynecol 1999; 13: 370–2.

32. Langer JC, Khanna J, Caco C, et al. Prenatal diagnosis of gastroschisis: development of objective sonographic criteria for predicting outcome. Obstet Gynecol 1993; 81: 53–6.

33. Pryde PG, Bardicef M, Treadwell MC, et al. Gastroschisis: Can antenatal ultrasound predict infant outcomes? Obstet Gynecol 1994; 84: 505–10.

34. Adra AM, Landy HJ, Nahmias J, et al. The fetus with gastroschisis: impact of route of delivery and prenatal ultrasonography. Am J Obstet Gynecol 1996; 174: 540–6.

35. Alsulyman OM, Monteiro H, Ouzounian JG, et al. Clinical significance of prenatal ultrasonographic intestinal dilatation in fetuses with gastroschisis. Am J Obstet Gynecol 1996; 175: 982–4.

36. Aina-Mumuney AJ, Fischer AC, Blakemore KJ, et al. A dilated fetal stomach predicts a complicated postnatal course in cases of prenatally diagnosed gastroschisis. Am J Obstet Gynecol 2004; 190: 1326–30.

37. Lenke RR, Persutte WH, Nemes J. Ultrasonographic assessment of intestinal damage in fetuses with gastroschisis: Is it of clinical value? Am J Obstet Gynecol 1990; 163: 995–8.

38. Babcook CJ, Hedrick MH, Goldstein RB, et al. Gastroschisis: Can sonography of the fetal bowel accurately predict postnatal outcome? J Ultrasound Med 1994; 13: 701–6.

39. Brun M, Grignon A, Guibaud L, et al. Gastroschisis: Are prenatal ultrasonographic findings useful for assessing the prognosis? Pediatr Radiol 1996; 26: 723–6.

40. McMahon MJ, Kuller JA, Chescheir NC. Prenatal ultrasonographic findings associated with short bowel syndrome in two fetuses with gastroschisis. Obstet Gynecol 1996; 88: 676–8.

41. Broth R, Sholssman P, Kaufmann M, et al. Increased incidence of stillbirth in fetuses with gastroschisis. Am J Obstet Gynecol 2001; 185: S246.

42. Robinson JN, Abuhamad AZ, Evans AT. Umbilical artery Doppler velocimetry waveform abnormality in fetal gastroschisis. Ultrasound Obstet Gynecol 1997; 10: 356–8.

43. Kalache KD, Bierlich A, Hammer H, et al. Is unexplained third trimester intrauterine death of fetuses with gastroschisis caused by umbilical cord compression due to acute extra-abdominal bowel dilatation? Prenat Diagn 2002; 22: 715–17.

44. Abuhamad AZ, Mari G, Cortina RM, et al. Superior mesenteric artery Doppler velocimetry and ultrasonographic assessment of fetal bowel in gastroschisis: a prospective longitudinal study. Am J Obstet Gynecol 1997; 176: 985–90.

45. Luton D, De Lagausie P, Guibourdenche J, et al. Prognostic factors of prenatally diagnosed gastroschisis. Fetal Diagn Ther 1997; 12: 7–14.

46. Luton D, de Lagausie P, Guibourdenche J, et al. Effect of amnioinfusion on the outcome of prenatally diagnosed gastroschisis. Fetal Diagn Ther 1999; 14: 152–5.

47. Sapin E, Mahieu D, Borgnon J, et al. Transabdominal amnioinfusion to avoid fetal demise and intestinal damage in fetuses with gastroschisis and severe oligohydramnios. J Pediatr Surg 2000; 35: 598–600.

48. Burc L, Volumenie JL, de Lagausie P, et al. Amniotic fluid inflammatory proteins and digestive compounds profile in fetuses with gastroschisis undergoing amnioexchange. Br J Obstet Gynaecol 2004; 111: 292–7.

49. Api A, Olguner M, Hakguder G, et al. Intestinal damage in gastroschisis correlates with the concentration of intraamniotic meconium. J Pediatr Surg 2001; 36: 1181–5.

50. Correia-Pinto J, Tavares ML, Baptista MJ, et al. Meconium dependence of bowel damage in gastroschisis. J Pediatr Surg 2002; 37: 31–5.

51. Bonilla-Musoles F, Machado LE, Bailao LA, et al. Abdominal wall defects: two- versus three-dimensional ultrasonographic diagnosis. J Ultrasound Med 2001; 20: 379–89.

52. Reid CO, Hall JG, Anderson C, et al. Association of amyoplasia with gastroschisis, bowel atresia, and defects of the muscular layer of the trunk. Am J Med Genet 1986; 24: 701–10.

53. Moir CR, Ramsey PS, Ogbrn PL, et al. A prospective trial of elective preterm delivery for fetal gastroschisis. Am J Perinatol 2004; 21: 289–94.

54. Huang J, Kurkchubasche AG, Carr SR, et al. Benefits of term delivery in infants with antenatally diagnosed gastroschisis. Obstet Gynecol 2002; 100: 695–9.

55. Burge DM, Ade-Ajayi N. Adverse outcome after prenatal diagnosis of gastroschisis: the role of fetal monitoring. J Pediatr Surg 1997; 32: 441–4.

56. Sakala EP, Erhard LN, White JJ. Elective cesarean section improves outcomes of neonates with gastroschisis. Am J Obstet Gynecol 1993; 169: 1050–3.

57. Rinehart BK, Terrone DA, Isler CM, et al. Modern obstetric management and outcome of infants with gastroschisis. Obstet Gynecol 1999; 94: 112–16.

58. How HY, Harris BJ, Pietrantoni M, et al. Is vaginal delivery preferable to elective cesarean delivery in fetuses with a known ventral wall defect? Am J Obstet Gynecol 2000; 182: 1527–34.

59. Strauss RA, Balu R, Kuller JA, et al. Gastroschisis: the effect of labor and ruptured membranes on neonatal outcome. Am J Obstet Gynecol 2003; 189: 1672–8.

60. Anteby EY, Yagel S. Route of delivery of fetuses with structural anomalies. Eur J Obstet Gynecol Reprod Biol 2003; 106: 5–9.

61. Segel SY, Marder SJ, Parry S, et al. Fetal abdominal wall defects and mode of delivery: a systematic review. Obstet Gynecol 2001; 98: 867–73.

62. Robilio D, Greve L, Towner D. Gastroschisis outcomes and site of delivery. Am J Obstet Gynecol 2001; 185: S244.

63. Kitchanan S, Patole SK, Muller R, et al. Neonatal outcome of gastroschisis and exomphalos: a 10-year review. J Paediatric Child Health 2000; 36: 428–30.

64. Kidd JN, Levy MS, Wagner CW. Staged reduction of gastroschisis: a simple method. Pediatr Surg Int 2001; 17: 242–4.

65. Schlatter M, Norris K, Uitvlugt N, et al. Improved outcomes in the treatment of gastroschisis using a preformed silo and delayed repair approach. J Pediatr Surg 2003; 38: 459–64.

66. Durfee SM, Downard CD, Benson CB, et al. Postnatal outcome of fetuses with the prenatal diagnosis of gastroschisis. J Ultrasound Med 2002; 21: 269–74.

67. Calzolari E, Bianchi F, Dolk H, et al. Omphalocele and gastroschisis in Europe: a survey of 3 million births 1980–1990. EUROCAT Working Group. Am J Med Genet 1995; 58: 187–94.

68. Botto LD, Mulinare J, Erickson JD. Occurrence of omphalocele in relation to maternal multivitamin use: a population-based study. Pediatrics 2002; 13: 620–1.

69. Ericson A, Kallen B. Congenital malformations in infants born after IVF: a population-based study. Hum Reprod 2001; 16: 504–9.

70. Pryde PG, Greb A, Isada NB, et al. Familial omphalocele: considerations in genetic counseling. Am J Med Genet 1992; 44: 624–7.

71. Lurie IW, Ilyina HG. Familial omphalocele and recurrence risk. Am J Med Genet 1992; 17: 541–3.

72. Hwang PJ, Koussef BG. Omphalocele and gastroschisis: an 18-year review study. Genet Med 2004; 6: 232–6.

73. Mann L, Ferguson-Smith MA, Desai M. Prenatal assessment of anterior abdominal wall defects and their prognosis. Prenat Diagn 1984; 4: 427–31.

74. Martin R. Screening for fetal abdominal wall defects. Obstet Gynecol Clin 1998; 24: 518–26.

75. Levine D, Callen PW, Goldstein RB, et al. Imaging the fetal abdomen: how efficacious are the AIUM/ACR guidelines? J Ultrasound Med 1995; 14: 335–41.

76. Benacerraf BR, Saltzman DH, Estroff JA, et al. Abnormal karyotype of fetuses with omphalocele: prediction based on omphalocele contents. Obstet Gynecol 1990; 75: 317–19.

77. De Veciana M, Major CA, Porto M. Prediction of an abnormal karyotype in fetuses with omphalocele. Prenat Diagn 1994; 14: 487–92.

78. Biard JM, Wilson RD, Johnson MP, et al. Prenatally diagnosed giant omphaloceles: short and long-term outcomes. Prenat Diagn 2004; 24: 434–9.

79. Pelizzo G, Maso G, Dell'Oste C, et al. Giant omphaloceles with a small abdominal defect: prenatal diagnosis and neonatal management. Ultrasound Obstet Gynecol 2005; 26: 786–8.

80. Blazer S, Zimmer EZ, Gover A, et al. Fetal omphalocele detected early in pregnancy: associated anomalies and outcomes. Radiology 2004; 232: 191–5.

81. Brantberg A, Blaas HGK, Haugen SE, et al. Characteristics and outcome of 90 cases of fetal omphalocele. Ultrasound Obstet Gynecol 2005; 26: 527–37.

82. Chen CP, Jan SW, Liu FF, et al. Prenatal diagnosis of omphalocele associated with umbilical cord cyst. Acta Obstet Gynecol Scand 1995; 74: 832–5.

83. Sepulveda W, Gutierrez J, Sanchez J, et al. Pseudocyst of the umbilical cord: prenatal sonographic appearance and clinical significance. Obstet Gynecol 1999; 93: 377–81.

84. Anandakumar C, Nuruddin Badruddin M, Chua MT, et al. First trimester prenatal diagnosis of omphalocele using three-dimensional ultrasonography. Ultrasound Obstet Gynecol 2002; 20: 635–7.

85. Chuang L, Chang CH, Yu CH, et al. Three-dimensional sonographic visualization of a fetal omphalocele at 14 weeks of gestation. Prenat Diagn 2000; 20: 517.

86. Snijders RJ, Brizot ML, Faria M, et al. Fetal exomphalos at 11 to 14 weeks of gestation. J Ultrasound Med 1995; 14: 569–74.

87. Snijders RJ, Sebire NJ, Souka A, et al. Fetal exomphalos and chromosomal defects: relationship to maternal age and gestation. Ultrasound Obstet Gynecol 1995; 6: 250–5.

88. Salomon LJ, Benachi A, Auber F, et al. Omphalocele: beyond the size issue. J Pediatr Surg 2002; 37: 1504–5.

89. Holland AJ, Ford WD, Linke RJ, et al. Influence of antenatal ultrasound on the management of fetal exomphalos. Fetal Diagn Ther 1999; 14: 223–8.

90. Kirk EP, Wah RM. Obstetric management of the fetus with omphalocele or gastroschisis: a review and report of one hundred twelve cases. Am J Obstet Gynecol 1983; 146: 512–18.

91. Sipes SL, Weiner CP, Sipes DR, et al. Gastroschisis and omphalocele: Does either antenatal diagnosis or route of delivery make a difference in perinatal outcome? Obstet Gynecol 1990; 76: 195–9.

92. Heider AI, Strauss RA, Kuller JA. Ophalocele: clinical outcomes in cases with normal karyotypes. Am J Obstet Gynecol 2004; 190: 135–41.

93. Lurie S, Sherman D, Bukovsky I. Omphalocele delivery enigma: the best mode of delivery still remains dubious. Eur J Obstet Gynecol Reprod Biol 1999; 82: 19–22.

94. Rizzo A, Davis PC, Hamm CR, et al. Intraoperative vesical pressure measurements as a guide in the closure of abdomina wall defects. Ann Surg 1996; 62: 192–6.

95. Ghidini A, Sirtori M, Romero R, et al. Prenatal diagnosis of pentalogy of Cantrell. J Ultrasound Med 1988; 7: 567–72.

96. Leon G, Chedraui P, San Miguel G. Prenatal diagnosis of Cantrell's pentalogy with conventional and three-dimensional sonography. J Matern Fetal Neonatal Med 2002; 12: 209–11.

97. Polat I, Gul A, Aslan H, et al. Prenatal diagnosis of pentalogy of Cantrell in three cases, two with craniorachischisis. J Clin Ultrasound 2005; 33: 308–11.

98. Kaplan LC, Matsuoka R, Gilbert EF, et al. Ectopia cordis and cleft sternum: evidence of mechanical teratogenesis following rupture of the chorion or yolk sac. Am J Med Genet 1985; 21: 187–99.

99. Klingensmith WC III, Cioffi-Ragan DT, Harvey DE. Diagnosis of ectopia cordis in the second trimester. J Clin Ultrasound 1988; 16: 204–6.

100. Knox L, Tuggle D, Knott-Craig CJ. Repair of congenital sternal clefts in adolescence and infancy. J Pediatr Surg 1994; 29: 1513–16.

101. Watterson KG, Wilkinson JL, Kliman L, et al. Complete thoracic ectopia cordis with double-outlet right ventricle: neonatal repair. Ann Thorac Surg 1992; 53: 146–7.

102. Sepulveda W, Weiner E, Bower S, et al. Ectopia cordis in a triploid fetus: first-trimester diagnosis using transvaginal color Doppler ultrasonography and chorionic villus sampling. J Clin Ultrasound 1994; 22: 573–5.

103. Bennett TL, Burlbaw J, Drake CK, et al. Diagnosis of ectopia cordis at 12 weeks gestation using transabdominal ultrasonography with color flow Doppler. J Ultrasound Med 1991; 10: 695–6.

104. Liang RI, Huang SE, Chang FM. Prenatal diagnosis of ectopia cordis at 10 weeks of gestation using two-dimensional and three-dimensional ultrasonography. Ultrasound Obstet Gynecol 1997; 10: 137–9.

105. Sanders RC. Structural Fetal Abnormalities: The Total Picture. St Louis, MO: Mosby. 1996.

106. Daskalakis G, Sebire NJ, Jurkovic D, et al. Body stalk anomaly at 10–14 weeks of gestation. Ultrasound Obstet Gynecol 1997; 10: 419–21.

107. Becker R, Runkel S, Entezami M. Prenatal diagnosis of body stalk anomaly at 9 weeks of gestation. Fetal Diagn Ther 2000; 15: 301–3.

108. Chen CP, Shih JC, Chan YJ. Prenatal diagnosis of limb–body wall complex using two- and three-dimensional ultrasound. Prenat Diagn 2000; 20: 1018–20.

109. Liu IF, Yu CH, Chang CH, et al. Prenatal diagnosis of limb–body wall complex in early pregnancy using three-dimensional ultrasound. Prenat Diagn 2003; 23: 513–14.

16 Urologic tract diseases: 2D versus 3D sonography and biochemical markers

Juan-Mario Troyano, Luis T Mercé, and Luis Martinez-Cortes

INTRODUCTION

Three-dimensional (3D) sonography is now being applied in the prenatal clinic for the investigation of the fetal kidney (Figure 16.1), and much work is currently being done to develop the technique further in this context. 3D reconstruction with power Doppler is very useful in examination of the vascularization of the kidney, the visualization of the spatial distribution of the renal vessels, and the determination of the presence of small vessels in the renal cortex (Figure 16.2). These observations can provide interesting signs of renal

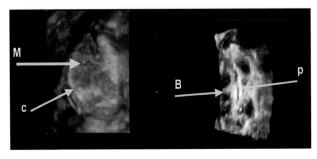

Figure 16.1 Normal kidney by 3D sonography. (M) Malpighi's pyramid; (B) Bertin's column; (c) limits of the renal capsule; (p) renal pelvis

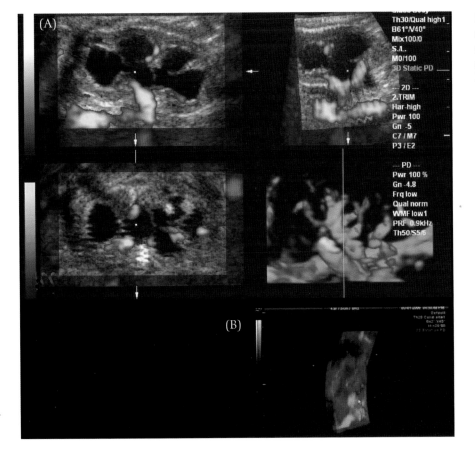

Figure 16.2 (A) Vessels in the renal cortex and renal vessels, associated with hydronephrosis – spatial distribution by 3D power Doppler. (B) Glassbody mode

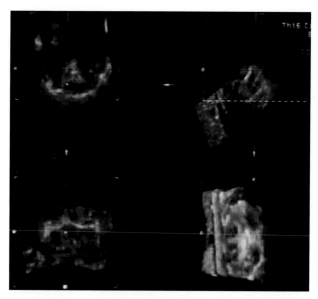

Figure 16.3 The multiplanar mode allows simultaneous observations of the *x*-, *y*-, and *z*-planes

obstruction, arterial stenosis, kidney infarction, venous thrombosis, and changes in the vascularization index (VI) in the presence of hemodynamic restriction in cases of intrauterine growth restriction (IUGR).

In addition, the use of multiplanar presentation allows observation of the *x*-, *y*-, and *z*-planes simultaneously, offering the picture of a virtual coronal scan that could not be obtained with conventional techniques. It is very useful in detecting solid or cystic tumor masses, as well as providing a detailed view of internal structure and the limits of the renal capsule (Figure 16.3).

Similarly, 3D sonography in the niche mode (Figure 16.4) can show longitudinal, transverse, and coronal cuts in the same image, providing an accurate exploration and a stereotactic view of the location and limits of a hydronephrosis or other kidney tissue pathology. It also allows the length and degree of any ureteral dilatation to be determined.

Volumetric reconstruction and the surface option are the only way of imaging the interior of a cystic injury, whether simple or tumoral (Figure 16.5).

It is important to take into account that, from the 2nd trimester of pregnancy, the scanning angle used to evaluate the fetal kidney cannot be greater than 35°–45° in transverse sections as well as in longitudinal sections.

NEPHROUROPATHIES: PRENATAL DIAGNOSIS AND ASSESSMENT

Nephrouropathies are among the main fetal diseases, amounting to 34% of all malformations detected at our research unit.[1] Of these, nearly 32% have shown isolated pathologies, 20% have been associated with other nephrourologic deseases, and 48% have resulted from tumor-related syndromes and chromosomal anomalies. Renal pathology in fetuses has been linked to a wide spectrum of non-nephrourologic diseases (Table 16.1), and its assessment, therefore, should always be addressed in terms of overall medical forecasting and therapeutic treatment.

When assessing the fetal kidney, a considerable degree of expertise is necessary regarding both how it works and the techniques to be employed in its sonographic imaging, given the need to obtain a diagnosis and implement therapeutic strategies during the early stages of fetal development (i.e., before the 20th week of gestation), whenever possible.

To start with, prenatal diagnosis of nephrouropathies (like that of cardiopathies) is handicapped by the fact that there is no high-risk population target in which to seek out renal desease. However, dilatation of excretory channels, whether obstructive or not, occurs in 87% of cases showing renal malfunction, so that basic sonographic experience should normally lead to chance diagnoses of renal abnormalities. It follows

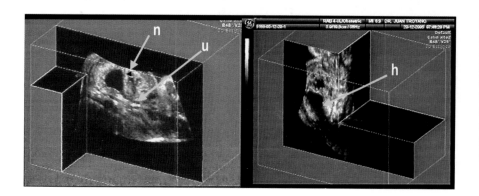

Figure 16.4 The niche mode can provide an accurate exploration and a stereotactic view of the location and limits of a hydronephrosis or other kidney pathology (h). It can also allow determination of the length of a ureteral dilatation or stenosis (u) and monitoring of a kidney biopsy (n)

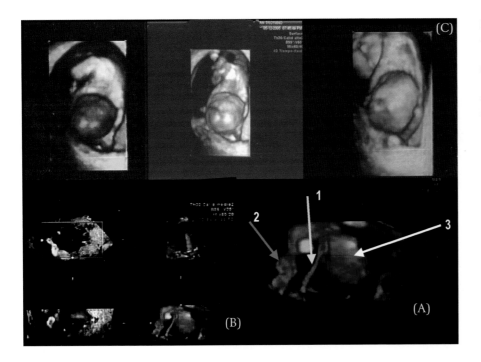

Figure 16.5 (A) (1) Hypogastric artery stenosis in megabladder; (2) umbilical cord; (3) bladder surface in prune belly syndrome. (B) Multiplanar scan. (C) 3D surface mode in a different deep scan

Table 16.1 Nephrourologic malformations

Ureter-hydronephrosis complex with megaureter
Vesicoureteral ebb
Unblocked megaureter
Megaureter–megabladder syndrome
Prune belly syndrome
Neurogenic bladder
Ureteral atresia
Ureteral–vesical stenosis
Ureterocele:
  Stenotic
  Sphincteral
  Mixed
  Blind
  Double pyeloureteral systems
  With ureterocele
  Without ureterocele

Megaureter
Pyeloureteral stenosis
Megacaliosis
Smith–Lemli–Opitz syndrome
Schwartz–Jampel syndrome
Ivemark syndrome
Lawrence–Bardet–Biedl syndrome
Miranda syndrome

Associated with X chromosome
Ehlers–Danlos syndrome
Oro-facio-digital syndrome

Non-Mendelian heredity
Lowe syndrome
Beckwith syndrome
Goldenhar syndrome
Dandy–Walker syndrome

Metabolic disorders
Tyrosinemia
Galactosemia:
  Von Gierke syndrome

Chromosomal anomalies
Trisomy 13, 18, 21
Turner syndrome

Non-genetic conditions
Multicystic dysplasia
Pyelic duplicity
Malrotations
Ectopies

Cystic kidney
Genetic
Polycystic desease (autosomal recessive: chromosome 16)
Prenatal–neonatal type
Childhood type
Juvenile type
Polycystic type (autosomal dominant)
Postnatal
Juvenile nephroptisis
Cyst–dysmorphism

Mendelian heredity
Autosomal dominant
Tuberous sclerosis
Von Hippel–Lindau syndrome
Peutz–Jeghers syndrome
Autosomal recessive
Meckel syndrome
Jeune (thoracic asphyxiating dysplasia) syndrome
Zelleweger (cerebro–hepatic–renal) syndrome
Goldston syndrome
Simple cyst
Multilocular cyst
Acquired cystic renal disease
Spongiomedullar kidney
Calicial diverticulosis (pyelogenic cyst)

Morphologic and positional pathologies
Renal agenesis:
  Bilateral
  Unilateral
Renal hypoplasia
Renal ectopy
Horseshoe kidney
Further malformations

Infections
Rubella
Parvovirus B19

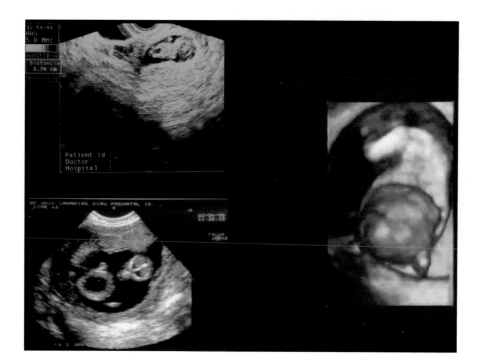

Figure 16.6 Ureteral obstruction resulting from prune belly syndrome with megabladder. The appearance of a vesicle on sonography before the 10th week of gestation is indicative of ureteral obstruction

that parenchymal disease without excretory dilatation occurs in only 13% of cases. As a guide, a transverse diameter of the excretory channels up to 0.5–0.8 cm by the 28th week of gestation and 0.8 cm by the end of gestation can both be regarded as normal.

It should be noted that any degree of dilatation of the excretory network is morphologically so obvious that further exploration will most often follow preliminary tests. For example, the discovery of a vesicle on sonography before the 10th week of gestation is indicative of ureteral obstruction, possibly resulting from a prune belly syndrome[2] (Figure 16.6). In contrast, under physiologic conditions, there will be an appearance of a vesicle because of the simultaneous production and excretion of fetal urine.

Thus, prenatal diagnosis of nephrourologic disease should be based upon a study of the parenchyma and the excretory tissues.

PATHOLOGY OF PARENCHYMAL SUBSTRATES

The most important problem in clinical diagnoses of prenatal nephrouropathies concerns those fetuses suffering from renal dysplasia.[3,4] This disease comprises the following (Figure 16.7):[2]

- islets in primordial tubules
- fibrous layers

- cartilaginous metaplasia
- fetal pathology (malformative or genetic).

The Potter classification concerning renal dysplasia defines a range of severity as follows:[3–8]

Type I cystic kidney:
- diffuse increase in cyst size
- branched collecting tubules
- tubular giantism–spongiform kidney
- infantile polycystic kidney disease (autosomal recessive).

Type II cystic kidney:
- irregular renal differentiation
- precocious induction of the renal blastema from the uteral primod of primitive ureter
- abnormal pan-nephrons (all nephrons) and collecting tubules
- slightly branched cysts
- non-hereditary external aggression.

Type III cystic kidney:
- obvious increase in cyst size
- various degrees of impact upon nephrons and collecting tubules
- undamaged concomita system
- non-hereditary: typical of newborn and breast-feeding children

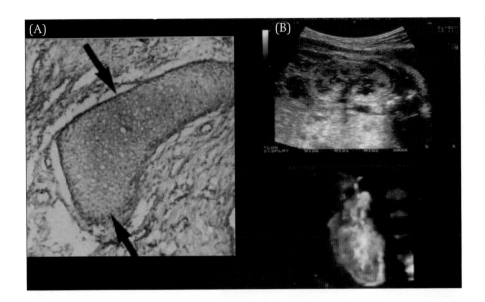

Figure 16.7 Renal dysplasia. (A) Islets in primordial tubules, fibrous layers, and cartilaginous metaplasia (arrows). (B) Corticomedullar dysplasia in 3D ultrasound, large surface option

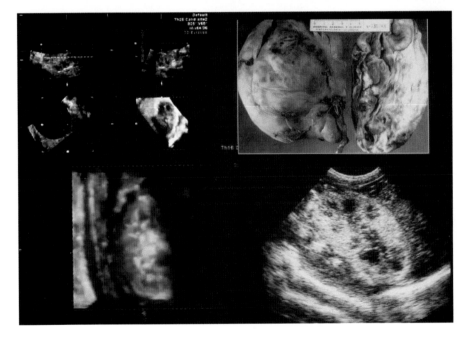

Figure 16.8 Renal dysplasia: renomegaly, capsular underdevelopment, loss of corticomedullar layers, and hyperechogenicity

- frequent association with chromosomal abnormality.

Type IV cystic kidney:
- cysts all subcapsular
- initial nephrogenesis normal (first cohorts of nephrons and tubules well developed and healthy)
- terminal portions of collecting tubules dilated, and nephronal development delayed (prune belly syndrome)
- ureteral obstruction
- vesical hypertrophia
- functionality of noxas delayed
- non-hereditary (in newborns).

Renal dysplasia: informative echographic records

It should be stressed that the complexity of the Potter classification factors may at times preclude straightforward prenatal assessment.[9–13] Thus, sonographic exploration can only detect renal dysplasia associated with parenchymal pathology in cases showing some of the following symptoms:

- renomegaly
- capsular underdevelopment
- loss of corticomedullar layers
- hyperechogenicity (Figure 16.8).

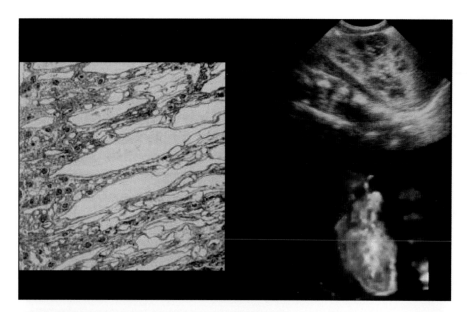

Figure 16.9 Multicystic dysplasia: corticomedullar cysts with patchy distribution

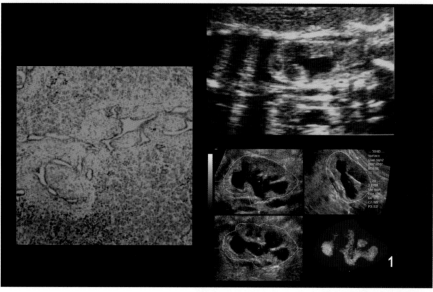

Figure 16.10 Dysplasia with pelvic dilatation: loss of corticomedullar layers and pathologic dilatation of the pelvis. (1) Inverse mode allows evaluation of the size of the hydronephrosis

Possible sonographic profiles resulting from renal dysplasia

Parenchymal pathologies can be of various forms according to the type of sonographic records sampled[1] (see below):

1. *Multicystic dysplasia (Potter type I)* (Figure 16.9):
   - increased echogenicity
   - loss of corticomedullar layers
   [a] corticomedullar cysts
2. *Dysplasia with pelvic dilatation (Potter type II)* (Figure 16.10):
   - loss of corticomedullar layers
   - undefined capsules
   - pathologic dilatation of the pelvis

3. *Severe dysplasia (Potter type III)* (Figure 16.11):
   - loss of corticomedullar layers
   - pelvic dilatation: moderate, precocious, and persistent
   - reversal of the nephroabdominal index (renomegaly)
   - oligohydramnion
4. *Dysplasia associated with dysmorphism (Potter type IV)* (Figure 16.12):
   - hydronephrosis
   - megaureter
   - atrophy of rectoabdominal muscles
   - cryptorchidism
   - vesical hypertrophy
   - megabladder
   - oligohydramnion.

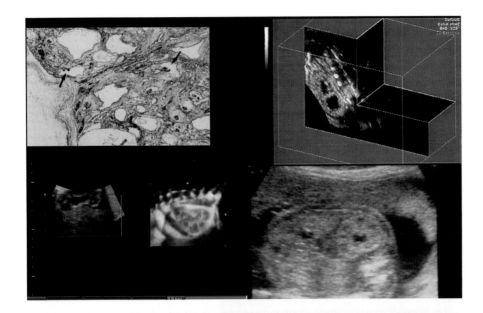

Figure 16.11 Severe dysplasia: pelvic dilatation is moderate, precocious, and persistent, with associated renomegaly. The size of the hydronephrosis can be determined in the niche mode

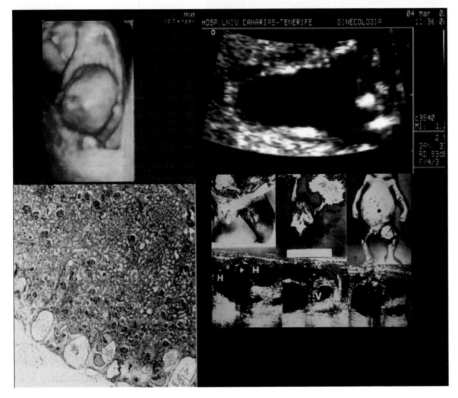

Figure 16.12 Dysplasia associated with dysmorphism: mega-ureter, hydronephrosis, bladder hypertrophy, megabladder, and oligohidramnion are frequent

Renal dysplasia can be also assessed in terms of the size and spread of the areas affected:[11]

- Bilateral agenesis (genuine Potter syndrome)
  - incidence 1/5000
  - lethal
  - pulmonary hypoplasia
  - precocious anhidramnion (by the 12th week of gestation)
- Unilateral agenesis:
  - 1/2000
  - no vital effects
- Hypoplasia
  - simple
  - oligomeganephron
  - segmentary (delayed impact on the child's health).

Finally, the study of renal dysplasia can be also undertaken in cystic pathologies by considering the morphology of the cyst:[5,13]

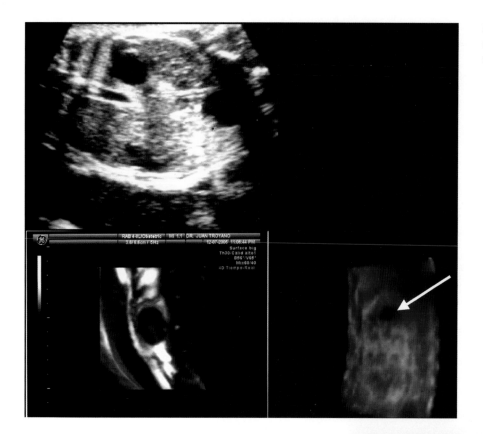

Figure 16.13 Simple cyst: the cyst body is isolated, with associated renal parenchyma (arrow)

- Simple cyst (Figure 16.13):
  - isolated cyst body
  - healthy renal parenchyma
  - cysts sometimes multilocular
- Multicystic (uni- or bilateral types)[8] (Figure 16.14):
  - most frequent
  - renomegaly
  - cysts merge with one another
  - variable size
  - walls thickened
  - associations include low obstructive pathology; pyeloureteral stenosis; posterior valves; ureteral atresia
- Polycystic:
  - renomegaly
  - loss of cortical structure of renal tissues
  - irregular cysts, of variable size
  - patchy distribution
  - hyperechogenicity.[5,7,13]

Initially, multicystic dysplasia does not necessarily entail renal malfunction. Thus, urine clearance and diuresis remain functional throughout the first two-thirds of postnatal life, as some quantity of renal parenchyma remains healthy between the fine-walled cystic layers.[9] On the contrary, the polycystic type

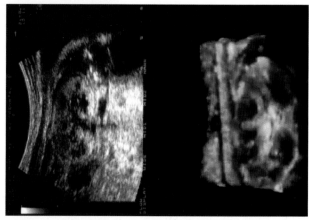

Figure 16.14 Multicystic kidney: the cysts merge with one another, with variable size and thickened walls

displays early functional alterations, even during the prenatal period.

DILATION OF EXCRETORY CONDUCTS: PATHOLOGY OF THE EXCRETORY SUBSTRATE

The renal pelvis has a cavity 5 mm in diameter by the 28th week of gestation. Renal blockages at the pyeloureteral level, or below, may trigger an initial

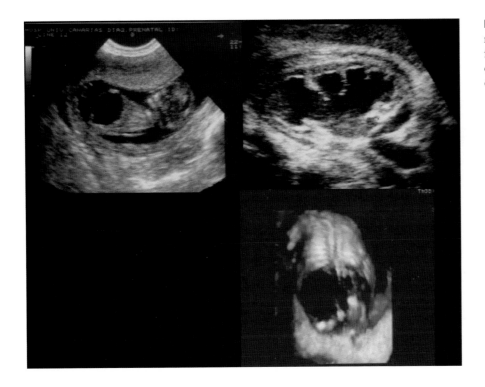

Figure 16.15 Severe hydronephrosis: in severely affected fetuses, the size of the renal pelvis exceeds that of the abdominal cavity

urinary ectasia and subsequently drift to retrograde hypertension, which in turn may evolve in three different ways:

- persistent dilatation
- gradual increase in the size of the dilated area
- changes in renal morphology.

In these cases, sonography shows an eccentric lacunary area within the renal parenchyma, even though the resulting dilatation is in fact extra-renal in origin. The morphology of the lacunary area is either lenticular or spherical, with a diameter normally no larger that 0.8 mm.[14] In severely affected fetuses, the size of the pelvic dilatation may reach 4–7 cm, exceeding the size of the abdominal cavity and causing digestive upset and other kinds of extrarenal cystic processes (Figure 16.15).[14,15]

Caliceal dilatation[1]

When the renal pelvis is subjected to increasing hypertension, the dilatation may affect the whole or only a part of the caliceal network, normally the superior area.[15,16]

Light hydronephrosis may also have a severe impact on the calicial system, which translates into renal malfunction. However, severe pelvic dilatation may not affect the calices or the overall renal physiology.

The size of the caliceal area and the thickness of the renal parenchyma of the calices are both key factors in the medical assessment of hypertension-derived alterations. Caliceal size increases with the severity of the dilatation, this expansion even displacing or destroying the parenchymatous area.[15]

Some fetuses experience a combined process of dilatation of the superior caliceal area (>1 cm) and a moderate dilatation of the renal pelvis (>15 mm). In these cases, the obstructive situation worsens throughout the first year after birth, and surgery is frequently necessary[1] (Figure 16.16).

Cystic pathology can be ruled out from examination of the position and evolution of abnormal tissues and the external appearance of the pelvic area in dilatation diseases.

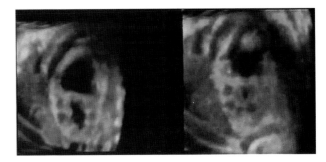

Figure 16.16 Dilatation of the superior caliceal area. An ectopic ureter is frequently associated

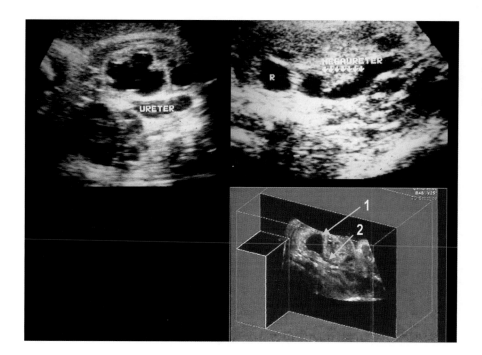

Figure 16.17 Ureteral dilatation and associated hydronephrosis. The 3D niche mode is adequate to evaluate this pathology: (1) hydronephrosis; (2) ureteral stenosis

Ureteral dilatation

Ureteral dilatation originates from obstructive processes in the ureter leading to increasing thickness of the prestenotic ureter. This is fairly obvious on exploration. The morphology of the dilated area varies according to its etiology.[1]

Static forms

- *Rectilinear:* there is a long lacunar area (cross-section >5 mm) on the renal pelvis, even reaching the bladder. This is an early condition leading to ureteral obstruction.
- *Winding:* the morphology is long and meandering, sometimes bent. It is often associated with pseudo-cystic sonographic images in the ureter between kidney and bladder. This is an advanced condition, with harmful effects on kidney function.
- *Lacunar:* there is a cystic lacuna filling most of the abdominal cavity of the fetus, even beyond the vertebral spine. There are similarities with other obstructive phenomena and extrarenal cysts, precluding easy differential diagnosis.
- *Sacular:* there are one or more cystic lacunae between the kidney and bladder (diverticula). It is infrequent, but when present is commonly associated with excretory deseases such as ureteral agenesis. Assessment is often precluded when overall renal function remains normal (Figure 16.17).

Dynamic forms

Changes in the pattern of pathologic stress induce changes manifested in the morphology of the ureter in two ways:

- *Episodic:* this is characteristic of pathologies such as vesico-ureteral reflux, but may possibly be confused with physiologic behavior and premicturitional dynamics. It is frequently associated with a moderately dilated renal pelvis.
- *Peristaltic:* the ureter is dilated, sometimes cylindrical, showing peristaltic waves from pelvis to bladder. Efficiency is low since the ureteral thickness varies considerably over pregnancy. It is frequently associated with initial phases of prestenotic megaureter.

As mentioned above, dilatation pathologies affecting excretory tissues are particularly harmful to the welfare of the fetus, because they may alter the whole renal system to the extent of causing severe or irreversible damage.

PATHOLOGY OF THE RENAL PARENCHYMA

Morbid processes involving some degree of dilatation of the excretory network may sometimes result in shrinkage of the renal parenchyma. Thus, both ectasia

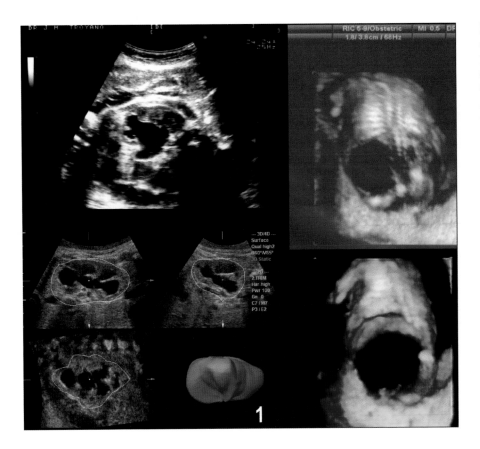

Figure 16.18 Extreme shrinkage of the renal parenchyma. The parenchyma is not visible on 3D sonography. (1) The VOCAL mode allows evaluation of the gradual evolution and extreme dilatation of the renal pelvis and caliceal system

and flow pressure decrease and so upset the parenchymal structure, even leading to a dysplasia that impacts overall renal functionality, particularly in fetuses suffering from the syndrome of pyelocaliceal dilatation.[1,15]

These mechanisms of retrograde hypertension may lead to a number of different parenchymal states:

- *Shrinking parenchyma:* calices grow in size and the pelvic volume is increased. There is overlapping between the calices and pelvis. Tissue shrinkage is concentrated around the dilated calices.
- *Laminate parenchyma:* there is extreme shrinkage of the parenchyma as a result of hyperpressure (severe hydronephrosis). The parenchyma cannot be seen on sonography. There is gradual evolution to final stages showing extreme dilatation of the pelvis and caliceal system (Figure 16.18).

Apart from the above, alterations in renal function may follow other patterns that merit a separate description. Partial destruction of the renal parenchyma by compressive dilatation is an outstanding example, with a varying amount of healthy parenchyma, calices and pelvis remaining functional. There are two kinds of renal compressive dilatation:

superior and *inferior*. The former is the more frequent and severe, and presents the following morphologic features:

- round or cluttered cysts on the superior pole
- laminated parenchyma due to compression
- stable renal volume.

These phenomena usually derive from abnormalities such as ureteral duplication, such that changes in the drainage of the affected ureter lead to dilatation of the superior pole of the renal tissue. A vesical cyst (ureterocele) may often be observed accompanying these duplicate systems (ectopic ureter), which can be confused with tumors at the supra-renal level (Figure 16.19).

Etiologic factors

Dilatation pathologies can be classified on the basis of two phenomena:

1. *Pyeloureteral stenosis.* This is a primary hydronephrosis consisting of functional/anatomic collapse at the pyeloureteral level. It is frequently

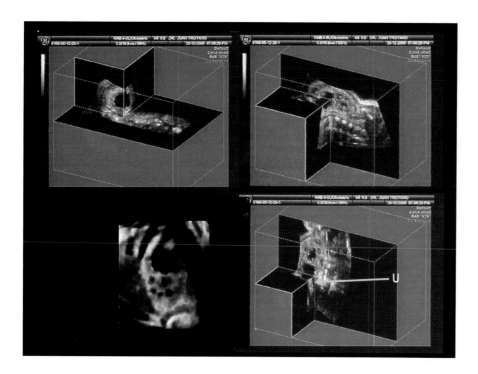

Figure 16.19 Niche mode sonography allows evaluation of two kinds of compressive renal dilatation: superior and inferior. Partial destruction of the renal parenchyma is caused by hyperpressure, with a varying amount of healthy parenchyma being present. Superior dilatations (the more frequent of the two types) present cysts around the superior pole, parenchymal shrinkage, and stable renal volume. (U) Ureteral stenosis

associated with extrarenal malformations (cloacal syndrome, and anal perforation), and even urogenital anomalies (hypospadias, renal malrotation, renal ectopy, etc.).[1]

2. *Ureteral alteration.* The pattern of the dilatation takes two forms:
   - Reflux dilatation:
     - primary (prune belly syndrome)[10]
     - secondary (ureteral duplication and megabladder)
   - Refluxless dilatation:
     - primary: obstructive (atresia, stenosis, and posterior valves) or non-obstructive
     - secondary (ectopia, ureterocele, vesical diverticula, and extrinsic compression).

It should be noted that sonographic detection of this kind of nephrourologic damage is more efficient when the dilatation of the ureter is very obvious and constant, and usually coincides with extreme retrograde dilatation processes. The size of the dilated area is in proportion to the degree of renal alteration.[14,15]

INTRAUTERINE TREATMENTS FOR OBSTRUCTIVE NEPHROUROPATHIES

Sonography can be very useful in assessing the complexities of prenatal nephrouropathies as a guide to possible therapy. The implementation of such therapy is not always easy, and, indeed, when treatment is technically feasible, it may not actually be necessary. Furthermore many patients are not eligible for intrauterine intervention, particularly in the case of severe or irreversible disease.[14-18] A very small group of affected fetuses are appropriate for prenatal therapy, neonatal treatment generally being called for (provided that the gestational age exceeds 32–34 weeks).

Renal obstructions do not necessarily trigger irreversible alteration of excretory functions. In this context, the amniotic volume can be employed as an indirect indicator of renal pathology. Normal values of the amniotic volume suggest maintained renal (excretory) function and normal physiologic pulmonary development. In contrast, severe excretory problems can be forecast in those cases with a high degree of oligohydramnion.[9,19]

Since intrauterine therapy should be used only for those fetuses suffering reversible damage to their kidneys,[15] careful selection of appropriate patients must be undertaken on the basis of fetal renal performance.[15,20,21] Irreversible damage results from renal dysplasia, the type and extent of the disease determining the degree of impact upon renal physiology. A number of tissue alterations coexist in dysplastic kidneys, namely fibrosis, cartilaginous dysplasia, and sometimes corticomedullar cysts. A total of 90% of dysplastic diseases are associated with obstructive problems – and this high percentage is enough to question the use of any treatment prior to birth.[15,22,23]

Table 16.2 Prenatal nephrouropathy: sonographic prediction

Indicator	Predictive power (%)	Tissue specificity (%)
Corticomedullar cysts	50	100
Hyperechogenicity	60	90
Hydronephrosis	35	70
Hydronephrosis + cysts	90	100

There is a 25–30% rate of false-negatives, i.e., obstructive uropathies displaying sonographical signals of normal tissue

Sonographic techniques are the main tools for the diagnosis of prenatal pathology. The resolving power of these techniques is reaching high standards, but must be developed further (Table 16.2).

Since dysplastic kidneys are not always detected sonographically, additional techniques are required in order to differentiate physiologic from pathologic conditions, and to forecast fetal obstructive uropathies that may be eligible for nephrostomy.[1,23–26] These alternative techniques should be tailored to the three kind of parameters described below.

Biometric parameters

These comprise the following (Figure 16.20):

- longitudinal renal diameter
- transverse renal diameter
- renal ellipse
- renal volume
- nephroabdominal index.

These parameters, taken together, complement the assessment of renal function, with a close relationship with gestational chronology.[20] Throughout gestation, there is a steady increase in all of the biometric parameters, with the scores being highest for longitudinal diameter and renal volume. The transverse diameter, however, stops growing by the 34th week of gestation.[20] The nephroabdominal index starts to increase from the 22th week of gestation. The rate of increase is higher for the abdomen than for the kidney up to the 22nd week of gestation, being equal from then onwards. Changes in this index are a good indicator of renomegaly and micro-renomegaly.

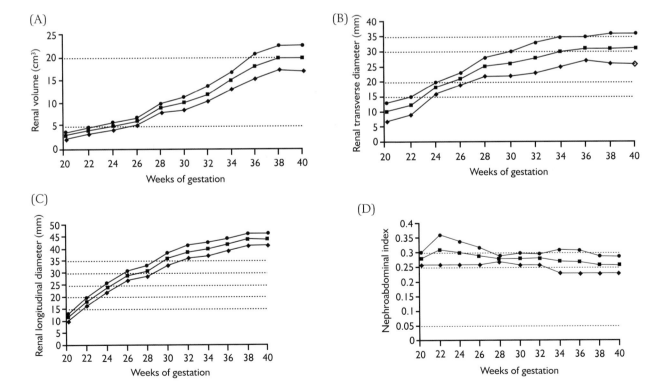

Figure 16.20 Biometric parameters: (A) renal volume; (B) renal transverse diameter; (C) renal longitudinal diameter; (D) nephroabdominal index

Week	cm³
24	9.0
26	9.0
28	9.6
30	10.2
32	11.0
34	11.8
36	12.6
38	13.0

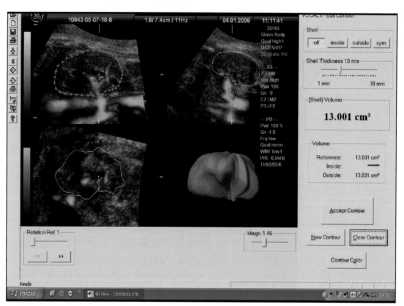

Figure 16.21 Determination of the mean volume of the kidney using the outside 'shell mode' under physiologic conditions

From the present point of view, renal volume measurement offers important advantages for biometric evaluation, since it gives accurate data about the true dimension, and it will probably allow detection of cases of hypoplasia and renomegaly.

Using the outside 'shell mode', performing 9 rotation steps on the kidney surface, the normal mean volume of the kidney lies between 9 cm³ in the 24th week and 13 cm³ in the 38th week (Figure 16.21).

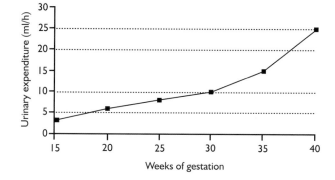

Figure 16.22 Fetal micturitational dynamics

Dynamic parameters

These comprise the following:

- urinary expenditure (micturitional dynamics) (Figure 16.22)
- Doppler velocimetry (Figure 16.23).

Some relative predictive power can be gained by assessing micturitional dynamics (diuresis).[9]

From the 2nd through the 3rd trimesters of gestation, active diuresis occurs at 25–30-minute intervals, while the micturitional volume per unit time increases with gestational age. *Clearance*, the most important intrinsic renal factor, is not clinically quantified when assessing urinary expenditure rates, so that micturitional dynamics, although informative, have a low predictive power in neophrourologic diagnoses. In this context, paradoxical cases of polyuria have been found, possibly resulting from a breakdown in the reabsorptive dynamics of the proximal tubules.[24,27,28]

Moreover, amniotic volume and fetal diuresis give complementary diagnostic information (i.e., the fetus is able to urinate).[29]

Velocimetry patterns of renal vessels can also be very useful in the assessment of renal functionality, particularly in IUGR, oligohydramnion, some malformative pathologies (mainly cardiopathies involving circulatory failure in the left ventricle), and hemodynamic responses to drugs (e.g., cardiotonics and prostaglandins).

For instance, the *resistance index* (*RI*) and the *pulsatility index* (*PI*) decrease with gestational age under physiologic conditions. This trend is due to the centrifugal nephrogenic development, which peaks in the 34th week of gestation when the fetus has already attained considerable functional maturity.[1,30,31]

Plasma flow normally amounts to 5% of the total cardiac expenditure of the fetus. It increases gradually

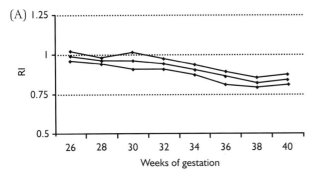

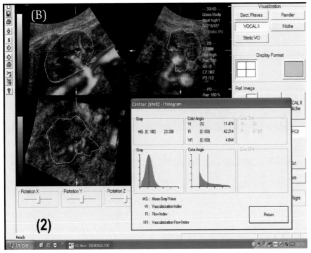

Figure 16.23 (A) Resistance index (RI) in the renal artery: the curve shows mean and 5th and 95th centiles. (B) The current status regarding fetal hemodynamic includes other parameters such us vascularization index (VI), flow index (FI), and vascularization flow index (VFI). These parameters represent the real 3D vascularization

with gestational age as the intrinsic vascular resistance decreases and the systemic resistance increases. Fetal nephrogenesis takes place from the 34th week of gestation onwards, the cortical flow being up to 12% of the cardiac expenditure by the end of pregnancy.

Hemodynamic records of renal flow from the middle third of the renal artery show a pattern of high systolic velocity and a lack of diastole for most of the gestational period. Diastolic flow can be first detected from the 34th week of gestation, as a consequence of the decrease in intraparenchymal resistance and of nephrogenic maturity. Interestingly, if birth occurs prior to the 34th week of gestation, the fetal kidneys continue to mature, achieving total functionality.[1]

Overlapping artery–vein images are not uncommon in velocimetry studies, but can be prevented by avoiding truncal movements of the fetus, and ensuring that the angle of measurement from the longitudinal axis of the renal artery is equal to or less than 40°.

IUGR-associated chronic hypoxia is normally associated with increased sympathetic tone, which subsequently leads to overall flow redistribution, noted as an increase in cerebral flow and a decrease in peripherical circulation.[1]

Vyas et al[32] applied funiculocentesis and a Doppler device to assess renal hypoxemia. Their results showed that the PI was significantly larger in pathologic than in physiologic cases, and was positively correlated with the levels of hypoxemia. Furthermore, increased PI values were recorded in cases of associated oligohydramnion.

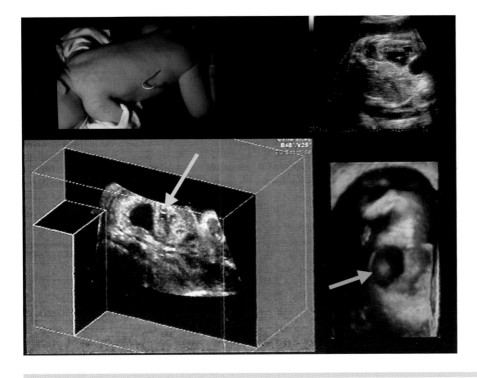

Figure 16.24 Aspirative nephrostomy with 4D sonographic monitoring and Niche mode (arrows), increasing the safety and efficiency of the puncture, and reducing the duration

Hemodynamic profiles encompassing cerebral and renal flows can be used to explore the severity of renal hypoxemia under the following guidelines:

- Cerebral PI *decreased* and renal PI *increased* → hypoxemia.
- Cerebral PI *normal* and renal PI *decreased* → physiologic renal condition.
- Cerebral PI *normal* and renal PI *increased* → renal disfunction.

Renal flows and glomerular filtration are regulated by prostaglandin E_2 (PGE_2) and $PGF_{2\alpha}$. Increases in the concentration of both of these modulators maintain physiologic renal flows (this has been observed in fetal urine samples obtained by intrauterine puncture).

PGE_2 acts as an antagonist to vasopressin in the proximal tubules, slowing down reabsorption of water and solutes. Moreover, severe parenchymal damage leads to a marked increase in vascular resistance.

This pattern is not general to all kinds of obstructive pathology. Thus, it has been suggested that extraparenchymal hemodynamic adaptations may play a role in slowing down vascular resistance and glomerular adaptation (Bowman's capsule and valves involving afferent and efferent arteries).

We have obtained a number of remarkable results with sonography of the middle third of the renal artery (between the aortic anastomosis and the parenchymal area) in situations of truncal stability and no overlapping venous images:[30,31]

- RI values decrease from the 32nd week of gestation owing to total centrifugal nephrogenesis.
- This hemodynamic trend correlates positively with the RI for both the medium cerebral artery (from the 22nd week of gestation) and the umbilical artery.
- There are significant differences in RI between the two renal arteries, its value being smaller in the right kidney, possibly under the influence of neighboring splanchnic vessels.
- The systole/diastole ratio in cases of IUGR associated with oligohydramnion is far lower than in cases of IUGR associated with euamniotic fetuses, the ratio in the latter being similar to that of a healthy fetus. The combination of IUGR and oligohydramnion is likely linked with renal hypoperfusion mechanisms and is indicative of corticomedullar hemodynamic failure in the context of visceral centralization.

- The arterial RI in severe hydronephrosis (dilatation >3 cm) is larger (although statistically not significantly) than that in mild hydronephrosis for fetuses suffering from nephrourologic disorders (hydronephrosis and/or corticomedullar dysplasia).
- There are significant differences in RI between severely hydronephrotic fetuses and those with healthy kidneys.
- The RI is significantly larger in cases of corticomedullar dysplasia associated with oligohydramnion than in healthy cases.

To sum up, renal perfusion constraints follow an increasing trend from healthy kidneys, through cases of hydronephrosis (even severe), to dysplastic kidneys (particularly in association with oligohydramnion). Even so, physiologic levels of both perfusion and diuresis are possible providing the corticomedullar system stays at least partly functional.[31]

Given the complexity existing in the vascular network of the fetus, however, it might still be asserted that, in response to stress, some fetal viscera experience important hemodynamic restrictions that favor and ensure the irrigation of essential tissues, such as myocardium, suprarenal tissues, and brain. It is known that reductions in renal perfusion result from situations of fetal distress and lead to typical oligohydramnios, often associated with IUGR.

Two main functions can be attributed to the vascular system of the kidneys: nourishment of the renal parenchyma and production and clearance of urine.

The complexity of renal vascularization patterns is in contrast to observations that, first, hemodynamic responses to stimuli are fairly variable, and, second, kidney function is regulated by up to five mechanisms:

- the sympathetic nervous system
- the arginine–vasopressin system
- levels of angiotensin
- levels of prostacyclin (PGI_2)
- heart blood reserve.

In response to chronic stress, the fetus is able to minimize water losses by reducing its diuretic effort. This is not a subsidiary event but a prime mechanism that governs the systemic perfusion of the fetus and, in particular, the perfusion of the renal parenchyma in situations of blood centralization.

In assessing renal hemodynamics, two principal factors must be taken into account. On the one hand, glomerular filtration is dependent on a number of parameters, including hydrostatic filtration, oncotic pressure, capillary permeability, and the total area of capillary glomerular tissue.

On the other hand, total renal flow is dependent on cardiac blood stores, the vascular tone of the renal interstitia, glomerular resistance, and tubular reabsorption.

Biochemical parameters

Biochemical parameters are the cornerstone of clinical assessment of fetal kidney function.

Fetal urine originates from ultrafiltration of fetal serum and is characteristically hypotonic owing to active reabsorption of sodium and chloride from the proximal area. This condition prevails throughout gestation and can aid in clinical predictions of function. In contrast, hypotonic or isotonic fetal urine is indicative of irreversible pathology in the proximal tubules.[1]

Unlike sodium and chloride, the fetal clearance of potassium and creatinine has very little clinical predictive value, because it overlaps with placental clearance and also because of the continuous changes in ionic charge of potassium over the course of pregnancy and because of the low potassium concentration in fetal blood due to insulin-mediated modulation. Therefore, potassium filtration and absorption levels are low and patchy in fetal kidneys.[33]

The reference threshold for the fetal kidney to be considered functionally operative should be at sodium <100 mmol/l, chloride <90 mmol/l, and osmolarity <200–210 mosmol/l, whereas potassium and creatinine concentrations have been shown to be indistinguishable for both pathologic and healthy groups.

Intrauterine monitoring of fetal urine is the best technique for assessing renal clearance.[1,33,34]

Aspirative puncture techniques are easy to implement by means of standard 18–20 gauge spinal needles in urinary exploration protocols. Two different methodologic approaches are possible, depending on the fetal posture. Dorsoposterior postures are best for vesical punctures, whereas aspirative nephrostomy is particularly suitable for dorsal anterior or lateral postures (Figure 16.24). As can be seen from sonographic monitoring of both techniques, nephrostomy-derived hematurias are rare (<4% of interventions), generally because of the ability and expertise of the practicioner.[33–36]

Even though 2D sonography remains irreplaceable in both obsteric and gynecologic punction techniques, 3D/4D sonography (in real time) is becoming a complementary procedure, increasing the safety and efficiency of the puncture, helping the 3D identification of the critical point puncture and consequently reducing the duration of the technique. In the future, this will be the way for invasive techniques within this speciality.

Sampling cylinders of 2 mm suffice to detect dysplastic disease. Nevertheless, technically feasible, renal byopsies are constrained by sampling efficiency. Satisfactory samples can be collected in 65% of attempts through 16-gauge needles, but in only 38% of attempts through 18-gauge needles.[35,36]

On the other hand, aspirative nephrostomy has a number of advantages in that it guarantees collection of urine samples, reassessment of dilated parenchyma, and parenchymal biopsies – always in a safe manner.[36]

Moreover, a number of biochemical indicators of tubuloproximal pathologies can be obtained from urine samples. They are all lysosomal proteins featuring two specific properties: either they are easily filtered and reabsorbed (e.g. β_2-microglobulin, β_2-M) or they are specific elements of tubular tissues (e.g. N-acetyl-D-glucosaminidase, NAG). Both groups are of low molecular weight and appear in large quantities in fetal urine and amniotic fluid.[34,36]

Our team has carried out a total of 93 urinary aspirations. In 82% of the punctures, nephrouropathies were associated with probable hydronephrosis. Medium- and long-term neonatal data are not yet available, so in the following we will present results from the first 38 punctures that have been undertaken.

Nephrourologic punctures were carried out from the 18th week of gestation and beyond the 32nd week. Out of the 38 aspirations, healthy and pathologic status were recorded in 25 and 13 cases, respectively (Table 16.3). The concentration of biochemical indicators is always markedly lower in physiologic cases than in irreversible pathologic cases. β_2-M and NAG behave in the same way over time[36] (Tables 16.4 and 16.5). There are no significant differences between healthy and pathologic fetuses in terms of ionic concentration (sodium and chloride) and osmolarity in both fetal urine and amniotic fluid. In contrast, the concentrations of NAG and β_2-M are significantly larger in the amniotic fluid of nephropathologic fetuses than in that of healthy fetuses (Tables 16.6 and 16.7).

Table 16.3 Punctures for nephrourologic aspiration: frequency distribution by gestational age

	Weeks of gestation		
	18–20	20–30	>32
Physiologic	6	16	3
Pathologic	2	9	2

Table 16.4 Concentrations of biochemical indicators from urine under physiologic conditions by nephrourologic aspiration

	Weeks of gestation		
	18–20	20–30	>32
Na$^+$ (mmol/l)	42±1.7	42±1.7	47±3.0
Cl$^-$ (mmol/l)	23±2.0	41±2.6	41±2.0
Osmolarity (mosmol/l)	96±1.2	102±1.6	102±2.1
NAG (units/l)	2.0±1.0	2.7±1.2	2.0±0.9
β$_2$-M (mg/l)	4.7±1.4	5.1±1.0	5.3±1.0

NAG, N-acetyl-D-glucosaminidase; β$_2$-M, β$_2$-microglobulin

Table 16.5 Concentrations of biochemical indicators from urine under pathologic conditions by nephrourologic aspiration

	Weeks of gestation		
	18–20	20–30	>32
Na$^+$ (mmol/l)	120.0	126.44±11.50	139.60
Cl$^-$ (mmol/l)	119.0	132.50±7.18	141.00
Osmolarity (mosmol/l)	240.0	261.50±7.18	281.00
NAG (units/l)	18.0	25.83±0.85	25.73
β$_2$-M (mg/l)	26.0	38.97±1.30	38.72
K$^+$ (mmol/l)	3.1	3.41±0.66	3.90
Creatinine (mg/l)	1.2	2.54±0.83	3.70

NAG, N-acetyl-D-glucosaminidase; β$_2$-M, β$_2$-microglobulin

It is our view that any increase in the concentration of lysosomal markers may well be caused by a concomitant increase in the volume of urinary excretion and also by a cumulative effect building up from the process of amniotic clearance. Lysosomal clinical techniques avoid physical invasion of the fetal kidneys, but further research is required before these can be routinely applied in the therapy of fetal nephrouropathy.

Concentrations of both potassium and creatinine have shown little predictive power due to the placental clearance effect and to continuous shifts in the ionic charge of potassium throughout gestation (along-

Table 16.6 Physiologic concentrations of biochemical indicators sampled from both urine and amniotic fluid (urinary value/amniotic fluid value)

	Weeks of gestation		
	18–20	20–30	>32
Na$^+$ (mmol/l)	42/37	42/140	47/140
Cl$^-$ (mmol/l)	23/109	47/109	41/108
Osmolarity (mosmol/l)	98/287	102/273	102/271
NAG (units/l)	2.0/3.6	2.7/3.62	2.0/4.69
β$_2$-M (mg/l)	4.7/4.5	5.1/5.0	5.3/5.8
K$^+$ (mmol/l)		41/140	
Creatinine (mg/l)		1.9/0.6	

NAG, N-acetyl-D-glucosaminidase; β$_2$-M, β$_2$-microglobulin

Table 16.7 Pathologic concentrations of biochemical indicators sampled from both urine and amniotic fluid (urinary value/amniotic fluid value)

	Weeks of gestation		
	18–20	20–30	>32
Na$^+$ (mmol/l)	120/132	126.4/140	139.6/140
Cl$^-$ (mmol/l)	119/107	132.5/149	141/158
Osmolarity (mosmol/l)	240/267	261.5/273	281/296
NAG (units/l)	18/16.9	25.8/20.3	25.73/20.8
β$_2$-M (mg/l)	26/22.3	38.9/28.7	38.72/30.0
K$^+$ (mmol/l)	3.1/138	3.4/140.6	3.9/148
Creatinine (mg/l)	1.2/0.7	2.54/0.82	3.7/0.9

NAG, N-acetyl-D-glucosaminidase; β$_2$-M, β$_2$-microglobulin

Table 16.8 Fetal urine: assessment of the nephrourologic status of the fetus at any gestational age by means of biochemical markers, sonography and quantification of amniotic volume

Prediction	Poor prognosis	Good prognosis
Sonography	Hyperechogenicity +cysts	Normal
Amniotic volume	Oligohydramnion	Normal
Fetal urine		
Na$^+$ (mmol/l)	>100	<100
Cl$^-$ (mmol/l)	>90	<90
Osmolarity (mosmol/l)	>210	<210
NAG (units/l)	>8	<8
β$_2$-M (mg/l)	>7	<7
K$^+$	Negligible	Negligible
Creatinine	Negligible	Negligible

side concomitant changes in glomerular filtration capacity and the low concentration of potassium in peripheral blood).

Nephrourologic assessment scores are summarized in Table 16.8.[36]

FURTHER ASPECTS RELATED TO KIDNEY FUNCTIONALITY

Diuresis

Administration of furosemide to the mother does not elicit diuretic responses in stressed fetuses, as shown by quantitative analysis of vesical storage velocity. In stressed neonates and IUGR cases, this pattern may be caused by an increase in the concentration of antidiuretic hormone, leading to water savings and maintainance of plasma volume.

Other hormones such as aldosterone and cortisol may play a role in the latter mechanism, since they mediate any increase in urinary flow and excretion rates of chloride, sodium, and potassium. This modulation is basically fetally based, not occurring in the adult kidney unless a high dosage is applied.

Losses of fetal sodium trigger polyhydramnion typical of chlorothiazide-treated mothers. Fetal hyponatremia could then account for polyhydramnion in cases of dilatation of the urinary system. Fetuses displaying losses of sodium experience a reduced capability for tubular absorption of water (polyuria), while fetal losses of water lead to natriuria.[1]

Both polyuria and polyhydramnion are indicators of heavy and irreversible tubulopathies (particularly in the proximal area).

Renal glomerular filtration (RGF)

Effective renal glomerular filtration occurs from 10–12 weeks of gestation onwards, the ranges being 0.32–0.24 ml/min up to the 24–26 weeks, 1.60–1.46 ml/min up to 32–34 weeks, and 4.67–1.72 ml/min up to 38–40 weeks.

It has been suggested that failure of placental activity in neonates leads to a physiologic adaptation involving IUGR. Such a pattern should be characteristic of neonates born after the 34th week of gestation, by which time the perfomance of an IUGR fetus is weak and stable. The process of nephrogenesis ends any time from the latter gestational age onwards, entailing a build-up of centrifugal (arterial) flows, which in turn enhance the maturation of cortical nephrons (the last nephrons to reach maturity).[1]

Tubular dynamics of sodium and chloride

A number of interesting results have been obtained from experimental animals subjected to saline overloading in their venous system. By dosing sodium chloride at 5–15 mmol/kg of animal weight in 30 minutes, and subsequently collecting the excreted urine over a 2-hour period, it was observed that less than 10% of the administered sodium chloride stayed within the intracellular space for longer than 5 minutes.[37]

Constraints on fetal excretion of saline excesses in the venous system are very obvious (with reabsorption rates of sodium and chloride from proximal tubules of >60%), but are not indicative of the actual fetal capacity for physiologic excretion.

Increases in glomerular filtration due to aqueous diuresis (i.e., administration of furosemide to the mother) bring about a decrease in proximal reabsorption of sodium, chloride, bicarbonate, calcium, phosphate, glucose, uric acid and β_2-M. The magnitudes of these changes can shift according to saline levels in both the fetus and the mother, the type of drugs employed, and the degree of fetal stress.[1]

Tubular dynamics of potassium

Plasma concentrations of potassium remain within a rather constant range throughout gestation and are modulated by two factors:

- the overall body content of potassium acting upon the external balance
- intra- and extracellular distribution of potassium acting upon the internal balance.

A total of 98% of fetal potassium load is found inside fetal cells (intracellular). Restricted potassium excretion takes place before the 35th week of gestation, while the overall potassium concentration is positively correlated with gestational time. The modulatory network is aided by insulin, which controls the entrance of potassium into the intracellular space, even when the concentration of aldosterone decreases.

Increases in the potassium concentration in fetal blood occur in situations of hyperkalemia, namely those resulting from renal failure, indomethacin administration, congenital renal hyperplasia involving saline losses, pseudohyperaldosteronism, obstructive uropathies, fetal renal thrombosis, and IUGR.

Tubular dynamics of calcium

Healthy fetuses can be considered to be in a condition of relative hypercalcemia combined with hypoparathyroidism counteracting the excess of calcium. Calcium concentrations are further enhanced by metabolic acidosis and increases in the fraction of ionic calcium.

Braun and Steranka[38] showed that excretion rates of urinary calcium are positively correlated with concentration and excretion rates of sodium, and negatively correlated with degree of calcemia. Furthermore, Goldsmith et al[37] showed that intravenous inputs of calcium triggered increases in the volume of urinary excretion, while furosemide led to a status of hypercalciuria (as a result of sodium excretion) and decreased reabsorption of calcium.

The degree of calcemia is reduced by the end of gestation compared with prenatal/neonatal maturity. This results in release of parathyroid hormone (PTH), which in turn activates the synthesis of vitamin D and digestive absorption of calcium from the intestines.

Calcium dynamics mirror those of sodium. In contrast, however, the reabsorption of calcium is greater than that of sodium in the pars recta of the proximal tubules, while the reverse pattern can be observed in the distal tubules.

Tubular dynamics of phosphorus

Reabsorption rates of phosphorus also vary with gestational time as shown in Table 16.9.

Phosphorus dynamics are opposite to those of calcium in that reabsorption rates increase towards the end of gestation. Phosphate savings seem to be directly related to PTH levels, as suggested by Mulroney et al.[39]

Tubular dynamics of uric acid

Uric acid dynamics are dependent on the extracellular volume present in the fetus. The uric acid concentration is normally in the range 7.7 ± 2.7 mg/dl (average) in immature fetuses and 5.2 ± 1.6 mg/dl in mature fetuses. Thus, uricosuria levels are lowest at early gestational ages, so that the release of uric acid increases towards the end of pregnancy.[1]

Table 16.9 Reabsorption of phosphorus

Reabsorption (%)	Week of gestation
85	28
93	34
98	40

Acid–base balance

Urine pH increases with gestational age, while net acid excretion decreases even in situations of metabolic acidosis. The threshold of bicarbonate excretion ranges between 14 and 18 mmol/l in preterminus fetuses, whereas it is around 20 mmol/l in terminus fetuses. Net acid excretion and plasmatic bicarbonate concentration levels are positively correlated with gestational age.

Tubular dynamics of glucose

The presence of physiologic concentrations of glucose (glucosuria) is a characteristic feature of the preterminus fetus. Furthermore, urine excretion volume is enhanced by physiologic increases in extracellular volume, whereas glucose tubular reabsorption decreases towards the end of gestation.

Tuvad[40] has shown that immature filtering capacity in the glomerulus results in decreased levels of tubular reabsorption, as well as transport of glucose.

Urinary concentration capacity

The capacity of the kidney for concentrating urinary fluid is modulated by three factors, all of which trigger decreased urine concentration responses. These factors are vasopressin (present from the 26th week of gestation), PGE_2 (acting upon the collecting tubules), and a weak corticomedullar gradient of both urea and sodium (resulting from a very short loop of Henle, underdevelopment of the chlorine pump causing low excretion rates of urea, and increased medullar blood flows).

Urine concentration mechanisms involve reabsorption of water from the collecting tubules, which becomes more permeable under vasopressin modulation, and are dependent on the occurrence and intensity of a corticomedullar osmotic gradient (which originates from the accumulation of urinary products in the medular interstitia in two ways: passive for urea and active for solutes such as chlorine and sodium).

Ine contrast, urinary dilution mechanisms (synthesis of free water) result from active reabsorption of chlorine and sodium in the descending loops and the proximal tubules, without vasopressin modulation.[1]

SUMMARY

Since only 25% of cases with renal dysplasia are detected sonographically, the biochemical assessment of fetal urine content represents a complementary tool for diagnosing and forecasting fetal nephrouropathy of any kind.

We are beginning a new era of investigation of fetal solid organs in general, and the anatomy and function of the kidney in particular, using 3D/4D sonography. There are several directions of research in this field, and the near future will see definitive outcomes.[41–43]

REFERENCES

1. Troyano JM, De la Fuente P. Prenatal Features of Fetal Kidney Physiopathology and Their Intra- and Extrauterine Treatment. A Multidisciplinary Problem. Santa Cruz de Tenerife: University Hospital of the Canary Islands, 1993: 35–9.

2. Alvarez-Argüelles F, Marín A, Domenech E, et al. Características clínico-patológicas del riñón quístico tipo II de Potter con especial referencia a las anomalías del desarrollo asociadas. Morfol Norm Patol Secc B 1981; 5: 117.

3. Ashey AC, Mostofy FK. Renal agenesis and dysgenesis. J Urol 1960; 82: 211.

4. Baxter TJ. Polycystic kidney of infants and children: morphology, distribution and relation of cysts. Nephron 1965; 10: 15–31.

5. Bernstein J. A classification of renal cysts. In: Gardner KD, Bernstein J, eds. The Cystic Kidney. Dordrecht, The Netherlands: Kluwer, 1990: 147–1.

6. Mottet NK, Jensen H. The anomalus embryonic development associated with trisomy 13–16. Am Clin Pathol 1965; 43: 334.

7. Potter EL. Normal and Abnormal Development of the Kidney. Chicago, IL: Year Book Medical, 1972.

8. Risdon RA. Renal dysplasia: 1. A clinicopathological study of 76 cases; 2. A necropsy study of 41 cases. J Clin Pathol 1971; 24: 57–65.

9. Campbell S, Wladimiroff JW, Dewhurst CJ. The antenatal measurement of foetal urine production. Br J Obstet Gynaecol 1973; 80: 680–5.

10. Christopher CR, Spinelli A, Servet D. Ultrasonic diagnosis of prune belly syndrome. Obstet Gynaecol 1982; 59: 391–4.

11. Dubbins PA, Kurtz AB, Wapner RJ, Goldberg BB. Renal agenesis: spectrum of in utero findings. J Clin Ultrasound 1981; 9: 189–93.

12. Fadel HE, Martin S. Realtime sonographic diagnosis of fetal dysplasic kidney. J Gynaecol Obstet 1980; 18: 140–3.

13. Friedberg JE, Mitnick JS, Davis DA. Antepartum ultrasonic detection of multicystic kidney. Radiology 1979; 131: 131–8.

14. Glick PL, Harrison MR, Golbus MS. Management of the fetus with congenital hydronephrosis. II. Prognostic criteria and selection for treatment. J Pediatr Surg 1985; 20: 376.

15. Golbus MS, Harrison MR, Filly RA. Prenatal diagnosis and treatment of fetal hydronephrosis. Semin Perinatol 1983; 7: 102.

16. Harrison MR, Anderson J, Rosen MS. Fetal surgery in the primate. I: Anesthesic, surgical and tocolytic management to maximize fetal–neonatal survival. J Pediatr Surg 1882; 17: 115.

17. Harrison MR, Golbus MS, Filly RA. Fetal surgical treatment. Pediatr Ann 1982; 11: 88–96.

18. Harrison MR, Golbus MS, Filly RA: Management of the fetus with a correctable defect. JAMA 1981; 246: 774.

19. Henderson SC, Van Kolken RJ, Rahatzad M. Multicystic kidney hydramnios. J Clin Ultrasound 1980; 8: 249–50.

20. Jeanty P, Dramaix-Wilment M, Elkazen N, Hibinot C, Van Regemorter GV. Measurement of fetal kidney growth on ultrasound. Radiology 1982; 144: 159–62.

21. Kurjak A, Kirkinen P, Latin V, Ivankovic D. Ultrasound assessment of fetal kidney function in normal and complicated pregnancies. Am J Obstet Gynecol 1981; 141: 266–70.

22. Mahoney BS, Filly RA, Callen PW, et al. Fetal renal dysplasia: sonographic evaluation. Radiology 1984; 152: 143–6.

23. Pedicelli G, Jequier S, Bowen A, Boisvert J. Multicystic dysplastic kidneys: spontaneous regression demostrated with ultrasound. Radiology 1986; 160: 23–6.

24. Smythe AR. Ultrasonic detection of fetal ascites and bladder dilation with resulting prune belly. J Pediatr 1981; 98: 978–80.

25. Stuck KJ, Koff SA, Silver TM. Ultrasonic features of multicystic dysplastic kidney: expanded diagnostic criteria. Radiology 1982; 143: 217–21.

26. Walzer A, Koenigsberg M. Prenatal evaluation of partial obstruction of the urinary tract. Radiology 1980; 135: 93–4.

27. Wladimiroff JW. Effect of furosemide on fetal urine production. Br J Obstet Gynaecol 1975; 82: 221–4.

28. Wladimiroff JW, Campbell S. Fetal urine production rates in normal and complicated pregnancy. Lancet 1974; i: 151–4.

29. Zerres K, Weiss F, Bulla M, Roth B. Prenatal diagnosis of an early manifestation of autosomal dominant adult-type polycystic kidney disease. Lancet 1982; ii: 988.

30. Troyano JM, Clavijo MT, Marco OY, et al. Velocimetry from renal vessels: techniques, results, assessment and interplay with other fetal vessels. 1: Techniques–results. Ultrasound Obstet Gynecol 1999; 14: 149.

31. Troyano JM, Clavijo MT, Marco OY, et al. Velocimetry patterns from the renal artery in a status of nephrological pathology. Ultrasound Obstet Gynecol 1999; 14: 151.

32. Vyas S, Nicolaides HK, Campbell S. Renal artery flow-velocity waveforms in normal and hypoxemic fetuses. Obstet Gynecol 1988; 6: 72–51.

33. Troyano JM, Padron E, Clavijo M. Fetal biopsy and puncture. Actual status. Balkan Ohrid's School of Ultrasound. In: Filipche DS, ed. Advanced Ultrasound II, Vol 9. OHRID (Macedonia Republic): 1996: 51–61.

34. Troyano JM, Clavijo M, Feo E, Laynez E, Gomez-Drieiro M. Paremeters of renal function by the obtention of fetal urine by intrauterine aspiration. Ultrasound Obstet Gynecol 2000; 16: 77.

35. Campbell WA, Yamase HT, Salafia CA, Vintzileos AM, Rodis JF. Fetal renal biopsy: technique development. Fetal Diagn Ther 1993; 8: 135–43.

36. Troyano JM. Fetal biopsy and puncture: actual status. In: Weiner S, Kurjak A, eds. Interventional Ultrasound. New York: Parthenon, 1999: 81–94.

37. Goldsmith MA, Bhatia SS, Kanto WP, Kutner MH, Rudman D. Gluconate calcium therapy and neonatal hypercalciuria. Am J Dis Child 1981; 135: 538–43.

38. Braun DR, Steranka BH. Renal cation excretion in the hypocalcemic premature human neonate. Pediatr Res 1981; 15: 1100.

39. Mulroney SE, Lumpking MD, Haramati A. Antagonist to growth hormone releasing factor inhibits growth and renal phosphate reabsortion in immature rats. Kidney Int 1988; 33: 344.

40. Tuvad F. Sugar reabsortion in prematures and full-term babies. Scand J Clin Lab Invest 1949; 1: 281.

41. Shields LE, Lowery C, Deforge C, Gustafson D. Technology and Early Clinical Experience with Real Time 3D Ultrasound. Electromedica, 1998; 66: No. 2.

42. Kurjak A, Kos M, Kalogjedra N. Three dimensional (3D) ultrasound in obstetrics. In: Kurjak A, Chervenak F (eds). Textbook of Ultrasound in Obstetrics and Gynecology. New Delhi: Jaypee Brothers, 2004: 462–79.

43. Bonilla-Musoles F, Machado LE, Raga F. Three dimensional visualization of fetal malformation. In: Kurjak A, Chervenak F, eds. Textbook of Ultrasound in Obstetrics and Gynecology. Oxford, UK: Taylor & Francis, 2004: 480–99.

17 Skeletal anomalies

Luiz Eduardo Machado, Fernando Bonilla-Musoles, and Newton Osborne

INTRODUCTION

Diagnosis of skeletal malformations using two-dimensional (2D) sonography is not always easy. Skeletal anomalies comprise a number of entities of low incidence (20 per 100 000 newborns). Half of these anomalies are lethal because of a narrow thorax with hypoplastic lungs. Lethal skeletal anomalies associated with hypoplastic lungs are responsible for 0.9% of all perinatal deaths.[1-3]

Thanatophoric dysplasia, the most common lethal osteochondrodysplasia has an estimated frequency of 5–6.9 cases per 100 000 newborns (i.e., one-fourth of all congenital skeletal anomalies are due to thanatophoric dysplasia). A recent study in Spain reported an incidence of achondroplasia of 2.53–2.70 cases per 100 000 newborns.

CLASSIFICATION OF SKELETAL DYSPLASIA

Skeletal dysplasia is frequently associated with limb malformations. Although they are usually divided into five different types, a universally accepted classification is still lacking, mainly because of a lack of uniformity in the criteria used for diagnosis. The types of skeletal dysplasia that are generally recognized are as follows:

- *Osteochondrodysplasia:* this involves alterations in the growth and development of bone and cartilage. The most frequent forms are osteogenesis imperfecta, achondroplasia, thanatophoric dysplasia, and achondrogenesis.
- *Dysostosis:* this refers to isolated malformations of single bones or combination of bones. Examples of this anomaly are craniosynostosis, craniofacial dysostosis or Crouzon's disease, mandibulofacial dysostosis, achiria, apodia, polydactyly, syndactyly, Poland syndrome, and brachydactyly.
- *Idiopathic osteolysis:* this is a disorder associated with multifocal bone resorption.
- *Skeletal disorders resulting from chromosomal defects:* these disorders may result either from de novo chromosomal mutations or from aneuploidy. In some cases, these disorders can result from dominant or recessive Mendelian inheritance.
- *Skeletal abnormalities resulting from primary metabolic disorders:* these include hypophosphatasia (i.e., osteogenesis imperfecta) in which severely demineralized bone secondary to congenital alkaline phosphatase deficiency leads to skeletal abnormalities that are incompatible with postnatal life.

THANATOPHORIC DYSPLASIA

Despite the reported low incidence of thanatophoric dysplasia, we have had the opportunity to examine nine cases of this malformation. In seven cases, polyhydramnion was present, improving the observation of the fetuses and allowing a more accurate diagnosis.

The typical cloverleaf-shaped skull image is usually seen in 14% of cases. This finding allows classification of thanatophoric dysplasia into two types. Type I, the most frequent, is characterized by:

- curved and short long bones
- a femur with the shape of an old-fashioned telephone receiver

- fibulas shorter than tibias
- platyspondylia resulting in mild kyphosis
- absence of a cloverleaf-shaped skull.

The narrow, short ribs along with flat vertebral bodies result in a short and narrow chest. The presence of midface hypoplasia, depressed nasal bridge, and a full forehead gives the appearance of a 'boxer's face'. Type II has in addition:

- a cloverleaf-shaped, trilobed skull, with
- straighter femurs and taller vertebral bodies than those seen in type I.

In both types, polyhydramnion is usually seen in the late 2nd and 3rd trimesters.

Without a family history of osteochondrodysplasia, or a 2D examination by an expert sonographer during the second half of pregnancy, these anomalies may be completely missed or may be erroneously diagnosed as intrauterine growth-restricted (IUGR) fetuses.

Because of the many types of skeletal malformations, definitive diagnosis of specific skeletal anomalies with 2D sonography can be difficult.

Sonographic diagnosis

At present, there are few references in the literature to skeletal dysplasia diagnosed prenatally with 3D sonography. Descriptions of phocomelia, thrombocytopenia with absent radius, platyspondylia, anomalies of the ribs, and Takayasu's disease, have been published.

The use of 3D transparency/X-ray mode allows visualization of the spine and thorax, evaluation of the curvature of the ribs, the observation of the vertebrae, medullar canal, clavicles, and scapulae, and completes the study with visualization of the form, angulations, and length of the long bones.[4-23]

In our experience, the best time to obtain good-quality 2D and 3D images is between weeks 18 and 32 of gestation, selecting an amniotic fluid sonic window that allows excellent 2D and 3D sagittal and frontal views of the fetus.

A presumptive sonographic diagnosis is based on the following (Figure 17.1):

- There is megacephaly with cloverleaf-shaped skull and progressive hydrocephaly.
- There is a hypoplastic thorax that is disproportionately small in relation to the abdomen (a bell-shaped thorax in the form of a 'champagne cork').
- The ribs and bones of the extremities are short and curved. Femurs often have a 'telephone receiver' shape.
- Excess skin confers a 'boxer's face' aspect.
- Flattened vertebrae with diminished intervertebral space give the vertebral body the form of an 'H' and enhancing the short and narrow appearance of the thorax.
- Polyhydramnion is present in most cases.

All of these characteristics can be observed, with greater or lesser frequency, using 2D sonography (Table 17.1).

Comments

Thanatophoric dysplasia is the most common of the lethal osteochondrodysplasias, and all newborns with this condition die during the first hours of life.

Prenatal diagnosis using the polymerase chain reaction (PCR) to analyze DNA from amniotic fluid

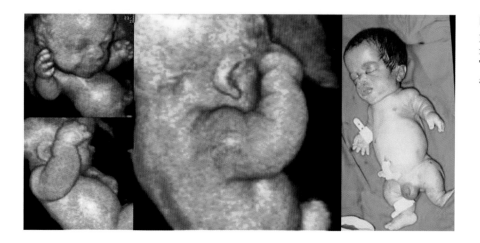

Figure 17.1 Thanatophoric dysplasia. Detail of hands, facies, nose, ears, and cloverleaf skull. The thorax is short and the abdomen is prominent

Table 17.1 Classical sonographic findings (2D or 3D) in thanatophoric dysplasia

Ultrasound findings	Frequency
Generalized micromelia	Always present
Small 'champagne cork' chest	Always present
Short or very short thorax	Always present
Prominent abdomen	Always present
Macrocephaly	High
Cloverleaf skull	Moderate
Frontal bossing	Moderate
Brachycephaly	Low
Depressed nasal bridge	Always present
Omphalocele	Very low
Bicuspid aortic valve	Very low
Atrial septal defect or single atrium	Very low
Short and/or thick ribs	High
Short femurs	Always present
Curved extremities	Always present
'Telephone receiver' femurs	Low
Angulations and deformities of long bones	High
Platyspondyly	Middle
Trident hand	Low
Excessive skin folds and edema	High
Polyhydramnios	High
'Boxer's face'	High

cells suggests that there is a mutation in the gene encoding fibroblast growth factor receptor 3 (*FGFR3*).

Although an autosomal recessive transmission has been suggested, the etiology of this disorder, which has an estimated recurrence rate of 2%, is likely to be multifactorial.

ACHONDROPLASIA

This is an autosomal dominant disorder related to a defect in the short arm of chromosome 4 that can be homozygous (always lethal) or heterozygous (mostly live newborns).

The diagnosis is made on the basis of family history (although most cases are due to de novo mutations) and by the following sonographic markers:

- There are short extremities – mainly rhizomelia. The femoral length is usually in the 50th percentile at 18 weeks, in the 30th percentile at 20 weeks, and below the 5th percentile at 22 weeks. The humerus is short by 22 weeks, and the other long bones display a moderate shortening.
- There is a long and narrow thorax and lumbar lordosis.
- The head is enlarged with frontal swelling (attention should be paid to the ratio of biparietal diameter to thoracic diameter). Sometimes, megalencephaly is observed through a disproportion between the base of the skull and the vault. For that reason, these cases can also present with hydrocephaly.

Joint hyperextension, especially of the knee, is also commonly observed.

OSTEOGENESIS IMPERFECTA TYPE II

This is an autosomal recessive disorder characterized by diffuse hypomineralization. It is distinguished by:

- shortening, angulations, curving, or multiple fractures of the long bones
- increased osseous transparency without posterior sonic shadow
- a demineralized and thin skull
- multiple fractures and costal fractures.

The combination of 2D and 3D sonography is ideal for providing diagnostic accuracy in this dysplasia. 2D sonography allows a better visualization and measurement of the long bones and internal organs, while 3D sonography provides more realistic surface visualization (Figures 17.2 and 17.3).

Figure 17.2 Osteogenesis imperfecta, lethal type II

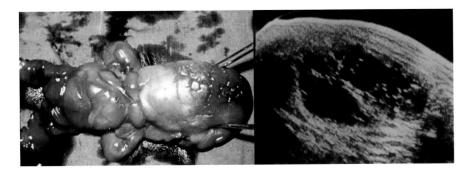

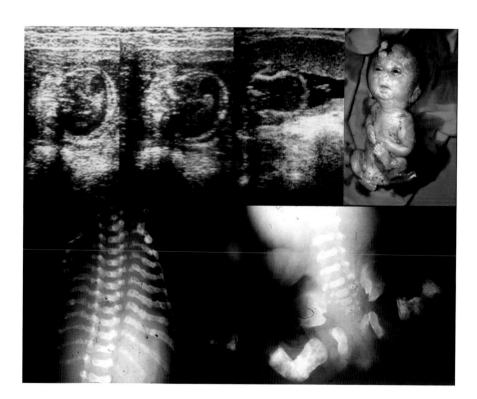

Figure 17.3 Osteogenesis imperfecta, lethal type II. 2D and X-ray examination.

INIENCEPHALY

Iniencephaly is a very rare and complex malformation, first described by van Saint Hilaire in 1836, consisting of an apertus or clausus neural tube defect, with a skull malformation in the areas of the occiput. The occipital bone is missing or has a large hole connecting it to the foramen magnum, making it extremely wide and irregular. The brain can protrude externally through this defect.

All the cases show neural tube defects at least affecting the cervical vertebrae, but cases have been reported in which the entire medullar canal is open. The cervical/cervicothoracic part of the spinal column exhibits extreme lordosis as a consequence of the disintegration of the affected vertebrae, which are reduced in size and number, fused to the cranium, and opened. These vertebral anomalies give rise to a reduction in the crown–rump length (CRL). The consequences of these vertebral defects include the following:

- an extremely extended head, which may be fixed, giving the affected fetuses (and newborns) their characteristic appearance
- an upward-looking face, in a so-called 'stargazing' position
- protrusion and torsion of the chest
- lung hypoplasia (occasionally)
- polyhydramnion (40%), due to difficulty in swallowing.

Iniencephaly is both rare and heterogeneous in terms of associated intracranial and skeletal anomalies. Female fetuses are more commonly affected.

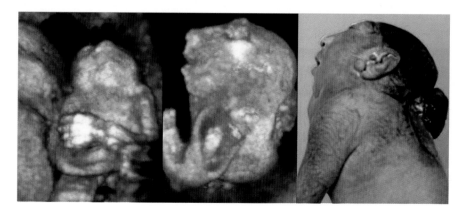

Figure 17.4 Iniencephaly, showing hyperextended head, 'star-gazing' face, short and fixed neck, occipital protruding mass, open mouth, cervical apertus neural tube defect, protrusion and torsion of the thorax, restricted CRL, and exophthalmia.

The etiology of iniencephaly is still unknown, but it has been associated with syphilis and intake of sedatives, tetracycline and related antibiotics, and vinblastine.

Sonographic diagnosis reveals the following (Figure 17.4):

- inability to locate the entire fetal spine on a longitudinal scan
- visualization of an occipital and cervical mass
- an extremely extended head ('stargazing') in sagittal view
- visualization of the head when scanning the thorax transversely (due to the hyperextended head)
- shortened neck, CRL, and spine.

The prognosis is generally fatal, although some reports of survival have been published.

Iniencephaly has been reported in some cases as an isolated anomaly, although in 84% of cases, it is associated with other malformations of the head (anencephaly, microcephaly, hydrocephaly, holoprosencephaly, agenesis of the corpus callosum, encephalocele, or cyclopia), as well as facial (cleft lip and palate), cardiovascular, and genitourinary malformations, abdominal wall defects, diaphragmatic hernia, and joint and limb anomalies.

NEURAL TUBE DEFECTS

The spine is an integrated system of bones, cartilage, joints, and membranous structures that protect the fundamental part of the nervous system and at the same time give support to the skeleton.

Reports of sonographic studies have been published over two decades, showing the origin of the three ossification centers: one at each lamina–pedicle junction and one in the vertebral body. Sonographic evaluation of the neural arch ossification centers of the distal fetal spine was reported in 1991,[24] and it was shown that this ossification occurred in a predictable pattern, in a caudal direction, and that an additional vertebral level became ossified every 2–3 weeks from L5, with S2 being ossified by 22 weeks.

Sonographic lesion level and pathologic level were in agreement in 64% of cases with spina bifida and were within one spinal level in 79% of cases, allowing accurate prediction of spina bifida lesion level and neuromotor handicap.[25]

Demonstration of spinal/vertebral structures using 3D sonography has been reported since 1996. Riccabona et al[26] demonstrated continuity of the spine and ribs. Mueller et al[27] described how the three orthogonal planes proved to be most helpful in delineating the exact nature and anatomic level of the defect, and how 3D reconstructions clarified and documented the true magnitude of the defects. Dyson et al[5] also set a high valuation on planar images derived from 3D sonographic volume datasets generally from the viewpoint of diagnosis, whereas rendered 3D images were more useful as a point of reference and were better appreciated by patients in understanding fetal abnormalities. Recent advanced 3D technology with higher-resolution imaging has contributed to more comprehensive and precise evaluation of the spine and vertebra. Blaas et al[6] and Bonilla-Musoles et al[7] reported the first cases of spina bifida as early as 9 weeks. Lee et al[8] evaluated spina bifida and described how the level of the defect on 3D images correlated well with that on 2D images and postnatal imaging studies. They concluded that 3D multiplanar views were more informative than rendered views for localizing bony defects of the fetal spine, and that this approach added diagnostic information complementary to the initial assessment by 2D sonography. Pooh also used 3D sonography for accurate prenatal diagnosis of fetal central nervous system (CNS) abnormalities.

Transvaginal 3D sonography has been useful for screening and evaluation of fetal spinal/vertebral lesions in the first half of pregnancy.

Of course, in cases with spina bifida, the existence of Chiari type II malformation, secondary hydrocephalus or ventriculomegaly, and deformities of the lower extremities (e.g., clubfoot) should be confirmed by sonography. Biggio et al[17] investigated the natural history of disease progression in utero in cases with open spina bifida, and found that most cases develop ventriculomegaly, with the majority doing so by 21 weeks of gestation, and that fetuses that develop ventriculomegaly later in gestation have less severe ventricular dilatation at birth.

Neuroimaging of normal vertebrae by 3D sonography

Demonstration of the spine and vertebrae by 3D sonography includes three orthogonal views and reconstruction of bony structure (Figures 17.5–17.8). Movement of the region of interest provides a 3D

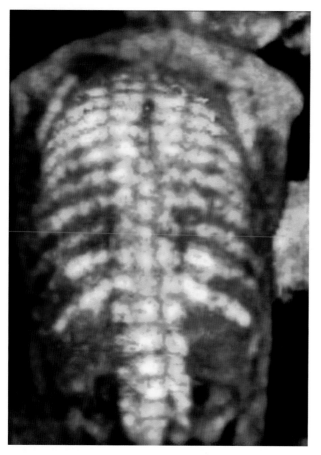

Figure 17.5 Normal development and morphology of the spine and ribs

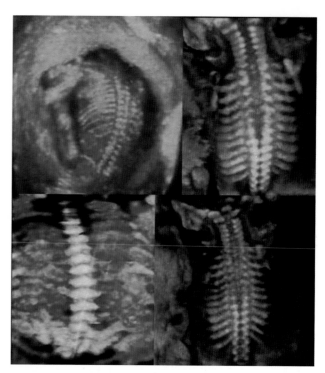

Figure 17.6 Normal fetal rachis with its closing process. When using maximum transparency and X-ray mode, it is possible to carry out the whole visualization of the medullar canal, vertebrae, and intervertebral space

reconstructed image of the surface, neural arch, and vertebral body levels. Figures 17.5–17.8 show the changing appearance of vertebral bony structure between 9 and 22 weeks of gestation; a transvaginal 3D transducer was used. By 13 weeks of gestation, vertebral bodies and intervertebral spaces and bilateral premature vertebral arches are clearly demonstrated. Until 15 weeks of gestation, bilateral laminae are completely separated at all vertebral levels; this condition is called 'physiologic spina bifida'. At the lumbosacral level, the median opening between the bilateral arches is wider than at the thoracic level. At 16 and 17 weeks, the right and left laminae grow toward a median line and closely approach each other at the thoracic level, but are still clearly separate at the lumbosacral level; thereafter, a gradual approach is seen. At 18 and 19 weeks, the lumbosacral vertebral laminae are still separated from each other in the median line, but before 23 weeks of gestation, the gaps between the bilateral laminae at lumbosacral levels are almost closed.[9,10]

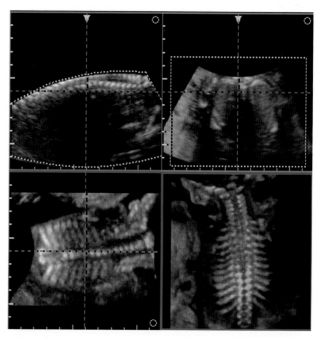

Figure 17.7 4D sonographic study of a normal spine

Vertebral column malformations are likely to have adverse sequelae or structural deformities that usually have a devastating effect on quality of life. Spinal

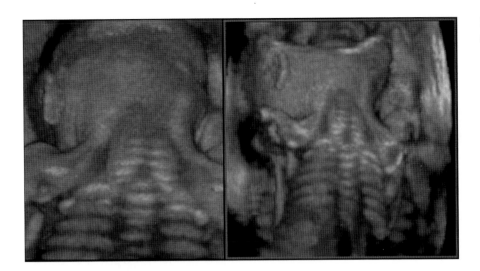

Figure 17.8 4D sonographic study of axis and atlas

defects with marrow externalization are among the most difficult malformations to diagnose, requiring considerable experience.

Many of these defects and anomalies are not diagnosed until well into the 2nd and 3rd trimesters with 2D sonography, with this frequently being prompted by the discovery of an abnormally elevated maternal serum α-fetoprotein (MS-AFP) level. Consequently, the majority of cases go unnoticed in routine prenatal sonographic check-ups.

However, sonographic diagnosis can be very difficult during the first half of pregnancy. Frequently, an experienced sonographer is needed to identify the subtle markers of medullar canal defects, which are often only found through the detection of indirect signs (polyhydramnion, hydrocephaly, banana sign, lemon sign, strawberry sign, etc.). Even the experienced eye at times may not readily detect small defects, or defects located in the inferior part of the lumbosacral region.

Currently, the combination of sonography and MS-AFP is considered the 'gold standard' for diagnosis.

Etiology and classification

Neural tube defects are malformations, starting early in pregnancy, that result from either a failure to close or a defective closure of the neural tube during the 4th week of embryonic development.

The most severe form of failure, craniorachischisis, is a lack of closure along the entire length of the medullar canal. It occurs when the brain and neural tube have not completed the neutralization process, remaining open. It has been imaged by 3D sonography.[28]

The mildest form is spina bifida occulta, which has also been reported with 3D sonography. Spina bifida occulta, no less dramatic than the other forms, is a spina bifida resulting when the two halves of the vertebral arch fail to fuse. This is referred to exclusively as a bone defect and not as a marrow protrusion.

Neural tube fusion starts in the area of the 4th somite and extends cephalad and caudad. Failure of primary closure results in upper-tube defects frequently associated with severe cephalic pole defects, while low thoracic, lumbar, and sacral defects result from failure of secondary closure. The most frequent location is in the lumbosacral region (60% of cases), followed by thoracolumbar (36% of cases), and sacral (4% of cases) (Figure 17.9).

Current classification

Neural tube defects have been divided into the following:

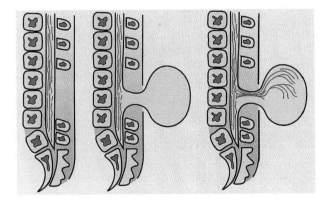

Figure 17.9 Longitudinal diagram of (from left to right); hidden spina bifida, open spina bifida meningocele, open spina bifida myelomeningocele.[16,17]

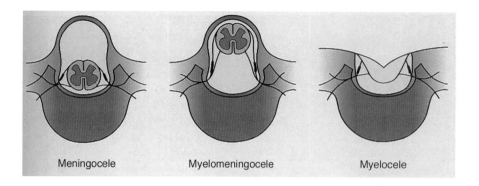

Figure 17.10 Diagram of different types of open spina bifida: meningocele, myelomeningocele and myelocele.[16,17]

- hidden spina bifida
- open spina bifida:
  - partial and complete rachischisis
  - cystic spina bifida: meningocele; myelomeningocele; myelocele (Figure 17.10).

Ultrasound diagnosis

Using sonography, especially 3D techniques, the spine is identified from week 8 on, and the spinal canal from week 10 on. Nevertheless, and with some exceptions, these defects are difficult to observe before week 16 (Figures 17.11–17.23).

With transvaginal 2D sonography, the dorsal ossification nuclei are observed as two parallel echogenic

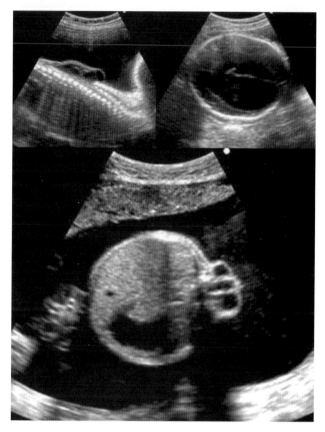

Figure 17.12 Myelomeningocele. This is the typical view. The fetus has also a hydrocephaly

lines separated by a narrow space that widens somewhat in the axis and atlas region. The three ossification nuclei surrounding the spinal marrow – two posterior and one anterior – are visualized in transverse sections.

Only 3D sonography allows visualization of the whole medullar canal, this being one of its advantages.

Ultrasound diagnosis of neural tube defects should also include the following parameters, to help predict perinatal outcome:

- identification of the defect, localization, extension, and degree of opening

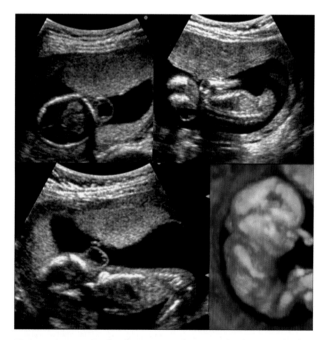

Figure 17.11 Early detection of a very high neural tube defect observed in week 14 of gestation. This is a cervical open neural tube defect affecting the axis, atlas, and cervical vertebrae

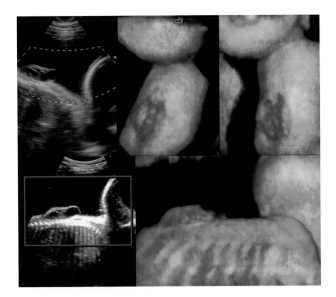

Figure 17.13 Comparison between 2D and 3D visualization of a high-located open spina bifida

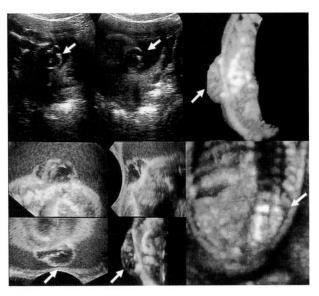

Figure 17.15 Lumbosacral myelomeningocele lumbar (the most common type), observed using maximum-transparency and X-ray modes

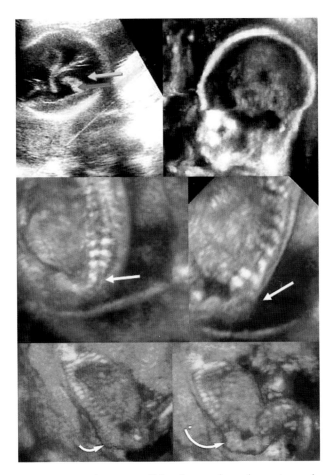

Figure 17.14 A very small lumbosacral myelomeningocele (the most common type). Although it is small, it is associated with hydrocephaly

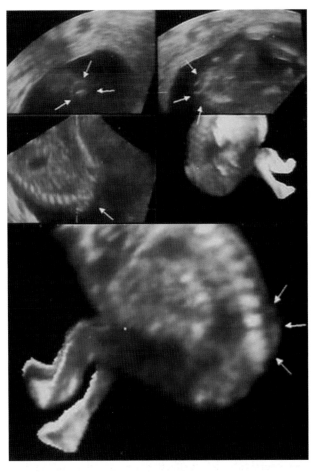

Figure 17.16 A very small myelomeningocele

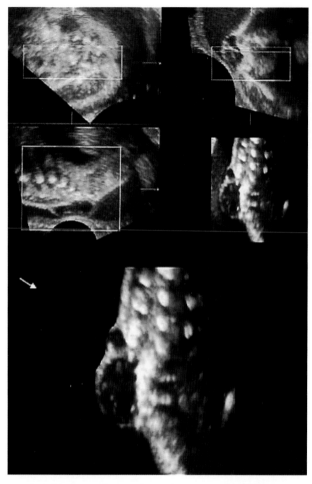

Figure 17.17 Lumbosacral myelomeningocele studied only with the X-ray mode

- a search for associated CNS lesions: more than 50% are associated with hydrocephaly, and with banana, lemon, and strawberry signs
- a search for associated lesions besides CNS lesions
- an estimate of the neurologic and functional consequences of the defect by observation of limb movements, presence of polyhydramnion, skull or brain abnormalities, and involvement of other organs.

In order to identify neural tube defects, especially minor defects, it is helpful to observe transverse cuts of each vertebra in the different sections of the vertebral column. Ideally, each vertebra should be visualized. However, with large defects, or with small defects in fetuses in the dorsal anterior position, axial cuts are preferable.

Meningocele results when the posterior neural arch fails to fuse and the herniated sack does not contain neural tissue. This defect is commonly associated with other malformations. In myelomeningocele, the most frequent open neural tube defect, the herniated sack does contain neural tissue.

The most frequently associated CNS malformation, accompanying 50–75% of cases, is ventriculomegaly, and hydrocephaly in the most severe forms. Occasionally, this is the initially detected anomaly that prompts the study of the spine and leads to the diagnosis.

Arnold–Chiari syndrome is nearly always accompanied by ventriculomegaly. This defect consists of a

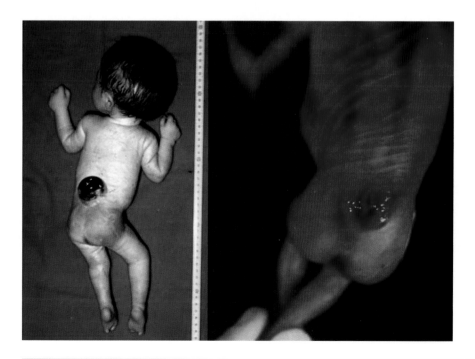

Figure 17.18 The case shown in Figure 17.17[16,17]

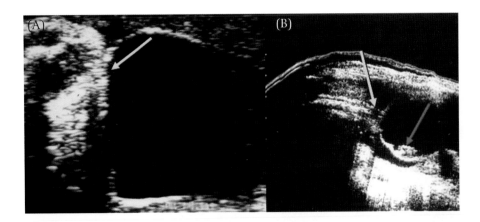

Figure 17.19 Old cases of myelo-meningoceles showing a very bright cyst (A) and medullar tissue (B: red arrow)

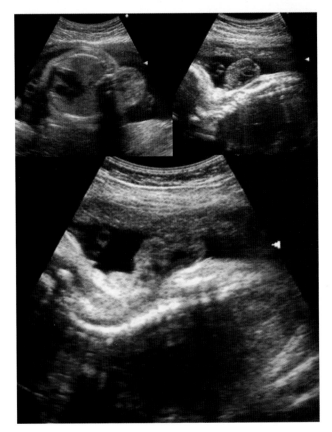

Figure 17.20 Myelomeningocele alta. This is an uncommon finding

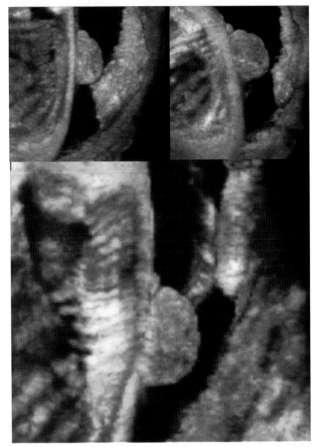

Figure 17.21 High-located myelomeningocele. 3D picture of Figure 17.20

posterior brain injury characterized by the displacement of a small portion of tissue from the cerebellar vermix. The displacement, in turn, causes the marrow and fourth ventricle to descend. Associated symptoms are typically neuromuscular, affecting the newborn's capacity to walk and retain urine. The most severe cases result in clubfoot, hip luxation, and paralysis of the lower extremities.

Although all neural tube defects have a poor prognosis, those located in the sacral region have shown relatively promising results with regard to ambulation when diagnosed in utero and when a pediatric surgery team is ready after birth. Nevertheless, urinary incontinence will affect 100% of cases. In our experience, these are among the most difficult malformations to diagnose with 2D sonography, and often the diagnosis comes either late or at birth.

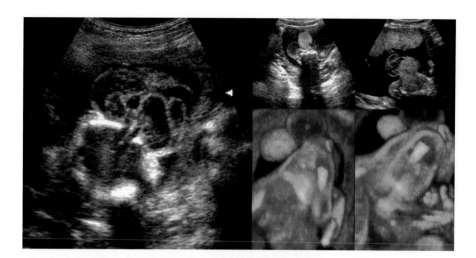

Figure 17.22 Major malformations with opening of the canal and protrusion of the external meninges and medullar mass

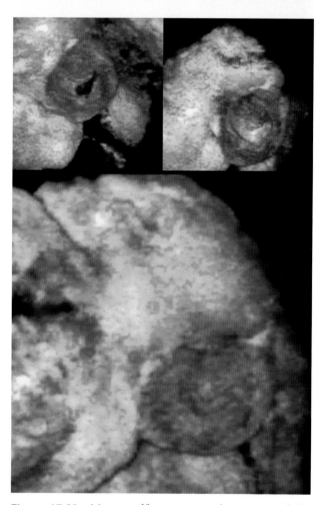

Figure 17.23 Major malformations with opening of the canal and protrusion of the external meninges from the medullar mass. 3D picture of Figure 17.22

3D sonography provides early and complementary information that helps establish the precise level and extent of the defect. Our experience suggests that the complicated and time-consuming 2D examinations can be facilitated by observing the whole vertebral column in surface and transparent 3D modes, and by studying the fetal behavior and motility with 4D sonography. When orthogonal planes with 3D rendering are used, a well-defined spatial image of high resolution can be obtained. We suggest that the major reason for using 3D is to precisely determine the level and extent of neural tube defects initially seen with 2D, and that 3D may also help establish a definitive diagnosis when elevated MS-AFP levels and inconclusive 2D scans suggest the possibility of a neural tube defect.

CAUDAL REGRESSION SYNDROME

This syndrome comprises a group of anomalies that associate vertebral agenesis and genitourinary and digestive malformations. Malformations can vary from anal atresia to sacral/lumbar or thoracic vertebral defects.

Caudal regression syndrome has been associated with mistreated maternal diabetes mellitus, given that the medial–posterior axis of the mesoderm is affected in these patients.

Even though some cases of this syndrome have been found to be of inherited nature, most appear de novo and the risk of recurrence is less than 3%.

SIRENOMELIA

Sirenomelia or mermaid syndrome is an extremely infrequent malformation, occurring in one out of 60 000 newborns, and is more frequent in males than

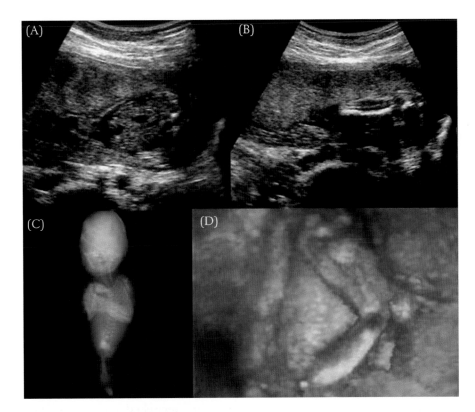

Figure 17.24 Sirenomelia. (A,B) 2D sonography of a single low extremity: only one femur can be seen; gender and pelvic structure are not depicted. (C) X-ray mode. (D) 3D picture. Compare these findings with the newborn in Figure 17.25

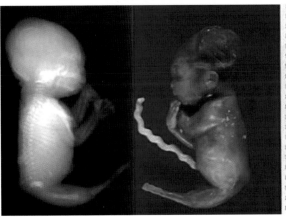
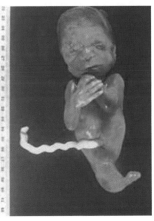

Figure 17.25 Sirenomelia. Radiographic and newborn findings of the case in Figure 17.24

in females (3:1). Although it was formerly described as the most severe form of caudal regression syndrome, recent studies have led to its categorization as a separate nosologic entity.

Even though the etiology of sirenomelia is unknown, it has been associated with maternal diabetes, cocaine consumption during the 1st month of gestation, and exposure to high doses of etretinate or cyclophosphamide (the evidence for the association with the latter two agents comes from animal experiments).

The diagnosis should be suspected from sonographic findings of oligohydramnion and bilateral renal agenesis during the 2nd trimester. Confirmation

is not always simple, because of the existence of a reduced amount of amniotic fluid (Figures 17.24 and 17.25). In fact, in some cases, only bilateral renal agenesis could be diagnosed in utero, and sirenomelia was found only after delivery.

Recently, diagnoses have been reported from week 14 of gestation, using transvaginal sonography. Amniotic fluid was slightly reduced, despite bilateral renal agenesis. This finding is not surprising, because at this gestational age amniotic fluid basically originates from the mother.

Severe oligohydramnion is a sonographic marker of renal agenesis or non-functioning kidneys in the second half of pregnancy. At week 16, fetal urine production proceeds basically from glomerular filtration. The amniotic fluid proceeds from urinary production, respiration, deglutition, and fetal skin transudation. Before this week, the amniotic fluid originates from the amniotic membrane, blood, and maternal transvasation. Nevertheless, even with a polyhydramnion, sonographic diagnosis is possible in the early 2nd trimester.

It has been suggested that amnioinfusion can improves prenatal diagnosis.

Morphologic alterations of lower limbs are of variable extension and are classified into three types, according to the number of feet observed during diagnosis:

- *Symelia apus:* this is the most frequent type; the fetus has no feet, not even rudimentary ones; it has one femur, one or two tibial bones, and no fibula.
- *Symelia unipus:* there is only one foot, which can have up to a full complement of 10 toes; the lower limb has a pair of femurs, as well as tibial and peroneal bones.
- *Symelia dipus:* both feet are present, giving the fetus a mermaid-like appearance.

Lower limb malformations are associated with other skeletal or visceral anomalies. The most frequent are:

- sacral agenesis
- anorectal atresia
- renal agenesis or renal cystic dysplasia
- internal and external dysplasia of the genitalia
- single umbilical artery.

Other anomalies that are usually associated include cardiovascular malformations, abdominal wall defects, severe scoliosis, and cerebral anomalies.

It has been suggested that this complex of malformations is caused by an early lesion in the caudal mesoderm that affects the normal development of the lower limbs of the fetus. Overdistension of the neural tube in this caudal portion could lead to lateral rotation of the mesoderm, causing fusion of the lower limbs and closure of the gut and urethra. Experiments with mice exposed to high doses of retinoic acid have confirmed an interference with mesoderm formation and a relationship with the pathogenesis of caudal digenesis.

Other proposals try to explain the defect by taking into consideration the accompanying vascular anomalies. Usually, there is a single umbilical artery, or one artery is normal and the other hypoplastic. These arteries come from the upper portion of the abdominal cavity; the vessels below this level are poorly developed. Therefore, tissues reliant on this hypoplastic vascular system do not show a normal development. It has been suggested that the single lower extremity in sirenomelia is caused by a lack of separation between two lateral masses, rather than a fusion of the inferior limbs.

Prenatal diagnosis of the mermaid syndrome must be suspected in cases of renal agenesis, single umbilical artery, and lack of visualization of two femurs. The lethal prognosis of this malformation makes early prenatal diagnosis very important, although some reports have been published of cases in which the fetus reached term with variable chances of survival.

CONJOINED TWINS

It is likely that in the near future 3D sonography will revolutionize prenatal diagnosis and that, combined with 2D techniques, it will be used systematically in any ultrasound examination, because it improves the diagnostic capability by 50–70% when compared with transabdominal and transvaginal 2D sonography. In subtle malformations such as nuchal translucency, phocomelia, ambiguous genitalia, and cleft lip, evidence is nowadays available. The earliest possible detection and most accurate diagnoses will influence obstetric decisions and perinatal outcome. Conjoined twins are an example of this.

Conjoined twins are variants of monozygotic twin gestation that occur through incomplete dissociation of cells from the internal cellular mass between days 9 and 13 of embryonic development (Figure 17.26).

The incidence of conjoined twins varies between 1 in 50 000 and 1 in 100 000 deliveries, with the highest frequency being observed in cases of multiple gestations resulting from the use of assisted reproduction technology. This incidence also seems to be higher in women during their later reproductive years than in younger women, presumably because of a thinner zona pellucida.

With assisted reproduction technology, diagnostic studies are justified early in the 1st trimester for several reasons:

- These pregnancies have a higher incidence of multifetal gestation.

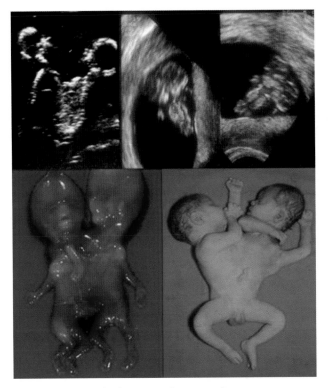

Figure 17.26 Early diagnosis of conjoined twins using transvaginal 2D sonography

- The incidence of fetal anomalies is higher with multiple gestations, especially if the twins are monozygotic.
- There is a better chance of uncomplicated embryo reduction with early detection of fetal malformations.

Etiology

The frequency of monozygotic twins is 0.3% of all pregnancies. Except for certain known situations and some variants of assisted reproduction technology, where it appears to be increased, this frequency is 'relatively constant' worldwide.

The time of production of monozygotic twins has been linked to a number of hypothetical mechanisms.

According to the latest knowledge, embryonic division should occur shortly after fertilization, but before pre-implantation, while the embryo is still within the zona pellucida. Also, it has been suggested that twinning should occur shortly after blastocyst implantation. These theories, however, are debatable.

The first hypothesis suggests that two divided embryos can remain within the zona pellucida. This suggestion was made before it was known that mammalian embryos can be artificially divided into halves or fourths before compaction, and still survive. For this to occur, it is crucial to cultivate these embryos separately in different zona pellucida, with the aim of avoiding subsequent aggregation and development of a simple chimera. This phenomenon occurs only in precompacted and compacted embryos, and implies that the first theory is incorrect.

The second hypothesis suggests that events of division are rare following implantation. This has not been confirmed by subsequent observations.

Recent observations have concentrated on the zona pellucida in monozygotic twins. According to this theory, monozygotic as well as dizygotic twins are produced during hatching, when embryos are trapped in the opening of the zona pellucida.

Twins can continue to develop when the internal cellular mass is halved. This can happen when the trophoblast remains integral or when it separates. In the first case, monoamniotic, monochorionic twins will result, of which conjoined twins would be a

Table 17.2 Relationship between the embryonic division, cause of twinning, and placentation

Days after ovulation	Type of placentation	Cause of twinning
Classical model		
1–3	Bichorial biamniotic	Preimplantation split
3–8	Monochorial biamniotic	Mixed causes
8–12	Monochorial monoamniotic	Embryonic disk split
13–15	Conjoined	Incomplete disk split
Hatching model		
6	Bichorial biamniotic	Trophoblastic split in gap
		Hatching
>6	Bichorial monoamniotic	Mixed causes
>6	Monochorial monoamniotic	Split cellular masses and conjoined internal but not trophoblast

Table 17.3 Classification of conjoined twinning

Class	Place of union
Thoracopagus	Thoracic region (Figure 17.27)
Xiphopagus	Xiphoid process of sternum
Omphalopagus	Umbilical region
Rachiopagus	Fusion of upper spinal column, back-to-back
Pygopagus	Sacrum; back-to-back most common
Pygodidymus	Cephalothoracic region; duplicate pelves and lower extremities
Pygomelus	Sacral or coccygeal region; additional limb or limbs at or near buttock
Ischiopagus	Pelvis, ischial region, end-to-end
Craniopagus	Head
Iniopagus (craniopagus occipitalis)	Head, at parasitic occipital region
Epicomus (craniopagus parasiticus)	Smaller, parasitic twin joined to larger auto site at occiput
Monocephalus	Single head with two bodies
Diprosopus	Single head and body with two faces
Dicephalus	Symmetric body with two heads (Figures 17.28 and 17.29)
Dipygus parasiticus	Head and thorax completely merged: pelvis and lower extremities duplicated (Figures 17.30 and 17.31)
Syncephalus	Face

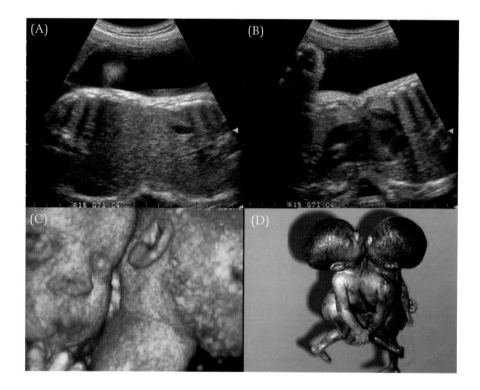

Figure 17.27 Thoracopagus. (A,B) 2D sonography showing the linkage, two thoraces, and one heart. (C) 3D image, with facing heads. (D) Newborn

variant, and would indicate a partial division of the internal cellular mass. This sets the time of most of these events at day 6, when the embryo does the hatching. For this reason, when artificial hatchings started to be performed, conjoined twinning was entertained as a possibility. Alternatively, conjoined twinning can occur when there is incomplete cleavage in the embryonic disc between days 13 and 15 following fertilization (Table 17.2).

Diagnosis

Although most referred cases are diagnosed in the 2nd and 3rd trimesters, the diagnosis can be made during the 1st trimester by performing a meticulous 2D transvaginal sonographic examination (Figure 17.26). The diagnostic accuracy and classification of conjoined twins can be improved with the use of color Doppler and 3D sonography and magnetic resonance imaging (MRI).

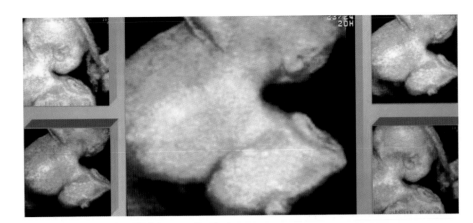

Figure 17.28 Dicephalus conjoined twins. This anomaly shows two separated heads, one or beginning of two rachis, one thorax and pelvis, and four extremities

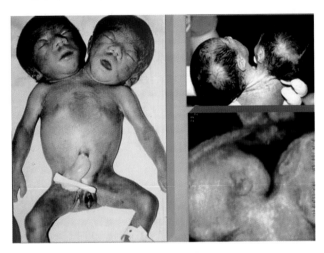

Figure 17.29 Dicephalus conjoined twins. Same case as in Figure 17.28

Although 2D sonography is adequate to establish a primary diagnosis, 3D techniques produce easily understood images that improve communication with patients, enhance their understanding of the abnormalities involved, and allow them to make better-informed decisions about subsequent management.

Comments

Although the prognosis for conjoined twins is extremely poor, meticulous exploration is necessary to determine which organs are shared and to establish an accurate classification.

Table 17.3 summarizes the classes of conjoined twinning that can occur. The most common unions occur at the trunk (thoracopagus, xiphopagus, and omphalopagus), but other forms have been observed. Accurate classification allows physicians to communicate more effectively with their patients and to discuss

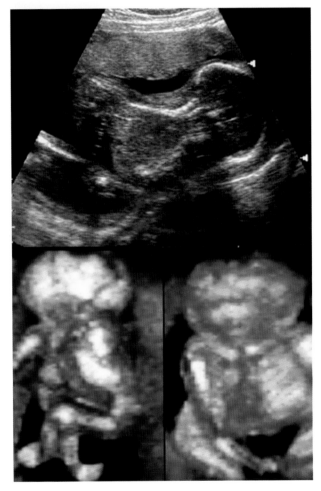

Figure 17.30 Dipygus parasiticus

with them the prognosis and options with greater objectivity.

During the 2nd and 3rd trimesters of pregnancy, it is difficult to clearly define the separation of fetal structures and organs (head, thorax, etc.) sonographically in cases of conjoined twins. In such cases, it is helpful to identify shared structures by provoking fetal

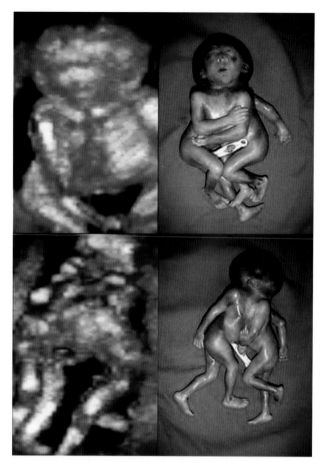

Figure 17.31 Dipygus parasiticus. 3D pictures and the newborn

movement with the transducer; this maneuver is easier during the first half of gestation.

The use of transvaginal 2D, color Doppler, and 3D sonography allows the diagnosis and classification of these devastating malformations during the 1st trimester of gestation. Color Doppler sonography is especially helpful during the 1st trimester for exploration of shared vessels and vascular organs.

2D sonography seems to allow a better assessment of internal anatomy or shared organs than 3D does, but 3D clearly provides images that are much easier for patients to understand than those from 2D.

If the gestation is multifetal, chorionicity and amnionicity are simpler to establish in the 1st trimester than they are later.

When conjoined twins or other fetal anomalies are identified, 3D sonography is likely to provide images that are easier for the physician and parents to understand than are those from 2D, therefore allowing them to make informed decisions on the basis of more comprehensible information.

REFERENCES

1. Menkes JH, Sarnat HE. Neuroembryology, genetic programming, and malformations. In: Child Neurology, 6th edn. Philadelphia, PA: Lippincott Williams and Wilkins, 2000: 316–35.

2. Gray DL, Crane JP, Rudloff MA. Prenatal diagnosis of neural tube defects: Origin of mid trimester vertebral ossification centers as determined by sonographic water-bath studies. J Ultrasound Med 1988; 7: 421–7.

3. Kollias SS, Goldstein RE, Cogen PH, Filly RA. Prenatally detected myelomeningoceles: sonographic accuracy in estimation of the spinal level. Radiology 1992; 185: 109–12.

4. Johnson DD, Pretorius DH, Riccabona M, et al. Three-dimensional ultrasound of the fetal spine. Obstet Gynecol 1997; 89: 434–8.

5. Dyson RL, Pretorius DH, Budorick NE, et al. Three-dimensional ultrasound in the evaluation of fetal anomalies. Ultrasound Obstet Gynecol 2000; 16: 321–8.

6. Blaas HG, Eik-Nes SH, Isaksen CV. The detection of spina bifida before 10 gestational weeks using two- and three-dimensional ultrasound. Ultrasound Obstet Gynecol 2000; 16: 25–9.

7. Bonilla-Musoles F, Machado LE, Osborne NG, et al. Two and three-dimensional ultrasound in malformations of the medullary canal: report of 4 cases. Prenat Diagn 2001; 21: 622–6.

8. Lee W, Chaiworapongsa T, Romero R, et al. A diagnostic approach for the evaluation of spina bifida by three-dimensional ultrasonography. J Ultrasound Med 2002; 21: 619–26.

9. Pooh RK, Pooh KH. Fetal neuroimaging with new technology. Ultrasound Review Obstet Gynecol 2002; 2: 178–81.

10. Pooh RK, Maeda K, Pooh KH. An Atlas of Fetal Central Nervous System Disease. Diagnosis and Management. London: Parthenon/CRC Press, 2003.

11. Biggio JR Jr, Wenstrom KD, Owen J. Fetal open spina bifida: a natural history of disease progression in utero. Prenat Diagn 2004; 24: 287–9.

12. Bonilla-Musoles F, Machado L, Osborne N. Malformations of the medullary canal. In: Bonilla-Musoles F, Machado L, Osborne N, eds. Three-Dimensional Ultrasound for the New Millenium. Text and Atlas. Madrid, Spain: Aloka, 2000: 193–204.

13. Bonilla-Musoles F, Machado L, Osborne N, et al. Neural tube defects. In: Bonilla-Musoles F, Machado L, eds. 3D–4D Ultrasound in Obstetrics. Madrid, Spain: Panamericana, 2004: 269–76.

14. Pooh RK, Pooh KH. Fetal vertebral structure detected by three-dimensional ultrasound. Ultrasound Rev Obstet Gynecol 2005; 5: 29–33.

15. Bonilla-Musoles F, Raga F, Villalobos A, Osborne N, Blanes J. First-trimester neck abnormalities: three-dimensional evaluation. J Ultrasound Med 1998; 17: 419–26.

16. Garjian KV, Pretorius D, Budorick N, et al. Fetal skeletal dysplasia: three-dimensional US – initial experience. Radiology 2000; 214: 717–23.

17. Johnson DD, Pretorius DH, Riccabona M, Budorick NE, Nelson TR. Three-dimensional ultrasound of the fetal spine. Obstet Gynecol 1997; 89: 434–8.

18. Ludomirski A, Khandelwal M, Uerpairojkit B, Reece EA, Chan L. Three-dimensional ultrasound evaluation of fetal facial and spinal anatomy. Am J Obstet Gynecol 1996; 174(Suppl): 318.

19. Nelson TR, Pretorius DH. Visualization of the fetal thoracic skeleton with three-dimensional sonography: a preliminary report. AJR Am J Roentgenol 1995; 164: 1485–8.

20. Schild RL. Fetal lumbar spine volumetry by three-dimensional ultrasound. Ultrasound Obstet Gynecol 1999; 13: 335–9.

21. Schild RL, Wallny T, Fimmers R, Hansmman M. The size of the fetal thoracolumbar spine: a three-dimen-sional ultrasound study. Ultrasound Obstet Gynecol 2000; 16: 468–72.

22. Steiner H, Staudach A, Zajc M, Wienerroither H. Verbesserte Diagnostik am fetalen Skelett mittels 3D-Sonographie. Ultraschall Klin Prax 1994; 8: 154.

23. Wallny TA. The fetal spinal canala three dimensional study. Ultrasound Med Biol 1999; 25: 1329–38.

24. Budorick NE, Pretorius DH, Grafe MR, et al. Ossification of the fetal spine. Radiology 1991; 181: 561–5.

25. Biggio JR, Owen J, Wenstrom KD, et al. Can prenatal ultrasound findings predict ambulatory status in fetuses with open spina bifida? Am J Obstet Gynecol 2001; 185: 1016–20.

26. Riccabona M, Johnson D, Pretorius DH, et al. Three dimensional ultrasound: display modalities in the fetal spine and thorax. Eur J Radiol 1996; 22: 141–5.

27. Mueller GM, Weiner CP, Yankowitz J. Three-dimen-sional ultrasound in the evaluation of fetal head and spine anomalies. Obstet Gynecol 1996; 88: 372–8.

28. Müller GM, Weiner CP, Yankowitz J. Three-dimen-sional ultrasound in the evaluation of fetal head and spine anomalies. Obstet Gynecol 1996; 88: 372–8.

18 Fetal tumors

Vincenzo D'Addario, Luca Di Cagno, and Armando Pintucci

INTRODUCTION

Fetal tumors are rare congenital anomalies that can be located in different parts of the fetal body. As in adults, tumors in the fetus may arise from any tissue as a consequence of developmental errors during embryogenesis. The 'cell rest' theory has been suggested as a possible explanation of fetal tumor development: according to this theory, more cells are produced than are required for the formation of an organ or tissue, and fetal tumors are the results of developmental errors in these surplus embryonic rudiments. A genetic mechanism has also been suggested as a possible factor in the complex pathogenesis of certain embryonic tumors.[1]

Because of their different location and histologic type, fetal tumors are consequently characterized by a variety of pathophysiologic findings. The histologic findings range widely from simple cyst to hamartoma, teratoma, and even complex sarcoma; the location can be in any compartment of the fetal body from the brain to the skin. The prognosis is variable, depending on the benign or malignant nature of the tumor, its location, and its size.

The prenatal diagnosis of a fetal tumor has important implications for fetal and neonatal, as well as maternal, outcome. Such a diagnosis, however, can sometimes be difficult or incomplete, due to limitations in identifying the type and/or the site of the tumor, thus precluding optimal perinatal management.

Three-dimensional (3D) sonography may help in a better identification of fetal tumors, both with surface rendering mode and with the multiplanar view mode. Surface rendering offers a clear view of the tumor in a photographic style, whereas the multiplanar view helps in evaluating the volume and infiltration of the tumor.

SACROCOCCYGEAL TERATOMA

Sacrococcygeal teratoma is one of the most common tumors in newborns, with a reported incidence of 1 in 35 000 to 1 in 40 000 live births. It is thought to develop from the totipotent cells in Hensen's node, the anchorage point of sexual cells. A 'twinning accident', with incomplete separation during embryogenesis and abnormal development of one fetus, has also been suggested as a possible etiology of sacrococcygeal teratoma. This hypothesis is supported by the fact that organoid elements are occasionally found in the tumor.

The size of these tumors is extremely variable, and unpredictable growths can occur in utero. Tumors as large as 20 cm have been reported to obstruct labor. As regards their location, sacrococcygeal teratoma may be entirely external, may have a partial intrapelvic extension, or may be completely intrapelvic. According to their site, they have been divided by the American Academy of Pediatrics Surgical Section (AAPSS) into four types:[2]

- *Type I:* predominantly exophytic
- *Type II:* mainly external, but with a significant intrapelvic retroperitoneal extension
- *Type III:* apparently external, but with the main part of the mass extending into the abdomen and displacing the abdominal structures
- *Type IV:* presacral, with no external presentation.

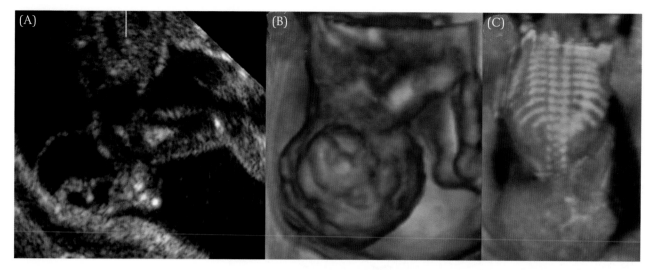

Figure 18.1 Large sacrococcygeal teratoma. (A) 2D sonography shows the mainly cystic internal structure of the tumor. (B) 3D surface rendering outlines the sacrococcygeal teratoma in a photographic way and helps in distinguishing it from other pathologic entities. (C) The transparent mode offers a better outline of the body structure, thus allowing a better view of the relation between the tumor and the spine

In the AAPSS survey of 405 cases, 46% were of type I, 36% of type II, 9% of type III, and 10% of type IV. Most sacrococcygeal teratomas are solid or mixed solid and cystic. Purely cystic forms are rare. In about 80% of cases, they are histologically benign. Malignancy is more common in males, in solid tumors, and in type III tumors. Other important factors influencing prognosis are the size and morphologic type of the tumor: large and mainly solid tumors carry a higher mortality rate, due to difficulty in resection and tumor hemorrhage. These considerations emphasize the importance of sonographic prenatal diagnosis, which reveals the internal structure as well as the size and intra-abdominal extent of the tumor.

The most common sonographic finding of a fetal sacrococcygeal teratoma is that of a mixed or predominantly solid mass located near the caudal region of the fetus. A mainly cystic appearance is rare. Calcifications may be present. Color Doppler study can demonstrate rich vascularization. The diagnosis can occasionally be made even in the 1st trimester.[3]

3D sonography makes it easier to evaluate the relation of the tumor with the surrounding structures and calculate the tumor volume by the multiplanar view mode. Surface rendering outlines sacrococcygeal teratomas in a photographic way and helps in distinguishing them from other pathologic entities. The transparent mode offers a better outline of the body structure, thus allowing a better view of the relation between the tumor and the spine[4] (Figures 18.1 and 18.2). 3D color Doppler sonography is of help in

visualizing the blood supply to the tumor[5] (Figure 18.3).

Polyhydramnios is present in most prenatally diagnosed sacrococcygeal teratomas, although the mechanism is not clear. Fetal hydrops can be a further complication associated with large tumors; it is secondary to fetal heart failure, which can be due to two possible mechanisms: either severe fetal anemia secondary to tumor hemorrhage or high cardiac output from arteriovenous shunting within the tumor. Fetal hydrops is always an ominous finding.

The differential diagnosis of sacrococcygeal teratoma mainly includes meningomyeloceles: however, these anomalies are virtually never solid, do not contain calcifications, and demonstrate the typical spinal defect. Other anomalies that can simulate a sacrococcygeal teratoma are lymphomas, retrorectal hamartomas, intracanicular epidermoid tumors, neuroblastomas, hemangiomas, gliomas, and many other rare conditions that can occur with skin-covered lesions in the sacrococcygeal region.

Associated anomalies are reported in 11–38% of cases. Some of the local abnormalities, such as rectovaginal fistula and imperforate anus, are thought to be directly related to tumor growth during fetal development. Association with aneuploidies is extremely rare.

The prognosis of sacrococcygeal teratoma is usually good after neonatal surgery; the only exceptions are represented by the rare cases of malignant teratomas and by type III lesions, due to the cranial displacement of abdominal organs, sometimes even resulting in lung

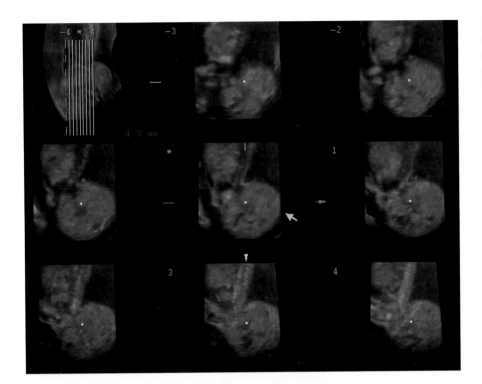

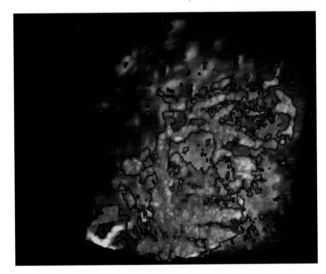

Figure 18.3 3D power Doppler of a sacrococcygeal teratoma demonstrating the high vascularity of the tumor

hypoplasia. The main complications that can occur in fetal sacrococcygeal teratomas are prematurity, fetal hydrops, and tumor hemorrhage in utero or during delivery.

Once the prenatal diagnosis has been made, serial sonographic examinations should be performed in order to assess tumor growth, amniotic fluid volume, and early evidence of fetal hydrops. Fetal renal and gastrointestinal functions should also be evaluated, since the tumor can cause compression of the urethra as well as of the bowel, causing hydronephrosis or intestinal tract obstruction.

The mode of delivery depends on the size of the tumor. Vaginal delivery may be possible with small tumors. In large tumors, however, since the main complication is represented by rupture or hemorrhage during delivery, cesarean section is recommended to avoid hemorrhage or dystocia. Prenatal sonographically guided aspiration of cystic sacrococcygeal teratomas can be performed in order to facilitate delivery. Fetal surgery has also been attempted in order to interrupt vascular shunting through the tumor and avoid fetal cardiac failure. The surgical procedures suggested are in utero tumor resection,[6] radiofrequency ablation,[7] and thermocoagulation.[8] The potential benefit of such prenatal surgery, however, must be balanced against the potential risks for the mother and the fetus. Delivery should be performed in a tertiary center, with neonatologists present and pediatric surgeons available for prompt surgical resection.

INTRACRANIAL TUMORS

Brain tumors are extremely rare congenital abnormalities, represented, in approximately 50% of cases, by teratomas; glial tumors (glioblastomas, astroblastomas, and spongioblastomas) are second in frequency. Independently of their benign or malignant attitude,

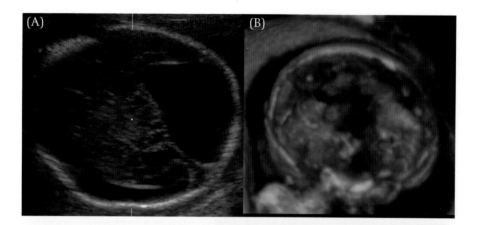

Figure 18.4 Brain teratoma: (A) 2D sonography; (B) 3D sonography. The tumor appears as an irregular predominantly solid mass distorting the brain anatomy and causing ventriculomegaly

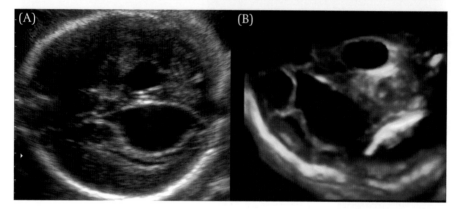

Figure 18.5 Large arachnoid cyst: (A) 2D sonography; (B) 3D sonography. The mass is located in the interhemispheric space and compresses the brain tissue

these tumors tend to have dramatic consequences for the developing fetal brain.

Teratomas appear as irregularly shaped, mixed solid and cystic masses distorting the brain anatomy (Figure 18.4). When the cystic component is prevalent, the differential diagnosis from an arachnoid cyst can be difficult. Glioblastoma may present as a diffusely hyperechoic mass with an appearance similar to that of a large hemorrhage. A definitive prenatal diagnosis of the tumor type, however, is limited.[9]

The tumors are more commonly supratentorial, although a precise location is not possible in cases of huge masses. Hydrocephalus is commonly associated as a consequence of the obstruction by the mass of the liquoral circulation. Macrocephaly can develop, due both to the size of the tumor mass and to increasing ventriculomegaly, and can make vaginal delivery impossible even after cephalocentesis. The prognosis of the prenatally detected fetal brain tumor is ominous; in most cases, babies are stillborn or die in the neonatal period.[10]

Other cystic tumors that can be ultrasonically detected in utero include arachnoid cysts.[11] These may be supratentorial or retrocerebellar. The former may present a more variable appearance, due to the larger

supratentorial compartment. They appear as cystic structures of variable size that cause pressure and a mass effect on the brain, and may result in hydrocephalus (Figure 18.5). For this reason, the prognosis of arachnoid cysts is better than that of teratomas and glial tumors, if they are treated before irreversible brain damage occurs.

The differential diagnosis of arachnoid cysts includes porencephalic cysts (mainly cystic teratomas), interhemispheric cysts associated with agenesis of the corpus callosum, cysts of the corpus callosum, and aneurysm of the vein of Galen. Unlike arachnoid cysts, porencephalic cysts usually communicate with the lateral ventricle. Cystic teratomas usually present some amount of solid tissue associated with the cystic components. Interhemispheric cysts associated with agenesis of the corpus callosum usually communicate with the third ventricle, due to the absence of the callosal fibers. Corpus callosum cysts show the typical C-shaped appearance in sagittal section. Finally, aneurysm of the vein of Galen is easily recognizable for the typical turbulent Doppler signal generated by the 'cystic' lesion. In this case, 3D color or power Doppler helps in evaluating the volume of the vascular mass (Figure 18.6).

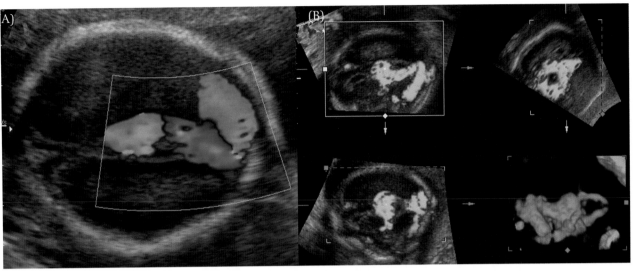

Figure 18.6 Vein of Galen. (A) Color Doppler shows the typical turbulent signal generated by the 'cystic' lesion. (B) 3D power Doppler helps in evaluating the volume of the vascular mass

TUMORS OF THE NECK

Tumors of the fetal neck are mainly represented by cervical teratomas and other differentiated soft tissue masses, such as lymphangiomas and hemangiomas.

Cervical teratomas are very rare tumors, composed of tissues foreign to a particular anatomic site, with all three germ layers being represented. Sonographically, they appear as unilateral, asymmetric masses located in the lateral and anterior regions of the fetal neck. They usually extend to the mastoid process and to the mandible, displacing the ear. Extension into the oral vault and the mediastinum has also been reported. Their structure is usually that of a complex mass, with solid and cystic components; color Doppler can visualize their rich vascularization. Their size can be extremely variable: tumor masses greater than the fetal head have been reported. Polyhydramnios is associated with 20–40% of cases, and is due to esophageal obstruction by the large cervical mass.[12]

The differential diagnosis mainly includes cystic hygroma. This is the cervical mass most commonly diagnosed in the prenatal period. It is not a true tumor, but a developmental abnormality of the lymphatic system characterized by a lack of jugular lymph sac drainage into the jugular vein with consequent formation of a cystic structure located in the posterior aspect of the fetal neck; the cyst is typically flaccid and presents thin borders with thin septa. Cystic hygroma can be recognized early in the 1st trimester using transvaginal sonography; association with hydrops, cardiac defects, and chromosomal abnormalities (mainly Turner syndrome) has been reported in up to 90% of cases.[13]

Other conditions mimicking a cervical teratoma, whose differential diagnosis is not always possible, are sarcomas, hemangiomas, lymphangiomas, congenital goiter, and, less frequently, branchial cysts, laryngoceles, thyroglossal cysts, and other very rare conditions.[14] Cervical teratomas should also be differentiated from epignathus, a teratoma arising from the oral cavity or pharynx, which is recognizable by its anterior location with respect to the fetal neck.

In all cases of neck tumors, 3D sonography is useful for precise location of the tumor and to determine the involvment of adjacent organs in order to predict the likelihood of upper-airways impairment; furthermore, it helps in providing evidence that the fetal face is not distorted.

Although rare cases of malignancies have been reported,[15] most cervical teratomas in fetuses, infants, and children are benign. The prenatal diagnosis of a large cervical teratoma represents an indication for cesarean section to avoid malpresentation and dystocia caused by hyperextension of the neck and large tumor size. Since the tumor can obstruct the upper airways, delivery should be planned in a tertiary care unit, where pediatric surgeons are ready for ex utero intrapartum tracheal intubation and subsequent intervention.[16]

CHEST TUMORS

Chest tumors are rare congenital anomalies arising from the lung, the mediastinal space, or the heart.

Lung tumors

The most common congenital lung tumor is cystic adenomatoid malformation. This is a hamartoma characterized by overgrowth of terminal bronchioles. A classification into three types of cystic adenomatoid malformation has been proposed by Stocker et al:[17] type I has large cysts; type II has multiple small cysts; type III is the microcystic variety, and involves the entire lobe with regularly spaced bronchiole-like structures, causing mediastinal shift. Adzick[18] has proposed two categories based on gross anatomy, sonographic findings, and prognosis: macro- and microcystic tumors. The former contain single or multiple cysts 5 mm or more in diameter; the latter appear as a solid mass, since the cysts are too small to be visualized by ultrasound, but produce an echo enhancement due to the innumerable interfaces. The macrocystic type is more common and has a more favorable prognosis, whereas the microcystic (solid) type is more severe because of the development of fetal hydrops and hypoplasia of the normal lung tissue, secondary to vena cava or cardiac compression.

The differential diagnosis includes bronchogenic cysts, pulmonary sequestration, and some very rare mediastinal masses, such as teratomas, pericardial cysts, thymus neoplasms, and neurogenic tumors. A bronchogenic cyst appears as an isolated regular hypoechoic area in the lung. Pulmonary sequestration is a mass of pulmonary parenchyma separated from the normal lung, usually not communicating with an airway, and receiving its blood supply from the systemic circulation.[19] It appears as a triangularly shaped hyperechogenic mass within the fetal chest, whose differentiation from the microcystic variety of cystic adenomatoid malformation remains difficult. The most characteristic sign of pulmonary sequestration is the visualization of its anomalous arterial supply arising from the aorta. 3D sonography with the use of multiplanar view or volume contrast imaging (VCI) may be useful for more precise differentiation.[20]

The prognosis of cystic adenomatoid malformation depends on the type and severity of the disease. Small lesions may also shrink or even disappear during pregnancy. Large lesions can produce a mass effect on the developing lungs, with subsequent pulmonary hypoplasia. Usually, the prognosis is worse in the microcystic type, which is frequently complicated by mediastinal shift, hydrops, and polyhydramnios. Hydrops is the most important sign predictive of an unfavorable outcome. It is probably secondary to vena cava obstruction or cardiac compression from the mediastinal shift caused by the lesion. The absence of hydrops until the end of pregnancy carries a good prognosis for the neonate. The delivery, however, should be planned in a tertiary care center, where immediate resuscitation and thoracic surgery can be planned. Prenatal treatment, consisting of intrauterine shunting of the lung cysts and/or of the associated pleural effusion has been performed with a successful outcome in several cases.[21,22]

Tumors of the heart

Congenital cardiac tumors are extremely rare lesions, mainly represented by rhabdomyomas. Teratomas, fibromas, myxomas, and hemangiomas are less common.[23] In most cases, the tumors are benign. Rhabdomyomas are typically associated in up to 85% of cases with tuberous sclerosis. However, despite the development of modern imaging, the typical brain and skin lesions of tuberous sclerosis cannot be detected in the fetal stage. Rhabdomyomas, on the other hand, as well as other cardiac tumors, are easily detectable in the prenatal period; they appear as hyperechoic masses occupying the cardiac area.[24,25] They can be isolated or, more frequently, multiple and can be located on any structure of the heart, including the septum. They can also be present as diffuse myocardial thickening. The prognosis depends on the number, size, and location of the tumors and on the association with tuberous sclerosis. Small tumors may undergo spontaneous reduction after delivery.[24] The presence of hydrops is a severe complication, indicating heart failure. This carries a very poor prognosis.

ABDOMINAL TUMORS

Abdominal tumors include both solid and cystic lesions arising from different intra-abdominal organs (liver, kidneys, adrenal glands, spleen, mesentery, omentum, ovaries, uterus, and retroperitoneal space).

Correct prenatal diagnosis of these abnormalities is not always possible with ultrasound, because of the difficulties in defining the organ from which the tumor originates. However, the location of the mass, its relation with other structures, and the normality of other organs may be helpful in suggesting a reliable diagnosis.

Hepatic tumors

These are easily identified by their location in the liver area. Primary liver tumors are very rare conditions, which can occasionally be seen in the prenatal period. They include hemangioma, mesenchymal hamartoma, adenoma, hepatoblastoma, metastatic neuroblastoma, and isolated cysts.

The sonographic appearance of hepatic hemangioma varies, depending on the degree of fibrosis and stage of involution of the tumor: it can be hypo-echogenic, hyperechogenic, or mixed in appearance. The size can vary from a few millimeters to some centimeters. The vascular nature of hemangioma can be confirmed by pulsed Doppler with color flow only in cases with large vessels and turbulent flow. Polyhydramnios can be associated in cases of large hemangiomas. A possible reduction in size or even disappearance in utero of small lesions is possible, as a consequence of the progressive fibrosis and involution of the tumor.[26]

Mesenchymal hamartomas may be solid and homogeneous, but also multicystic with a hetereogeneous echogenicity similar to that of hepatoblastoma and adenoma.[27,28]

For this reason, a prenatal differential diagnosis among the above different pathologic conditions is not possible.

Isolated hepatic cysts appear as well-defined anechoic lesions in the liver area; their differential diagnosis from a choledochal cyst could be difficult. This can be suspected when tubular structures referred to dilated hepatic ducts can be seen, adjacent or leading to the cyst.

The management of a fetus affected by a hepatic tumor is expectant, with monitoring of the size and evolution of the tumor. Huge hemangiomas associated with arteriovenous shunting can cause fetal heart failure; small hemangiomas, on the other hand, may undergo no change or even spontaneous resolution. Very large tumors may represent an indication for cesarean section, to avoid rupture or dystocia during vaginal delivery. After delivery, once the diagnosis has been confirmed by computed tomography or magnetic resonance imaging, surgical resection is indicated in cases of large tumors; if the tumor is small and the neonate is asymptomatic, no treatment is indicated.

Renal tumors

The most common renal mass identified sonographically during prenatal life is multicystic kidney; however, this space-occupying lesion cannot be considered as a true tumor, but rather as a cystic dysplasia resulting from arrest of the complex embryogenetic process, which, starting from the serial dichotomous branching of the ureteric bud, leads to formation of the tubules and consequent induction of nephron development.

The most common renal tumor developing during prenatal life is mesoblastic nephroma, also known as mesenchymal hamartoma. Although the tumor is not encapsulated, it is a benign neoplasm, which in very rare instances may show a malignant pattern. The sonographic appearance of mesoblastic nephroma is that of a solid mass in one of the upper quadrants of the fetal abdomen, replacing the normal kidney; cystic areas may occasionally be seen in the case of hemorrhage and consequent cystic degeneration.[29] 3D sonography allows evaluation of all three orthogonal planes of the tumor in detail and accurate estimation of the volume of the lesion.[30] The tumor may also appear as a diffuse enlargement of the kidney. Polyhydramnios is frequently associated. Possible mechanisms of the polyhydramnios are compression by the tumor of the gastrointestinal tract, and an increase in renal blood flow or impaired renal concentrating ability.

The differential diagnosis should include Wilms' tumor and other congenital tumors such as teratomas and rhabdoid tumors, as well as multicystic kidney. Although Wilms' tumor tends to have a well-defined capsule, it may be indistinguishable from mesoblastic nephroma. The appearance of the rhabdoid tumor is similar, but it is characterized by a rapid growth.[31] Multicystic kidney can be differentiated by its typical cystic appearance.

Tumors from adjacent organs such as the adrenal glands should be included in the differential diagnosis. The most common tumor of the adrenal glands is neuroblastoma, the sonographic appearance of which is not dissimilar from that of mesoblastic nephroma. However, a careful examination can allow recognition of the kidney compressed and displaced caudally by

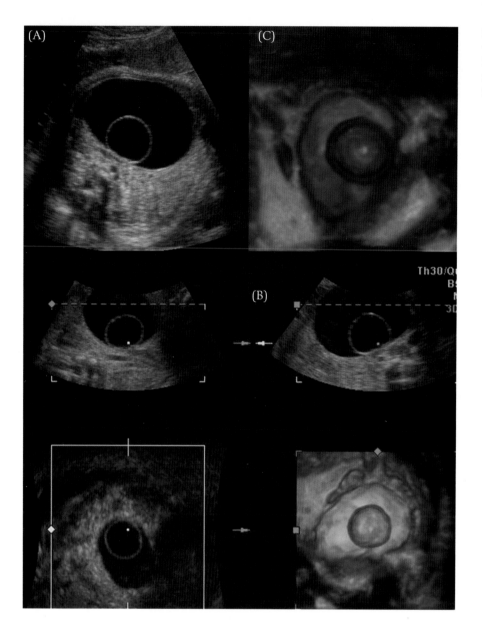

Figure 18.7 Fetal ovarian cyst with a daughter cyst inside: (A) 2D sonography; (B) 3D muliplanar view; (C) 3D surface rendering

the adrenal mass, which can also present a rich vascularization on color Doppler examination.[32] The differential diagnosis of adrenal neuroblastoma includes adrenal hemorrhage[33] and subdiaphragmatic extralobar pulmonary sequestration.[34]

The diagnosis of renal and adrenal tumors requires serial sonography to monitor the tumor growth and the onset of complications such as polyhydramnios. Surgical treatment can be planned in the neonatal period.

Intra-abdominal cysts

These may arise from different organs, and frequently a specific diagnosis cannot be made. Fetal ovarian cysts

are the most common intra-abdominal cysts detected in the prenatal period. This is not surprising when one considers that ovarian follicular cysts are found in about one-third of newborns at autopsy, although they are usually small and asymptomatic. Most fetal ovarian cysts are of follicular origin. Granulosa cell tumors, teratomas, and mesonephromas have been reported in the neonatal period, but are extremely rare in comparison with the cysts of Graafian origin. Fetal ovarian cysts are hormone-sensitive and usually develop in the late 2nd and 3rd trimesters of pregnancy, following completion of functional maturation of the fetal gonads.[35]

The sonographic diagnosis of a fetal ovarian cyst should be suspected when a well-defined cystic mass is detected in the lower abdomen of a female fetus with normally structured and functioning

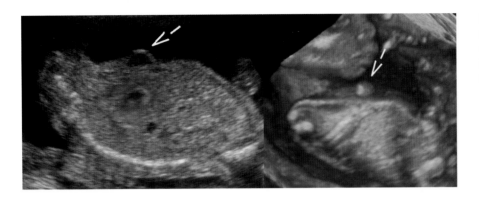

Figure 18.8 Small lymphangioma of the skin located on the anterior wall of the fetal thorax: (A) 2D sonography; (B) 3D surface rendering

intra-abdominal organs (Figure 18.7). Fetal ovarian cysts are of extremely variable size: up to 10 cm in diameter and more. They can be unilateral or, less frequently, bilateral; thin septa or daughter cysts may occasionally be seen inside the cystic structure. Sometimes, the cysts contain irregular echoes and debris. These are signs of complications in the cyst, such as torsion and hemorrhage, as confirmed by the occurrence of such findings during monitoring with serial sonography of cysts that were originally transonic. Association with polyhydramnios can be possible, perhaps as a consequence of intestinal compression by the mass.

The prognosis of fetal ovarian cysts is usually good. Simple uncomplicated cysts frequently undergo spontaneous resolution by the end of pregnancy or in the first few months of life, thus confirming their functional origin. Complicated cysts will need surgery after delivery, although spontaneous resolution in utero has been reported even in these cases. Very large cysts may cause dystocia; to prevent this complication, a cesarean section can be planned. An alternative approach is sonographically guided needle aspiration of the cyst.

Other cystic structures inside the fetal abdomen are urachal cysts, enteric duplication, duodenal atresia, bowel obstruction, hydrometrocolpos, and mesenteric and omental cysts. Urachal cysts are tubular in shape and extend from the bladder to the umbilicus. Enteric duplication tends to present a tubular more than a round shape. Duodenal atresia shows the typical double-bubble appearance with the 'cysts' located in the upper abdomen. Bowel obstruction shows multiple dilated loops and increased peristalsis. In hydrometrocolpos, the cyst is located on the middle pelvis between the bladder and the sacrum, and may present low-level echoes inside. Mesenteric and omental cysts or lymphangiomas are usually located in the middle area of the abdomen, but may be indistinguishable from those of ovarian origin.[36]

TUMORS OF THE SKIN

Tumors of the skin that can be detected prenatally by sonography are hemangiomas and related angiomatous malformations. These lesions may occur as isolated tumors, frequently located on the scalp, ear, eyelid, or extremities, or may be part of more complex syndromes, such as Klippel–Trenaunay–Weber syndrome (large cutaneous hemangiomas and hypertrophy of the related bones and soft tissues), Sturge–Weber syndrome (nevus flammeus of the face and angiomas of the meninges), and von Hippel–Lindau syndrome (angiomas of the retina and cerebellum). Sonographically, they appear as septated cystic areas on the fetal surface. 3D sonography is an excellent tool to demonstrate the extension of the lesions with the use of the surface rendering mode, even in the case of small lesions[37] (Figure 18.8).

REFERENCES

1. Meizner I. Perinatal oncology – the role of prenatal ultrasound diagnosis. Ultrasound Obstet Gynecol 2000; 16: 507–9.

2. Altmann RP, Randolph JG, Lilly JR. Sacrococcygeal teratoma: an American Accademy of Pediatrics Surgical Section survey. J Pediatr Surg 1974; 9: 389–95.

3. Roman AS, Monteagudo A, Timor-Tritsch I, Rebarber A. First trimester diagnosis of sacrococcygeal teratoma: the role of three-dimensional ultrasound. Ultrasound Obstet Gynecol 2004; 23: 612–14.

4. Bonilla-Musoles F, Machado LE, Raga F, Osborne NG, Bonila F Jr. Prenatal diagnosis of scarococcygeal teratomas by two- and three-dimensional ultrasound. Ultrasound Obstet Gynecol 2002; 19: 200–5.

5. Chih-Ping C, Jin-Chung S, Jon-Kway H, Wayseen W, Chin-Yuan T. Second trimester evaluation of fetal sacroccygeal teratoma using three-dimensional color

Doppler ultrasound and magnetic resonance imaging. Prenat Diagn 2003; 23: 602–3.

6. Graf JL, Albanese CT. Fetal sacrococcygeal teratoma. World J Surg 2003; 27: 84–6.

7. Paek BW, Jennings RW, Harrison MR. Radiofrequency ablation of human sacroccygeal teratoma. Am J Obstet Gynecol 2001; 184: 503–7.

8. Lam YH, Tang MHY, Shek TWH. Thermocoagulation of fetal sacrococcygeal teratoma. Prenat Diagn 2002; 22: 99–101.

9. D'Addario V, Pinto V, Meo F, Resta M. The specificity of ultrasound in the detection of fetal intracranial tumors. J Perinat Med 1998; 2: 480–5.

10. Schlembach D, Bornemann A, Rupprecht T, Beider E. Fetal intracranial tumors detected by ultrasound: a reprt of two cases and review of the literature. Ultrasound Obstet Gynecol 1999; 14: 407–18.

11. Bannister CM, Russel SA, Rimmer S, Mowle DH. Fetal arachnoid cysts: their site, progress, prognosis and differential diagnosis. Eur J Pediatr Surg 1999; 9(Suppl 1): 27–8.

12. Roodhoot AM, Delbeke L, Vaneerdeweg W. Cervical teratoma: prenatal detection and management in the neonate. Pediatr Surg Int 1987; 2: 181–4.

13. Azar G, Snijders RJM, Gosden CM, Nicolaides KH. Fetal nuchal cystic hygromata: associated malformations and chromosomal defects. Fetal Diagn Ther 1991; 6: 46–57.

14. Sepulveda W, Muhlhausen G, Flores X, Gutierrez J. Giant hemangiopericitoma of the fetal neck – prenatal two- and three-dimensional ultrasound. J Ultrasound Med 2003; 22: 831–5.

15. Yoshino K, Takeuchi M, Nakayama M, Suehara N. Congenital cervical rhabdomyosarcoma arising in one fetus of a twin pregnancy. Fetal Diagn Ther 2005; 20: 291–5.

16. Bouchard S, Johnson MP, Flake AW. The EXIT procedure: experience and outcome in 31 cases. J Pediatr Surg 2002; 37: 418–26.

17. Stocker T, Madewell J, Drake R. Congenital cystic adenomatoid malformation of the lung: classification and morphological spectrum. Hum Pathol 1975; 8: 155–66.

18. Adzick NS. The fetus with a cystic adenomatoid malformation. In: Harrison MR, Golbus MS, Filly RA, eds. The Unborn Patient. Philadelphia, PA: WB Saunders, 1990: 320–9.

19. Becmeur F, Horta-Geraud P, Donato L, Sauvage P. Pulmonary sequestrations: prenatal ultrasound diagnosis, treatment, and outcome. J Pediatr Surg 1998; 33: 492–6.

20. Ruano R, Benachi A, Aubry MC, Dumez Y, Dommergues M. Volume contrast imaging: a new approach to identify fetal thoracic structures. J Ultrasound Med 2004; 23: 403–8.

21. Adzick NS. Management of fetal lung lesions. Clin Perinatol 2003; 30: 481–92.

22. Nicolini U, Cerri V, Groli C, Poblete A, Mauro F. A new approach to prenatal treatment of extralobar pulmonary sequestration. Prenat Diagn 2000; 20: 758–60.

23. Tongson T, Sirichotiyakul S, Sittiwangkul R, Wanapirak C. Prenatal sonographic diagnosis of cardiac hemangioma with postnatal spontaneous regression. Ultrasound Obstet Gynecol 2004; 24: 207–8.

24. D'Addario V, Pinto V, Dinaro E, et al. Prenatal diagnosis and postnatal outcome of cardiac rhabdomyomas. J Perinat Med 2002; 30: 170–5.

25. Geipel A, Krapp U, Germer U, Becker R, Gembruch U. Perinatal diagnosis of cardiac tumors. Ultrasound Obstet Gynecol 2001; 17: 17–21.

26. Gembruch U, Baschat AA, Gloeckner-Hoffmann K, Gortners L, Germer U. Prenatal diagnosis and management of fetuses with liver hemangiomata. Ultrasound Obstet Gynecol 2002; 19: 454–60.

27. Bessho T, Kubota K, Komori S, et al. Prenatally detected hepatic amartoma: another cause of non-immune hydrops. Prenat Diagn 1996; 16: 337–41.

28. Kazzi NJ, Chang C, Roberts EC, Shankaran S. Fetal heatoblastoma presenting as non-immune hydrops. Am J Perinatol 1989; 6: 278–80.

29. Apuzio JJ, Unwin W, Adhate A, Nichols R. Prenatal diagnosis of fetal renal mesoblastic nephroma. Am J Obstet Gynecol 1986; 154: 636–7.

30. Schild RL, Plath H, Hofstaetter C, Hansmann M. Diagnosis of fetal mesoblastic nephroma by 3D-ultrasound. Ultrasound Obstet Gynecol 2000; 15: 533–6.

31. Fuchs IB, Henrich W, Kalache KD, Lippek F, Dudenhausen JW. Prenatal sonographic diagnosis of a rhabdoid tumor of the kidney. Ultrasound Obstet Gynecol 2004; 23: 407–10.

32. Jennings RW, La Quaglia MP, Leong K, Hendren WH, Adzik NS. Fetal neuroblastoma: prenatal diagnosis and natural hystory. J Pediatr Surg 1993; 28: 437–43.

33. Schwarzler P, Bennard JP, Sebat MV, Ville Y. Prenatal diagnosis of fetal adrenal masses: differentiation between hemorrage and solid tumor by color Doppler sonography. Ultrasound Obstet Gynecol 1999; 13: 351–5.

34. Curtis MR, Mooney DP, Vaccaro TJ, et al. Prenatal ultrasound characterization of the suprarenal mass: distinction between neuroblastoma and subdiphragmatic extralobar pulmonary sequestration. J Ultrasound Med 1997; 16: 272–8.

35. D'Addario V, Volpe G, Kurjak A, Lituania M, Zmijnac J. Ultrasonic diagnosis and perinatal management of complicated and uncomplicated fetal ovarian cysts: a collaborative study. J Perinat Med 1990; 18: 375–81.

36. Signorelli M, Cerri V, Groli C, et al. Cystic lymphangioma of the greater omentum and ascites: an unusual combination. Prenat Diagn 2004; 24: 746–7.

37. Hosli I, Holzgreve W, Danzer E, Tercanli S. Two case reports of rare fetal tumors: an indication for surface rendering? Ultrasound Obstet Gynecol 2001; 17: 522–6.

19 IUGR fetus studied by 3D and 4D sonography

Wiku Andonotopo, Asim Kurjak, and Radoslav Herman

INTRODUCTION

It is well known that intrauterine growth restriction (IUGR) can lead to significant fetal or neonatal complications. A number of studies have reported a 5–27% incidence of congenital abnormalities associated with IUGR, as compared with a 0.1–4% anomaly rate in control groups of normally grown neonates.[1] The incidence of chromosomal abnormalities in IUGR infants is 4–5 times that of appropriate-for-gestational-age (AGA) infants (2% vs 0.4%); and intrauterine infection, especially cytomegalovirus, has been reported in 0.3–3.5% of IUGR infants.[1] In addition, growth-restricted infants have up to an 8–10-fold increase in stillbirth and neonatal mortality.[1] This, in part, is due to a higher incidence of hypoxia, asphyxia, meconium aspiration, and a generally poorer ability to tolerate labor with IUGR.[1] Other developmental problems such as necrotizing enterocolitis, intraventricular hemorrhage (IVH), and neonatal encephalopathy, can also be related to IUGR. Those infants who survive the immediate perinatal period are still at risk for hypothermia, hypoglycemia, polycythemia, and other complications.[1,2] Animal studies have also shown an increased risk for cardiovascular and renal problems later in life.[3]

IUGR results mostly from chronic placental insufficiency, and IUGR fetuses are recognized by the occurrence of umbilical artery Doppler aberrations, frequently associated with the reduced amniotic fluid index. Abnormal small-for-gestational-age (SGA) fetuses are individuals with abnormal constitution on comprehensive ultrasound scan, abnormal chromosomes on karyotyping, or confirmation of genetic syndrome or fetal diseases. Normal SGA fetuses are those documented by a negative screening for abnormal structure and chromosomes, fetal diseases, and genetic syndromes, and by a normal umbilical artery Doppler examination and a normal amniotic fluid volume.[4]

IUGR fetuses are connected with high rates of low ponderal indices at birth, hypoglycemia, and admittances to nurseries.[4,5] Many babies are simply genetically small and are otherwise normal.[5] Some women have a tendency to have constitutionally small babies. Although both parents' genes affect childhood growth and final adult size, maternal genes mainly influence birthweight.[6] Parity, age, and socioeconomic status are intercorrelated, and may also influence the pregnancy and the infant's birthweight. There is no basis for the recommendation that monitoring at more regular intervals would diminish perinatal morbidity in this group of fetuses,[7] with outpatient monitoring being a safe alternative.[8]

CONSEQUENCES OF IUGR

According to some data, severely IUGR fetuses suffer from intellectual impairment in the long term, particularly if neonatal management is less than adequate.[4] Consequently, it is essential to recognize these fetuses – and the earlier in fetal life, the better. Kurjak et al[9] illustrated two different patterns of IUGR that may be of significance for the short- and long-term prognosis of the fetus using antenatal ultrasonic assessment by measurement of fetal dimensions. They concluded that the late IUGR pattern is frequently associated with conditions that cause reduced placental perfusion, such as hypertension. A typical wasted look and low weight for height is the main characteristic of this group.[9] In these fetuses, there is a predisposition to perinatal asphyxia and the Apgar score is low, with an increased brain-to-liver ratio. This type is probably the result of uteroplacental vascular insufficiency.[9,10] The symmetric IUGR pattern, which occurs in 20% of SGA fetuses, results from prolonged growth impairment beginning early in the 2nd trimester, even from 18 weeks. There is a proportionate reduction in the fetal head, body length, and body weight, but growth does not generally stop. This type is not typically linked with hypertension or intrapartum asphyxia. Such growth failure has been realized in experimental animals by restriction of the mother's protein or calorie intake.[11] Some of these fetuses have genetic or chromosomal abnormalities and could be examples of reduced growth potential. Long-term follow-up of these fetuses has shown that prolonged IUGR causes stunting of growth in childhood and most likely up to adulthood, and a considerably reduced general development proportion.[9]

In infancy, low birthweight is associated with childhood mortality from causes including infectious diseases and congenital anomalies, such as central nervous system and cardiovascular anomalies.[12,13] Numerous adult cardiovascular diseases, including coronary heart disease, hypertension, type II diabetes mellitus, dyslipidemia, and stroke, have been linked with low birthweight;[14] the evidence for the link between risk of coronary heart disease and IUGR comes from the fact that it is independent of gestational age.[15] SGA is connected with major psychiatric sequelae in later years. Birthweight less than 3 kg is linked with an increased risk of depression at age 26 years and over, in women but not in men.[16] SGA is also connected with an increased risk of suicide and suicide attempts in later life.[17]

IUGR AS AN ANTENATAL RISK FACTOR FOR CEREBRAL PALSY

IUGR entails an increased risk of neonatal morbidity and mortality and also seems to affect brain development.[18,19] Some specific alterations in the brains of IUGR infants, including restriction of the volume of gray matter, a reduced amount of total DNA in glial cells and neurons, and changes in cerebral hemodynamics, have been reported.[20] This is also supported by animal studies showing the reduced oxygen delivery to the brain and restricted growth of the forebrain

and cerebellum.[21] Therefore, IUGR has been hypothesized to be related to brain injury and cerebral palsy (CP). A 'brain-sparing mechanism' has been suggested to prevent or reduce the severity of brain injury in growth-restricted children.[22] Several mechanisms have been suggested for the relation between IUGR in term babies and CP. The abnormal growth might play a direct role in causing CP or in utero brain injury, and could trigger abnormal growth. Alternatively, a separate process, such as placental insufficiency, could cause both the growth retardation and brain injury.

There are several concepts of IUGR, and information on true IUGR is often missing from retrospective studies. The most common proxy for IUGR is SGA, often defined as smaller than 2 standard deviations from the mean birthweight or from intrauterine growth curves based on ultrasonically estimated fetal weights.[23] However, SGA is a heterogeneous category, including not only growth-restricted infants but also infants with chromosomal abnormalities, and small healthy infants as well. There are at least three ways to obtain information on true intrauterine growth restriction: (1) by serial ultrasound estimates during pregnancies in which a decreased growth is detected; (2) by anthropometric measures postnatally; and (3) by using individualized or customized growth standards.

Some studies have found a dose–response-like relationship between SGA and CP in term infants.[24] No such clear association has been found in preterm infants,[24] but there are some indications of a similar relationship between SGA and CP in two large preterm studies.[25] No data are available for true IUGR, but preliminary data from a Swedish study that used Gardosi's customized percentiles to the full extent indicate such an association between children born at term with a history of IUGR and CP.[26] As described by Jacobsson et al,[26] children with severe IUGR at term have an 8-fold higher risk of CP. In contrast, preterm infants suffering from IUGR were not at risk. These findings highlight the need for close antenatal monitoring of fetal growth.[26]

FETAL WEIGHT ESTIMATION BY 3D SONOGRAPHY

Fetal growth is a complex developmental process that involves anatomic changes over time. IUGR and macrosomia are usually identified from sonographic measurements of one or more anatomic parameters.

For many years, fetal weight has been assessed by taking a combination of standard two-dimensional (2D) measurements that are all related to three anatomic sites: the fetal head, the fetal abdomen, and the femur. However, none of the established formulae,[27,28] considers soft tissue thickness, despite evidence that abnormal tissue content may be a reliable indicator of fetal growth aberrations.[29] Such aberrations may not be detected if soft tissue abnormalities are the earliest manifestation of pathologic growth unless these measurements are sensitive to subtle changes in muscle or fat. Relatively few measurements, such as those from the fetal thigh[30,31] and abdomen, have been evaluated for the prenatal assessment of soft tissue mass.[31,32]

As 2D measurements cannot precisely assess 3D body dimensions, it is reasonable to further investigate the role of 3D volumetry of different parts of the fetal body.[33] Diagnosis of fetal growth restriction due to placental insufficiency and fetal malnutrition depends mainly on measurement of the fetal abdominal circumference, which is predominantly affected by fetal liver size. Therefore, direct measurements of fetal liver size may enhance the early detection of the fetus at risk of growth restriction. Many efforts have been made to assess fetal liver dimensions directly. It was suggested that the measurement of fetal liver volume has the potential to contribute to early assessment of fetal growth.[34] 3D sonography has been proposed for accurate determination of fetal organ volume.[35] Recently, it has been recommended that 3D instead of 2D sonography should be used for reaching an accurate assessment of fetal liver volume.[36]

3D sonography can provide more accurate and precise volume measurements of small, irregular objects.[37,38] Volume measurements by conventional sonography can be technically difficult if the organ does not conform to a regular geometric shape.

Several investigators have used 3D sonography to demonstrate a significant correlation between fetal limb volume and birthweight.[39,40] Unfortunately, the application of this technique has been limited by the excessive time required for making volume measurements.[41] Furthermore, acoustic shadowing near the joints can hinder accurate assessment of soft tissue borders, which is necessary for reliable volume calculations. Most weight prediction models, however, have not emphasized the relationship of soft tissue changes to fetal weight. Thigh volume is a new soft tissue parameter that addresses these technical limitations. This parameter is easily acquired and rapidly

measured, and is reproducible among blinded observers.[42] A useful thigh volume parameter should also be capable of detecting soft tissue changes during pregnancy. Measurements from an individual fetus are usually compared with those from other pregnancies by referring to a population-based nomogram. Accurate and precise fetal weight predictions using thigh volume have been reported during the late 2nd and early 3rd trimesters of pregnancy. This new parameter may allow earlier detection and improved monitoring of fetal soft tissue abnormalities such as IUGR.[31]

Liver volume measurement

Early detection of fetal growth restriction is important because this condition carries a risk for the fetus. At present, the best sonographic predictor of fetal growth restriction is measurement of the abdominal circumference. The fetal liver comprises most of the abdomen measured by the abdominal circumference. In normal fetuses, glycogen reserves in the liver increase towards the end of gestation. However, growth-restricted fetuses have severely reduced hepatic glycogen stores because of fetal malnutrition. Reduction of liver weight in the growth-restricted fetus is more profound than reduction of brain weight. This is due to the so-called 'brain-sparing effect', so often observed in growth restriction caused by uteroplacental insufficiency.[43]

Consequently, accurate assessment of liver size may contribute to the early detection of the growth-restricted fetus. The development of 3D sonography has introduced a new and accurate means of volume measurement, which is fast and easy to perform and has high patient acceptability (Figure 19.1).[34]

Thigh volume measurement

Although fetal limb volume has been proposed to be associated with fetal growth and nutrition,[30] many researchers have attempted to use limb circumference to predict fetal weight with unsatisfactory results. With the erroneous assumption that the fetal thigh is a cylinder,[30] or using the thigh circumference indirectly to replace the real thigh volume, inaccurate results are to be expected. With the advent of 3D sonography, Chang et al[39] showed its primary use in obstetrics. In addition, the accuracy of 3D sonography

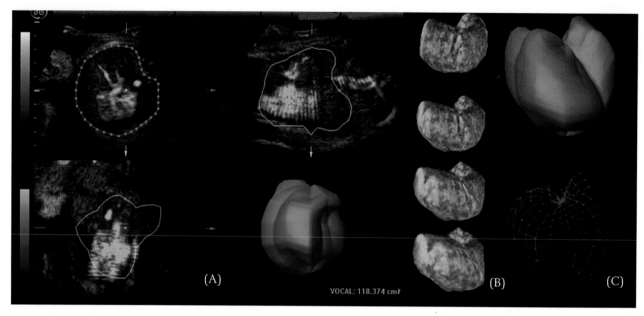

VOCAL: 118.374 cm³

Figure 19.1 (A) 3D volume calculation of fetal liver using VOCAL software. (B) Surface rendering image of fetal liver. (C) Reconstruction of fetal liver using VOCAL software

in volumetry has been validated extensively in many organ systems, either in vitro or in vivo. Riccabona et al[38] concluded that 3D sonography provides accurate volume measurements of regular and irregular objects and can offer improved accuracy compared with 2D methods. Hence, the accurate assessment of limb volume becomes feasible using 3D sonographic volumetry. In a previous study by Liang et al,[44] they showed that fetal upper-arm volume assessed by 3D sonography can achieve satisfactory results in birth weight prediction. Chang et al[39] conducted a prospective study to correlate the 3D sonographically assessed thigh volume with the actual birthweight and to compare its accuracy in predicting birthweight with that of the traditional weight-estimating formulae using 2D techniques. They concluded that the thigh-volume formula is valid at least for the low-for-gestational-age (LGA) and SGA categories, with the birthweight ranging from 1194 to 4425 g in the formula-generating group and from 2310 to 4110 g in the validation group. However, further studies with more SGA and LGA cases are needed to confirm this point. There are several disadvantages of 3D thigh volumetry. For instance, 3D sonography is relatively expensive and is not available in many centers. The thigh-volume assessment is relatively sophisticated, meticulous, and time-consuming compared with that using 2D sonography. In the future, computer-assisted programs for automatic volumetry will be more objec-

tive than is possible manually (Figure 19.2). Nevertheless, 3D sonographic assessment of thigh volume can accurately predict fetal weight and deserves a large-scale prospective study.[45] Fetuses that weigh at the extremes (i.e., <2500 g and >4000 g) are very important in clinical practice.[45]

3D ASSESSMENT OF HOURLY URINARY PRODUCTION RATE

Sonographic measurement of fetal urinary flow is an indirect method of assessing fetal urinary production to clinically assess fetal behavior and well-being in both normal and abnormal pregnancies.[46,47] However, the methods used for evaluating fetal urinary flow are controversial as they continue to evolve. The reliability of the method is of utmost concern because there is no direct method of assessing fetal renal function. Above all, fetal micturition behavior is poorly understood; its study is undergoing its own evolutionary process. The human urinary bladder was one of the first fetal organs to be readily visualized when sonography was used in a clinical setting.

Campbell et al[48] were the first to describe visualization of the human fetal bladder and estimate fetal urinary flow rates using static longitudinal and transverse images from a compound B-scan sonogram. This technique was the first glimpse of human fetal urinary

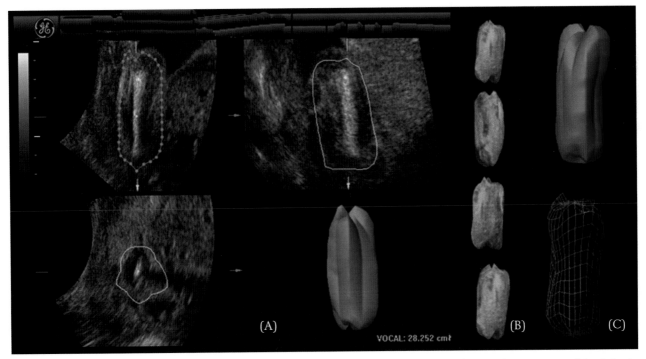

Figure 19.2 (A) 3D volume calculation of fetal thigh using VOCAL software. (B) Surface rendering image of fetal thigh. (C) Reconstruction of fetal thigh using VOCAL software

flow and micturition behavior. They felt that a non-invasive method of assessing fetal urinary function would increase our understanding of fetal physiology and its response to medical conditions affecting pregnancy.

A change in the hourly fetal urinary production rate (HFUPR) has been demonstrated in pregnancies when the fetuses are subjected to hypoxia.[49] Nevertheless, the normal HFUPR is low for premature fetuses[50] and even lower when the fetus is growth-restricted.[51] However, at present, this estimation is plagued with methodologic problems. Methods with high measurement precision are therefore mandatory in order to detect these small changes in HFUPR in complicated pregnancies.

Because of the difficulty in performing serial, shorter-interval compound B-scans, Campbell et al[48] measured the sonographic images every 15 and 30 minutes and established a cross-sectional study of predicted HFUPR for each week of gestation from 32 to 41 weeks. Using 2D real-time sonography 8 years later, Kurjak et al[46] measured these images every 30 minutes with the same method described earlier by Campbell et al.[48]

Conventionally, calculation of the HFUPR is based on repeated 2D sonograms of the bladder during the filling phase. Volumes are calculated by using the diameters of the longitudinal and transverse bladder images and the formula for ellipsoids.[47] Two assumptions are made. The first is that the bladder has an ellipsoidal shape. However, the bladder shape changes from ellipsoidal to superellipsoidal (almost cylindrical) during the filling phase, which could result in an underestimate of the bladder volume and the HFUPR. The second assumption is that the urinary bladder has rotational symmetry, which was supported in a previous study in which the diameters in the transverse section were shown to be equal.[52] This means that only longitudinal bladder images are needed for volume calculation. Human fetal urinary production in normal and complicated pregnancies has been investigated.[46,48] Previous studies of urinary production rate during the last two decades have shown very different results, ranging from 2.2 ml/h at 22 weeks of gestation to 26.3 ml/h at 40 weeks.[46] Only a few papers have thoroughly evaluated potential human and technical sources of inaccuracy when carrying out such measurements.[52] In principle, there are two different and incoherent varieties of measurement error: (1) imprecision due to the selection of an unsuitable image, and (2) imprecision due to inaccuracy when measuring on the selected image.[52]

We have examined the accuracy of 3D sonographically obtained fetal bladder volume predictions under

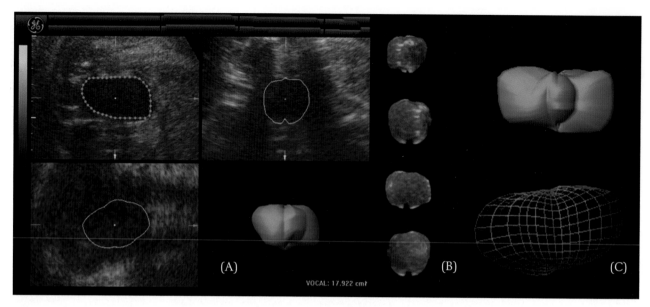

VOCAL: 17.922 cm³

Figure 19.3 (A) 3D imaging of bladder volume for HFUPR calculation using VOCAL software. (B) Surface rendering image of fetal bladder. (C) Reconstruction of fetal bladder using VOCAL software

conditions similar to a clinical setting. A simpler but equally accurate method was suggested requiring fewer measurements, which translated to a shorter observation time for the fetal micturition behavior. Using the 3D sonographic technique, a longitudinal bladder image without disturbing shadows and at its largest appearance was first visualized using tissue harmonic imaging, which yields a clear contrast between adjacent tissue structures (Figure 19.3). These advantages of 3D sonography overcome the inaccuracy of conventional 2D sonographic assessment of fetal bladder volume. In the sectional plane mode, three orthogonal planes were simultaneously displayed on the screen. Once the scan was completed, the volume data were stored on the internal hard drive of the system.

OBJECTIVE GOALS OF FETAL NEUROBEHAVIORAL ASSESSMENT

Clinical fetal assessment is oriented toward identifying markers of fetal distress to detect conditions that threaten pregnancy outcome and are amenable to obstetric intervention, thereby optimizing outcome.[53] As such, it requires designation of performance criteria that can successfully distinguish between outcomes in order to inform management decisions. The current focus of antenatal neurobehavioral assessment is different in that its goal is to gather information that reveals neural continuity from fetus to child. Such knowledge can provide basic scientific information regarding normal human ontogeny and identify antenatal factors that influence the trajectory of development. Thus, neurobehavioral assessment measures performance along a continuum so as to distinguish among individuals within as well as beyond the normal range. The ultimate clinical application of fetal neurobehavioral assessment will be to identify functional characteristics of the fetus that predict a range of subsequent developmental dysfunction. Establishing this link will require demonstration of positive and negative predictability to outcomes significantly beyond the immediate perinatal period. Many clinical fetal assessment tools, such as the biophysical profile, non-stress test,[54] and fetal movement counting, rely on aspects of fetal neurobehavior. Indeed, much of the existing knowledge about fetal neurobehavioral development has its origins in obstetric research. Despite this overlap, determining the precursors of perinatal mortality and morbidity is among a circumscribed subset of the broader goals of fetal neurobehavioral assessment.

4D SONOGRAPHY FOR FETAL BEHAVIORAL ASSESSMENT

Over the last few years, ultrasound techniques have enabled direct visualization of the fetus in utero, as well as real-time assessment of fetal activity, and have provided dynamic information arising from fetal motion.[55] Analysis of the dynamics of fetal behavior in comparison with morphologic studies has led to the conclusion that fetal behavioral patterns directly reflect developmental and maturational processes of the fetal central nervous system (CNS).[56–58] Therefore, it was suggested that the assessment of fetal behavior and developmental processes in different periods of gestation[59] may allow a distinction between normal and abnormal brain development, as well as early diagnosis of various structural or functional abnormalities.[60]

4D sonography enables continuous monitoring of the fetal face and other surface features of the fetus, such as fetal extremities. This permits exciting new possibilities for the study of fetal behavior. 4D sonography provides a tool for observation of the fetal face. Simultaneous imaging of complex facial movements was not possible using real-time 2D sonography. 4D sonography integrates the advantage of the spatial imaging of the fetal face with the addition of time. Therefore, this new technology allows the appearance and duration of each facial movement and expression to be determined and measured.[61,62]

4D sonography enables visualization of more details regarding the dynamics of small anatomic structures. Therefore, body and limb movements can be visualized a week earlier than with 2D.[56] 4D sonography can enhance the fetal–maternal bond by showing real-time fetal movements to the mother. There is no question that visualization of fetal movements confirms viability to parents. It should be emphasized that image quality and rendering speed will continuously increase.[61] It is to be expected that this ultrasound modality will significantly impact on quality assessment of fetal intrauterine activity.[59]

In a relatively short period of time, 4D sonography has stimulated multicenter studies of fetal behavior and even fetal awareness, with more convincing imaging and data than those obtained by conventional ultrasound and non-ultrasound methods.[63] The visualization of fetal activity in utero by 4D sonography could allow a more precise distinction between normal and abnormal behavioral patterns and could make possible the early recognition of fetal brain impairment.[64]

COMBINATION OF MORPHOLOGIC AND DYNAMIC ASSESSMENT

Fetal organ volumetry by 3D sonography has already been introduced into clinical practice. Several studies support the superior role of 3D sonography in estimating fetal weight close to delivery. The idea of direct fetal organ volumetry compares favorably with other techniques using 2D measurements, since the fetal organ is not a perfect cylinder, nor can fetal organ circumference replace the real fetal organ volume. Estimating fetal weight by 3D sonography is a more time-consuming process than using standard 2D methods, but the extra time spent on measuring volumes is justified in cases in which accurate weight determination is of importance.[33]

A change in HFUPR has been demonstrated in pregnancies when the fetuses are subjected to hypoxia.[46] Takeuchi et al[51] had proved that the normal HFUPR is low for premature fetuses and even lower when the fetus is growth-restricted. Therefore, methods with high measurement precision are mandatory in order to detect these dynamic changes in HFUPR in complicated pregnancies.

The possibility of studying fetal motor behavior by 4D sonography has provoked research on its potential application for better assessment of prenatal neurologic conditions. Some recent studies have investigated whether the quality or the quantity of fetal movements correlated with other clinical variables during complicated pregnancies, and whether they provided prognostic information for the neurologic outcome.[59,62,64] The quality of fetal movements appeared to be strongly correlated with parameters of fetal clinical condition in individual cases and fullfilled several prerequisites for serving as a reliable diagnostic tool for prediction of the fetal condition and for assessment of the integration of the CNS.[65]

The concept of combining assessment of fetal growth with morphologic examination of volumetric measurements and fetal motor behavior in the management of high-risk patients is new. The clinical spectrum of IUGR is wide, in both presentation and progression. Gestational age, differential fetal maturation, maternal condition, and therapeutic interventions modulate the presentation and manifestation of fetal disease in various testing modalities. Therefore, no single test provides well-validated cut-offs to accurately depict fetal status in IUGR. If acute intervention is not mandated, the timeframe for ongoing surveillance can be tailored based on the severity of the condition. This may include transfer to a referral center with the highest level of perinatal care, admission for daily inpatient monitoring, and administration of steroids in anticipation of preterm delivery.[66] The goal of comprehensive fetal assessment tailored to the condition can be achieved using widely available technology.

MORPHOLOGIC AND DYNAMIC ASSESSMENT OF FETAL GROWTH RESTRICTION BY 3D AND 4D SONOGRAPHY

Methodology and sampling characteristics

A prospective study was conducted in 50 uncomplicated healthy women with reliably dated pregnancies as a control group with AGA fetuses of gestational age 210–280 days (30–40 weeks). The study group consisted of 50 pregnant women with IUGR fetus identified by abnormal 2D B-mode biometric measurements or abnormal 2D color Doppler hemodynamics in the 3rd trimester of pregnancy (gestational age 210–280 days (30–40 weeks)). The same 3D and 4D recording procedures were performed at one time, and the gestational age at the time of the recording was matched to that of the study group. The duration of the 4D recordings was 30 minutes in all groups.

Pregnancy outcome and neonatal follow-up were obtained in all cases from review of patient records. Adverse neonatal outcome included admission to the neonatal intermediate care unit for indications other than low weight alone, i.e., hypoglycemia, hypocalcemia, respiratory distress requiring ventilatory support for more than 24 hours, intraventricular hemorrhage, need for total parenteral nutrition, sepsis, disseminated intravascular coagulation, or generalized hypotonia. Absence of the above criteria defined good outcome.

Fetal liver volume measurement

Assessment of fetal liver volume by 3D sonography was based on the method described by Laudy et al[34] (Figure 19.1). For the fetal liver volume measurement, a transverse cross-section of the liver immediately anterior to the stomach was positioned on the screen as a reference measurement was completed (Figure 19.1). The next step was to calculate the surface geometry of the liver by rotating the transverse plane around the vertical axis and defining 2D liver contours on each plane. The liver was traced manually from its upper limit at the diaphragm to its distal rim as the lower limit. These two landmarks were visualized in each of six planes obtained by counterclockwise rotation of the liver via the vertical axis. The 2D

contours were defined manually, and a rotation step of 30° was arbitrarily chosen. A 3D volume model of the liver was generated and reviewed for possible inconsistencies (Figure 19.1). The liver volume was calculated after all contours were considered to be adequately traced.

Fetal thigh volume measurement

Assessment of fetal thigh volume by 3D sonography was based on the method described by Chang et al[41] (Figure 19.2). The transducer was placed to display the femur closer to the transducer while the fetus was at rest in the traditional plane for measuring the femur length. Care was taken that the whole contour of the thigh could be clearly seen on the screen. This demonstrated the area of interest, with the size of the volume box adjusted accordingly. Each scan sweep took approximately 8 seconds, and volume data were stored on removable digital media for subsequent analysis. Thigh volume values were obtained by a sagittal sweep that included both ends of the femoral diaphysis (Figure 19.2). A fast sweep speed was selected to avoid motion artifacts. The rendered volume was displayed in three orthogonal planes on the screen and subsequently stored on a magneto-optic disk for later analysis. After retrieval from storage, the dataset was rotated to standard anatomic orientations with the sagittal, transverse, and frontal views positioned in upper left, upper right, and lower left planes, respectively. For final review, the area of interest was rotated into the optimal position. Subsequent volume measurements were performed with the femur in the longitudinal plane as a reference measurement. This plane was rotated around the z-axis until the proximal diaphysis of the femur was up and the distal diaphysis was down. Starting from the upper to the lower end of the femoral shaft, the contour of the thigh was outlined with a cursor and stored. The 2D contouring procedure was repeated manually whenever the shape of the thigh changed. A rotation step of 30° was arbitrarily chosen. Area tracing was carefully performed until completion of a 180° rotation. The built-in computer calculated the 3D volume of the thigh automatically by integrating the area and thickness of each slice (Figure 19.2).

Fetal hourly urinary production rate

Fetal urinary production rate may be used as a non-invasive test of fetal well-being.[47] However, at present

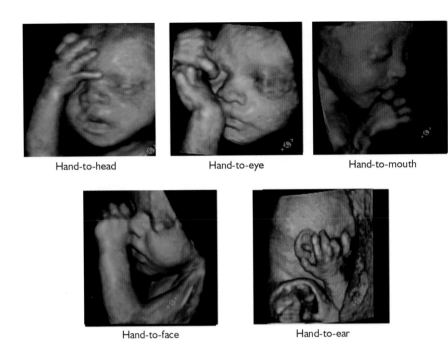

Hand-to-head   Hand-to-eye   Hand-to-mouth

Hand-to-face   Hand-to-ear

Figure 19.4 The visualization of hand movement directions by 3D surface rendering used in our study

there are methodologic problems with this estimation.[52] Fetal urinary production can be calculated using serial ultrasound registrations of bladder volume during the filling phase. The product of three orthogonal bladder diameters estimated by longitudinal and transverse scans is directly proportional to the volume.[48] Healthy fetuses have a small urinary production rate range, which increases with fetal age.[46,48] Nevertheless, SGA fetuses and fetuses with hypoxemia display a reduced urinary production rate.[46]

For the fetal bladder volume calculation, we preferred to select the longitudinal plane as a reference. The next step was to calculate the surface geometry of the bladder by rotating the longitudinal plane around the vertical axis and defining 2D bladder contours on each plane. The 2D contours were defined manually, and the rotation step for each contour plane was selected with an angle ranging to 30°. A 3D volume model of the bladder was generated and reviewed for possible inconsistencies. The bladder was then measured by a single observer at each increment with electronic calipers after 30 minutes and after 1 hour to obtain the hourly urinary production rate. Bladder volume was calculated after all contours were considered to be adequately traced (Figure 19.3).

4D sonographic parameters of fetal behavioral patterns

We have recently published normal standards for fetal neurodevelopmental parameters.[62] These establish reference ranges with gestational age for suggested fetal behavioral parameters in 100 normal singleton pregnancies. Standard of movement pattern and facial expression pattern curves are constructed through all trimesters of pregnancy.[62] We analyzed parameters of fetal movement and facial expression by transabdominal 4D sonography from the 2nd to the 3rd trimester. From the preliminary reports, it was obvious that the study of fetal behavior should be standardized as much as possible. An objective analysis with strict application techniques and the use of valid reference ranges appropriate for the gestational age are essential. Without these, comparisons with previous or future measurements of patients and studies cannot be made.[62]

We have focused on observation of fetal behavior in a study group and compare it with that in a control group. We analyzed quantitatively 14 parameters of fetal movements and facial expressions on 30 minutes' observation by 4D sonography (Figures 19.4–19.6). The definitions of the types of analyzed movement pattern and facial expressions focused upon in this study were given by Prechtl[67] and de Vries et al.[68] Pregnant women were asked not to eat within 2 hours before the beginning of the investigation.

We have presented a modification of the qualitative scoring system for the single aspects of head and hand movement pattern (Table 19.1).[69] Five criteria dealing with amplitude, speed, movement character, fluency and elegance, and onset and offset of movements are given a score of 2 for every optimal aspect, while the

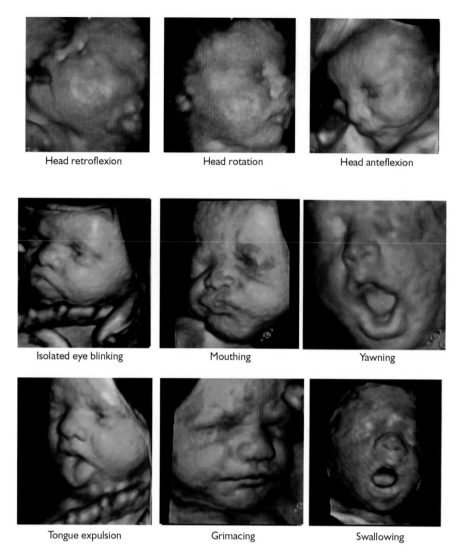

Head retroflexion   Head rotation   Head anteflexion

Figure 19.5 The visualization of head movement pattern by 3D surface rendering used in our study

Isolated eye blinking   Mouthing   Yawning

Tongue expulsion   Grimacing   Swallowing

Figure 19.6 The visualization of fetal facial expression patterns by 3D surface rendering used in our study

non-optimal aspects are given a score of 1. Therefore, the optimal score ranges from a maximum of 10 to a minimum of 5 points. Normal movements are defined as synchronized movements showing fluency and elegance and creating an impression of complexity and variability. Three categories of abnormal movements are distinguished: (1) *poor repertoire* – the sequence of successive components is monotonous and movements do not occur in the complex manner observed in normal movements; (2) *cramped–synchronized* – movements look rigid and lack the normal smooth and fluent character; limb and muscles contract and relax almost simultaneously; (3) *chaotic* – movements look chaotic in their sequence with neither fluency nor smoothness; they consistently appear to be abrupt.[69]

Variables of maternal and fetal characteristics, including gestational age, fetal movement patterns, and fetal facial expression patterns, were included in the construction of the behavioral parametric charts from data obtained from these pregnancy groups.

Results

3D volumetric measurements

Technically adequate 3D volumetric measurements were obtained in both groups (Table 19.2). 3D volumetric measurements of liver volume (LV) were taken using the method described by Laudy et al.[34] A statistically significant increase in normal fetal LV was found with advancing gestational age (GA) ($p < 0.05$), (Figure 19.7A) and with increasing estimated fetal weight (EFW) ($p < 0.05$, Figure 19.7B). The relationship between LV and GA is defined by the regression equation

$$LV = -108.18 + 5.97 \, GA \qquad (r = 0.82)$$

Table 19.1 Modification of scoring system for analysis of head and hand movement quality[69]

Type of quality analysis	Score	Description
Amplitude	1	Predominantly small range
	1	Predominantly large range
	1	Small and large, no intermediate range
	2	Variable in full range
Speed	1	Monotonously slow
	1	Monotonously fast
	1	Slow and fast, no intermediate
	1	Invariable
	2	Variable
Movement character	1	Cramped
	1	Floppy
	1	Flapping
	1	Tremulous
	1	Poor repertoire
	2	Variable and complex
Fluency and elegance	1	Not fluent, no rotations
	1	Not fluent, few rotations
	2	Fluent and elegant, many rotations
Onset–offset of movements	1	Abrupt
	1	Minimal fluctuations in intensity
	2	Smooth crescendo and decrescendo

Global evaluation	• Normal (synchronized movements of head and head)
	 • Abnormal:
	   – Poor repertoire of movements
	   – Cramped–synchronized movements
	   – Chaotic movements
		Optimal score: maximum 10

and the relationship between LV and EFW by the equation

$$LV = 12.89 + 0.03 \text{ EFW} \qquad (r = 0.98)$$

The thigh volume (TV) measurements were obtained by 3D sonography using the technique described by Chang et al.[41] A linear relationship was found between GA and TV (Figure 19.7C). The optimal model for TV is

$$TV = -185.54 + 7.39 \text{ GA} \qquad (r = 0.82; \ p <0.05)$$

The relationship between TV and EFW (Figure 19.7D) was given by

$$TV = -35.66 + 0.04 \text{ EFW} \qquad (r = 0.97; \ p <0.05)$$

The correlation coefficient of TV with GA was almost equal to that of LV with GA ($r = 0.82$).

Abnormal liver/thigh volume ratio was defined as a ratio greater than the 90th percentile in the normal group. However, the results of liver/thigh volume ratio analysis were not used for patient management. The normal fetal liver/thigh volume ratio demonstrated a significant decrease with advancing gestational age ($r = 0.83$; $p <0.05$) (Figure 19.7E). We found that the ratio of liver to thigh volume is normally about 1.3 : 1, but in the presence of fetal growth restriction, this ratio was increased to 1.8 : 1 or more during the 3rd trimester of pregnancy. In this study, the fetal liver/thigh volume ratio was plotted above the 90th percentile in 49 of 50 (98%) IUGR fetuses.

3D sonographic measurement of fetal urinary production

We reassessed the urinary production rate in normal fetuses from different gestational ages in comparison

Table 19.2 Comparison between 3D volumetric measurements in the two groups

	Normal group			IUGR group			Significance
	25th centile	Median	75th centile	25th centile	Median	75th centile	(p)
Gestational age at examination (weeks)	37	38.1	40.2	37.2	38.1	39.4	0.73 (NS)
Estimated fetal weight (g)	2850	3246	3400	2000	2400	2600	<0.05
Liver volume (ml)	110	119.6	130	78.5	88	100	<0.05
Thigh volume (ml)	82.5	96.5	110.5	40	52.6	65	<0.05
Liver/thigh volume ratio	1.2	1.3	1.3	1.5	1.8	1.9	<0.05
HFUPR[a] (ml/h)	42	47.6	52	36.5	38.3	42	<0.05

[a]Hourly fetal urinary production rate

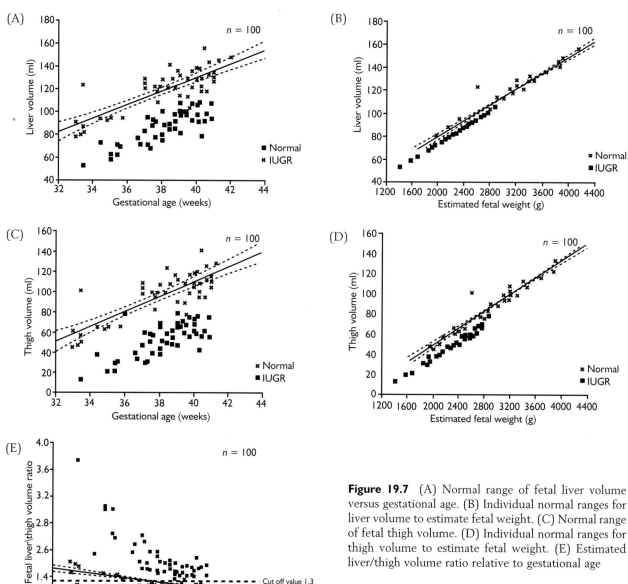

Figure 19.7 (A) Normal range of fetal liver volume versus gestational age. (B) Individual normal ranges for liver volume to estimate fetal weight. (C) Normal range of fetal thigh volume. (D) Individual normal ranges for thigh volume to estimate fetal weight. (E) Estimated liver/thigh volume ratio relative to gestational age

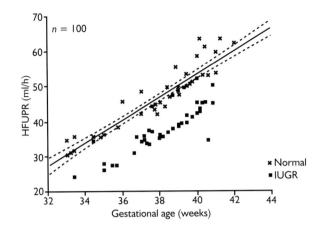

Figure 19.8 Relationship between gestational age and hourly fetal urinary production rate (HFUPR)

Figure 19.9 Scatterplot and multiple regression analysis of the 3rd-trimester frequency of hand movement patterns versus gestational age in the formula-generating group: (A) hand-to-head pattern; (B) hand-to-mouth pattern; (C) hand-to-eye pattern; (D) hand-to-face pattern; (D) hand-to-face pattern; (E) hand-to-ear pattern

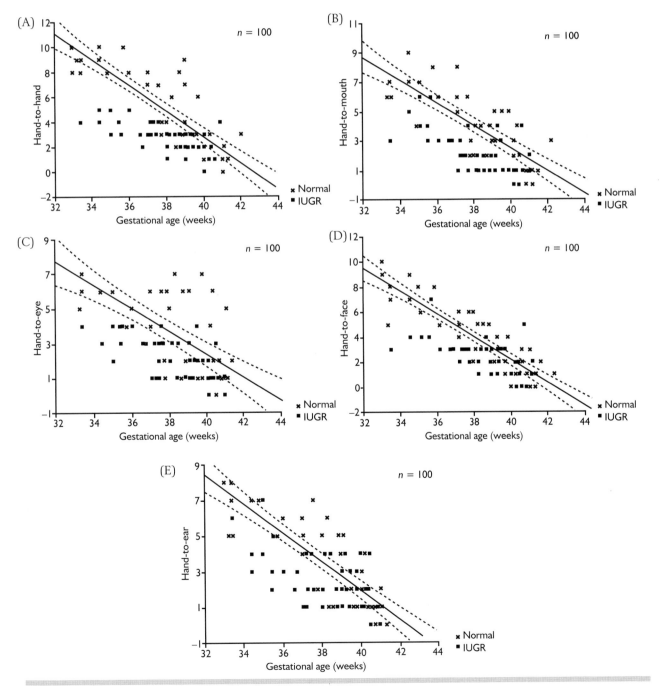

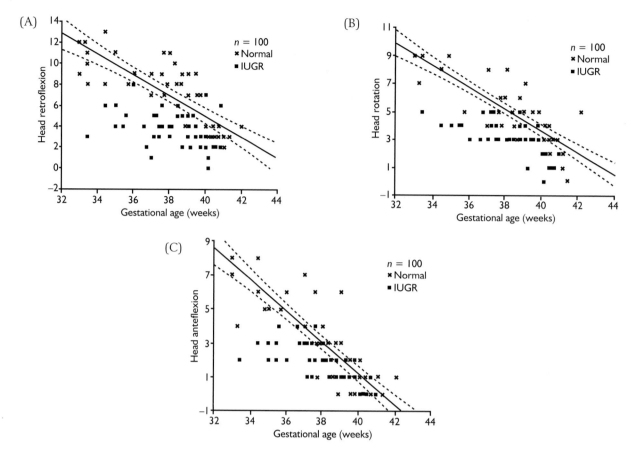

Figure 19.10 Scatterplot and multiple regression analysis of the 3rd-trimester frequency of head movement pattern versus gestational age in the formula-generating group: (A) head retroflexion; (B) head rotation; (C) head anteflexion

with IUGR fetuses using a 3D sonographic volume calculation (VOCAL) to estimate fetal bladder volume. This method takes account of the actual bladder shape but is not dependent on whether or not it is ellipsoidal. 3D sonographic assessment of fetal bladder is an accurate and convenient alternative to rotating the ultrasound transducer for a transverse scan as in 2D sonography. Using this technique, a single 3D image is obtained in which the fundus and bladder neck can be properly visualized.

Measurements were obtained in the manner proposed by Kurjak et al.[46] The bladder volumes were regressed against known gestational age. The VOCAL software consistently predicted the bladder volume. The relationship between HFUPR and gestational age (GA) is defined by the regression equation

$$HFUPR = 77.98 + 3.29\ GA \qquad (r = 0.94;\ p < 0.05)$$

In Figure 19.8, a scattergram of the relationship illustrates this prediction. We found an increase in HFUPR from 30.44 ml/h at 33 weeks to approxi-

mately 63.54 ml/h at 40 weeks in normal fetuses, while the HFUPR in IUGR fetuses varied from 24.23 ml/h at 33 weeks to around 52.18 ml/h at 40 weeks. All IUGR cases have demonstrated lower HFUPR (below the normal regression line) compared with the normal fetus.

The prediction using the 3D volume calculation may indeed have an effect on previous calculations of fetal urinary flow rates, particularly late in gestation when the fetal bladder can accommodate larger volumes of urine. Some errors might be caused by the changing shape of the fetal bladder as it is filled and emptied. Using real-time sonography, it may be observed that frequently the fetal bladder image appears as an irregularly shaped ellipse, ranging from a teardrop- or pear-shaped image to an occasionally almost spherical image.

Fetal behavioral assessment

From the 32nd week of gestation onwards, head and hand movements decline quantitatively with gestational

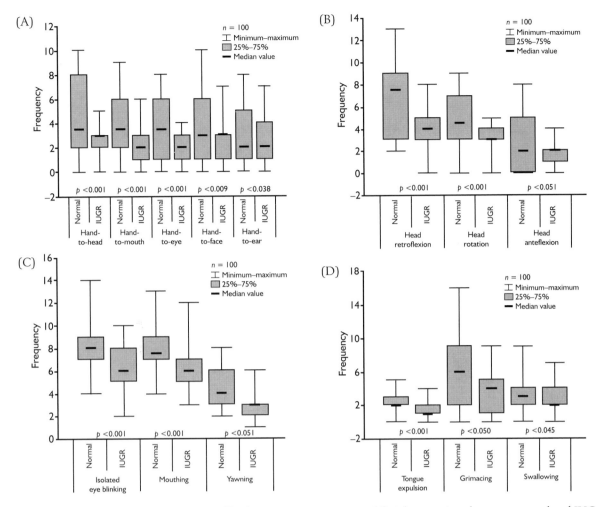

Figure 19.11 Comparison of frequency of body movement patterns and facial expressions between normal and IUGR fetuses in the 3rd trimester of pregnancy, measured for 30 minutes with 50 fetuses: (A) hand movement patterns; (B) head movement patterns; (C) isolated eye blinking, mouthing, and yawning patterns; (D) tongue expulsion, grimacing, and swallowing pattern. *p*-values indicate differences for Wilcoxon rank-sum test between normal and IUGR results

age (Figures 19.9 and 19.10). These trends were confirmed after relating the head and hand movements to gestational age in IUGR fetuses in relatively uncomplicated conditions. The highest incidence was registered for the head retroflexion pattern, followed by hand-to-head and hand-to-face movements. Among facial expressions, the highest incidence was found for grimacing, followed by isolated eye blinking and mouthing. A comparison of facial expressions and hand movements in the 3rd trimester of normal and IUGR fetuses is presented in Figure 19.11. During the 3rd trimester, the median value of all movement patterns in the normal fetuses differed apparently from that in fetuses with IUGR (Figure 19.11). Statistical evaluation (Wilcoxon rank-sum test) revealed significant differences in the distribution of the movements between these groups (*p*

<0.05). We noted a tendency for IUGR fetuses to have less behavioral activity than normal fetuses in all of the observed movement patterns. Spearman rank-order correlation reached statistical significance between the normal fetuses and IUGR fetuses in the 3rd trimester in hand-to-head and hand-to-face movements and head retroflexion (Table 19.3).

During the 3rd trimester, multiple regression and polynomial regression revealed statistically significant changes in all hand-to-body contact movement, head movements, yawning, tongue expulsion, grimacing, and swallowing (*p* <0.05) (Figures 19.9, 19.10, and 19.12). All head and hand movements showed a negative slope between frequency and gestational age (caused by a decline in the number of movements) (Figures 19.9 and 19.10). At the 3rd trimester, the fetuses began to display decreasing (yawning,

Table 19.3 Correlation of median frequencies of behavioral patterns in the 3rd trimester between normal and IUGR fetuses

Movement pattern	Frequency of behavior patterns per 30 minutes[a]		R^b	p
	Normal	**IUGR**		
Hand-to-head	0–5–10	0–3–5	0.44	<0.05
Hand-to-eye	0–4–8	0–2–4	−0.05	0.68 (NS)
Hand-to-mouth	0–4–9	0–2–6	−0.70	0.62 (NS)
Hand-to-face	0–4–10	0–2–7	0.29	<0.05
Hand-to-ear	0–3–8	0–2–7	−0.20	0.15 (NS)
Head retroflexion	2–7–13	0–3–8	0.49	<0.05
Head rotation	0–5–9	0–3–5	−0.06	0.64 (NS)
Head anteflexion	0–3–8	0–2–4	−0.03	0.82 (NS)
Isolated eye blinking	4–8–14	2–6–10	0.19	0.17 (NS)
Mouthing	4–8–13	3–6–12	0.24	0.09 (NS)
Yawning	2–4–8	1–3–6	−0.12	0.37 (NS)
Tongue expulsion	0–2–5	0–1–4	−0.06	0.66 (NS)
Grimacing	0–6–16	0–3–9	−0.07	0.59 (NS)
Swallowing	0–3–9	0–2–7	−0.07	0.51 (NS)

[a]Minimum–median–maximum
[b]R = Spearman rank-order correlation

grimacing, and swallowing) or constant (isolated eye blinking, mouthing, and tongue expulsion) incidence of fetal facial expression, as shown in the scatterplot (Figure 19.12). Only the isolated eye blinking and mouthing pattern demonstrated no significant correlation, as shown by the large dispersion of scatterpoints around the regression line.

Comparison of the median values of the qualitative scores of head and hand movements showed different trends during deterioration of the fetal condition (Figure 19.13). The median values of head and hand movements varied from 5 to 10 for IUGR, while the median values of the qualitative scores in a normal fetus varied from 8 to 10. Statistically significant differences (Wilcoxon rank-sum test) could be shown in the distribution of the median values of observation over the five qualitative categories of head and hand movements (p <0.05).

In the normal fetus, movements are complex and variable in composition, speed, and intensity. We noted a poor repertoire of movement patterns in 11 cases of IUGR, 4 being affected by pre-eclampsia, 3 being affected by non-reassuring cardiotocogram (CTG), one being affected by meconium staining, and one being affected by periventricular hemorrhage (PVH) (Table 19.4). The movements were monotony and lack of complexity of the sequence of successive movement components. Although parameters such as amplitude and speed were reduced, it must be empha-

sized that the overall monotony slow and predominantly small range of amplitude were the most impressive feature in this group. We also noted normal quality of general movements during complicated IUGR, 7 being complicated by pre-eclampsia, 1 being affected by non-reassuring CTG, one being complicated by PVH, one being complicated by IVH, and one being complicated by meconium staining (Table 19.4). Movements of the head and hand, varying in amplitude, speed, and intensity, were seen only in the normal fetuses. Those movements were performed slowly with small amplitude in the IUGR fetuses. The position of the fetus did not seem to influence the quality of movement. Positional changes, such as rotations around the longitudinal axis, were seen more often in the control group than in the IUGR group.

DISCUSSION

Early detection of IUGR is important because this condition carries a risk for the fetus. At present, the best sonographic predictor of IUGR is measurement of the abdominal circumference. The fetal liver comprises most of the abdomen as measured by the abdominal circumference. In normal fetuses, glycogen reserves in the liver increase towards the end of gestation. However, growth-restricted fetuses have severely reduced hepatic glycogen stores[10] because of fetal

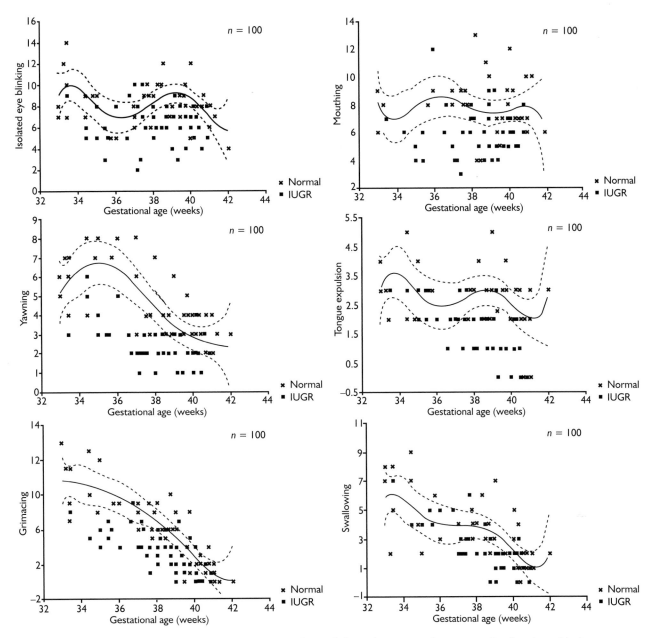

Figure 19.12 Scatterplot and polynomial regression analysis of the 3rd-trimester frequency of isolated eye blinking pattern versus gestational age in the formula-generating group: (A) isolated eye blinking; (B) mouthing; (C) yawning; (D) tongue expulsion; (E) grimacing; (F) swallowing

malnutrition. Reduction of liver weight in a growth-restricted fetus is more profound than reduction of brain weight. This is due to the so-called 'brain-sparing effect', so often observed in growth restriction caused by uteroplacental insufficiency.[10] Consequently, accurate assessment of liver size may contribute to the early detection of a growth-restricted fetus.[33]

The development of 3D sonography has introduced a new and accurate means of volume measurement, which is fast and easy to perform and has high patient acceptability. With respect to fetal liver volume measurement, Chang et al[36] showed that 3D sonography was superior to 2D sonography in a reproducibility test of fetal liver volume assessment.

Laudy et al[34] reported acceptable fetal liver volume measurement using 3D sonography in 25 patients. However, the number of measurements reported in their study was small, and subjects included AGA and large-for-gestational-age (LGA) fetuses. Therefore, the usefulness of their standard growth curve for fetal liver

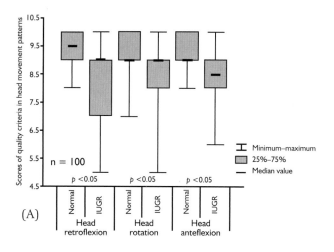

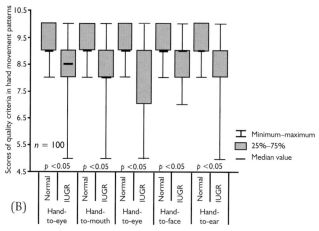

Figure 19.13 Comparison of quality scores of head movement patterns (A) and hand movement patterns (B) between normal and IUGR fetuses. *p*-values indicate differences for Wilcoxon rank-sum test between normal and IUGR results

volume may be unconvincing for detection of the fetus at risk of IUGR. In our study, we selected singleton IUGR fetuses as subjects to avoid this bias, and we tried to generate a normal range of liver volume measurement for estimating the growth of the fetal liver during normal pregnancy. Consequently, fetal liver volume was increased in a curvilinear manner with advancing gestation. The results show a close correlation between fetal liver volume and gestational age, similar to that observed by Chang et al,[36] with an approximately 2-fold increase in fetal liver volume from the beginning to the end of the 3rd trimester. The success rate of obtaining acceptable volume measurements was 100%. Possible recording difficulties seemed mainly to be determined by fetal (breathing) movements. The most unfavorable fetal position was with the back anterior, which caused considerable shadowing.

We can use the thigh volume alone as a single index to predict the birthweight accurately, given the assumption that the amount of subcutaneous tissue in the limbs can accurately assess the degree of obesity in adults.[31,42] Because the thigh volume as estimated by 3D sonography may reflect the real status of fetal growth, nutrition, and weight, the formula for 3D thigh volumetry predicted birthweight significantly better than the traditional 2D formulae using biparietal diameter, abdominal circumference (AC), and femur length.

In normal fetuses, the estimated liver/thigh volume ratio decreased significantly with advancing gestational age (Figure 19.7E). The estimated liver/thigh volume ratio is impaired in IUGR fetuses due to placental insufficiency, which may result in diminished glucose transfer and hepatic storage.[10] With regard to postmortem data on growth-restricted fetuses, the necropsy diagnosis of immaturity depends on the recognition of characteristic abnormalities of organ weight and composition. An approach was adopted in the present study in which the liver/thigh volume ratio rather than the head/abdominal circumference ratio was determined to ensure a more reliable reflection of change in organ size associated with fetal growth restriction. Our fetal data revealed a mean liver/thigh volume ratio of 1.3 : 1 in normal fetuses, and 1.8 : 1 in the IUGR fetuses.

All fetuses with IUGR have an estimated fetal liver/thigh volume ratio above the 90th centile (Figure 19.7E). This strongly indicates that liver/thigh volume ratio can predict fetal condition for fetuses in the 3rd trimester. We speculate that asymmetry of the fetal liver/thigh volume ratio indicates pronounced growth impairment secondary to uteroplacental insufficiency.

Campbell et al[48] and Kurjak et al[46] estimated HFUPR using static longitudinal and transverse images from a compound B-scan sonogram. Urinary flow rates were calculated from changes of bladder volume over a period of time. Campbell et al[48] found that the HFUPR was not significantly different between fetuses scanned at different hours of the day and showed that it increased linearly with advancing gestational age. With this technique, several studies have correlated variations in fetal urinary flow rates with normal and abnormal pregnancies.[46,48,50,70] This technique was based on static scanners, which limited bladder measurements to intervals of 15–30 minutes. With the advent of real-time sonography, fetal behavior may be assessed continuously and the bladder may be measured as frequently as possible. Refining the original technique of Campbell et al, Rabinowitz et al[50] measured bladder volumes every 2–5 minutes regressed during 1 hour to calculate HFUPR. Because of the frequency of bladder measurements, the calculated HFUPR was more than doubled in the 24-hour period for a term fetus (from 655 ml daily to 1224 ml daily).[50] However, because actual human fetal bladder volumes at different gestational ages were not known, the confidence limits associated with this technique were unknown.[71]

Because obvious reasons prevent the use of invasive methods for measuring human HFUPR, these ultrasound techniques have not been adequately validated in true clinical settings. Despite numerous studies of bladder volume estimations and calculations of flow rates, the confidence limits of a single, optimally obtained rate estimate are not known; therefore, assessment of reliable changes and differences in rate is not possible. This prompted us to repeat our study as a direct 3D sonographic fetal bladder volumetry, simulating the original text of their technique by Campbell et al. Figure 19.8 shows fetal urinary flow rate estimates by linear regression in a representative fetus using 3D VOCAL calculations for bladder volume.

Campbell et al[48] noted that there was no diurnal variation of bladder volume. However, complete bladder cycles and the calculated bladder volumes varied widely. The cycles ranged from 50 to 155 minutes and the volumes from 1.7 to 31 ml towards term gestation. Chamberlain et al[70] found similar widely varying volumes of 24–58 ml; however, a significant diurnal pattern was noted when bladder volumes were measured after midnight. The decreased bladder volume after midnight was speculated to be due to the diurnal decrease of fetal heart rate at these late gestations that occurred at about the same time of day. This finding suggested that the decrease in bladder volume may be secondary to a decrease in blood flow rate to the fetal bladder. Visser et al[72] noted that bladder emptying was associated with cyclic variation of the fetal heart rate. Micturition was noted in 95% of their observations to occur within 30 minutes after an increase in fetal heart rate. Similarly, stress from vibroacoustic instrument use likewise elicited fetal micturition corresponding to fetal heart rate accelerations.[73]

As previously discussed, the in vivo human fetal bladder volume is unknown. Unless it can be determined, accurate calculation of HFUPR will continue to be controversial. The closest we can calculate the in vivo bladder volume is to simulate bladder filling in a recently born dead fetus.[48,71] Campbell et al[48] validated their assumption of a fetal bladder closely resembling an ellipsoid in a single-term fetal cadaver. Hedriana and Moore[74] developed a simpler and more accurate method that required fewer measurements than described above. The bladder was filled with a controlled saline solution infusion, and an average error of 0.7 ± 0.6 ml was reported. The mean error was reported to be similar throughout the range of volumes assessed indicating that the greater the volume, the greater was the relative accuracy. Because of the controversy,[48,50] the same method was repeated with carefully selected fetal cadavers ranging from 22 to 40 weeks of gestation.[74]

There was a positive correlation between growth-restricted fetuses and lower HFUPR. Lower HFUPR values were found when the pregnancy was complicated with pre-eclampsia or placental insufficiency. However, the common denominator seems to be the presence of growth restriction.[48] Aside from a decrease in HFUPR, Kurjak et al[46] found a decrease in glomerular filtration rate (GFR <2.66 ml/min) and tubular water reabsorption (TWR <60%). Furosemide increased HFUPR, regardless of fetal size, to an average of 110% ± 24% from controls. The increase in HFUPR was not consistent with advancing gestation, changes in fetal heart rate, or maternal blood pressure and pulse rate. In pregnancies complicated by preterm premature rupture of membranes,[75] there was no correlation between HFUPR and the amount of residual amniotic fluid volume. Unexpectedly, in a fetus with Potter syndrome secondary to renal hypoplasia, the HFUPR was 7 ml/h, with a sharp increase to 21 ml/h at 31 weeks and to 16 ml/h at 33 weeks.[76] However, where hypoplasia is absent but the kidneys are small such as those found in a growth-restricted fetus, the HFUPR is low and correlates positively with kidney size;[77] this may be due to hypoperfusion of the kidneys in growth-restricted fetuses.

The principal source of existing knowledge about the development of fetal motor behavior has been 4D sonography, which basically relies on observation periods of 30 minutes.[56,59,62] Coding of fetal movement can be done in real time by trained observers, or the session may be videotaped for later review.[59,62] Accurate visualization involves a significant degree of expertise. However, the selection of the method to measure fetal motor behavior should be guided by the research question and the nature of the fetal movement information necessary to obtain the best answer.

Our previous reports on fetal 4D sonographic examination set out to determine whether dynamic observations of the fetus were possible in the 1st and 2nd trimester.[59,62,78,79] Now, using 4D sonographic techniques, it is possible to perform dynamic 3D observations of fetal behavior. Moreover, it is possible to obtain better image quality, since the whole fetus can be visualized (Figures 19.4–19.6).[59,61,62]

The complexities of neurobehavioral assessment of the fetus, which cannot be viewed directly or manipulated, cannot be understated. Identification of measurable indicators of fetal functioning that reflect the development of the peripheral and central nervous system is the primary goal of fetal neurobehavioral research.[80] No unified neurobehavioral assessment methods for the fetus currently exist. It has long been recognized that features of neurobehavioral functioning that have been measured extensively in the full-term neonate and infant and that are integral to current theories of development do not originate at term or with birth.[81] Instead, most investigators focus on one or more aspects of functioning within four general domains, comprising fetal heart rate, motor activity, behavioral state, and responsivity to stimulation. However, construction of a unified fetal neurobehavioral scale is premature until a sufficient amount of normative data is available and the predictive validity of specific aspects of fetal neurobehavior for child developmental outcomes is better established.[53]

Successive maturational transformations are orderly, and progressively and gradually enriched at identical stages of development, although neurologic assessments are strictly comparable. Thus, maturative phenomena are intimately and exclusively a function of age.[82] Although this assumption was the impetus for devising postnatal strategies for assessing gestational age, several validation studies of various methods observed groups of infants with aberrant measures of gestational age, suggesting alteration of their rate of maturation. This was especially true of infants born with IUGR or after stressed or complicated pregnancies.[83] Dubowitz and Dubowitz[84] recognized that neurologic scores overestimated gestational age in SGA infants.

Amiel-Tison et al[83] concluded that factors that lead to IUGR also accelerate neuromaturation and that this is not an 'all-or-nothing' phenomenon but rather a 'progressive response by variable degree'. Evidence of accelerated neuromaturation 'as a progressive response by variable degree' in stressed or IUGR pregnancies is also seen with auditory evoked responses. Pettigrew et al[85] found significantly shorter mean conduction times in brainstem auditory evoked responses (i.e., a higher degree of neuromaturation) in 25 preterm SGA infants compared with 76 preterm AGA infants.

The linear and polynomial regression reached statistical significance in all hand-to-body contact movements, head movements, yawning, and tongue expulsion, grimacing, and swallowing. Only the isolated eye blinking and mouthing patterns revealed no significant correlation, as shown by the large dispersion of scatterpoints. This is concordant with the findings of other authors. Roodenburg et al[86] stated that inhibition is a hallmark of neurologic development, and most longitudinal studies report that the fetus becomes less active as gestation advances. Although estimates vary, in the latter half of gestation fetuses move approximately once per minute and are active between 10% and 30% of the time.[87] Discrepancies in the literature may be explained by procedural variation in defining movement onset and offset and other differences in quantification.[88] This type of developmental trend may be depicting the adaptability of the organism to changing environmental and intrinsic challenges. However, the linear decrease in the occurrence of the fetal movements during gestation in our study is difficult to compare with the findings of other studies because of methodologic differences.[86,89]

Some movement patterns occurred more frequently than the others in this study. Large fluctuations of incidence of movement were noted in each fetus. Still, we had the impression that a 30-minute observation in the morning was representative of the rest of the day. This was confirmed by observations performed at different periods of the day, as has been described earlier.[86]

Fetal behavior is a continuation of the activities shown in the fetal period.[78] One of the mysterious behavioral patterns observed prenatally is yawning. There is no explanation why a human fetus should yawn, but it appears to have some purpose.[90] The literature fails to define yawning in a fetus, which has led to far too many interpretations of open mouths as yawns. The range of variation includes, for example, a single, continuous opening of the mouth lasting 3 minutes and a set of five repetitive openings of the mouth for 4–6 seconds each.[90] It has been proposed that yawning is a complex arousal defense mechanism, the center of which is located in the reticular brainstem, and its function is to reverse brain hypoxia and

Table 19.4 Characteristics, obstetrics, and neonatal outcome in the study population

Characteristic	Normal quality of movements (n = 39)	Abnormal quality of movements		
		Poor repertoire (n = 11)	Cramped–synchronized	Chaotic
Mean gestational age at examination (weeks)	38.39 ± 1.64	37 ± 2.25	–	–
Pre-eclampsia	7	4	–	–
Abnormal fetal testing	1	3	–	–
Meconium	1	1	–	–
Induced labor	2	0	–	–
Cesarean section	32	11	–	–
Cesarean section for fetal distress	1	3	–	–
Estimated birthweight (g)	2458.97 ± 362.74	2152.72 ± 461.84	–	–
5-minute Apgar score <7	0	1	–	–
Neonatal hospital stay (days)	8.32 ± 5.45	10.8 ± 5.06	–	–
Admission to intermediate care unit	3	5	–	–
Neonatal complication:				
Hypoglycemia	1	0	–	–
Hyperbilirubinemia	5	1	–	–
Respiratory distress syndrome	2	0	–	–
Periventricular hemorrhage	1	1	–	–
Intraventricular hemorrhage (2nd-grade)	1	0	–	–

improve brain oxygenation. However, its role in only primary respiratory purposes has been questioned.

Significant trends in fetal eye movement organization can also be observed during the second half of pregnancy, especially during the 3rd trimester, and eye movement patterns are a sensitive reflection of the activity of the neural control system. The earliest eye movements appear during the 16th to 18th weeks of gestation, as sporadic movements with a limited frequency. However, in our study, we did not perform observation of fetal eye movement patterns separately. From our previous study, we already knew that isolated eye blinking patterns appear more frequently and begin to consolidate during the 24th to 26th weeks of gestation.[62] In this study, we found a slight difference in frequency of isolated eye blinking between normal and IUGR fetuses. IUGR fetuses seem to blink their eyes less frequently than normal fetuses (Figure 19.11C).

We noted a typical quality of fetal behavioral patterns in our IUGR cases. A poor repertoire of behavioral patterns was revealed in 11 cases of IUGR, 4 being affected by pre-eclampsia, 3 by non-reassuring CTG, one by meconium staining, and 1 by PVH. It must be emphasized that a slowly varying and predominantly small amplitude was the most impressive feature in these fetuses. However, we did not

perform continuous neurologic observation during the infancy period and our study group consisted mostly of non-hypoxic IUGR fetuses (with normal cerebroplacental Doppler ratio), and this fact might influence our findings.

According to Ferrari and Prechtl, a poor repertoire is characterized by monotony and lack of complexity of the sequence of successive movement components. From previous studies of fetal movements of preterm and term infants affected by brain lesions of perinatal origin – i.e. IVH, PVH, or periventricular leukomalacia in preterm infants[69,91] and hypoxic–ischemic lesions in full-term infants,[91] we know that a poor repertoire of movements is the most common motor abnormality. Poor repertoire is the least extreme form of abnormal movement quality, with the complexity, variability, and fluency of movements being somewhat poorer than normal, and the outcome of these infants is unpredictable with respect to their future development. As shown in Table 19.4, 3 out of 39 neonates admitted to the neonatal intermediate care unit had normal quality of movement, while 5 out of 11 who were also admitted exhibited a poor repertoire. In this condition, poor repertoire might be a sign that these infants are affected by brain impairment.

A qualitative scoring system based on a 4D view of 3D movement might enhance the credibility of the data (Table 19.1). Since we did not perform inter-observer reliability testing, it is possible that we did not score true behavior or that behavior was modified by the imaging procedure. Reliability must be based on extensive training in the future.

The number of subjects in this study was relatively small. Because of this, we did not perform separate quantitative and qualitative analyses between hypoxic and non-hypoxic IUGR fetuses. Although significance was achieved for some movements using non-parametric statistics, the actual amount of data used for analysis was specified, and a variety of subjects were included over the course of pregnancy, with appropriate follow-up, there is still a need for a larger subject pool. In this study, we have assessed fetal behavior and scored fetal movements only when the fetus is in the 'wake' period during the morning.

In 39 out of 50 growth-restricted fetuses, no abnormalities in the quality of general movements were observed. These results indicate that uncomplicated IUGR as such does not necessarily affect the quality of general movements. Furthermore, the presence of an increase of the umbilical artery resistance in these fetuses clearly showed that this phenomenon precedes changes in the quality of movement. Under the condition of a reduced fetal supply of oxygen and nutrients, a decrease in the carotid artery resistance is supposed to have an adaptive function, favoring blood supply to the fetal CNS.[92–94] Such a redistribution could indicate that an early reduction in the supply to the fetus has no influence on the quality of fetal movements, either due to the capacity of the CNS to adapt to such circumstances or due to a compensatory redistribution of blood flow from the fetal body to the CNS.

In this study, the characteristics of reduced speed and amplitude were found in the IUGR group. However, impairment of neurologic development cannot be ruled out, since extensive blood flow redistribution is likely to be associated with a markedly reduced supply of nutrients. The same holds for the association that was found with a poor repertoire of fetal movements. It is reasonable to speculate that oxygen deprivation is at least partly responsible for the poor movement repertoire.[95] Therefore, the poor movement repertoire may also be an expression of impaired neurologic development. Support for this reasoning is rendered by the morphologic findings in human growth-restricted infants and in animal models where a smaller brain size, fewer neurons, deficits in synapse-to-neuron ratios, and reduced dendritic growth have been found.[96,97] Moreover, even if the

poor repertoire was due to hypoxemia alone, restoration of movements would be expected to occur directly after birth when the oxygen supply is restored. However, the poor repertoire continued for some time after birth. It also has been found that neonatal neurologic morbidity in IUGR fetuses is largely restricted to those who antenatally showed signs of hypoxemia and malnutrition.[97]

Using 2D real-time sonography, Bekedam et al[95] have pioneered qualitative and quantitative study of various movement patterns between IUGR and normal fetuses. Recording for a duration of 1 hour, qualitative analysis was carried out during replay of video recordings. They proved that there were reductions in both number and duration of fetal movements in the IUGR group. Qualitative analysis of fetal movements revealed a reduction in the faster components, leading to slow and monotonous movement patterns. There was also a marked reduction of variability of speed and intensity within each movement.

Almost after two decades, we have confirmed what Bekedam et al[97] found in their pioneering study on the IUGR fetuses using 4D sonography. Although we have performed our study of fetal movement pattern in the same group of IUGR fetuses, the results are still conflicting. In our study, the quantity of movement patterns and facial expressions differed slightly (as shown by the median values) from those in the control fetuses. According to Bekedam et al,[95] the reduction in fetal movements was due to hypoxemia. However, we have found reduced quality and quantity of fetal movement patterns as shown by Bekedam et al, although almost all of our IUGR cases are non-hypoxic fetuses. A number of points that can explain the discrepancies among them should be considered. The most important point is the heterogeneity of the group of fetuses with growth restriction. Bekedam et al have performed their study on 10 severe IUGR fetuses, almost all of whom were subjected to hypoxic conditions and had birthweight below the 5th percentile. Nevertheless, in this study, different criteria are used to define IUGR, as a birthweight below the 10th percentile on a curve of birthweight versus gestational age. Particularly when the broadest criterion is applied, many of these fetuses would not qualify as IUGR at all: they just happen to fall into the lower range of the normal population distribution. In addition, within the IUGR group, due to placental dysfunction, the onset and severity of the growth restriction add to the heterogeneity of the IUGR fetuses.

Using 4D sonography, our study has opened for the first time the possibility of visualizing the full range of facial expressions in the IUGR condition. The median frequency of all facial expressions in the IUGR group was slightly lower compared with the control group. Contrary to the declining trend of body and limb movements, an almost constant frequency of fetal facial expression patterns was noted during the 3rd trimester. This impressive finding, however, raises a number of questions, many of which are yet to be answered. Precise criteria to distinguish between these facial expressions in the fetus should be established and the exact onset of facial expressions should be determined.

Furthermore, in contrast to progressing gestation, which goes together with a reduction in the number of fetal movements, fetal deterioration caused only a reduction in the frequency of fetal movements. No clear explanation can be given, as in the IUGR condition, fetal movements appear short in duration and small in amplitude. This qualitative description is in agreement with the study by Bekedam et al.[95]

This study indicates that in non-hypoxic IUGR, as shown mostly in our study group, the quantities of fetal movements and facial expression were not in the same range as those found in control fetuses. Since the number of subjects in this study was relatively small, it is not possible to perform separate analyses of hypoxic and non-hypoxic IUGR. In our study, alterations in the quality of fetal movements were accompanied by considerable decreases in the quantity of fetal movements. However, the quantity of fetal movements and facial expressions showed an intra-individual variation.

Using combination techniques with 3D and 4D sonography, we have proved that differences in motor performance between IUGR and normal fetuses may be attributable to several causes. Possible explanations include reductions in the glycogen store as shown in the liver volume, then of muscle bulk as shown in the thigh volume, and of urinary production as shown in the bladder volume, with or without impairment of the movement pattern.

The reduced muscle bulk in the IUGR fetus might be responsible for the lack of power in the behavior patterns; nevertheless, it is unlikely to be responsible for the small amplitude, reduced speed, reduced variability, and poor repertoire of the movements. Likewise, spatial restriction might reduce the amplitude of fetal movements, but is most unlikely to affect the other parameters. Metabolic deprivation, such as that associated with hypoxemia, might be responsible for the type of abnormal patterns found in this study.

REFERENCES

1. Ott WJ. An update on the ultrasonic diagnosis and evaluation of intrauterine growth restriction. Ultrasound Rev Obstet Gynecol 2005; 5: 111–24.

2. Neligan GA, Kolvin I, Scott D. Born too Soon or Born too Small. A Follow-up Study to Seven Years of Age. Spastic International Medical Publications. London: William Heinemann Medical Books, 1978: 66.

3. Briscoe TA, Rehn AE, Dieni S, et al. Cardiovascular and renal disease in the adolescent guinea pig after chronic placental insufficiency. Am J Obstet Gynecol 2004; 191: 847–55.

4. Tan TY, Yeo GS. Intrauterine growth restriction. Curr Opin Obstet Gynecol 2005; 17: 135–42.

5. McCowan LM, Harding JE, Stewart AW. Umbilical artery Doppler studies in small for gestational age babies reflect disease severity. Br J Obstet Gynaecol 2000; 107: 916–25.

6. Neerhof MG. Causes of intrauterine growth restriction. Clin Perinatol 1995; 22: 375–85.

7. McCowan LM, Harding JE, Roberts AB, et al. A pilot randomized controlled trial of two regimens of fetal surveillance for small-for-gestational-age fetuses with normal results of umbilical artery Doppler velocimetry. Am J Obstet Gynecol 2000; 182: 81–6.

8. Nienhuis SJ, Vles JS, Gerver WJ, et al. Doppler ultrasonography in suspected intrauterine growth retardation: a randomized clinical trial. Ultrasound Obstet Gynecol 1997; 9: 6–13.

9. Kurjak A, Latin V, Polak J. Ultrasonic recognition of two types of growth retardation by measurement of four fetal dimension. J Perinat Med 1978; 6: 102–8.

10. Ott WJ. Intrauterine growth restriction and Doppler ultrasonography. J Ultrasound Med 2000; 19: 661–5.

11. Ergaz Z, Avgil M, Ornoy A. Intrauterine growth restriction–etiology and consequences: What do we know about the human situation and experimental animal models? Reprod Toxicol. 2005; 20: 301–22.

12. Gilbert WM, Danielsen B. Pregnancy outcomes associated with intrauterine growth restriction. Am J Obstet Gynecol 2003; 188: 1596–9.

13. Li CI, Daling JR, Emanuel I. Birthweight and risk of overall and cause-specific childhood mortality. Paediatr Perinat Epidemiol 2003; 17: 164–70.

14. Barker DJ. Intrauterine programming of adult disease. Mol Med Today 1995; 1: 418–23.

15. Barker DJ, Osmond C, Simmonds SJ, et al. The

relation of small head circumference and thinness at birth to death from cardiovascular disease in adult life. BMJ 1993; 306: 422–6.

16. Gale CR, Martyn CN. Birthweight and later risk of depression in a national birth cohort. Br J Psychiatry 2004; 184: 28–33.

17. Mittendorfer-Rutz E, Rasmussen F, Wasserman D. Restricted fetal growth and adverse maternal psychosocial and socioeconomic conditions as risk factors for suicidal behaviour of offspring: a cohort study. Lancet 2004; 364: 1135–40.

18. Baschat AA. Doppler application in the delivery timing of the preterm growth restricted fetus: another step in the right direction. Ultrasound Obstet Gynecol 2004; 23: 111–19.

19. Jacobsson B, Hagberg G. Antenatal risk factors for cerebral palsy. Best Pract Res Clin Obstet Gynaecol 2004; 18: 425–36.

20. Toft PB, Leth H, Ring PB, et al. Volumetric analysis of the normal infant brain and in intrauterine growth retardation. Early Hum Dev 1995; 43: 15–29.

21. Rees S, Mallard C, Breen S, et al. Fetal brain injury following prolonged hypoxemia and placental insufficiency: a review. Comp Biochem Physiol A Mol Integr Physiol 1998; 19: 653–60.

22. Scherjon SA, Costing H, Smolders-DeHaas H, et al. Neurodevelopmental outcome at three years of age after fetal 'brain-sparing'. Early Hum Dev 1998; 52: 67–79.

23. Marsal K. Intrauterine growth restriction. Curr Opin Obstet Gynecol 2002; 14: 127–35.

24. Jacobsson B, Hagberg G, Hagberg B, et al. Cerebral palsy in preterm infants: a population-based case–control study of antenatal and intrapartal risk factors. Acta Paediatr 2002; 91: 946–51.

25. Thorngren-Jerneck K. Cerebral Injury in Perinatal Asphyxia. Lund: Lund University, 2002.

26. Jacobsson B, Francis A, Hagberg G, et al. Cerebral palsy is strongly associated with severe intrauterine growth restriction in term but not in preterm cases. Am J Obstet Gynecol 2003; 189: S74.

27. Bahado-Singh RO, Kovanci E, Jeffres A, et al. The Doppler cerebroplacental ratio and perinatal outcome in intrauterine growth restriction. Am J Obstet Gynecol 1999; 180: 750–6.

28. Hirata GI, Medearis AL, Horenstein J, et al. Ultrasonographic estimation of fetal weight in the clinically macrosomic fetus. Am J Obstet Gynecol 1990; 162: 238–42.

29. Deter RL, Nazar R, Milner LL. Modified neonatal growth assessment score: a multivariate approach to the detection of intrauterine growth retardation in the neonate. Ultrasound Obstet Gynecol 1995; 6: 400–10.

30. Jeanty P, Romero R, Hobbins JC. Fetal limb volume: a new parameter to assess fetal growth and nutrition. J Ultrasound Med 1985; 4: 272–82.

31. Lee W, Deter RL, McNie B, et al. Individualized growth assessment of fetal soft tissue using fractional thigh volume. Ultrasound Obstet Gynecol 2004; 24: 766–74.

32. Bethune M, Bell R. Evaluation of the measurement of the fetal fat layer, interventricular septum and abdominal circumference percentile in the prediction of macrosomia in pregnancies affected by gestational diabetes. Ultrasound Obstet Gynecol 2003; 22: 586–90.

33. Schild RL, Fimmers R, Hansmann M. Fetal weight estimation by three-dimensional ultrasound. Ultrasound Obstet Gynecol 2000; 16: 445–52.

34. Laudy JAM, Janssen MMM, Struyk PC, et al. Fetal liver volume measurement by three-dimensional ultrasonography: a preliminary study. Ultrasound Obstet Gynecol 1998; 12: 93–6.

35. Lee AL, Kratochwil A, Stumpflen I, Deutinger J, Bernaschek G. Fetal lung volume determination by 3D ultrasonography. Am J Obstet Gynecol 1996; 175: 588–92.

36. Chang FM, Hsu KF, Ko HC, et al. Three-dimensional ultrasound assessment of fetal liver volume in normal pregnancy: a comparison of reproducibility with two-dimensional ultrasound and a search for a volume constant. Ultrasound Med Biol 1997; 23: 381–9.

37. Berg S, Torp H, Blaas HG. Accuracy of in-vitro volume estimation of small structures using three-dimensional ultrasound. Ultrasound Med Biol 2000; 26: 425–32.

38. Riccabona M, Nelson TR, Pretorius DH. Three-dimensional ultrasound: accuracy of distance and volume measurements. Ultrasound Obstet Gynecol 1996; 7: 429–34.

39. Chang FM, Liang RI, Ko HC, et al. Three-dimensional ultrasound-assessed fetal thigh volumetry in predicting birthweight. Obstet Gynecol 1997; 90: 331–9.

40. Song TB, Moore TR, Lee JI, Kim YH, Kim EK. Fetal weight prediction by thigh volume measurement with three-dimensional ultrasonography. Obstet Gynecol 2000; 96: 157–61.

41. Chang CH, Yu CH, Chang FM, Ko HC, Chen HY. Three-dimensional ultrasound in the assessment of normal fetal thigh volume. Ultrasound Med Biol 2003; 29: 361–6.

42. Lee W, Deter RL, Ebersole JD, et al. Birthweight prediction by three-dimensional ultrasonography: fractional limb volume. J Ultrasound Med 2001; 20: 1283–92.

43. Evans MI, Mukherjee AB, Schulman JD. Animal models of intrauterine growth retardation. Obstet Gynecol Surv 1983; 3: 183–92.

44. Liang RI, Chang FM, Yao BL, et al. Predicting birth weight by fetal upper-arm volume with use of three-dimensional ultrasonography. Am J Obstet Gynecol 1997; 177: 632–8.

45. Chang CH, Yu CH, Ko HC, Chen CL, Chang FM. The efficacy assessment of thigh volume in predicting intrauterine fetal growth restriction by 3D ultrasound. Ultrasound Med Biol 2005; 31: 883–7.

46. Kurjak A, Kirkinen P, Latin V, et al. Ultrasonic assessment of fetal kidney function in normal and complicated pregnacies. Am J Obstet Gynecol 1981; 141: 266–70.

47. Fagerquist M, Fagerquist U, Oden A, Blomberg SG. Estimation of fetal urinary bladder volume using the sum-of-cylinders method vs. the ellipsoid formula. Ultrasound Obstet Gynecol 2003; 22: 67–73.

48. Campbell S, Wladimiroff JW, Dewhurst CJ. The antenatal measurement of fetal urine production. J Obstet Gynaecol Br Commonw 1973; 80: 680–6.

49. Nicolaides KH, Peters MT, Vyas S, et al. Relation of rate of urine production to oxygen tension in small-for-gestational-age fetuses. Am J Obstet Gynecol 1990; 162: 387–91.

50. Rabinowitz R, Peters MT, Vyas S, Campbell S, Nicolaides KH. Measurement of fetal urine production in normal pregnancy by real-time ultrasonography. Am J Obstet Gynecol 1989; 161: 1264–6.

51. Takeuchi H, Koyanagi T, Yoshizato T, et al. Fetal urine production at different gestational age: correlation to various compromised fetuses in utero. Early Hum Dev 1994; 40: 1–11.

52. Fagerquist M, Fagerquist U, Oden A, Blomberg SG. Fetal urine production and accuracy when estimating fetal urinary bladder volume. Ultrasound Obstet Gynecol 2001; 17: 132–9.

53. DiPietro JA. Neurobehavioral assessment before birth. Ment Retard Dev Disabil Res Rev 2005; 11: 4–13.

54. Devoe L, Jones C. Nonstress test: evidence based use in high-risk pregnancy. Clin Obstet Gynecol 2002; 45: 986–92.

55. Velazquez M, Rayburn W. Antenatal evaluation of the fetus using fetal movement monitoring. Clin Obstet Gynecol 2002; 45: 993–1004.

56. Kurjak A, Vecek N, Hafner T, et al. Prenatal diagnosis: What does four-dimensional ultrasound add? J Perinat Med 2002; 30: 57–62.

57. Kurjak A, Carrera JM, Medic M, et al. The antenatal development of fetal behavioral patterns assessed by four-dimensional sonography. J Matern Fetal Neonatal Med 2005; 17: 401–16.

58. Kurjak A, Carrera JM, Andonotopo W, et al. The role of 4D sonography in the neurological assessment of early human development. Ultrasound Rev Obstet Gynecol 2004; 4: 148–59.

59. Kurjak A, Stanojevic M, Andonotopo W, et al. Fetal behaviour assessed in all three trimesters of normal pregnancy by 4D ultrasonography. Croat Med J 2005; 46: 772–80.

60. Kurjak A, Pooh RK, Merce LT, et al. Structural and functional early human development assessed by three-dimensional and four-dimensional sonography. Fertil Steril 2005; 84: 1285–99.

61. Andonotopo W, Stanojevic M, Kurjak A, Azumendi G, Carrera JM. Assessment of fetal behavior and general movements by four-dimensional sonography. Ultrasound Rev Obstet Gynecol 2004; 4: 103–14.

62. Kurjak A, Andonotopo W, Hafner T, et al. Normal standards for fetal neurobehavioral developments – longitudinal study by 4D sonography. J Perinat Med 2006; 34: 56–65.

63. Kurjak A, Stanojevic M, Azumendi G, Carrera JM. The potential of four-dimensional (4D) ultrasonography in the assessment of fetal awareness. J Perinat Med 2005; 33: 46–53.

64. Ahmed B, Kurjak A, Andonotopo W, et al. Fetal behavioral and structural abnormalities in high risk fetuses assessed by 4D sonography. Ultrasound Rev Obstet Gynecol 2005; 5: 275–87.

65. Sival DA. Studies on fetal motor behaviour in normal and complicated pregnancies. Early Hum Dev 1993; 34: 13–20.

66. Baschat AA, Harman CR. Antenatal assessment of the growth restricted fetus. Curr Opin Obstet Gynecol 2001; 13: 161–8.

67. Prechtl HF. Ultrasound studies of human fetal behaviour. Early Hum Dev 1985; 12: 91–8.

68. de Vries JI, Visser GHA, Prechtl HFR. The emergence of fetal behaviour I. Qualitative aspects. Early Human Dev 1982; 7: 301–22.

69. Ferrari F, Prechtl HF, Cioni G, et al. Posture, spontaneous movements, and behavioral state organisation in infants affected by brain malformations. Early Hum Dev 1997; 50: 87–113.

70. Chamberlain PF, Manning FA, Morrison MB, Lange IR. Circadian rhythm in bladder volumes in the term human fetus. Obstet Gynecol 1984; 64: 657–60.

71. Hedriana HL. Ultrasound measurement of fetal urine flow. Clin Obstet Gynecol 1997; 40: 337–51.

72. Visser GHA, Goodman JDS, Levine DH, et al. Micturition and the heart period cycle in the human fetus. Br J Obstet Gynaecol 1981; 88: 803–5.

73. Zimmer EZ, Chao CR, Guy GP, et al. Vibroacoustic stimulation evokes human fetal micturition. Obstet Gynecol 1993; 81: 178–80.

74. Hedriana HL, Moore TR. Accuracy limits of ultrasonographic estimation of human fetal urinary flow rate. Am J Obstet Gynecol 1994; 171: 989–92.

75. Watson WJ, Katz VL, Seeds JW. Fetal urine output does not influence residual amniotic fluid volume after premature rupture of membranes. Am J Obstet Gynecol 1991; 164: 64–5.

76. Fagerquist M, Sillen U, Oden A, et al. Fetal urine production estimated with ultrasound. The lower limit of normality is illustrated in a case with severe hypoplasia of the kidneys. Ultrasound Obstet Gynecol 1996; 7: 268–71.

77. Deutinger J, Bartl W, Pfersmann C, et al. Fetal kidney volume and urine production in cases of fetal growth retardation. J Perinat Med 1987; 15: 307–15.

78. Kurjak A, Stanojevic M, Andonotopo W, et al. Behavioral pattern continuity from prenatal to postnatal life – a study by four-dimensional (4D) ultrasonography. J Perinat Med 2004; 32: 346–53.

79. Andonotopo W, Medic M, Salihagic-Kadic A, et al. The assessment of fetal behavior in early pregnancy: comparison between 2D and 4D sonographic scanning. J Perinat Med 2005; 33: 406–14.

80. Vindla S, James D, Sahota D. Computerised analysis of unstimulated and stimulated behaviour in fetuses with intrauterine growth restriction. Eur J Obstet Gynecol Reprod Biol 1999; 83: 37–45.

81. Comparetti AM. The neurophysiologic and clinical implications of studies on fetal motor behavior. Semin Perinatol 1981; 5: 183–9.

82. Allen MC. Assessment of gestational age and neuro-maturation. Ment Retard Dev Disabil Res Rev 2005; 11: 21–33.

83. Amiel-Tison C, Cabrol D, Denver R, et al. Fetal adaptation to stress. Part I: Acceleration of fetal maturation and earlier birth triggered by placental insufficiency in humans. Early Hum Dev 2004; 78: 15–27.

84. Dubowitz V, Dubowitz LM. Inadequacy of Dubowitz gestational age in low birthweight infants. Obstet Gynecol 1985; 65: 601–2.

85. Pettigrew AG, Edwards DA, Henderson-Smart DJ. The influence of intra-uterine growth retardation on brainstem development of preterm infants. Dev Med Child Neurol 1985; 27: 467–72.

86. Roodenburg PJ, Wladimiroff JW, van Es A, Prechtl HF. Classification and quantitative aspects of fetal movements during the second half of normal pregnancy. Early Hum Dev 1991; 25: 19–35.

87. Roberts AB, Griffin D, Mooney R, et al. Fetal activity in 100 normal third trimester pregnancies. Br J Obstet Gynaecol 1980; 87: 480–4.

88. ten Hof J, Nijhuis IJM, Mulder EJH, et al. Quantitative analysis of fetal generalized movements: methodological considerations. Early Hum Dev 1999; 56: 57–73.

89. de Vries JI, Visser GHA, Prechtl HFR. The emergence of fetal behaviour II. Quantitative aspects. Early Human Dev 1985; 12: 99–120.

90. Walusinski O, Kurjak A, Andonotopo W, et al. Fetal yawning assessed by 3D and 4D sonography. Ultrasound Rev Obstet Gynecol 2005; 5: 210–17.

91. Cioni G, Ferrari F, Einspieler C, et al. Comparison between observation of spontaneous movements and neurologic examination in preterm infants. J Pediatr 1997; 130: 704–11.

92. Baschat AA. Integrated fetal testing in growth restriction: combining multivessel Doppler and biophysical parameters. Ultrasound Obstet Gynecol 2003; 21: 1–8.

93. Baschat AA, Gembruch U, Reiss I, et al. Relationship between arterial and venous Doppler and perinatal outcome in fetal growth restriction. Ultrasound Obstet Gynecol 2000; 16: 407–13.

94. van Eyck J, Wladimiroff JW, Noordam MJ, Tonge HM, Prechtl HF. The blood flow velocity waveform in the fetal descending aorta; its relationship to behavioural states in the growth-retarded fetus at 37–38 weeks of gestation. Early Hum Dev 1986; 14: 99–107.

95. Bekedam DJ, Visser GH, de Vries JJ, Prechtl HF. Motor behaviour in the growth retarded fetus. Early Hum Dev 1985; 12: 155–65.

96. Sival DA, Visser GHA, Prechtl HFR. The effect of intrauterine growth retardation on the quality of general movements in the human fetus. Early Hum Dev 1992; 28: 119–32.

97. Smart JL. Vulnerability of developing brain to undernutrition. Ups J Med Sci 1990; 48(Suppl 1): 21–41.

20 Volumetric fetal organ measurements by 3D sonography

Wiku Andonotopo, Asim Kurjak, and Berivoj Miskovic

INTRODUCTION

For many years, fetal weight has been assessed by taking a combination of standard two-dimensional (2D) measurements that are all related to three anatomic sites: the fetal head, the fetal abdomen, and the femur. However, none of the established formulae,[1–4] consider soft tissue thickness despite evidence that abnormal tissue content may be a reliable indicator of fetal growth aberration.[5,6]

3D sonography has been proposed for accurate determination of fetal organ volume.[7] It has been recommended that 3D instead of 2D sonography should be used for reaching an accurate assessment of fetal organ volume.[8] This chapter reviews several applications of 3D sonography in measuring fetal organ volume during the second half of pregnancy.

FETAL VOLUME

In the 1st trimester of pregnancy, assessment of gestational age and fetal growth, as well as diagnosis of early-onset fetal growth restriction in association with fetal abnormalities, are essentially based on 2D sonographic measurement of the fetal crown–rump length (CRL).[9–11] The introduction of 3D ultrasound has now made it possible to measure fetal volume, and two studies (on a combined total of 106 fetuses) have reported on the relation between this measurement and gestational age at 6–12 weeks.[12,13] Measurement of fetal nuchal translucency (NT), as an effective method of early screening for chromosomal defects, has led to the widespread introduction of routine ultrasound scanning at 11–14 weeks of gestation.[14,15]

Falcon et al[16] have established a reference range of fetal volume at 11–14 weeks that could form the basis for a new approach to the early diagnosis of impaired fetal growth. The inclusion criteria for their study were singleton pregnancy, live fetus with CRL between 45 and 84 mm, and normal fetal karyotype. The same 3D volumes were previously used to measure placental volume and gestational sac volume.[17,18]

The built-in VOCAL (<u>v</u>irtual <u>o</u>rgan <u>c</u>omputer-aided <u>a</u>nalysis) software in the Voluson 730 Expert machine (GE Medical Systems) was used to obtain a sequence of six longitudinal sections of the fetus around a fixed axis, each after a 30° rotation. The contour of the fetus (excluding the limbs and the NT) was drawn manually in each of the six different planes to obtain the 3D volume measurement (Figure 20.1). Every measurement can be done offline after the scan by the operator without the presence of the patient.

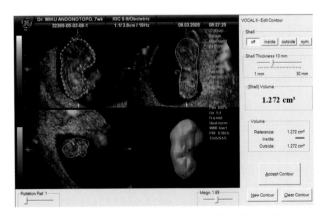

Figure 20.1 3D trunk and head volume of the fetus obtained using the virtual organ computer-aided analysis (VOCAL) technique

Falcon et al[16] have demonstrated that 3D sonography can provide a reproducible measurement of the fetal volume, which increases linearly with gestation between 11 and 14 weeks. Two previous studies of fetal volume by 3D sonography examined 34 patients at 7–10 weeks of gestation and 72 fetuses at 6–12 weeks, respectively.[12,13] In both of these studies, the scans were carried out transvaginally, and volumes, which included the limbs, were calculated using the VOCAL technique in the first study and the multiplanar method in the second study. However, using transabdominal scanning, Falcon et al[16] were able to obtain sufficiently good images to calculate the fetal volumes. In their study, they excluded the limbs from the volume measurements because at 11–14 weeks the legs are usually crossed over each other and the hands are often in contact with the face, which would make volume calculation too complex and probably less reproducible.[16]

It has previously been demonstrated that the VOCAL and multiplanar techniques are equally accurate and reliable for in vitro measurements of objects greater than 20 ml.[19] Although there are no studies demonstrating the accuracy of these methods for smaller objects, Falcon et al[16] showed that in 95% of cases the differences between measurements performed by the same and by different observers were less than 4 ml, which is actually much less than most fetal volumes calculated from 11–14 weeks.

The findings of the Falcon et al study provide in vivo evidence of a biphasic pattern of fetal growth in early pregnancy. Several 2D sonographic studies have reported the S-shaped pattern of fetal growth with gestation, with a linear component at 10 and 30 weeks.[9,10,20] This has also been reported in postmortem pathologic studies, which demonstrated a biphasic pattern in fetal growth, with a mean embryonic/fetal weight of approximately 1, 8, and 45 g at the respective gestations of 8, 11, and 14 weeks.[21] Thus, the first 10 weeks of gestation, which is the embryonic period, are primarily devoted to embryogenesis with establishment of all major organ systems.[22] Subsequently, with the onset of the fetal period, there is a shift in emphasis towards growth and maturation.

According to Falcon et al,[16] the fetal volume increased linearly with gestation from a mean of 5.8 ml at 11 weeks to 33.3 ml at the beginning of 14 weeks, with a standard deviation (SD) of 4.4 ml. There was also a significant linear association between fetal volume and CRL, from a mean of 5.1 ml at a CRL of 45 mm to 37.5 ml at a CRL of 84 mm, with

SD of 2.7 ml. However, within this gestational range, a doubling in CRL, from a mean of 48 mm at 11 weeks to 79 mm at 14 weeks, was associated with a 5–6-fold increase in fetal volume. The mean difference in fetal volume between paired measurements by the same sonographer was –0.87 ml (95% limits of agreement, –2.31 to 4.05 ml) and the mean difference between paired measurements by two sonographers was –1.09 ml (–5.49 to 3.32 ml).[16] However, the extent to which this additional information provided by 3D sonography can potentially allow a better understanding of the patterns of fetal growth in normal and pathologic pregnancies remains to be determined.

LUNG VOLUME

Pulmonary hypoplasia occurs frequently, being found in 7–10% of neonatal autopsies and in up to 50% of cases in which other associated congenital abnormalities are present.[23] The clinical presentation ranges from acute respiratory distress with neonatal death to various degrees of chronic respiratory failure, and complications include pulmonary hemorrhage, bronchopulmonary dysplasia, and transient respiratory distress. The causes of pulmonary hypoplasia are numerous and varied, and include thoracic compression, lack of fetal movement, and severe oligohydramnios. These disorders can occur when there are renal, skeletal, or muscular abnormalities, in the presence of congenital diaphragmatic hernia, or when membranes rupture prematurely. There are several pathologic definitions of pulmonary hypoplasia: decreased dry weight of the lung, decreased rato of lung to body weight, decreased radial alveolar count, and/or decreased DNA content of the lung.[24]

In practice, it is difficult to predict which fetuses are going to have a fatal outcome as a result of lung hypoplasia. Lung height, lung diameter, thoracic circumference, rib length, pulmonary surface area, pulmonary-to-abdominal surface area ratio, and Doppler velocimetry of pulmonary vessels have been proposed as indirect estimates of pulmonary volume.[25,26] However, none of these parameters has been shown to be accurate or specific. Although magnetic resonance imaging (MRI) may overcome the limitations of sonographic evaluation for fetal pulmonary hypoplasia,[27] this technique is limited by its cost, poor patient compliance, and artifacts related to fetal movements. 3D sonography has been advocated as a valid alternative to estimate fetal pulmonary volume.[28,29] This new technique is better tolerated by patients than is MRI, and has been shown to measure fetal organ volumes accurately, both in vivo and in vitro.[30] However, there are no ultrasound-based nomograms that can be used reliably to define a risk threshold for pulmonary hypoplasia, and 3D sonography is currently limited by the fact that it is not yet available to all practitioners. The assessment of organ volumes can also be obtained from equations that use 2D measurements. These values, calculated by 3D sonography, make it possible to improve the accuracy of 2D equations.

For rotational-based volume measurements, the VOCAL software was used. Using this rotational technique, the volume of a lung object is obtained by contouring its surface. The volume of each lung can be measured separately, and the total lung volume was obtained by addition of these two values. We used the frontal view as plane of acquisition, which is already obtained for the multiplanar technique. This plane was rotated around the z-axis until the lung apex was above and the diaphragm was below. The next step was to calculate the surface geometry of the lung by rotating the longitudinal plane around the vertical axis and defining 2D lung contours on each plane. The 2D contours can be defined automatically or manually, and the rotation step for each contour plane can be selected with an angle ranging from 6° to 30°. A rotation step of 30° was chosen arbitrarily. The upper and lower contour points were then positioned automatically at the level of the clavicle and mid-diaphragm, respectively, after the first manual traces. These two landmarks were visualized in each of six planes obtained by counterclockwise rotation of the lung via the vertical axis. Area tracing was carefully performed,

excluding the fetal heart, mediastinal structures, ribs, and spine, until a rotation of 180° was completed. A 3D volume model of the lung was generated and reviewed for possible inconsistencies (Figure 20.2). The lung volume was calculated after all contours were considered to have been adequately traced.[23]

The VOCAL mode seems to have advantages, however: it allows finer contouring of the lung and subsequent modification of the contour. This is of particular interest when the outline of the lung is irregular, such as in congenital diaphragmatic hernia. In practice, however, extrapolating pulmonary volume from a 2D scan is more convenient compared with using 3D, as it is quicker and easier (Figure 20.2).

When studying the fetal lung using a 3D technique, the thoracic volume is best estimated by starting the data acquisition on a transverse view of the thorax.[31] Lee et al[32] have obtained the pulmonary volume by subtracting the heart volume from the thoracic volume. The thoracic volume is obtained by adding together the areas of several slices of thorax (transverse views), excluding the ribs and vertebrae. The heart volume is measured by contouring the shape of the heart on the same slices. The mediastinal structures (thymus, trachea, esophagus, and great vessels) are included in the measurement when using this method, and it therefore tends to overestimate the pulmonary volume. Measuring the volume of each lung individually has been proposed as a way of reducing the error. It is of note, however, that when these authors excluded the mediastinal volume from their measurements, they also failed to include the lower-most part of the lung bases, situated below the apex of the diaphragm.

Moeglin et al[23] stated that there was no demonstrable difference between the volumes obtained using

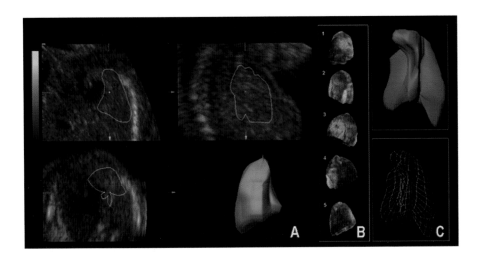

Figure 20.2 (A) Volume calculation of the lung can be exactly measured by 3D VOCAL software. (B) 3D rotational image of the lung. (C) 3D surface rendering of the lung

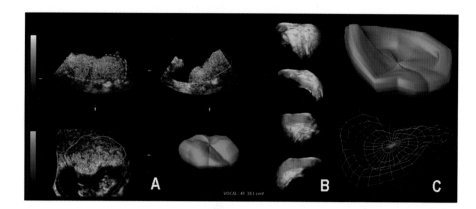

Figure 20.3 (A) 3D volume calculation of placenta. (B) 3D volume rendering showing the placenta from different angles. (C) 3D reconstruction of the placenta

either 3D technique, and it can be imagined that the small portion of the lung not included when measuring the lung height from the apex of the diaphragm to the clavicle is pretty much equivalent to the mediastinal volume included in the technique of Lee et al.[32] The multiplanar technique allowed satisfactory estimation of pulmonary volume, with much shorter measurement and calculation times compared with using a frontal surfacing technique such as the VOCAL mode. The VOCAL mode may, however, be more accurate, as the whole of the lung volume is included in the measurement, and subsequent modifications of the initial contouring are possible.

PLACENTAL VOLUME

Placental and neonatal weights are closely related.[33] To investigate a complex system, it is first necessary to look at its parts. In the present context, one of these parts is placental and fetal growth and size at the beginning of the 2nd trimester of pregnancy, a period when many pathogenetic mechanisms (e.g. smoking and inadequate uterine blood circulation) are potentially not yet relevant to fetal development.[34] The measurement of fetal growth by assessment of sonographic transverse and longitudinal diameters and circumferences is a satisfactory method, in contrast to 2D sonographic measurement of the placenta. Nevertheless, some studies have been performed that calculated the placental volume and evaluated the sensitivity and specificity regarding fetal growth restriction in the 3rd trimester.[35]

With the introduction of 3D sonography, volume calculation was simplified considerably. The 3D size of structures such as the placenta and the fetus can be easily observed over a specific period of time (Figure 20.3). This time period is limited due to the defined size of the volume box in which the 3D sonographic picture is built up and stored. From week 19 onward, the size of the placenta may exceed the capacity of the equipment. Hafner et al[36] demonstrated that the method is easily reproducible but the measurement is of limited value for the prediction of small-for-gestational age (SGA) babies.

The measurement of the placental volume was performed as follows. The placental site was determined by 2D sonography with a 3.5 MHz volume transducer. The scanning plane parallel to the placental attachment area was chosen. The placental volume was then constructed with the same transducer in volume mode around a plane in the central part of the placenta stored automatically. The scanning procedure was repeated until a satisfactory image of the entire placenta was obtained, which was generally possible in the majority of cases at the first trial (Figure 20.3). The placental border was traced by an electronic caliper and the rotational volume every 30° was calculated by the VOCAL software. The ultrasound machine calculates the volume automatically after completing all traces.

According to Hafner et al,[34] placental volume increased slightly (from 111.1 ml at 15 weeks of gestation to 114 ml at the end of the 17th week). The random variation of placental volumes around the mean in all three gestational weeks was considerably higher than the volume of the fetus, indicating that in this early period of gestation there is little correlation between fetal and placental sizes.

High sensitivity and specificity of placental volumes for the detection of intrauterine growth restriction performed with a complex calculation program and a series of 2D scans in the 3rd trimester have not been replicated in the 2nd trimester.[35] Nevertheless, a clear correlation between the placental volume in the 2nd trimester and the birth of an SGA infant has been demonstrated.[34,36] It was obvious from the beginning that placental volume calculation in the 2nd and 3rd trimesters could not compete with the well-established method of fetal biometry for the diagnosis of growth restriction.[34] However, placental volume in the 2nd trimester could provide important information about the reserve capacity of the placenta, which means that a large 2nd-trimester placenta will be better able to cope with its task of fetal support in the 3rd trimester. This calculation can be performed at an earlier period of gestation and cannot be substituted with fetal biometry. The limitation of the size of the volume box of the current technology necessitates the performance of volumetry in the 2nd trimester (e.g. weeks 14–18 for placental measurements with a transabdominal transducer). Future advances in medical therapy to enhance placental development suggest that the optimal time for therapeutic intervention may be at this early period of gestation.[34]

Placental volume is apparently different in the same period of time. Due to its slow increase and its wide variation, it is unsuitable for the calculation of gestational age. The main characteristic of placental volume appears to be its variation of size even at this early period of gestation. Hafner et al[34] stated that small placental size may be indicative of both fetal growth restriction and placental insufficiency in late pregnancy. Large fetuses are usually associated with big placentas. The time of major placental growth has already been reached by weeks 15–17, with placental volume increasing 4-fold until the end of pregnancy, whereas the fetal volume demonstrates a 50-fold increase.[34]

Hafner et al[34] suggested that placental volume measurements are reproducible. However, the predictive value of placental volume measurement for adverse pregnancy outcome should be evaluated. The main advantage of placental volume assessment is that it gives early information on the development of a structure that is difficult to assess later in pregnancy. In combination with assessment of the fetal volume, conclusions might be drawn on early placental pathologic changes leading to fetal macrosomia or an SGA neonate. Thus, placental volume measurement could be a viable addition to the routine sonographic examination.[34]

FETAL SPINE VOLUMETRY

Sonographic evaluation of the fetal spine is an essential part of any fetal survey aiming at the timely diagnosis of structural malformations, with special emphasis on neural tube defects.[37,38] Examination of the fetal spine depends on visualization of the three primary ossification centers within each vertebra: one in the vertebral body and one in each transverse process.[39] The pattern of ossification of the vertebral bodies is independent of that of the neural arches.[40] In the former, ossification starts at the thoracolumbar junction and from there proceeds in a cephalocaudad direction.[40] In the latter, two patterns of ossification have been proposed: originating in three spinal regions (thoracolumbar, cervicothoracic junction, and upper cervical region) or in the midthoracic spine.[37]

Usually, two planes of imaging are used to assess the integrity of the spine: transverse and parasagittal. On the former view, the spine is seen to consist of three echogenic foci arranged in a triangular fashion, corresponding to the respective ossification centers.[41] On the parasagittal view, the spine can be seen as 'interrupted railroad tracks' with the distance between the two lines similar to the interpediculate distance of the adult spine.[41] Although the fetal spine has been extensively researched with conventional 2D sonography, and in postmortem studies, few data exist about its intrauterine volume growth and that of its thoracolumbar junction in particular.

For the purpose of spine volumetry, single readings were used. The size of the acquired volume was determined by selecting the sweep speed and range as well as by defining the region of interest on the 2D image. The transducer was then initiated to perform a mechanical sweep through the outlined object. Subsequently, the automatically rendered volume was displayed in three orthogonal planes on the screen. Postprocessing rendering used maximum-intensity mixed with X-ray weighted rendering to create a translucent image. In the next step, the volume was rotated to a standard anatomic orientation, with a multiplanar image showing the frontal, parasagittal, and transverse views. For final review, the area of interest (lower thoracic spine and lumbar spine) was rotated into an optimal position (Figure 20.4).

The 12th thoracic vertebral body was identified in the A-plane by scrolling through the rendered volume until the origin of the lowest ribs was seen. Subsequent volume measurements were performed in the C-plane with the spine in transverse view. From the apical to the lower pole, the contour of the three ossification centers of the 12th thoracic vertebra and the 1st and 5th lumbar vertebrae was outlined with a cursor and stored. The contouring procedure was

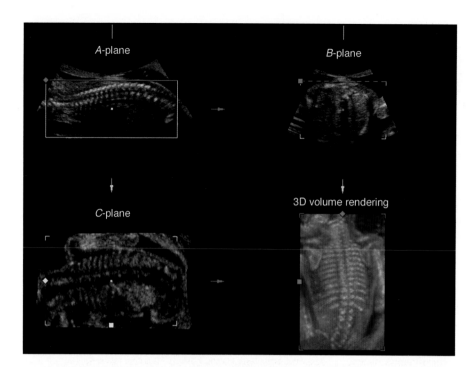

Figure 20.4 Multiplanar 3D image of the lower thoracic spine and lumbar spine. The region of interest is illustrated in the frontal (C-plane), parasagittal (A-plane), and transverse (B-plane) views

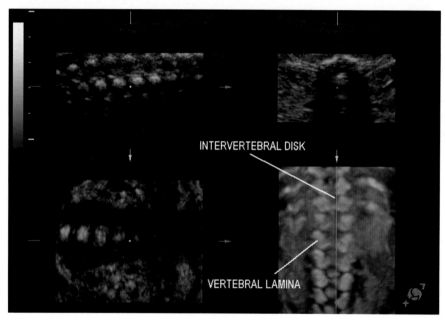

Figure 20.5 3D image of the lower thoracic spine and lumbar spine. The region of interest is illustrated in the frontal view

repeated whenever the shape of the vertebrae changed. In a similar procedure, starting from the upper pole of the 1st lumbar vertebra and proceeding to the caudal pole of the 5th lumbar vertebral body, the volume of the lumbar spine was calculated, including the intervertebral disk spaces (Figure 20.5).

Schild et al[37] have shown an increase in lumbar vertebrae (L1–L5) volume from 0.652 ml at 16 weeks to approximately 3.8 ml at 25 weeks, while the thoracic vertebral (T12) volume varied from 0.093 ml at 16 weeks to around 0.497 at 26 weeks. This finding

was collaborated again by Schild et al,[38] after refining the method by increasing the samples.

Sonographic evaluation of the spine, however, is operator-dependent, and difficulties may arise when, for a number of reasons, display of the sectional planes is inappropriate. The recent introduction of 3D sonography into clinical practice may alleviate some of these problems. Not only has fetal organ volumetry and surface rendering become possible, but 3D sonography is also less operator-dependent, resulting in a superior display of complex anatomy.[38] Imaging of the

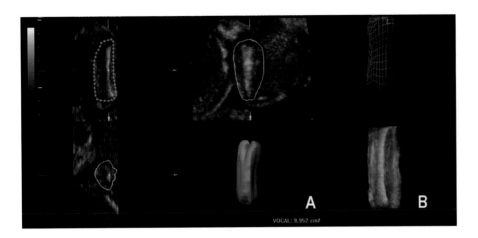

Figure 20.6 (A) Volume calculation of the upper arm using VOCAL software. (B) illustration of 3D mesh structure of the upper arm (above) and 3D surface rendering imaging (below)

fetal spine (Figure 20.5), in particular, benefits from this new technique, since the spine cannot be completely examined in a single plane in 2D sonography.[37] Furthermore, 3D volume measurements have proved to be superior to conventional 2D volume calculations, this benefit being most obvious when volumetry is performed on irregularly shaped objects.[37,38] However, there are no data available relating to volume changes of the fetal thoracolumbar section in utero.[37,38]

Schild et al[38] were able to provide preliminary results for each set of volumes between 16 and 37 completed weeks of gestation. Their data may be used in the assessment of fetal spinal anatomy and possibly of fetal size. Spinal abnormalities, such as hemivertebrae, scoliosis, and neural tube defects, or skeletal dysplasias can be analyzed on the basis of their reference values. Their preliminary data demonstrate that 3D sonography allows direct volume calculations on the fetal thoracolumbar spine. There is an increase in all volumetric measurements with gestational age.

UPPER-ARM VOLUME

Liang et al[42] have reported the primary use of 3D sonography in obstetrics to assess fetal upper-arm volume and have correlated it with birthweight. In brief, they used the upper-arm volume as a single parameter in predicting fetal weight, and the efficacy of this new modality was compared with those of traditional 2D sonographic formulae published previously.

The upper-arm volume was measured with a 3D sonographic scanner with a 5.0 MHz transabdominal transducer. Liang et al[42] performed the 3D sonography with the fetus at rest. The transducer was placed to identify the traditional plane for measuring humerus length (Figure 20.6). When the whole contour of the humerus and the upper arm could be clearly seen on the screen, the upper arm of the side closer to the transducer, either the right or the left side, was chosen for assessment. Then, the 3D scanning began with the normal velocity mode (which swept 30° automatically within 4 seconds), and the scanned volume of the whole upper arm was stored into the built-in computer for further analysis.[42]

Liang et al[42] performed 3D sonographic measurements of both arms. Their study was based predominantly on normal-weight term fetuses and may not be applicable or as accurate in fetuses weighing less than 2000 g or more than 4000 g. The mean absolute difference (±1 SD) between the right and left upper-arm volumes was 0.40 (±0.25) ml and the correlation coefficient between the right- and left upper-arm volumes was 0.99 ($p < 0.001$). They found that there is no significant difference between the right- and left-side upper-arm volumes ($n = 30$, $t = -0.61$, $p = 0.55$, not significant). Hence both sides of the upper arms were randomly used to assess upper-arm volume in their study.

With the 3D assessed upper-arm volume, the new formula results in a significant improvement in the prediction of fetal weight over the traditional 2D formulae. Liang et al[42] also stated that their formula is depended on ethnic factors. However, 3D measurement achieves an even higher accuracy with the smallest mean error and mean absolute error, and their difference is statistically significant (most $p < 0.001$ and all $p < 0.05$). On the basis of these data, they believed that the population differences may contribute less than the systemic technical measurement differences. In addition, their formula gives the lowest SD for both the error and the absolute error.

Furthermore, the same results can be replicated in another validation group. Liang et al[42] suggested that 3D-assessed upper-arm volume can accurately predict fetal weight without the common limitations such as fetal position.

FETAL URINARY PRODUCTION

Fetal urinary production can be calculated using serial sonographic registrations of bladder volume during the filling phase.[43] The product of three orthogonal bladder diameters estimated by longitudinal and transverse scans is directly proportional to the volume (Figure 20.7).[43] Healthy fetuses have a narrow urine production rate range, which increases with fetal age.[43,44] However, SGA fetuses and fetuses with hypoxemia display a reduced urine production rate.[43,45] Fetuses with bladder dysfunction (e.g., spina bifida) can have cyclical intervals of bladder filling and emptying that deviate from the norm.[46]

Previous studies of urine production rate during the last decade have shown very divergent results, ranging from 2.2 ml/h at 22 weeks to 26.3 ml/h at term,[43] in spite of using similar methods. The difference might reflect methodologic problems. Unfortunately, very few papers have rigorously evaluated potential human and technical sources of inaccuracy when carrying out such measurements.[47,48] According to Fagerquist et al,[44] there are two different and disjointed kinds of measurement error: (1) inaccuracy due to the selection of an inappropriate image, and (2) inaccuracy due to errors when measuring on the selected image.

Selection of appropriate images involves moving the ultrasound transducer correctly to scan the appropriate longitudinal and transverse sections (to avoid so-called 'freezing' error), and finding the appropriate image for assessment by playing the videotape recording backwards and forwards or by using the cine-loop function.[44]

Fagerquist et al[44] found some technical issues to be of very little importance quantitatively; i.e., the difference between ultrasound velocity in urine and that used in the ultrasound computer (1535 m/s vs 1540 m/s), measurements of vertical versus horizontal distances, the distortion of the videotape with time, and inter-operator variability.

Using unpublished data, we have reassessed the urinary production rate for fetuses of different gestational ages using 3D volume calculation (VOCAL) measurement to estimate fetal bladder volume.

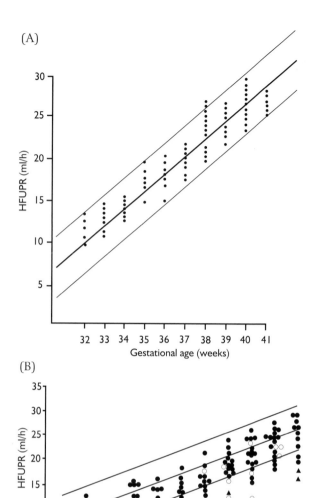

Figure 20.7 Hourly fetal urinary production rates (HFUPR) calculated by Kurjak et al in normal pregnancy (A) and growth-restricted fetuses (B) using 2D-US formula. Adapted from reference 43 with permission

Measurement of sonographic examinations of one urinary bladder filling phase documented on video clip was then undertaken (Figure 20.8). The longitudinal bladder image without disturbing shadows and at its largest appearance was first visualized using tissue harmonic imaging, which yields a clear contrast between adjacent tissue structures. The volume box was adjusted for the region of interest. The volume sweep angle was set between 45° and 75°. The slowest scan duration was adjusted to obtain the best resolution. In the sectional plane mode, three orthogonal

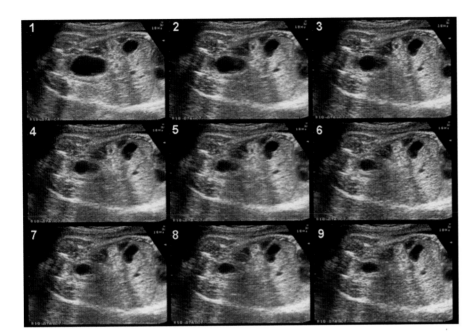

Figure 20.8 2D video clip imaging showing emptying of the fetal bladder

planes were simultaneously displayed on the screen. Once the scan was completed, the volume data were stored on the internal hard drive of the system. We selected the longitudinal plane as a reference for fetal bladder volume calculation. The next step was to calculate the surface geometry of the bladder by rotating the longitudinal plane around the vertical axis and defining 2D bladder contours on each plane. The 2D contours were defined manually, and the rotation step for each contour plane selected with an angle ranging to 30°. A 3D volume model of the bladder was generated and reviewed for possible inconsistencies. Bladder volume was calculated after all contours were considered to be adequately traced (Figure 20.9).

3D sonographic assessment of fetal bladder volume can be used to accurately predict fetal urinary production rate, but needs to be justified in a large-scale prospective study. We believe that computer-assisted programs for automatic volumetry will provide more objectivity than we were able to do manually.

CONCLUSIONS

This chapter has demonstrated the use of 3D sonography as a new modality in estimating fetal growth by volumetric measurement. The 3D technique is superior to traditional 2D biometry, without the common limitations of the latter, such as fetal position. However, 3D sonography is not available everywhere. Hence, the traditional 2D methods are still important in estimating fetal growth for most obstetricians. The advent of 3D volume sonography is enormously exciting and gives us control over the subject we are imaging, which goes much further than 2D imaging. We can manipulate that volume, rescan the fetus using the volume, and display any part of it. However, we have much to learn to determine where the applications will be as this technology leaps forward in the future. It is equally important to use this technique properly and maintain responsible use of 3D sonography as we explore its new and exciting capabilities.

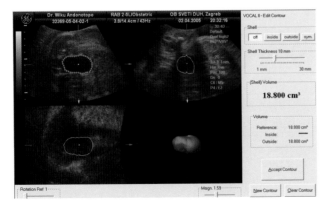

Figure 20.9 3D volume calculation measurement of the fetal bladder volume using VOCAL software

REFERENCES

1. Kurjak A, Hafner T, Kos M, Kupesic S, Stanojevic M. Three-dimensional sonography in prenatal diagnosis: a luxury or a necessity? J Perinat Med 2000; 28: 194–209.

2. Hadlock FP, Harrist RB, Sharman RS, Deter RL, Park SK. Estimation of fetal weight with the use of head, body, and femur measurements – a prospective study. Am J Obstet Gynecol 1985; 151: 333–7.

3. Shepard MJ, Richards VA, Berkowitz RL, Warsof SL, Hobbins JC. An evaluation of two equations for predicting fetal weight by ultrasound. Am J Obstet Gynecol 1982; 142: 47–54.

4. Thurnau GR, Tamura RK, Sabbagha R, et al. A simple estimated fetal weight equation based on real-time ultrasound measurements of fetuses less than thirty-four weeks' gestation. Am J Obstet Gynecol 1983; 145: 557–61.

5. Deter RL, Nazar R, Milner LL. Modified neonatal growth assessment score: a multivariate approach to the detection of intrauterine growth retardation in the neonate. Ultrasound Obstet Gynecol 1995; 6: 400–10.

6. Vintzileos AM, Campbell WA, Rodis JF, Bors-Koefoed R, Nochimson DJ. Fetal weight estimation formulas with head, abdominal, femur, and thigh circumference measurements. Am J Obstet Gynecol 1987; 157: 410–14.

7. Lee AL, Kratochwil A, Stümpflen I, Deutinger J, Bernaschek G. Fetal lung volume determination by three-dimensional ultrasonography. Am J Obstet Gynecol 1996; 175: 588–92.

8. Chang FM, Hsu KF, Ko HC, et al. Three-dimensional ultrasound assessment of fetal liver volume in normal pregnancy: a comparison of reproducibility with two-dimensional ultrasound and a search for a volume constant. Ultrasound Med Biol 1997; 23: 381–9.

9. Hadlock FP, Shah YP, Kanon OJ, Lindsey JV. Fetal crown–rump length: reevaluation of relation to menstrual age (5–18 weeks) with high-resolution real-time ultrasound. Radiology 1992; 182: 501–5.

10. Deter RL, Buster JE, Casson PR, Carson SA. Individual growth patterns in the first trimester: evidence for difference in embryonic and fetal growth rates. Ultrasound Obstet Gynecol 1999; 13: 90–8.

11. Kuhn P, Brizot ML, Pandya PP, Snijders RJ, Nicolaides KH. Crown–rump length in chromosomally abnormal fetuses at 10 to 13 weeks' gestation. Am J Obstet Gynecol 1995; 172: 32–5.

12. Blaas HG, Eik-Nes SH, Berg S, Torp H. In-vivo three-dimensional ultrasound reconstructions of embryos and early fetuses. Lancet 1998; 352: 1182–6.

13. Aviram R, Shpan DK, Markovitch O, Fishman A, Tepper R. Three-dimensional first trimester fetal volumetry: comparison with crown–rump length. Early Hum Dev 2004; 80: 1–5.

14. Nicolaides KH, Azar GB, Byrne D, Mansur CA, Marks K. Nuchal translucency: ultrasound screening for chromosomal defects in the first trimester of pregnancy. BMJ 1992; 304: 867–9.

15. Snijders RJ, Noble P, Sebire N, Souka A, Nicolaides KH. UK multicentre project on assessment of risk of trisomy 21 by maternal age and fetal nuchal-translucency thickness at 10–14 weeks of gestation. Fetal Medicine Foundation First Trimester Screening Group. Lancet 1998; 352: 343–6.

16. Falcon O, Peralta CFA, Cavoretto P, Faiola S, Nicolaides KH. Fetal trunk and head volume measured by three-dimensional ultrasound at 11 + 0 to 13 + 6 weeks of gestation in chromosomally normal pregnancies. Ultrasound Obstet Gynecol 2005; 26: 263–6

17. Falcon O, Wegrzyn P, Faro C, Peralta CFA, Nicolaides KH. Gestational sac volume measured by three-dimensional ultrasound at 11 to 13 + 6 weeks of gestation: relation to chromosomal defects. Ultrasound Obstet Gynecol 2005; 26: 546–50.

18. Wegrzyn P, Faro C, Falcon O, Peralta CFA, Nicolaides KH. Placental volume measured by three-dimensional ultrasound at 11 to 13 + 6 weeks of gestation: relation to chromosomal defects. Ultrasound Obstet Gynecol 2005; 26: 28–32.

19. Raine-Fenning NJ, Clewes JS, Kendall NR, et al. The interobserver reliability and validity of volume calculation from three-dimensional ultrasound datasets in the in-vitro setting. Ultrasound Obstet Gynecol 2003; 21: 283–91.

20. Snijders RJM, Nicolaides KH. Fetal biometry at 14–40 weeks' gestation. Ultrasound Obstet Gynecol 1994; 4: 34–8.

21. Streeter GL. Weight, sitting height, head size, foot length and menstrual age of the human embryo. Contrib Embryol 1920; 11: 143–70.

22. Sadler TW. Langman's Medical Embryology. Philadelphia, PA: Lippincott Williams and Wilkins, 2004.

23. Moeglin D, Talmant C, Duyme M, Lopez AC. Fetal lung volumetry using two- and three-dimensional ultrasound. Ultrasound Obstet Gynecol 2005; 25: 119–27.

24. Wigglesworth JS, Desay R. Use of DNA estimation for growth assessment in normal and hypoplastic fetal lungs. Arch Dis Child 1981; 56: 601–5.

25. Wladimiroff JW. Predicting pulmonary hypoplasia: assessment of lung volume or lung function or both? Ultrasound Obstet Gynecol 1998; 11: 164–6.

26. Fuke S, Kanzaki T, Mu J, et al. Antenatal prediction of pulmonary hypoplasia by acceleration time/ejection time ratio of fetal pulmonary arteries by Doppler blood flow velocimetry. Am J Obstet Gynecol 2003; 188: 228–233.

27. Rypens F, Metens T, Rocourt N, et al. Fetal lung volume: estimation at MR imaging-initial results. Radiology 2001; 219: 236–41.

28. Chang CH, Yu CH, Chang FM, Ko HC, Chen HY. Volumetric assessment of normal fetal lungs using three-dimensional ultrasound. Ultrasound Med Biol 2003; 29: 935–42.

29. Ruano R, Benachi A, Joubin L, et al. Three-dimensional ultrasonographic assessment of fetal lung volume as prognostic factor in isolated congenital diaphragmatic hernia. Br J Obstet Gynaecol 2004; 111: 423–9.

30. Riccabona M, Nelson TR, Pretorius DH. Three-dimensional ultrasound: accuracy of distance and volume measurements. Ultrasound Obstet Gynecol 1996; 7: 429–34.

31. Pohls UG, Rempen A. Fetal lung volumetry by three dimensional ultrasound. Ultrasound Obstet Gynecol 1998; 11: 6–12.

32. Lee A, Kratochwil A, Stumpflen L, Deutinger J, Bernaschek G. Fetal lung volume determination by three-dimensional ultrasonography. Am J Obstet Gynecol 1996; 175: 588–92.

33. Kloosterman GJ. On intrauterine growth, the significance of prenatal care. Int J Gynecol Obstet 1970; 8: 985.

34. Hafner E, Schuchter K, Van Leeuwen M, et al. Three-dimensional sonographic volumetry of the placenta and the fetus between weeks 15 and 17 of gestation. Ultrasound Obstet Gynecol 2001; 18: 116–20.

35. Wolf H, Oosting H, Treffers PE. Sonographic placental volume measurement – prediction of fetal outcome. Am J Obstet Gynecol 1989; 160: 121–6.

36. Hafner E, Philipp T, Schuchter K, et al. Second trimester measurement of placental volume by 3D ultrasound to predict SGA-infants. Ultrasound Obstet Gynecol 1998; 12: 97–102.

37. Schild RL, Wallny T, Fimmers R, Hansmann M. Fetal lumbar spine volumetry by three-dimensional ultrasound. Ultrasound Obstet Gynecol 1999; 13: 335–9.

38. Schild RL, Wallny T, Fimmers R, Hansmann M. The size of the fetal thoracolumbar spine: a three-dimen-

39. Filly RA, Golbus MS. Ultrasonography of the normal and pathologic fetal skeleton. Radiol Clin North Am 1982; 20: 311–23.

40. Budorick NE, Pretorius DH, Grafe MR, Lou KV. Ossification of the fetal spine. Radiology 1991; 181: 561–5.

41. Raghavendra BN. Ultrasonography of the spine and the spinal cord. Normal anatomy. Fetal spine. In: Sanders RC, Hill MC, eds. Ultrasound Annual 1985. New York: Raven Press, 1985: 227–9.

42. Liang RI, Chang FM, Yao BL, et al. Predicting birth weight by fetal upper-arm volume with use of three-dimensional ultrasonography. Am J Obstet Gynecol 1997; 177: 632–8.

43. Kurjak A, Kirkinen P, Latin V, Ivankovic D. Ultrasonic assessment of fetal kidney function in normal and complicated pregnancies. Am J Obtet Gynecol 1981; 141: 266–70.

44. Fagerquist M, Fagerquist U, Oden A, Blomberg SG. Fetal urine production and accuracy when estimating fetal urinary bladder volume. Ultrasound Obstet Gynecol 2001; 17: 132–9.

45. Nicolaides KH, Peters MT, Vyas S, et al. Relation of rate of urine production rate to oxygen tension in small-for-gestational age fetuses. Am J Obstet Gynecol 1990; 162: 387–91.

46. Nicolaides KH, Rosen D, Rabinowitz R, Campbell S. Urine production and bladder function in fetuses with open spina bifida. Fetal Ther 1988; 3: 135–40.

47. Hedriana HL, Moore TR. Ultrasonographic evaluation of human fetal urinary flow rate: accuracy limits of bladder volume estimations. Am J Obstet Gynecol 1994; 170: 1250–4.

48. Hedriana HL, Moore TR. Accuracy limits of ultrasonographic estimation of human fetal urinary flow rate. Am J Obstet Gynecol 1994; 171: 989–92.

21 Recent advances in neurophysiology

Aida Salihagic Kadic, Marijana Medic, and Asim Kurjak

INTRODUCTION

Physiology teaches us the wisdom of creating harmony and balance not only at the level of cells, tissues, and organs, but also in ourselves, and in relation to the world and environment where we live. Even in the fascinating world of intrauterine life, many fetal organ systems function in order to develop and maintain homeostasis. Only recently have we come to understand just how significantly our life outside the uterus is determined by our 40 or so weeks within it. There is a growing pool of evidence that many severe neurologic disorders, as well as the minimal cerebral dysfunctions, originate from the intrauterine rather than the perinatal or postnatal period.[1,2] Although developmental processes are genetically determined, only in the optimal intrauterine environment can the fetus reach its full genetic potential. Therefore, one should not be surprised by the diversity of the fetal mechanisms that have evolved to protect and defend the interior milieu. For example, the physiologic control mechanisms that are activated in the fetal organism in response to hypoxia include the cardiovascular, endocrine, and metabolic systems. As is well known, fetal cardiovascular adaptation to hypoxia is manifested by the redistribution of blood flow primarily toward the fetal brain. However, our latest investigations have shown that severe brain damage can develop despite the fetal blood flow redistribution and increased brain perfusion[3–5] (and personal unpublished data). These results indicate that the border between physiologic adaptation and pathophysiologic processes is extremely fragile and needs to be determined precisely in order to prevent brain damage, as well as lesions in other organ systems. Fortunately, our preliminary results indicate that in the case of chronic fetal hypoxia, this border can be determined by the use of a new vascular score, the hypoxia index. It is our belief that this new vascular score could represent a significant advance in the prevention of hypoxic brain damage, which is one of the most frequent causes of perinatal morbidity and mortality[6] (and personal unpublished data).

Nevertheless, in many cases, perinatal brain damage cannot be explained by the existence of fetal hypoxia. There is also an increasing number of results showing that a wide spectrum of neurologic problems, such as minimal cerebral dysfunction, schizophrenia, epilepsy, and autism, result at least in part from prenatal neurodevelopmental problems.[1] Epidemiologic studies have shown that cerebral palsy most frequently results from prenatal rather than perinatal or postnatal causes.[2] Presently, despite significant advances in prenatal and perinatal care, there is no means to detect or predict the development of these disorders. Hence, the development of diagnostic strategies to prevent and reduce the burden of perinatal brain injury has become one of the most important tasks of modern perinatal medicine. The development of any such strategy requires an understanding of normal neurodevelopmental processes and their influence on fetal functional and behavioral patterns, detectable by modern diagnostic methods.

STRUCTURAL DEVELOPMENT OF THE HUMAN CENTRAL NERVOUS SYSTEM

A detailed review of the complex of neurodevelopmental processes in the human fetus would exceed the

Table 21.1 Dynamics of the most important progressive processes in the development of the human brain (with permission from reference 10)

Process	Beginning	Most intensive activity	Ending
Neurogenesis	Early embryonic period (4th week)	8th–12th weeks	Approximately 20 weeks
Migration	Simultaneously with proliferation	18th–24th weeks	38th week
Synaptogenesis	6th–7th week for spinal cord 8th week for cortical plate	13th–18th weeks, after 24th week, 8th month–2nd year of postnatal life	Puberty

limits of this chapter. Since it has been extensively discussed elsewhere, we will present a brief overview of structural neurodevelopmental events, important for understanding of fetal neurophysiology and behavior.

Development of the central nervous system (CNS) begins approximately at the end of gastrulation. Generation of the neuroectoderm from the ectoderm during the 3rd postconceptional week results in the formation of the neural plate. Thus, the neural epithelium of the embryo, which is a precursor of neurons and glia, is virtually the first part of that organism that acquires a separate identity from other cells (for references, see reference 7). Formation of the neural plate is succeeded by folding of its edges and the formation of a neural tube, whose further growth and reshaping results in the formation of the structures of the CNS. According to O'Rahilly and Muller,[8] the forebrain (prosencephalon), midbrain (mesencephalon), and hindbrain (rhombencephalon) can be distinguished in the rostral portion of the unfused neural folds earlier than is usually referred to – at approximately the 22nd postconceptional day. In rapid succession, during the 4th postconceptional week, the forebrain components – diencephalon and telencephalon – can be detected. The cerebral hemispheres begin to evaginate from the neural tube at around the 35th day,[9] whereas the telencephalon medium appears a week earlier.[8] Obviously, the rostral regions of the neural tube proliferate extensively and fold up to form the brain, while the more caudal regions proliferate less so and form the spinal cord. The early formation of the structures of the CNS is a direct reflection of complicated histogenetic processes, generally represented by neurogenesis, migration, and cytodifferentiation. These three processes show a significant overlap in embryonic and fetal life. Neurogenesis predominates during the embryonic and early fetal period, migration occurs most intensively during midgestation, while cytodifferentiation, including myelination, occurs mainly in late fetal life (3rd trimester) and in the postnatal period

(Table 21.1, for references, see reference 10). Moreover, the fetal brain has a number of transitory structures that cannot be observed in the adult human brain. Three embryonic zones – ventricular, intermediary, and marginal zones (seen from the ventricular to the pial surface) – are present in all parts of the neural tube, whereas the telencephalon contains an additional two zones – the subventricular and subplate zones.[11,12] The ventricular and subventricular zones of the telencephalon are the sites of neurogenesis, and all the future neurons and glia are born in these structures. During migration towards the pial surface, they form other transitional zones before reaching their genetically predetermined final destinations. These destinations are the cortical plate or different nuclei in the brainstem, diencephalon, and basal forebrain.[11,13,14] One of the transitional structures – a subplate zone that is a site for transient synapses and neuronal interactions – can play a major role in developmental plasticity following perinatal brain damage.[12]

The early appearance of interneuronal connections (Table 21.1) implies the possibility of early functional development. However, these first synapses exist only temporarily and disappear due to normal reorganization processes. Most embryonic zones, types of neurons and glia, and early synapses, which play a crucial role in certain periods of fetal brain development, eventually disappear, significantly changing the structure and function of the brain. Reorganization processes include apoptosis (programmed cell death), disappearance of redundant synapses, axonal retraction and transposition, and transformation of the neurotransmitter phenotype.[12]

Obviously, the development of human brain is not complete at the time of delivery. In an infant born at term, characteristic cellular layers can be observed in motor, somatosensory, visual, and auditory cortical areas. Although proliferation and migration are completed in a term infant, synaptogenesis and neuronal differentiation continue very intensively.[15] The brainstem demonstrates a high level of maturity, whereas all histogenetic processes actively persist in the cerebellum.[16] Therefore, only the subcortical formations and primary cortical areas are well developed in a newborn. The associative cortex, barely visible in a newborn, is scantily developed in a 6-month-old infant. Postnatal formation of synapses in associative cortical areas, which intensifies between the 8th month and the 2nd year of life, precedes the onset of the first cognitive functions, such as speech. Following the 2nd year of life, many redundant synapses are eliminated. Elimination of synapses begins very rapidly, and continues slowly until puberty, when the same number of synapses as seen in adults is reached.[16]

FUNCTIONAL DEVELOPMENT OF THE NERVOUS SYSTEM AND THE ORIGINS OF FETAL BEHAVIOR

Fetal behavior can be defined as fetal activities observed or recorded with ultrasound equipment. As it is not yet possible to assess the functional development of the CNS directly, investigators have started to analyze fetal behavior as a measure of neurologic maturation.[17] A turning point in the assessment of fetal behavior was the introduction of real-time sonography. Ultrasound studies have revealed the fascinating diversity of fetal intrauterine activities. It has been shown that fetal activity occurs far earlier than a mother can register it, in fact as early as the late embryonic period. Furthermore, the qualitative and quantitative spectra of behavioral patterns expand rapidly as pregnancy progresses, and the random movements of the fetal body, which are the earliest signs of fetal activity, change into the well-organized behavioral patterns that are observed late in gestation. Analysis of the dynamics of fetal behavior has lead to the conclusion that fetal behavioral patterns directly reflect developmental and maturational processes of the fetal CNS. However, sonographic findings and their relevance in the assessment of the development of the CNS can be interpreted only in comparison with structural developmental events in the particular period of gestation. Therefore, understanding the relation between fetal behavior and developmental processes in different periods of gestation would make possible a distinction between normal and abnormal brain development, as well as early diagnosis of various structural and functional abnormalities.

Early embryonic development is characterized by immobility of the embryo. A prerequisite for the generation of embryonic and fetal motility is the existence of interneuronal and neuromuscular connections. This includes the ingrowth of axons, development of synapses, and formation of postsynaptic dendrites. Studies in vitro have shown that neurons begin to generate and propagate action potentials as soon as they interconnect.[18] The interconnected neurons will generate patterned activity because of the endogenous properties of neurons.[19] Generally, it seems that patterned activity emerges in networks of interacting neurons, due to interactions of intrinsic membrane properties and synaptic interactions (for references, see reference 20). The earliest synapses can be detected in the spinal cord shortly before the onset of embryonic motility, at 6–7 postconceptional weeks.[21] Therefore, the neural activity leading to the first detectable movements is considered to originate from spinal motor neurons.[21] Another prerequisite for motility is the development and innervation of muscle fibers. It is well known that primitive muscle fibers (myotubes) are able to contract as soon as they are innervated by motor neurons.[22] Between 6 and 8 postconceptional weeks, muscle fibers have formed by fusion of myoblasts, efferent and afferent neuromuscular connections have developed, and spontaneous neural activity causing motility can begin. The first spontaneous fetal movements can be observed with conventional two-dimensional (2D) sonography around the 8th postconceptional week, while the newly developed 4D sonography allows visualization of fetal motility 1 week earlier.[23,24]

Approximately at the 7th postconceptional week, the brainstem begins to develop and mature. In the subsequent weeks, it gradually begins to take control over fetal movements and behavioral patterns, which results in expansion of the motor and behavioral repertoires. This structure contains the nuclei of the cranial nerves, descending motor pathways into the spinal cord, and structures that mediate heart rate patterns and sleep–wake cycles. Until delivery, subunits of the brainstem will remain the main regulators of all fetal behavioral patterns.[25] The brainstem, which consists of the medulla oblongata, pons, and midbrain, forms and matures in a caudal-to-rostral direction. This means that the fillogenetically older structures, such as the medulla oblongata, will form and mature earlier in gestation. The major structures of the medulla oblongata are fashioned by the 7th and 8th postconceptional weeks, and are completely matured by 7 postconceptional months (for references, see reference 25). In addition to its many subnuclei, the medulla gives rise to a variety of descending spinal motor tracts that reflexively trigger limb and body movements. It also hosts the five cranial nerves (VIII–XII) that exert tremendous influences on gross body movements, heart rate, respiration, and head-turning. As the medulla matures in advance of more rostral structures of the brainstem, reflexive movements of the head, body, and extremities, as well as breathing movements and alterations in heart rate, appear in advance of other functions. Formation of the pons begins almost simultaneously, but its maturation is more prolonged. The structures of the pons include cranial nerves V–VIII (vestibular nuclei of cranial nerve VIII) and the medial longitudinal fasciculus (MLF), pontine tegmentum, raphe nucleus, and locus ceruleus, which exert widespread influences on arousal, including the sleep–wake cycles. Facial movements, which are also controlled by cranial nerves V and VII, appear around 10–11 weeks, while delayed onset of more specific functions, such as selective response to sounds and vibration, can be explained by the prolonged pontine maturation. Therefore, high levels of pontine arousal, including the perception of loud sounds, can trigger head-turning, whole-body movement, and the startle reaction in the 3rd trimester. Although the midbrain begins to form at almost the same time as the pons, its maturation does not even begin until the 2nd trimester. It consists of the dopamine-producing substantia nigra, the inferior-auditory and superior-visual colliculus, and cranial nerves III–IV, which, together with the MLF and cranial nerve VI, control eye movements. This explains the delayed onset of the latter, which cannot be registered before the 16th postconceptional week. Late in gestation, the fetus becomes increasingly responsive to sound, and reflexively orients, turns the head, and reacts with lateral eye movements if sufficiently stimulated. Many investigators agree that eye movement in response to light stimulation is even more delayed and appears only shortly prior to term (for references, see reference 25).

Generally, the basic structures of the diencephalon and cerebral hemispheres are formed by the end of the 8th postconceptional week.[7] The remarkable expansion of the cerebral hemispheres resulting from the above histogenetic processes proceeds during the remainder of gestation. Although the development of synapses in the human cerebral cortex begins after the formation of the cortical plate, at the end of the 8th week of gestation,[26,27] the number of synapses during the 1st trimester is miniscule. Development of the subplate zone, between the 13th and 15th weeks is

accompanied by an increase in the number of cortical synapses, which probably form the substrate for the earliest cortical electric activity at 19 weeks of gestation.[28] The spinothalamic tract is established at the 20th week and myelinized by the 29th week of gestation,[29] and thalamocortical connections penetrate the cortical plate at 24–26 weeks.[30,31] At the 29th week, evoked potentials can be registered from the cortex, indicating that the functional connection between periphery and cortex operates from that time onwards.[29] The establishment of thalamocortical connections seems to be a prerequisite for cortical analysis of sensory inputs. Approximately between 24 and 34 weeks, cortical areal differentiation begins and continues until the end of gestation (for a review, see reference 12). Neuronal differentiation and the laminar distribution of thalamocortical axons lead to the appearance of six-layered lamination throughout the neocortex after 32 weeks of gestation.[11] However, it should be noted that the cerebral cortex is still very immature, despite the appearance of an adult-like lamination pattern and initial areal differentiation.

The complexity of the structural development of the CNS is reflected in the complexity of motor, sensory, cognitive, affective functions and behavior patterns.[13,14,16,32]

FETAL MOTOR DEVELOPMENT

The first spontaneous fetal movements can be observed at 7–7.5 postconceptional weeks. These movements, consisting of slow flexion and extension of the fetal trunk, accompanied by the passive displacement of the arms and legs,[33] and appearing in irregular sequences, have been described as 'vermicular'.[34] In a short time, they are replaced by various well-organized general movements, which include head, trunk, and limb movements, such as 'rippling' seen at the 8th week, 'twitching' and 'strong twitching' at the 9th and 9.5th weeks, respectively, and 'floating', 'swimming', and 'jumping' at the 10th week.[35] Isolated limb movements appear almost simultaneously with the generalized movements. It is very important to note that even at this early stage of development, fetal movement appears in recognizable temporal sequences, without any amorphous or random movement. The explanation for this fascinating phenomenon lies in the previously described intrinsic properties of neurons. Even monocellular layers of cultured neural cells generate intrinsic, rhythmic bursts of action potential.[18] Although findings from simple in vitro experiments can hardly be paralleled with the complex neural structures of the human fetus, these observations indicate the important intrinsic properties of the developing neurons, consistent with the observation of embryonic and fetal endogenous motor patterns.

Simultaneously with the onset of spontaneous movements, at 7.5 postconceptional weeks, the earliest motor reflex activity can be observed, allowing an assumption to be made of the existence of the first afferent–efferent circuits.[36] At that time, head-tilting has been noted after perioral stimulation. The first reflex movements are massive, and indicate a limited number of synapses in a reflex pathway. During the 8th week of gestation, these massive reflex movements are replaced with local movements, probably owing to an increase in the number of axodendritic synapses. The hands become sensitive at 10.5 weeks and the lower limbs begin to participate in these reflexes at approximately the 14th week.[36–39]

From 10 weeks onwards, the number and frequency of fetal movements increase and the repertoire of movements begins to expand. The isolated limb movements seen at the 9th week are followed by the appearance of movements in the elbow joint at 10 weeks, changes in finger position in the 11th week, and easily recognizable clenching and unclenching of the fist at 12–13 weeks. Finally, at 13–14 weeks, isolated finger movements can be seen, as well as increases in the activity and strength of the hand/finger movements.[40] By 14–19 weeks, fetuses are highly active, with the longest period between movements being only 5–6 minutes. In the 15th week, 15 different types of movement can be observed. Besides the general body movements and isolated limb movements, retroflection, anteflection, and rotation of the head can easily be seen. Moreover, facial movements such as mouthing, yawning, hiccups, suckling, and swallowing, can be added to the wide repertoire of fetal motor activity in this period.[41] Finally, at 16–18 postconceptional weeks, slow rolling eye movements can be observed.[42,43] The further development of these movements and their relation to the sensory stimulation and circadian rhythms will be described later in this chapter. Using 4D sonography, Kurjak et al[44] have found that from 13 gestational weeks onwards, a 'goal orientation' of hand movements appears and a target point can be recognized for each hand movement. They classified hand movements into several subtypes according to spatial orientation: hand-to-head (Figure 21.1), hand-to-mouth (Figure 21.2), hand-near-mouth (Figure 21.3), hand-to-face, hand-near-face, hand-to-eye (Figure 21.4), and hand-to-ear. They investigated the

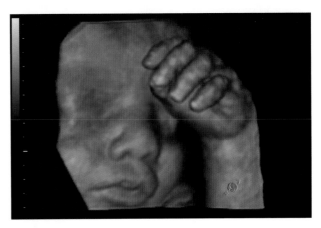

Figure 21.1 Fetal hand-to-head movement as seen by 3D/4D sonography

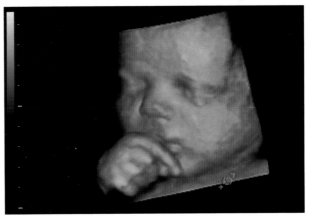

Figure 21.2 Fetal hand-to-mouth movement as seen by 3D/4D sonography

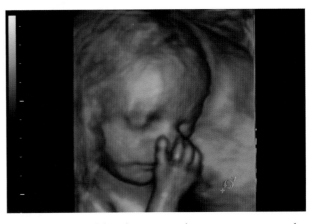

Figure 21.3 Fetal hand-near-mouth movement as seen by 3D/4D sonography

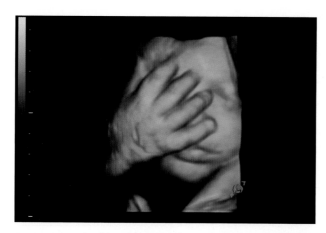

Figure 21.4 Fetal hand-to-eye movement as seen by 3D/4D sonography

frequency of each movement pattern in the period between 13 and 16 weeks, in an interval of 15 minutes, and found that the incidence of all movement patterns decreases slightly in this period. These findings are in slight contradiction to the previous observations by de Vries et al,[41] who described a constant increase in the frequency of hand movements until 18–19 weeks of pregnancy. This difference could be attributed to the technical limitation of 4D sonography, but it should also be noted that the classification of movement patterns as well as the length of the observation period differed between these two studies, which complicates their comparison.

The active and diverse fetal motor behavior in this period is related to the development of neuronal connections, through axonal ingrowth, synaptogenesis, and dendrite proliferation. However, it must be emphasized that despite the great diversity of fetal motor patterns in the first half of pregnancy, and a dynamic pattern of neuronal production and migration, the cerebral circuits are too immature for cerebral involvement in motor behavior (for a review, see reference 12). Nevertheless, studies of anencephalic fetuses have provided apparent evidence for the influence of supraspinal structures on motor behavior at around the 20th week of gestation. In these fetuses, the incidence of movements was normal or even increased, but the complexity of movement patterns changed dramatically and movements were stereotyped and simplified.[45] Similar qualitative changes were described at the 17th week of gestation in fetuses with cerebral aplasia, and at the 18th week in fetuses with hydrocephalus.[46]

The second half of pregnancy is characterized by organization of fetal movement patterns. The periods of fetal quiescence begin to increase, and rest–activity cycles become recognizable. Hardly any new movement pattern emerges in this period. The number of general body movements, which tends to increase from the 9th week onwards, gradually declines during the last 10 weeks of pregnancy.[47–49] By term, the average number of general movements per hour was found to be 31 (range 16–45), with the longest period between movements ranging from 50 to 75 minutes.[50] Although this decrease was initially explained as a consequence of the decrease in amniotic fluid volume, it is now considered to be a result of cerebral maturation processes. As the medulla oblongata matures, myelinates, and stabilizes, these spontaneous movements are less easily triggered, and begin to be controlled by more stable intrinsic activities generated within the brainstem.[25] Using 4D sonography, it was possible to confirm the declining trend in the frequency of fetal body and limb movements as pregnancy progresses. The median frequency of all body movements is slightly lower in the 2nd than in the 1st trimester, whereas the lowest frequency is noted in the 3rd trimester.[51] Simultaneously with the decrease in the number of general movements, an increase in facial movements, including opening/closing of the jaw, swallowing, and chewing, was observed using 2D sonography. These movements appeared mostly in the periods of absence of generalized movements, and this pattern was considered to be a reflection of the normal neurologic development of the fetus.[47] However, a revolutionary improvement in the study of fetal facial movements came with the development of 3D and 4D sonography (Figure 21.5). The application of 4D sonography to the examination of fetal facial movements has revealed the existence of a full range of facial expressions, including smiling, crying, and eyelid movements,[51–53] similar to emotional expressions in adults, in the 2nd and 3rd trimesters (Figures 21.6–21.8). Other facial movements, such as yawning, suckling, swallowing, and jaw opening, can also be observed in this period by 4D sonography. In our recent investigation of fetal motor activity,[51] the most frequent facial movement patterns in the 2nd trimester were isolated eye blinking, grimacing, suckling, and swallowing, whereas mouthing, yawning, tongue expulsion, and smiling could be seen less frequently. Longitudinal analysis of the frequencies of these facial movements in the 2nd and 3rd trimesters revealed some interesting results. A constant increase in the frequencies of almost all movement types was observed during the 2nd

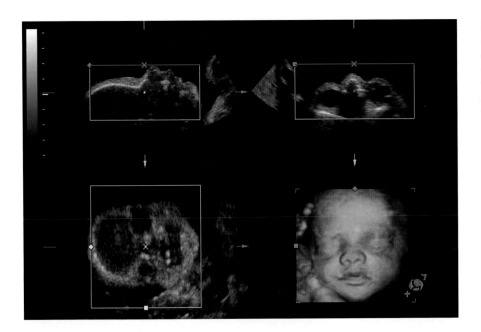

Figure 21.5 Three 2D sections are integrated by the computer to create a 3D image, which significantly improves visualization of fetal facial anatomy. Dynamic 3D scanning enables the analysis of all facial movements

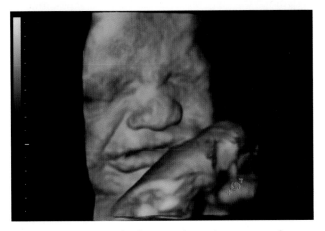

Figure 21.6 Image of a fetus in the 3rd trimester of gestation, taken by 3D/4D sonography, showing fetal grimacing

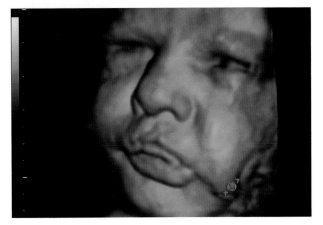

Figure 21.8 Image of the fetus in the 3rd trimester of gestation, taken by 3D/4D sonography: opened eyelids are clearly visible

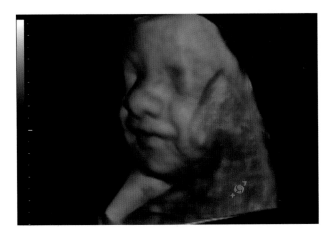

Figure 21.7 Image of a fetus in the 3rd trimester of gestation, taken by 3D/4D sonography, showing a smiling movement

trimester, which was followed by a brief plateau around the 24th–28th weeks, and a more or less prominent decline during the reminder of pregnancy (Figure 21.9).[52] Obviously, this developmental trend provides yet another example of the maturation of the medulla oblongata, pons, and midbrain, or perhaps even the establishment of control by more cranial structures. These impressive findings have, however, raised a number of questions, many of which are yet to be resolved. First of all, precise criteria for distinction of these facial expressions in the fetus should be established. The earliest appearance of different facial expressions has not yet been determined, and it is still unclear whether there are any gestational age-related trends in their onset. The nuclei of the facial nerve, a

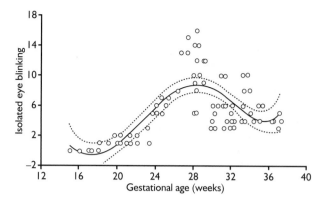

Figure 21.9 Scatterplot and polynomial regression analysis of the frequency of isolated eye blinking pattern in the 2nd–3rd trimesters of gestation (with permission from reference 52)

structure that controls these motor patterns, are developed by the end of 1st trimester, indicating that some facial grimaces could appear rather early in gestation. Nevertheless, the possibility of studying such subtle movements provided by this advanced ultrasound technique certainly opens a completely new area of investigation. One potential value of the observation of facial expressions could be the possibility of detecting facial nerve paresis in utero.[53] To what extent fetal facial motor patterns reveal the function and integrity of the CNS remains to be determined. Nevertheless, the facts that even in the embryonic period the same inductive forces that cause the growth and reshaping of the neural tube influence the development of facial structures, and that many genetic disorders affecting the CNS are also characterized by dysmorphology and dysfunction of facial structures, emphasize the importance of these investigations.[7,54] Obviously, the story of fetal intrauterine activity is far from complete; the development of new recording techniques should enrich our perspective on intrauterine life.[52,53]

Significant trends in fetal eye movement organization can also be observed during the second half of pregnancy, especially during the 3rd trimester. The earliest eye movements appear at 16–18 weeks of gestation, as sporadic movements with a limited frequency. At 24–26 weeks of gestation, they appear more frequently and begin to consolidate, so that periods of eye movement begin to alternate with those without eye movement. During the last 10 weeks of gestation, both switching and maintaining mechanisms responsible for this rhythm mature, and constant mean values of duration of eye movement (EM) and non-eye-movement (NEM) periods are achieved by 37–38 weeks. At that time, these periods

last 27–29 and 23–24 minutes, respectively, which is similar to the values in the neonate. From 33 weeks of gestation onwards, two types of eye movements can be distinguished during the EM periods. Rapid eye movements (REM) alternate with slow eye movements (SEM). At 36–38 weeks of gestation, they become integrated with other parameters of fetal activity, such as heart rate and fetal movements, into organized, coherent behavioral states.[42,43]

The diverse repertoire of fetal movements present during intrauterine life raises the question of their function and significance for normal fetal development. The finding that intrauterine motor activity exists in different animal species, even including invertebrates, implies their importance in neurodevelopment. The 'neuronal group selection' theory suggests the existence of genetically determined neural networks at the onset of development.[55] These networks undergo substantial variations through dynamic epigenetic regulation of histogenetic processes. Development then proceeds with selection on the basis of afferent information produced by the movements, and this selection is accomplished by the retention of the most favorable neural networks and motor patterns.[56] According to this theory, fetal movements could be important for the regulation of some histogenetic processes in the brain and spinal cord, such as programmed cell death (apoptosis), or fine-tuning of connectivity in the nervous system. For instance, breach presentation at the end of pregnancy may have long-lasting effects on the motility of the lower limbs. Mechanical restriction of fetal leg movement in these cases can affect the neurologic maturation of the leg reflexes and later motility.[56–58] Hence, fetal motor activity appears to be crucial for the development of most parts of the nervous system and the muscles.

The fine interaction between external influences and endogenous fetal activity is revealed in the fact that fetal behavior may be influenced by a number of external factors. Cigarette smoking or injection of corticosteroids for fetal lung maturation have been shown to decrease the number of spontaneous fetal movements.[59] Furthermore, fetal activity is increased in mothers suffering emotional stress.[60] It is known that qualitative alterations of spontaneous general movements can be observed in preterm and term newborns with cerebral impairment. Their movements seem to lose the characteristic fluency and complexity, and become cramped and unsynchronized. Similar qualitative alterations in fetal general movements have been observed in several conditions,

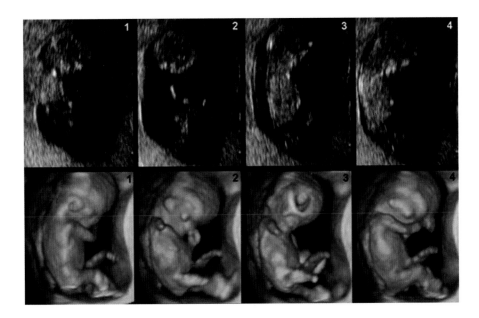

Figure 21.10 A sequence of images of fetus in the 11th week of gestation exhibiting general movements, taken by 2D and 4D sonography. Fetal head, trunk, and all extremities can be visualized simultaneously by 4D but not by 2D sonography

including maternal diabetes mellitus, fetal anencephaly, and intrauterine growth restriction (IUGR) (for references, see reference 61). In fetuses suffering IUGR, fetal movements become slower and monotonous, resembling cramps, and their variability in strength and amplitude is reduced. The alterations in amplitude and complexity of movements in these fetuses do not appear to be due to the oligohydramnios. In cases of premature rupture of fetal membranes and a subsequently reduced volume of amniotic fluid, movements occur less frequently, but their complexity resembles that of movements performed in the normal volume of amniotic fluid (for references, see reference 61). Unfortunately, despite the rapidly expanding pool of evidence that the qualitative assessment of general movements has a high predictive value for cerebral dysfunctions, the precise criteria for prenatal neurologic assessment have not yet been defined, mainly due to a lack of appropriate technology. Assessment of neonatal behavior often seems more informative about brain function than functional testing does, despite the availability of various neurologic, physiologic, and other methods of investigation.[62] A comprehensive description of spontaneous motor assessment as a diagnostic tool for detection of brain dysfunction in newborns was given by Einspieler et al.[62] The application of 4D sonography might facilitate the development of such diagnostic method in the prenatal period. According to the study of Andonotopo et al,[63] spatial imaging using 4D sonography, which allows simultaneous visualization of all fetal extremities, head, and trunk, might enable a good qualitative assessment of general movements even in

the 1st trimester of pregnancy (Figure 21.10). However, one of the possible limitations to such an assessment might be the fact that 4D imaging occurs in near-real time. Nevertheless, our recent study, performed on 50 embryos and fetuses in the 1st trimester of normal pregnancies, has shown that this technical limitation do not represent an obstacle to the assessment of general movements.[64] The median frequency of this movement pattern recorded by 4D sonography was similar to that obtained using 2D sonography, and there was a significant correlation between the number of movements observed by the two techniques, as shown in Figure 21.11. General movements were the most frequent movement

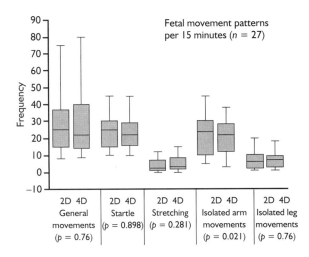

Figure 21.11 Comparison of frequencies of body movements and isolated limb movements between the 9th and 14th week of gestation as observed by 2D and 4D sonography (with permission from reference 64)

pattern in the 1st trimester of normal pregnancies. The possible relation between the qualitative and/or quantitative alterations of these movements and brain dysfunction remains to be determined.

The possibility of obtaining good-quality dynamic scans of fetal hand and facial motility allows comparison of fetal motor activity with the motor activity of neonates during the 1st week of life. In order to determine to what proportion of fetal movements in the 3rd trimester of pregnancy resemble those seen in preterm and term infants, we recorded fetal movements by 4D sonography in 10 term pregnancies, and also recorded neonatal spontaneous motor activity.[65] Interestingly, we found no statistically significant differences in either quality or quantity of fetal hand-to-face movements or fetal facial movements. No movements were observed in fetal life that were not present in neonatal life, whereas a Moro reflex was present only in neonates.[65] This study confirmed the existence of prenatal–neonatal continuity even in subtle, fine movements such as facial mimics. However, extensive investigations are required in order to determine whether and to what extent this recording modality can be used for the prenatal evaluation of the integrity of the central nervous system.

DEVELOPMENT OF SPECIALIZED MOVEMENTS

Studies on animals, especially various mammalian species, as well as comparisons with the sonograms of human fetuses, have revealed that some specialized movement patterns, crucial for the survival of newborns, such as swallowing or rhythmic respiratory movements, develop and mature during gestation (Figure 21.12). Although these patterns differ somewhat from adult patterns, in near-term fetuses they are developed sufficiently to enable the survival of the fetus. Furthermore, the results of studies on human fetuses and animal models have shown that these movements have very important functions during intrauterine life.

FETAL BREATHING

The rhythmic respiration-related neuronal network has been located within the hindbrain, in the pons and medulla oblongata.[66] In vertebrates, the hindbrain is one of the vesicles appearing at the cranial end of the neural tube. During the early embryonic period, the hindbrain neuroepithelium becomes partitioned into

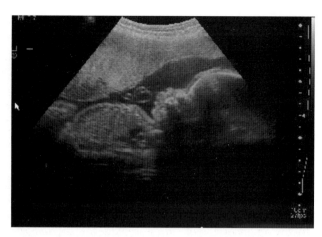

Figure 21.12 Image of a fetus, taken by 2D sonography. Fetal lungs and diaphragm are easily recognized, which facilitates assessment of breathing movements

several cellular segments, called rhombomeres. In the human embryo, this transient segmentation occurs during the second half of the 1st postconceptional month (in the chick embryo between stages 9 and 24), and is believed to regulate the spatial distribution of neurons.[66] At the end of the segmentation period, the hindbrain neuronal network in a chick embryo exhibits a consistent organized electric activity, composed of simultaneous burst discharges that occur spontaneously in the different cranial nerves.[66] The onset of breathing movements in the human fetus coincides partly with the end of the segmentation period and occurs around the 10th week of gestation.[67] Early in gestation, fetal breathing activity is present almost continually and is associated with activity in the postural muscles of the neck and limb. However, the frequency and complexity of the breathing patterns change as pregnancy progresses. It has been reported that at 24–28 weeks of gestation, fetuses breathe about 14% of the time in a 24-hour period, and by weeks 32–40, the breathing period increases to about 30% of the time.[68,69] From the 25th to the 32nd week, episodes of breathing lasting less than 10 seconds decrease, whereas episodes lasting longer than 30 seconds increase. Moreover, episodes of breathing are interspersed with apneic periods, which vary in length from 14 minutes in premature fetuses to 122 minutes at term.[68,69] Changes in breathing patterns are considered to result from maturation of the fetal lungs as well as the respiratory and sleep centers in the fetal CNS. At the 38th and 39th weeks of gestation, the frequency of movements decreases to 41 respirations per minute and the movements become as regular as in the postnatal period.[70]

A number of internal and external factors have been shown to influence fetal breathing movements during the last trimester of pregnancy. For instance, a decrease in fetal breathing has been observed following premature rupture of membranes,[71,72] during the 3 days prior to the initiation of labor.[73,74] Conversely, an increased number of fetal movements following the elevation of the glucose concentration in the maternal blood has been noted at the 34th week of gestation.[75,76] Furthermore, the level of carbon dioxide influences fetal respiratory movements from the 30th week of gestation onwards; the number of respirations increases following an excess of carbon dioxide in the maternal blood.[77,78] This sensitivity to alterations in the plasma carbon dioxide level is connected to the maturation of fetal respiratory neural centers, which is thought to occur during the last 10 weeks of pregnancy.[73] Kisilevsky et al[79] compared body movements and breathing patterns in normal 24–33-week-old fetuses and fetuses threatening to deliver prematurely. High-risk fetuses had a reduced level of body movements and an earlier onset of extended amounts of breathing, which occurred at 30 weeks, in contrast to their occurrence at 33 weeks in the control group. However, accelerated maturation of breathing was not observed in the presence of ruptured membranes. In this group, fetuses delivered prematurely had less breathing than those delivered at term.[79] Maternal consumption of alcohol, methadone, and, according to some authors, even cigarette smoking, is also known to decrease the incidence of breathing movements.[80–82] On the other hand, aminophylline, used for the treatment of bronchial asthma, as well as conjugated estrogens and betamethasone, increased the frequency of breathing.[83,84] The functions of breathing movements during prenatal life are the development of respiratory muscles and widening of the alveolar spaces. Experiments on animal models have shown that absence of respiratory movements (due to destruction of the brainstem nuclei above the phrenic nucleus) results in hypoplasia of the lungs. Therefore, respiratory movements, as well as lung liquid, are essential for normal lung development.

FETAL SWALLOWING AND DEVELOPMENT OF DIPSOGENIC MECHANISMS, APPETITE, AND SATIETY

Swallowing is a primary physiologic function that provides for the ingestion of food and fluid. In the human fetus, swallowing was noted as early as 11 weeks of gestation,[85] with daily swallowing rates near term of 500–1000 ml.[86] Swallowing movements are likely developed during intrauterine life in all species in which there is significant fetal fluid excretion (urine and lung liquid) into an amniotic cavity.[86,87] It might be suggested that fetal development of this physiologic function serves only to provide acquisition of water and food intake during the neonatal period. However, fetal swallowing and ingestive behavior contribute importantly to the regulation of the amniotic fluid volume and composition, acquisition and potential recirculation of solutes from the fetal environment, and maturation of the fetal gastrointestinal tract.[86]

Fetal swallowing serves as a major route for amniotic fluid resorption, recirculating water and solutes to the fetus.[86] In some, although not all, fetuses with esophageal atresia, the volume of amniotic fluid is increased. However, this anomaly is often accompanied by tracheoesophageal fistula, a shortcut to the gastrointestinal tract. Thus, intake of liquid during respiratory movements might explain the absence of polyhidramnios in some of these cases (for a review, see reference 86). Furthermore, polyhidramnios sometimes, although not always, develops in anencephalic fetuses. However, some of these fetuses have an intact swallowing reflex, whereas cases with normal amniotic fluid volume and decreased fetal swallowing were described. Recent studies suggest that fetal swallowing activity may be modulated in accordance with neurobehavioral state changes (stimulation of swallowing with shifts from quiet to active sleep) and influenced by the volume of amniotic fluid, hypoxia, hypotension, and plasma osmolality changes (for a review, see reference 86).

Experiments in animal models, especially fetal lambs, have shown that dipsogenic mechanisms begin to regulate swallowing during intrauterine life. For instance, in fetal lambs, swallowing and arginine-vasopressin (AVP) secretion increase following central administration of hypertonic saline and angiotensin II.[88,89] In recent investigations, hypertonicity-activated neurons were detected by determination of the Fos protein in dipsogenic hypothalamic nuclei in near-term ovine fetus. Intensive production of Fos protein, indicating activation of c-fos genes, was detected in putative dipsogenic nuclei, parvocellular and magnocellular divisions of the paraventricular nucleus (PVN), and the supraoptic nucleus (SON).[86,90–92] The findings that the fetus swallows 5–10 times more liquid in comparison with an adult, according to the results of these authors, can be explained by the persistence of tonic activation of angiotensin II receptors and the production of nitric oxide.[93,94] The fetus also appears to have a significantly reduced sensitivity to osmotic stimuli when compared with the adult,[95–97] despite the intact dipsogenic nuclei. Furthermore, reduced swallowing during systemic hypotension, despite elevated plasma renin levels, provides further evidence that the fetal dipsogenic response differs significantly from that of the adult.[98] It is possible that dipsogenic responses develop in utero in the human fetus, potentially to provide thirst stimulation for appropriate water intake during the immediate neonatal period.[86] Recent studies have indicated that an altered osmotic environment may modulate not only swallowing activity in utero but also the development of adult sensitivities for thirst, AVP secretion, and AVP responsiveness.[86,99]

Ingestive behavior during intrauterine life is manifested as swallowing and intake of amniotic fluid. Amniotic fluid proteins and growth factors contribute to the growth and maturation of the fetal gastrointestinal tract, and possibly to fetal somatic growth.[100] Amniotic fluid proteins provide 10–15% of the nitrogen requirement in the normal fetus, and esophageal atresia is often associated with a lower birthweight.[101] It is generally believed that appetite and satiety mechanisms develop during the intrauterine period in all precocious species. Human embryos demonstrate taste buds by 7 weeks of gestation.[102] Sweet taste, such as that of a low-concentration sucrose solution, stimulates swallowing in the human fetus, whereas the incidence of swallowing movements decreases following the injection of Lipiodol, a bitter extract of poppy seeds used as a contrast, into the amniotic fluid.[102] The main feeding regulatory factors – neuropeptide Y (NPY) and leptin – are secreted as early as 16 and 18 weeks, respectively, in the human fetus, but the ontogeny and functions of their regulatory pathways have not been delineated in the human fetal brain.[103–105] NPY is the most potent known inducer of food intake and a leptin is a primary satiety factor. Experiments in animals have shown an increase in fetal swallowing upon NPY administration.[106] Interestingly, fetal swallowing activity was significantly increased following the injection of leptin, which is opposite to the function of leptin in adults.[107] Therefore, some investigators have postulated that the absence of leptin-inhibitory responses might potentiate feeding and facilitate weight gain in newborns, despite high body fat levels.[100] Recent studies have

also suggested that the potential in utero imprinting of appetite and satiety mechanisms may influence infant, childhood, and ultimately adult appetite 'set-points'. Thus, disturbances of appetite regulation, and perhaps obesity, may result from maternal environmental influences during critical stages of development (for a review, see reference 100).

DEVELOPMENT OF THE FETAL SENSORY SYSTEM

Fetal tactile sensations, such as pain and touch, are among the first to be developed during intrauterine life. In monochorionic twins, movements evoked by tactile stimulation can be registered around the 8th postconceptional week,[108] while specific sensory receptors, the Maissner and Paccini bodies, are well developed by the 24th week of gestation. Evoked movements in early pregnancy can be explained only as motor reflexes, driven by the spinal cord. Thalamocortical pathways, important for the perception of sensory impulses, appear in the somatosensory cortex around the 23rd week, correlating with the development of synapses in the cortical plate.[27] These events are followed by the areal differentiation of the primary somatosensory cortex, as well as other primary cortical areas, between the 24th and 34th weeks (for reviews, see references 12 and 28).

During the past decade, fetal perception of pain has been not only an object of interest for scientists but also an important issue in public debates regarding late abortions and the increasing number of intrauterine operations. The concept that the fetus is a patient in its own right has also led to increasing interest in the subject of fetal pain. According to the International Association for the Study of Pain, pain is 'an unpleasant sensory and emotional experience associated with actual or potential tissue damage'. This definition obviously puts the emphasis on previous injury-related experience. In that sense, pain consists of two components: (i) perception of a stimulus and (ii) an emotional reaction, an unpleasant feeling of a noxious stimulus. Each component occurs in anatomically and physiologically distinct regions of the brain. Furthermore, reactions to pain can be analyzed at three different levels: a somatosensory response, pain-induced physiologic (autonomic and endocrine) reactions, and pain-related behavior.[109]

The first nociceptors appear at 7 weeks of gestation, and by the 20th week these are present all over the body. This suggests that already early in life, pain is a very important signal. Upon the development of nociceptors, peripheral afferents make synapses to the spinal cord, during approximately weeks 10–30,[110] which is followed by myelination of these pathways.[111] Functional spinal reflex circuitry develops simultaneously with the growth of peripheral afferents into the spinal cord.[112,113] Higher parts of the pain pathways include the spinothalamic tract, established at 20 weeks of gestation and myelinated by 29 weeks,[114] and thalamocortical connections, which begin to grow into the cortex at 24–26 weeks.[30,31] Finally, at 29 weeks, evoked potentials can be registered from the cortex, indicating that a functionally meaningful pathway from the periphery to the cerebral cortex starts to operate from that time onwards.[38,113]

The earliest reactions to painful stimuli, appearing early in gestation, are motor reflexes, resembling withdrawal reflexes. Reflex threshold is remarkably low, and various kinds of stimuli may induce very holistic and unspecific reactions. It is important to emphasize that these reactions are completely reflexive, directed by the spinal cord, and higher perception or processing of painful sensation does not exist at this stage (for a review, see reference 109). However, some investigators have indicated that facial reflexes in response to somatic stimuli, which could indicate an emotional reaction to pain, develop rather early in gestation.[39] These reflexes are thought to be coordinated by subcortical systems and probably reflect development of these lower brain circuitries.[114] With regard to the autonomic and endocrine responses to pain, an elevation of noradrenaline (norepinephrine), cortisol, and β-endorphin plasma levels, in response to needle pricking of the innervated hepatic vein for intrauterine transfusion, was registered in a 23-week-old fetus. Pricking of the non-innervated placental cord insertion for the same purpose had no effect.[115,116] Later, alterations in cerebral blood flow (i.e., blood flow redistribution) were noted during invasive procedures in an 18-week-old fetus.[117] This redistribution of blood flow may be mediated by the sympathetic system or by other undetermined mechanisms.[117] Obviously, painful stimuli trigger a wide spectrum of reactions in the CNS, such as activation of the hypothalamo-hypophysial axis, or autonomic reflexes, without reaching the cortex. Furthermore, it is interesting to note that the hormonal, autonomic, and metabolic responses can be suppressed by analgesics. For instance, fentanyl suppressed autonomic and hormonal reactions to surgical operations in 28-week

fetuses.[117,118] These findings are extremely important if we bear in mind the relations of early pain experiences to later behavioral variables or to later developmental outcomes, which have been confirmed in many studies.[119] One of the most important effects of a painful experience is the prolonged stress response.[120] This includes marked fluctuations in blood pressure and cerebral blood flow and hypoxemia, which may predispose to intracranial hemorrhage.[117] Furthermore, animal experiments have confirmed that elevated cortisol levels, equivalent to those secreted during the stress response in humans, were associated with degenerative changes in the fetal hippocampus.[121] Finally, long-term follow-up studies of infants treated in intensive care units and exposed to pain and/or stress have demonstrated correlations between the length of stay in the intensive care unit and altered pain thresholds as well as abnormal pain-related behavior later in life.[120,122] Even a short-term painful experience, namely neonatal circumcision without analgesia, was shown to intensify subsequent pain-related behavior (following vaccination 4–6 months later) in comparison with the findings in non-circumcised infants.[123] All of these findings underline the importance of a stress-free environment for the normal physiologic and psychologic development of the fetus and the neonate. Thus, from a clinical perspective, the findings that harmful stress responses and their sequelae can be prevented by adequate pain treatment[113,118] are extremely important. Certainly, the crucial precondition for the treatment of pain and prevention of stress is the ability to recognize pain responses. In premature neonates born after the 28th week of gestation, the most promising pain indicators are changes in facial activity, shifts in infant sleep/wake state, and physiologic changes of heart rate and oxygen saturation.[124,125]

The development of fetal hearing is described more extensively in Chapter 22 and will be addressed only briefly here. It is generally accepted that reflexes of the brainstem, including vestibular, olfactory, and auditory reflexes, develop early in gestation.[126] Vestibular ganglionic cells mature earlier than the neurons of the lateral and inferior vestibular nuclei, which are functional from 9 weeks of gestation onwards.[127] Vestibular stimulation is thought to contribute to the development of fetal movements. The gravity-free environment in the uterus appears to promote the development of vestibular reflexes.[128]

According to electrophysiologic examinations of evoked potentials in prematurely delivered healthy infants, cochlear function develops between 22 and 25 weeks of gestation, and its maturation continues during the first 6 months after delivery.[129–131] Maternal heartbeats and motility of the gastrointestinal tract during digestion appear to generate 60–90 decibels of sound in utero.[132] However, fluid in the fetal ear as well as the immaturity of the cochlea complicate the transmission of sound, so that only strong acoustic stimuli can be registered by the fetus. Reflex movements, such as startles of trunk and/or extremities, accompanied by changes in heart rate, can be observed during or soon after vibroacoustic stimulation.[131] By the 26th week of gestation, the fetus will react reflexively not only to vibration but also to exceedingly loud sounds 60% of the time, whereas the same response can be elicited 80% of time in a 32-week-old fetus. The response to vibratory and acoustic stimulation of a 29-week-old fetus includes not only startle but also fetal heart rate acceleration (for a review, see reference 25). As the brainstem continues to mature, it becomes increasingly responsive to sounds. During the last weeks of pregnancy (weeks 36–38), the fetus can respond to external noises, even to the sound of the mother's voice, with reflexive body movements, head-turning, and heart rate acceleration. However, these sounds have to be rather loud and high in frequency to overcome the attenuation of the uterus and amniotic fluid (for a review, see reference 25). Cortical auditory evoked potentials, which indicate the development of the primary auditory cortex, can be registered in a 28-week premature infant and are dominantly surface-negative. Maturation of the auditory cortex is characterized by the appearance of surface-positive evoked potentials, which happens between the 36th and 40th weeks and after birth (for references, see reference 12).

The intrauterine environment is not completely deprived of light. Moreover, some experimental results have indicated that the development of visual and auditory organs could not be possible without any light or acoustic stimulation.[133,134] Although the structural development of sensory pathways is a prerequisite for functional development, the final organization of brain circuitries relies predominantly on guidance from external inputs.[12] In cortical area 17, synaptogenesis persists between 24 weeks of gestation and 8 months after delivery,[133] whereas myelination of the optical tract begins at 32 weeks of gestation.[134] However, cones of the central foveola do not reach adult proportions until late in childhood.[135] The primary visual cortex can be clearly delineated in the occipital lobe by immunohystochemical staining even before the 25th week. Visual evoked potentials change in the same fashion as auditory evoked potentials, gradually becoming surface-positive between 36 and 40 weeks (for a review, see reference 12).

CYCLIC BEHAVIOR AND THE DEVELOPMENT OF CIRCADIAN RHYTHMS

The circadian system allows predictive adaptation of individuals to the reproducible 24-hour day/night alternations of our planet. Specific physiologic functions are distributed in given segments of the 24 hours, creating an internal temporal order. The circadian system can be described as a biologic clock that receives information from the environment and sends efferent outputs that orchestrate endocrine, biophysical (temperature), and behavioral (activity–rest and sleep–wake) circadian rhythms.[136] In mammals, the major role in orchestration of these rhythms is played by the suprachiasmatic nucleus (SCN) of the hypothalamus, which oscillates with a period of close to 24 hours.

In the human fetus, as well as other mammalian species, the SCN is developed by midgestation, but its maturation continues after birth, as shown by the increase in the number of neurons containing AVP and vasoactive intestinal peptide (VIP) during the 1st year of postnatal life (for a review, see reference 137). Circadian rhythms in behavior, cardiovascular function, and hormones are present in human fetuses, as well as in the fetal sheep and monkey, and are synchronized with the light/darkness cycle. However, the question of whether these rhythms are generated by the fetus itself or influenced by maternal rhythms remains to be resolved, although some animal experiments have indicated the importance of the maternal SCN. In this case, transmission of the signal to the fetus would necessarily require an endocrine mediator, but no such molecule has yet been identified. The latest results suggest the maternal pineal hormone melatonin plays a role. This hormone is present in humans, as well as in other mammals, and its plasma concentrations exhibit daily variations, with a peak during the night. Therefore, its role in sleep induction has been suggested.[136] Seasonal alterations in melatonin concentrations have also been reported. Daily oscillations of melatonin concentrations in the fetal plasma are present throughout gestation, and various human tissues, including the CNS, express some types of melatonin receptor.[138,139] However, the role of melatonin in the orchestration of fetal circadian rhythms remains to be confirmed. Nevertheless, we can state that fetal life in utero is organized in cyclic patterns. From midgestation onwards, periods of activity begin to alternate with periods of rest. As stated earlier, generalized body movements, which occur randomly during early pregnancy, from midgestation begin to appear in clusters alternating with episodes of fetal quiescence. As pregnancy progresses, the rest–activity cycles gradually become integrated with specific fetal heart rate patterns and to the absence or presence of REMs. Finally, they develop into fetal behavioral states, including sleep–wake episodes, with stable temporal organization near the end of pregnancy.[140,141] It is important to point out that sleep and wake patterns in EEGs become distinguishable at 30 weeks of gestation.[109]

In fetal animals, simultaneous measurements of fetal electrocortical activity and eye and body movements have shown that deep sleep, characterized by high-voltage waves and decreased fetal activity, occur during 54% of the day. The total length of the REM sleep period, characterized by low-voltage waves and REMs, lasts 40% of the day. The waking state (6% of a day) is characterized by low-voltage waves.[142] In human premature newborns, born 4 weeks prior to term, 60–65% of the total sleeping period is REM sleep, whereas in term newborns, the REM sleeping period includes 50% of the total 16 hours of sleep.[143] The intensive activity of neuronal circuits during REM sleep is thought to contribute to the development of the CNS.[143]

FETAL STRESS AND ITS LONG-TERM EFFECTS ON BEHAVIOR

Fetal stress has been a hot topic for decades, but it has recently become clear that the effects of fetal stress can have long-term consequences for adult health. Experimental findings and studies of human fetuses have shown that early life experience can have long-term phenotypic consequences.[144] Furthermore, there is evidence that phenotypic expression is strongly influenced by the actions of stress hormones produced during development. Overall, fetal development can be regarded as a trade-off between growth opportunity and mortality risk in the developmental environment. Physiologic sensors compute this trade-off as a function of energy balance and environmental stress,

and effectors initiate physiologic, developmental, and behavioral responses to these factors. The process that underlies all of the modifications of morphology, physiology, and behavior in response to the changing environment is known as phenotypic plasticity. This fascinating process is not the exclusive property of human beings, but can be observed in almost every plant and animal species.

The intrauterine environment has important effects on fetal growth and development and the timing of birth. A great number of environmental factors can trigger the fetal stress response. For example, maternal undernutrition or placental insufficiency can change the intrauterine environment and cause fetal stress. The effects of responses to painful stimuli have already been mentioned. According to some authors, even maternal emotional stress can influence the fetal environment.[145,146] Although the primary role of stress is protection of the organism, exposure to stress may affect fetal neurodevelopment, as well as the development of many other organ systems, and have lifelong consequences. It should be emphasized that the stress hormonal axis, acting both centrally and peripherally, can transduce environmental signals into developmental responses. Many adaptive changes induced by stress, which increase the chance of survival and thus can be regarded as short-term protection, may also leave profound modifications in the structure and functions of the organism (Figure 21.13). For a long time, it has been well known that brain and lung maturation may be accelerated as an adaptation to intrauterine stress (for a review, see reference 147). New experimental findings have also suggested an active participation of the fetus in the initiation of parturition.[148] Fetal as well as placental corticotropin-releasing hormone (CRH) has been shown to influence the timing of birth.[144] Altogether, these findings may explain the fact that high-risk pregnancies often end with premature delivery and that these infants are often functionally more mature than it could be expected considering their gestational age. Unfortunately, recent investigations have indicated that corticosteroids, which accelerate lung maturation and enable survival of premature infants, may have a negative influence on growth of the lungs, development of secondary alveolar septa, and even to growth of the whole organism (for a review, see reference 149).

Accelerated maturation of the brain is also associated with structural as well as behavioral changes, as shown in Figure 21.13. Behavioral changes associated

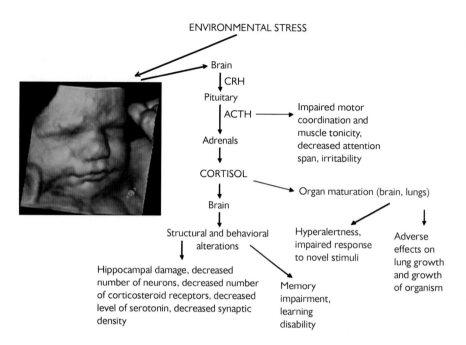

ENVIRONMENTAL STRESS

Brain
↓ CRH
Pituitary
↓ ACTH ——→ Impaired motor coordination and muscle tonicity, decreased attention span, irritability
Adrenals
↓
CORTISOL ——→ Organ maturation (brain, lungs)
↓
Brain
↓
Structural and behavioral alterations

Hyperalertness, impaired response to novel stimuli

Adverse effects on lung growth and growth of organism

Hippocampal damage, decreased number of neurons, decreased number of corticosteroid receptors, decreased level of serotonin, decreased synaptic density

Memory impairment, learning disability

Figure 21.13 The effects of environmental stress and stress hormones on fetal neurodevelopment and organ maturation. A detailed description is given in the text. CRH, corticotropin-releasing hormone; ACTH, adrenocorticotropic hormone

with acceleration of brain maturation include hyperalertness and impaired fetal responsiveness to novel stimuli, possibly due to the effects of CRH and stress hormones.[150] A few studies in very low-birthweight (VLBW) infants have indicated that selective impairment of memory could explain the high incidence of learning disabilities observed in this population, even in the group considered neurologically normal (for a review, see reference 147). Recent experiments have shown profound impairment of hippocampal functioning in the offspring of mothers exposed to prenatal stress (for a review, see reference 151). Prenatally stressed animals show lower performance in hippocampally mediated learning tasks, especially during aging.[152–157] They also have a higher propensity to develop drug abuse[153] and exhibit higher levels of drug-induced adaptations involved in the development of drug dependence.[158,159] Stress-induced structural changes of the hippocampus, obtained from animal experiments, include a decreased number of neurons and corticosteroid receptors, decreased levels of serotonin, and decreased synaptic density in distinct regions of the hippocampus.[160–162] A reduction in the neurotropin brain-derived neurotrophic factor (BDNF) has also been discovered in the fetal hippocampus.[163] Environmental factors can also change fetal cerebral levels of biogenic amines, which have the function of facilitating the formation and maintenance of synapses in diverse regions of the CNS.[164] The normal number of synapses maintained by biogenic amines is crucial to the acquisition of learning and memory.

Alterations in the endocrine response to stressful environment and novelty have also been observed, suggesting a more general impairment of their capability to cope with external challenges.[164–167] In general, the above-mentioned adverse effects of prenatal stress have been attributed to increased glucocorticoid secretion,[168] which impairs hippocampal plasticity, accelerates loss of memory during aging,[154–157] and increases the propensity to develop drug abuse.[169] Furthermore, adrenocorticotropic hormone (ACTH) itself impairs motor coordination and muscle tone, reduces attention span, and increases irritability.[170]

Retrospective studies on children whose mothers experienced severe psychologic stress or adverse life events during pregnancy have suggested long-term neurodevelopmental effects on the infant.[171–174] Attention deficit hyperactivity disorder (ADHD), sleep disturbances, and unsociable and inconsiderate behavior, as well as psychiatric disorders, including schizophrenic episodes, depressive and neurotic symptoms, drug abuse, mood, and anxiety (for a review, see reference 151), can be recognized in these children. Fortunately, there is recent evidence that increased maternal care and environmental enrichment can compensate for prenatal stress-induced effects.[175,176]

It has been shown that disruption of the fetal environment by maternal cocaine abuse can cause neurodevelopmental defects and predispose the fetus to behavioral alterations and neuropsychiatric disorders later in life.[177] Our results have shown that long-term exposure to cocaine leads to uterine and umbilical blood flow disorders, fetal growth restriction, and hypoxia. It reduces the capability of cerebral blood vessels to vasodilate and the heart rate to increase during acute hypoxia.[178] Recent studies have shown that cocaine exposure can also alter neurotransmitter function. The dopamine-rich anterior cingulate cortex is a target of in utero cocaine. Consequently, the ability to exhibit normal attention to the informational content of competing stimuli is reduced.[173]

It is very important to note that chronic adult diseases are also programmed in utero.[179] Adaptation to malnutrition during intrauterine life has definite effects on metabolism and organ structure that determine the occurrence of coronary heart diseases, hypertension, and diabetes in adulthood. The explanation for these diseases should be sought in the hyperresponsive neuroendocrine stress axis, which includes magnified or prolonged responses of CRH and cortisol to acute stressors, increased food intake associated with higher probabilities of obesity, and metabolic dysfunction. It is also possible that increased prenatal exposure to corticosteroids can affect the development of CNS feeding centers (by elevating the set point), and thus permanently alter feeding behavior later in life. Obviously, early survival benefits come at a cost.

SUMMARY

Functional development of the fetal brain begins as early as the late embryonic period. During the 9 months of gestation, the repertoire of fetal activities constantly expands, correlating precisely with structural development of the CNS. Major developmental events, such as the establishment of neural connections in different regions of the brain, are accompanied by new patterns of fetal activities and by the transformation of existing patterns. The integration of random and abundant fetal activity into organized behavioral states indicates the maturation of the control centers in the CNS. Another sign of advancing maturation is fetal ability to respond to a variety of vibratory, acoustic, and metabolic external stimuli, acquired during the 3rd trimester. Unfortunately, the ability to receive and respond to the external environment can have many adverse effects. Although the

intrauterine world provides optimal conditions for fetal development, in many situations the fetus is insufficiently protected from harmful external influences. Fetal hypoxia, infections, or maternal substance abuse have been recognized as possible causes of the brain damage, including the most severe disorder, cerebral palsy. Furthermore, fetal exposure to stress or even severe maternal stress can also interfere with fetal neurodevelopment and result in long-term and profound consequences on brain structure and function. A variety of neuropsychiatric diseases are nowadays considered to originate at least partly from prenatal incidents. In most of these conditions, there is no reliable parameter for detection or prediction of cerebral lesions. On the other hand, the severity of the consequences indicates the need to develop any strategy that would enable early detection of cerebral lesions or indications that such lesions might occur.

The investigation of fetal behavior and the development of new, advanced imaging techniques open a new perspective for the development of such strategies. According to the present results, 4D sonography represents a significant advance in the study of fetal behavioral patterns and understanding of the functional development of the fetal CNS. Knowing that fetal behavioral patterns correlate fairly well with the development of the CNS and that the quality of fetal movements reveals the integrity of the CNS, this technique could facilitate the development of a diagnostic strategy for the early detection of cerebral dysfunctions. Prevention of brain dysfunctions and structural lesions would enable the necessary initial preconditions for an untroubled and happy childhood.

REFERENCES

1. Blair E, Stanley FJ. Intrapartum asphyxia: a rare cause of cerebral palsy. J Pediatr 1988; 112: 515–19.

2. Harrison PJ. The neuropahology of schizophrenia. A critical review of the data and their interpretation. Brain 1999; 122: 593–624.

3. Fignon A, Salihagic A, Locatelli S, et al. Twenty-day umbilical and cerebral Doppler monitoring on a growth retarded and hypoxic fetus. Eur J Obstet Gynecol Reprod Biol 1996; 66: 83–6.

4. Salihagic A, Fignon A, Locateli S, et al. New advances in understanding fetal hypoxia. In: Chervanek F, Kurjak A, eds. Current Perspectives on the Fetus as a Patient. New York: Parthenon, 1996: 359–78.

5. Salihagic A, Georgescus M, Perrotin F, et al. Daily Doppler assessment of the fetal hemodynamic response to chronic hypoxia: a five case report. Prenat Neonat Med 2000; 5: 35–41.

6. Arbeille P, Perrotin F, Salihagic A, et al. Fetal Doppler hypoxic index for prediction of abnormal fetal heart rate at delivery in chronic fetal distress. Eur J Obstet Gynecol Reprod Biol 2005; 121: 171–7.

7. Pomeroy SL, Volpe JJ. Development of the nervous system. In: Polin RA, Fox WW, eds. Fetal and Neonatal Physiology. Philadelphia, PA: WB Saunders, 1992: 1491–509.

8. O'Rahilly R, Muller F. Minireview: Summary of the initial development of the human central nervous system. Teratology 1999; 60: 39–41.

9. Muller F, O'Rahilly R. The first appearance of the neural tube and optic primordium in the human embryo at stage 10. Anat Embryol (Berl) 1985; 172: 157–69.

10. Salihagic-Kadic A, Kurjak A, Medic M, et al. New data about embryonic and fetal neurodevelopment and behavior obtained by 3D and 4D sonography. J Perinat Med 2005; 33: 478–90.

11. Kostovic I, Judas M, Rados M, Hrabac P. Laminar organization of the human fetal cerebrum revealed by histochemical markers and magnetic resonance imaging. Cereb Cortex 2002; 12: 536–44.

12. Kostovic I, Judas M, Petanjek Z, Simic G. Ontogenesis of goal-dyrected behavior: anatomo-functional considerations. Int J Psychophysiol 1995; 19: 85–102.

13. Lightman SL, Insel TR, Ingram CD. New genomic avenues in behavioral neuroendocrinology. Eur J Neurosci 2002; 16: 369–72.

14. Hanganu IL, Kilb W, Luhmann HJ. Functional synaptic projections onto subplate neurons in neonatal rat somatosensory cortex. J Neurosci 2002; 22: 7165–76.

15. Jessell T. Development of the nervous system. In: Kandel ER, Schwartz JH, Jessell T, eds. Essentials of Neural Science and Behaviour. Norwalk, CT: Appleton & Lange, 1995: 89–107.

16. Kostovic I. Prenatal development of nucleus basalis complex and related fibre system in man: a histochemical study. Neuroscience 1986; 17: 1047–77.

17. Nijhuis JG, ed. Fetal Behaviour: Developmental and Perinatal Aspects. Oxford: Oxford University Press, 1992.

18. Stafstrom CE, Johnston D, Wehner JM, Sheppard JR. Spontaneous neural activity in fetal brain reaggregate culture. Neuroscience 1980; 5: 1681–9.

19. Streit J. Regular oscillations of synaptic activity in spinal networks in vitro. J Neurophysiol 1993; 70: 871–8.

20. Marder E, Calabrese R. Principles of rhythmic motor pattern generation. Physiol Rev 1996; 76: 687–717.

21. Okado N, Kojima T. Ontogeny of the central nervous system: neurogenesis, fibre connection, synaptogenesis and myelination in the spinal cord. In: Prechtl HFR, ed. Continuity of Neural Functions from Prenatal to Postnatal Life. Oxford: Blackwell Science, 1984: 31–5.

22. Landmesser LT, Morris DG. The development of functional innervation in the hind limb of the chick embryo. J Physiol (Lond) 1975; 249: 301–26.

23. De Vries JIP, Visser GHA, Prechtl HFR. Fetal motility in the first half of the pregnancy. In: Prechtl HFR, ed. Continuity of Neural Functions from Prenatal to Postnatal Life. Oxford: Blackwell Science, 1984: 44–64.

24. Kurjak A, Vecek N, Hafner T, et al. Prenatal diagnosis: What does four-dimensional ultrasound add? J Perinat Med 2002; 30: 57–62.

25. Joseph R. Fetal brain and cognitive development. Dev Rev 1999; 20: 81–98.

26. Kostovic I. Zentralenrvensystemen. In: Hinrichsen KV, ed. Humanembryologie. Berlin: Springer-Verlag, 1990; 381–448.

27. Molliver ME, Kostovic I, Van der Loos H. The development of synapses in cerebral cortex of the human fetus. Brain Res 1973; 50: 403–7.

28. Kostovic I, Rakic P. Developmental history of the transient subplate zone in the visual and somatosensory cortex of the macaque monkey and human brain. J Comp Neurol 1990; 274: 441–70.

29. Anand KJS, Hickey PR. Pain and its effects on human fetus. N Engl J Med 1987; 317: 1321–9.

30. Kostovic I, Rakic P. Development of prestriate visual projections in the monkey and human fetal cerebrum revealed by transient cholinesterase staining. J Neurosci 1984; 4: 25–42.

31. Kostovic I, Goldman-Rakic PS. Transient cholinesterase staining in the mediodorsal nucleus of the thalamus and its connections in the developing human and monkey brain. J Comp Neurol 1983; 219: 431–47.

32. Buhta AT, Anand KJ. Vulnerability of the developing brain. Neuronal mechanisms. Clin Perinatol 2002; 29: 357–72.

33. Prechtl HFR. Ultrasound studies of human fetal behaviour. Early Hum Dev 1985; 12: 91–8.

34. Ianniruberto A, Tajani E. Ultrasonographic study of fetal movements. Semin Perinatol 1981; 4: 175–81.

35. Goto S, Kato TK. Early movements are useful for estimating the gestational weeks in the first trimester of pregnancy. In: Levski RA, Morley P, eds. Ultrasound '82. Oxford: Pergamon Press, 1983: 577–82.

36. Okado N. Onset of synapse formation in the human spinal cord. J Comp Neurol 1981; 201: 211–19.

37. Okado N. Development of the human cervical spinal cord with reference to synapse formation in the motor nucleus. J Comp Neurol 1980; 191: 495–513.

38. Lloyd-Thomas AR, Fitzgerald M. Reflex responses do not necessarily signify pain. BMJ 1996; 313: 797–8.

39. Humphrey T. Some correlations between the appearance of human fetal reflexes and the development of the nervous system. Prog Brain Res 1964; 4: 93–135.

40. Pooh RK, Ogura T. Normal and abnormal fetal hand positioning and movement in early pregnancy detected by three and four-dimensional ultrasound. Ultrasound Rev Obstet Gynecol 2004; 4: 46–51.

41. de Vries JIP, Visser GHA, Prechtl HFR. The emergence of fetal behavior I. Qualitative aspects. Early Hum Dev 1982; 7: 301–22.

42. Awoust J, Levi S. Neurological maturation of the human fetus. Ultrasound Med Biol 1983; 9: 583–7.

43. Inoue M, Koyanagi T, Nakahara H. Functional development of human eye-movement in utero assessed quantitatively with real-time ultrasound. Am J Obstet Gynecol 1986; 155: 170–4.

44. Kurjak A, Azumendi G, Vecek N, et al. Fetal hand movements and facial expression in normal pregnancy studied by four-dimensional sonography. J Perinat Med 2003; 31: 496–508.

45. Visser GHA, Laurini RN, Vries JIP, et al. Abnormal motor behaviour in anencephalic fetuses. Early Hum Dev 1985; 12: 173–83.

46. Visser GHA, Prechtl HFR. Perinatal neurological development. Proceedings of the Third International Conference on Fetal and Neonatal Physiological Measurements III, 1989: 335–46.

47. D'Elia A, Pighetti M, Moccia G, Santangelo N. Spontaneous motor activity in normal fetus. Early Hum Dev 2001; 65: 139–44.

48. Natale R, Nasello-Paterson C, Turlink R. Longitudinal measurements of fetal breathing, body movements, and heart rate accelerations, and decelerations at 24 and 32 weeks of gestation. Am J Obstet Gynecol 1985; 151: 256–63.

49. Eller DP, Stramm SL, Newman RB. The effect of maternal intravenous glucose administration on fetal activity. Am J Obstet Gynecol 1992; 167: 1071–4.

50. Patrick J, Campbell K, Carmichael L, et al. Patterns of gross fetal body movements over 24-hour observation intervals during the last 10 weeks of pregnancy. Am J Obstet Gynecol 1982; 142: 363–71.

51. Kurjak A, Stanojevic M, Andonotopo W, et al. Fetal behavior assessed in all three trimesters of normal pregnancy by four dimensional (4D) ultrasonography. Croat Med J 2005; 46: 770.

52. Kurjak A, Andonotopo W, Salihagic-Kadic A, et al. Normal standards for fetal neurobehavioural developments – longitudinal quantifications by four-dimensional sonography. J Perinat Med 2006; 34: 56–65.

53. Kozuma S, Baba K, Okai T, et al. Dynamic observation of the fetal face by three-dimensional ultrasound. Ultrasound Obstet Gynecol 1999; 13: 283–4.

54. Merz E, Weller C. 2D and 3D ultrasound in the evaluation of normal and abnormal fetal anatomy in the second and third trimesters in a level III center. Ultraschall Med 2005; 26: 19.

55. Sporns O, Edelman GM. Solving Bernstein's problem: a proposal for the development of coordinated movement by selection. Child Dev 1993; 64: 960–81.

56. Changeux JP. Variation and selection in neural function. Trends Neurosci 1997; 20: 291–3.

57. Prechtl HFR, Knol AR. Der Einfluß der Beckenendlage auf die Fußsohlenreflexe bein neugeborenen Kind. Arch Psychiatr Zeitschr Neurol 1958; 196: 542–53.

58. Sival DA, Prechtl HFR, Sonder GHA, Touwen BCL. The effect of intrauterine breech position on postnatal motor functions of the lower limbs. Early Hum Dev 1993; 32: 161–76.

59. Graca LM, Cardoso CG, Clode N, Calhaz-Jorge C. Acute effects of maternal cigarette smoking on fetal heart rate and fetal movements felt the mother. J Perinat Med 1991; 19: 385–90.

60. Katz M, Meizner I, Holcberg G, et al. Reduction of cessation of fetal movements after administration of steroids for enhancement of lung maturation. Isr J Med Science 1988; 24: 5–9.

61. Prechtl HFR, Einspieler C. Is neurological assessment of the fetus possible? Eur J Obstet Gynecol Reprod Biol 1997; 75: 81–4.

62. Einspieler C, Prechtl HF, Ferrari F, et al. The qualitative assessment of general movements in preterm, term and young infants – review of the methodology. Early Hum Dev 1997; 50: 47–60.

63. Andonotopo W, Stanojevic M, Kurjak A, Azumendi G, Carrera JM. Assessment of fetal behavior and general movements by four-dimensional sonography. Ultrasound Rev Obstet Gynecol 2004; 4: 103.

64. Andonotopo W, Medic M, Salihagic-Kadic A, Milenkovic D. The assessment of fetal behaviour in early pregnancy; comparison between 2D and 4D sonographic scanning. J Perinat Med 2005; 33: 406–14.

65. Kurjak A, Stanojevic M, Andonotopo W, et al. Behavioral pattern continuity from prenatal to postnatal life – a study by four-dimensional (4D) ultrasonography. J Perinat Med 2004; 32: 346–53.

66. Champagnat J, Fortin G. Primordial respiratory-like rhythm generation in the vertebrate embryo. Trends Neurosci 1997; 20: 119–24.

67. Patrick J, Gagnon R. Fetal breathing and body movement. In: Creasy RK, Resnik R, eds. Maternal–Fetal Medicine: Principles and Practice, 2nd edn. Philadelphia, PA: WB Saunders, 1989: 268–84.

68. Natale R, Nasello-Paterson C, Connors G. Patterns of fetal breathing activity in the human fetus at 24 to 28 weeks of gestation. Am J Obstet Gynecol 1988; 158: 317–21.

69. Patrick J, Campbell K, Carmichael L, et al. Patterns of human fetal breathing during the last 10 weeks of pregnancy. Obstet Gynecol 1980; 56: 24–30.

70. Patrick J, Campbell K, Carmichael L, et al. A definition of human fetal apnea and the distribution of fetal apneic intervals during the last 10 weeks of pregnancy. Am J Obstet Gynecol 1978; 136: 371–7.

71. Roberts AB, Goldstein I, Romero R, et al. Fetal breathing movements after preterm rupture of membranes. Am J Obstet Gynecol 1991; 164: 821–5.

72. Kivikoski A, Amon E, Vaalamo PO, et al. Effect of third-trimester premature rupture of membranes on fetal breathing movements: a prospective case–control study. Am J Obstet Gynecol 1988; 159: 1474–7.

73. Richardson B, Natale R, Patrick J. Human fetal breathing activity during induced labour at term. Am J Obstet Gynecol 1979; 133: 247–55.

74. Besinger RE, Compton AA, Hayashi RH. The presence or absence of fetal breathing movements as a predictor of outcome in preterm labor. Am J Obstet Gynecol 1987; 157: 753–7.

75. Natale R, Patrick J, Richardson B. Effects of maternal venous plasma glucose concentrations on fetal breathing movements. Am J Obstet Gynecol 1978; 132–41.

76. Patrick J, Natale R, Richardson B. Patterns of human fetal breathing activity at 34 to 35 weeks gestational age. Am J Obstet Gynecol 1978; 507–13.

77. Ritchie K. The response to changes in the composition of maternal inspired air in human pregnancy. Semin Perinatol 1980; 4: 295–9.

78. Richardson B, Campbell K, Campbell L, et al. Effects of external physical stimulation on fetuses near term. Am J Obstet Gynecol 1981; 139: 344–52.

79. Kisilevsky BS, Hains SMJ, Low JA. Maturation of body and breathing movements in 24–33 week old fetuses threatening to deliver prematurely. Early Hum Dev 1999; 55: 25–38.

80. Fox HE, Steinbrecher M, Pessel D, et al. Maternal ethanol ingestion and occurence of human breathing movements. Am J Obstet Gynecol 1978; 132: 354–61.

81. Richardson B, O'Grady JP, Olsen GD. Fetal breathing movements in response to carbon dioxide in patients on methadone maintenance. Am J Obstet Gynecol 1984; 150: 400–4.

82. Manning FA, Wym Pugh E, Boddy K. Effect of cigarete smoking on fetal breathing movements in normal pregnancy. BMJ 1975; 1: 552–8.

83. Ishigava M, Yoneyama Y, Power GG, et al. Maternal teophylline administration and breathing movements in late gestation human fetus. Obstet Gynecol 1996; 88: 973–8.

84. Cosmi EV, Cosmi E, La Torre R. The effect of fetal breathing movements on the utero-placental circulation. Early Pregnancy 2001; 5: 51–2.

85. Diamant NE. Development of esophageal function. Am Rev Respir Dis 1985; 131: S29–32.

86. Ross MG, Nijland JM. Development of ingestive behavior. Am J Physiol 1998; 274: R879–93.

87. Abramovich DR. Fetal factor influencing the volume and composition of liquor amnii. J Obstet Gynaecol Br Commonw 1970; 77: 865–77.

88. Ross MG, Kullama LK, Ogundipe OA, et al. Ovine fetal swallowing response to intracerebroventricular hypertonic saline. J Appl Physiol 1995; 78: 2267–71.

89. Ross MG, Kullama LK, Ogundipe OA, et al. Central angiotensin II stimulation of ovine fetal swallowing. J Appl Physiol 1994; 76: 1340–5.

90. McDonald TJ, Li C, Nijland MJM, et al. Fos response of the fetal sheep anterior circumventricular organs to an osmotic challenge in late gestation. Am J Physiol 1998; 275: 609–14.

91. Xu Z, Nijland MJ, Ross MG. Plasma osmolality dypsogenic tresholds and c-fos expression in the near-term ovine fetus. Pediatr Res 2001; 49: 678–85.

92. Caston Balderrama A, Nijland MJM, McDonald TJ, et al. Central Fos expression in fetal and adult sheep following intraperitoneal hypertonic saline. Am J Physiol 1999; 276: 725–35.

93. El Haddad MA, Chao CR, MA SX, et al. Neuronal NO modulates spontaneous ANG II-stimulated fetal swallowing behavior in the near-term ovine fetus. Am J Physiol Regul Integr Comp Physiol 2002; 282: R1521–7.

94. El Haddad MA, Chao CR, Sayed AA, et al. Effects of central angiotensin II receptor antagonism on fetal swallowing and cardiovascular activity. Am J Obstet Gynecol 2001; 185: 828–33.

95. Davison JM, Gilmore EA, Durr J. Altered osmotic thresholds for vasopressin secretion and thirst in human pregnancy. Am J Physiol 1984; 246: 105–9.

96. Ross MG, Sherman DJ, Schreyer P, et al. Fetal rehydration via amniotic fluid: contribution of fetal swallowing. Pediat Res 1991; 29; 214–17.

97. Nijland MJM, Kullama LK, Ross MG. Maternal plasma hypo-osmolality: effects on spontaneous and stimulated ovine fetal swallowing. J Mater-Fetal Med 1998; 7: 165–71.

98. Ross MG, Sherman DJ, Ervin MG, et al. Fetal swallowing: response to systemic hypotension. Am J Physiol 1990; 257: R130–4.

99. Nicolaidis S, Galaverna O, Meltzer CH. Extracellular dehydration during pregnancy increases salt appetite of offspring. Am J Physiol (Regul Integr Comp Physiol) 1990; 258; 281–3.

100. Ross MG, El Haddad M, DeSai M. Unopposed orexic pathways in the developing fetus. Physiol Behav 2003; 79: 79–88.

101. Pitkin RM, Reynolds WA. Fetal ingestion and metabolism of amniotic fluid protein. Am J Obstet Gynecol 1975; 123: 356–63.

102. Bradley RM, Mistretta CM. The developing sense of taste. In: Denton DA, Coghlan JP, eds. Olfaction and Taste. New York: Academic Press, 1975: 91–8.

103. Kawamura K, Takebayashi S. The development of noradrenaline-, acetylcholinesterase-, neuropeptide Y- and vasoactive intestinal polypeptide-containing nerves in human cerebral arteries. Neurosci Lett 1994; 175: 1–4.

104. Cetin I, Morpurgo PS, Radaelli T, et al., Fetal plasma leptin concentrations: relationship with different intrauterine growth patterns from 19 weeks to term. Pediatr Res 2000; 48: 646–651.

105. Jaquet D, Leger J, Levy-Marchal C, et al. Ontogeny of leptin in human fetuses and newborns: effect of intrauterine growth retardation on serum leptin concentrations. J Clin Endocrinol Metab 1998; 83: 1243–6.

106. Roberts TJ, Caston-Balderrama A, Nijland MJ, et al. Central neuropeptide Y stimulates ingestive behavior and increases urine output in the ovine fetus. Am J Physiol Endocrinol Metab 2000; 279: E494–500.

107. Roberts TJ, Nijland MJ, Caston-Balderrama A, et al. Central leptin stimulates ingestive behavior and urine flow in the near term ovine fetus. Horm Metab Res 2001; 33: 144–50.

108. Arabin B, Bos R, Rijlaarsdam R, et al. The onset of inter-human contacts: longitudinal ultrasound observations in early twin pregnancies. Ultrasound Obstet Gynecol 1996; 8: 166–73.

109. Vanhatalo S, van Nieuvenhuizen O. Fetal pain? Brain Dev 2000; 22: 145–50.

110. Fitzgerald M. Development of pain mechanisms. Br Med Bul 1991; 47: 667–75.

111. Okado N, Kojima T. Ontogeny of central nervous system: neurogenesis, fibre connections, synaptogenesis and myelination in the spinal cord. In: Prechtl HFR, ed. Continuity of Neural Functions from Prenatal to Postnatal Life. Oxford: Blackwell Science 1984: 31–45.

112. Anand KJS, Hickey PR. Pain and its effects in the human neonate and fetus. N Engl J Med 1987; 317: 1321–9.

113. Anand KJ, Carr DB. The neuroanatomy, neurophysiology, and neurochemistry of pain, stress and analgesia in the newborns and children. Pediatr Clin North Am 1989; 36; 795–822.

114. Holstege G. Descending motor pathways and the spinal motor system: limbic and non-limbic components. Prog Brain Res 1991; 87: 307–421.

115. Giannakoulopoulos X, Sepulveda W, Kourtis P, et al. Fetal plasma cortisol and beta endorphin response to intrauterine needling. Lancet 1994; 344: 77–81.

116. Giannakoulopolous X, Teixeira J. Fisk N, et al. Human fetal and maternal noradernaline responses to invasive procedures. Pediatr Res 1999; 45: 494–9.

117. Smith RP, Gitau R, Glover V, et al. Pain and stress in the human fetus. Eur J Obstet Gynecol Reprod Biol 2000; 92: 161–5.

118. Anand KJS, Sippell WG, Aynsley-Green A. Randomized trial of fentanyl anaesthesia in preterm babies undergoing surgery: effects of the stress response. Lancet 1987; 1: 62–6.

119. Guinsburg R, Kopelman BI, Anand KJS, et al. Physiological, hormonal and behavioural responses to a single fentanyl dose in intubated and ventilated preterm neonates. J Pediatr 1998; 132: 954–9.

120. Anand KJS. Clinical importance of pain and stress in preterm neonates. Biol Neonate 1998; 73: 319–24.

121. Uno H, Lohmiller L, Thieme C, et al. Brain damage induced by prenatal exposure to dexamethasone in fetal rhesus macaques. I. Hippocampus. Brain Res Dev Brain Res 1990; 53: 157–67.

122. Grunau RVE, Whitfield MF, Petrie JH, et al. Early pain experience, child and family factors, as precursors of somatization: a prospective study of extremely premature infants and full-term children. Pain 1994; 56: 353–9.

123. Taddio A, Katz J, Ilerich Al, et al. Effect of neonatal circumcisiion on pain response during subsequent routine vaccination. Lancet 1997; 349: 599–603.

124. Stevens BJ, Johnston CC, Grunau RVE. Issues of assessment of pain and discomfort in neonates. J Obstet Gynecol Neonat Nurs 1995; 24: 849–55.

125. Stevens B, Johnston CC, Petryshen P, Taddio A. The premature infant pain profile. Clin J Pain 1996; 12: 13–22.

126. Humphrey T. The embryologic differentiation of the vestibular nuclei in man correlated with functional development. In: Proceedings of International Symposium on Vestibular and Ocular Problems. Tokyo: Society of Vestibular Research, University of Tokyo, 1965: 51–6.

127. Hooker D. Fetal reflexes and instinctual processes. Psychosom Med 1942; 4: 199–220.

128. Starr A, Amlie RN, Martin WH, Saunders S. Development of auditory function in newborn infants revealed by auditory brainstem potentials. Pediatrics 1991; 60: 831–8.

129. Morlet T, Collet L, Solle B, et al. Functional maturation of cochlear active mechanisms and of the medial olivocochlear system in humans. Acta Otolaryngol (Stockholm) 1993; 113: 271–7.

130. Morlet T, Collet L, Duclaux R, et al. Spontaneous and evoked otoacustical emissions in preterm and full term neonates: Is there a clinical application? Int J Ped Otorhinolaryngol 1995; 33: 207–11.

131. Leader LR, Baille P, Martin B, et al. The assessment and significance of habituation to a repeated stimulus by human fetus. Early Hum Dev 1982; 7: 211–18.

132. Liley AW. Fetus as a person. Speech at 8th Meeting of Psychiatric Societies of Australia and New Zealand. Fetal Ther 1986; 1: 8–17.

133. Huttenlocher PR, deCourten CH. The development of synapses in striate cortex of man. Hum Neurobiol 1987; 6: 1–9.

134. Magoon EH, Robb RM. Development of myelin in human optic nerve tract. A light and electron microscopic study. Arch Ophthalmol 1981; 99: 655–9.

135. Hendrickson AE, Youdelis C. The morphological development of the human foveola. Ophthalmology 1981; 91: 603–12.

136. Seron Ferre M, Torres C, Parraguez VH, et al. Perinatal neuroendocrine regulation. Development of the circadian time-keeping system. Mol Cell Endocrinol 2002; 186: 169–73.

137. Seron-Ferre M, Ducsay CA, Valenzuela GJ. Circadian rhythms during pregnancy. Endocr Rev 1993; 14: 594–609.

138. Vanececk J. Celluler mechanisms of melatonin action. Physiol Rev 1998; 78: 687–721.

139. Yie SM, Niles LP, Younglavi EV. Melatonin receptors on human granulosa cell membranes. J Clin Endocrinol Metab 1995; 80: 1747–9.

140. Visser GHA, Mulder EJH, Prechtl HFR. Studies on developmental neurology in the human fetus. Dev Pharmacol Ther 1992; 18: 175–83.

141. Mulder EJH, Visser GHA, Bekedan DJ, Prechtl HFR. Emergence of behavioural states in fetuses of type-1 diabetic women. Early Hum Dev 1987; 15: 231–52.

142. Ruckenbush Y, Gaujoux M, Eghbali B. Sleep cycles and kinesis in the fetal lamb. Electroenceph Clin Neurophysiol 1977; 42: 226–33.

143. Kelly DD. Sleep and dreaming. In: Kandell ER, Schwartz JH, eds. Principles of Neural Science, 2nd edn. New York: Elsevier Science, 1985: 651–62.

144. Crespi EJ, Denver RJ. Ancient origins of human developmental plasticity. Am J Hum Biol 2005; 17: 44–54.

145. Monk C, Fifer WP, Myers MM, et al. Maternal stress responses and anxiety during pregnancy: effects on fetal heart rate. Dev Psychobiol 2000 36: 67–77.

146. DiPietro JA, Hilton SC, Hawkins M, et al. Maternal stress and affect influence fetal neurobehavioral development. Dev Psychol 2002; 38: 659–68.

147. Amiel-Tison C, Cabrol D, Denver R, et al. Fetal adaptation to stress. Part I: Acceleration of fetal maturation and earlier birth triggered by placental insufficiency in humans. Early Hum Dev 2004; 78: 15–27.

148. Howe DC, Gertler A, Challis JR. The late gestation increase in circulating ACTH and cortisol in the fetal sheep is suppressed by intracerebroventricular infusion of recombinant ovine leptin. J Endocrinol 2002; 174: 259–66.

149. Hundertmark S, Ragosch V, Zimmermann B, et al. Effect of dexamethasone, triiodothyronine and dimethyl-isopropyl-thyronine on lung maturation of the fetal rat lung. J Perinat Med 1999; 27: 309–15.

150. Sandman CA, Wadhwa PD, Chicz-Demet A, et al. Maternal corticotropin-releasing hormone and habituation in human fetus. Dev Psychobiol 1999; 34: 163–73.

151. Amiel-Tison C, Vabrol D, Denver R, et al. Fetal adaptation to stress. Part II. Evolutionary aspects; Stress induced hippocampal damage; long-term effects on behavior; consequences on adult health. Early Hum Dev 2004; 78: 81–94.

152. Lemaire V, Koehl M, Le Moal M, Abrous DN. Prenatal stress produces learning deficits associated with an inhibition of neurogenesis in the hippocampus. Proc Natl Acad Sci USA 2000; 97: 11032–7.

153. Deminiere JM, Piazza PV, Guegan G, et al. Increased locomotor response to novelty and propensity to intravenous amphetamine self-administration in adult offspring of stressed mothers. Brain Res 1992; 586: 135–9.

154. McEwen BS, Sapolsky RM. Stress and cognitive function. Curr Opin Neurobiol 1995; 5: 205–16.

155. Sapolsky RM, Krey LC, McEwen BS. The neuroendocrinology of stress and aging; the glucocorticoid cascade hypothesis. Endocr Rev 1986; 7: 284–301.

156. Sapolsky RM. Stress, the Aging Brain, and the Mechanisms of Neuron Death. Cambridge, MA: MIT Press, 1992.

157. Lupien SJ, de Leon M, de Santi S, et al. Cortisol levels during human aging predict hippocampal atrophy and memory deficits. Nat Neurosci 1998; 1: 69–73.

158. Henry C, Guegant G, Cador M, et al. Prenatal stress in rats facilitates amphetamine induced sensitization and

induces long-lasting in dopamine receptors in the nucleus accumbens. Brain Res 1995; 685: 179–86.

159. Koehl M, Bjijou Y, Le Moal M, Cador M. Nicotine-induced locomotor activity is increased by preexposure of rats to prenatal stress. Brain Res 2000; 882: 196–200.

160. Uno H, Lohmiller L, Thieme C, et al. Brain damage induced by prenatal exposure to dexamethasone in fetal rhesus macaques: I. Hippocampus. Dev Brain Res 1990; 53: 157–67.

161. Barbazanges A, Piazza PV, Le Moal M, Maccari S. Maternal glucocorticoid secretion mediates long-term effects of prenatal stress. J Neurosci 1996; 16: 3943–9.

162. Hayashi A, Nagaoka M, Yamada K, et al. Maternal stress induces synaptic loss and developmental disabilities of offspring. Int J Dev Neurosci 1998; 16: 209–16.

163. Rees S, Harding R. Brain development during fetal life: influences of the intra-uterine environment. Neursci Lett 2004; 361: 111–14.

164. Fride E, Weinstock M. Prenatal stress increases anxiety related behavior and alters cerebral lateralization of dopamine activity. Life Sci 1988; 42: 1059–65.

165. Fride E, Dan Y, Feldon J, et al. Effects of prenatal stress on vulnerability to stress in prepubertal and adult rats. Physiol Behav 1986; 37: 681–7.

166. Wakshlak A, Weinstock M. Neonatal handling reverses behavioral abnormalities induced in rats by prenatal stress. Physiol Behav 1990; 48: 289–92.

167. Valee M, Mayo W, Dellu F, et al. Prenatal stress induces high anxiety and postnatal handling induces low anxiety in adult offspring: correlation with stress-induced corticosterone secretion. J Neurosci 1997; 17: 2626–36.

168. Koehl M, Lemaire V, Mayo W, et al. Individual vulnerability of substance abuse and affective disorers: role of early environmental influences. Neurotoxicity Res 2002; 4: 281–96.

169. Piazza PV, Le Moal ML. Pathophysiological basis of vulnerability to drug abuse: role of an interaction between stress, glucocorticoids and dopaminergic neurons. Annu Rev Pharmacol Toxicol 1996; 36: 359–78.

170. Schneider ML, Coe CL, Lubach GR. Endocrine activation mimics the adverse effects of prenatal stress on the neuromotor development of the infant primate. Dev Psychobiol 1992; 25: 427–39.

171. Glover V. Maternal stress or anxiety in pregnancy and emotional development of the child. Br J Psychiatry 1997; 171: 105–6.

172. Graham YP, Heim C, Goodman SH, et al. The effects of neonatal stress on brain development: implications for psychopathology. Dev Psychopathol 1999; 11: 545–65.

173. Weinstock M. Does prenatal stress impair coping and regulation of hypothalamic–pituitary–adrenal axis? Neurosci Biobehav Rev 1997; 21: 1–10.

174. Weinstock M. Alterations induced by gestational stress in brain morphology and behaviour of the off-spring. Prog Neurobiol 2001; 65: 427–51.

175. Cladji C, Dioro J, Meaney MJ. Variations in maternal care in infancy regulate the development of stress reactivity. Biol Psychiatry 2000; 48: 1164–74.

176. Francis DD, Diorio J, Plotsky PM, Meaney MJ. Environmental enrichment reverses the effects of maternal separation on stress reactivity. J Neurosci 2002; 22: 7840–3.

177. Levitt P, Reinoso B, Jones L. The critical impact of early cellular environment on neuronal development. Prev Med 1998; 27: 180–3.

178. Arbeille P, Maulik D, Salihagic A, et al. Effect of long-term cocaine administration to pregnant ewes on fetal hemodynamics, oxygenation, and growth. Obstet Gynecol 1997; 90: 795–802.

179. Barker DJP. Fetal origins of coronary heart disease. BMJ 1995; 311: 171–4.

22 Normal standards for fetal neurobehavioral developments

Asim Kurjak, Guillermo Azumendi, and Wiku Andonotopo

INTRODUCTION

Fetal motility is considered to reflect the developing nervous system but also involves functional and maturational properties of fetal hemodynamics and the muscular system. The introduction of four-dimensional (4D) sonography was a turning point in the assessment of fetal behavior by providing the capability of simultaneous spatial imaging of the entire fetus and its movements[1-9] (Figure 22.1). Indeed, sonographic studies have revealed the fascinating diversity of fetal intrauterine activities. It has been shown that fetal activity occurs far earlier than a mother can perceive – in fact as early as the late embryonic period. Furthermore, the qualitative and quantitative ranges of behavioral patterns expand rapidly as pregnancy progresses, and random movements of the fetal body, which are the earliest signs of fetal activity, change into well-organized behavioral patterns observed late in gestation. From the analysis of the dynamics of fetal behavior, it has been concluded that fetal behavioral patterns directly reflect the developmental and maturational processes of the fetal central nervous system.

de Vries et al[10-12] were the first to provide a systematic and detailed classification and quantitative longitudinal analysis of fetal behavior during the first half of pregnancy using 2D sonography. They distinguished 21 different movement patterns, 14 of which were extensively analyzed. Our group has performed several studies of the physiology of fetal movements during all three trimesters of pregnancy. This longitudinal study establishes reference ranges for gestational ages. Standard of movement pattern and facial expression pattern curves are constructed through all trimesters of pregnancy.

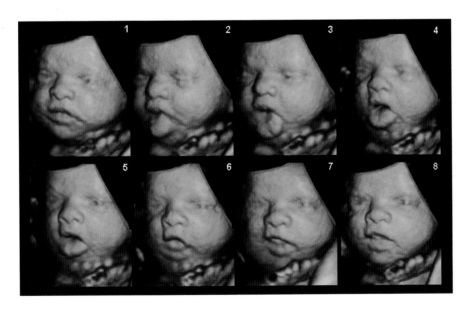

Figure 22.1 4D imaging sequences demonstrating isolated eye blinking parallel with tongue expulsion during the 3rd trimester of pregnancy

In a population of 1st-trimester uncomplicated singleton gestations and using transvaginal 4D sonography, we focused on eight fetal movement parameters: general movements, startle, stretching, isolated arm movements, isolated leg movements, head retroflexion, head rotation, and head anteflexion. In the second part of our study, 14 parameters of fetal movement and facial expression were analyzed by transabdominal 4D sonography from the 2nd to the 3rd trimester.

Recently, multicenter studies of fetal brain function have been published.[11,13-17] The preliminary reports obviously suggest that the study of fetal behavior should be standardized as much as possible. An objective analysis with strict application techniques and the use of valid reference ranges appropriate for gestational age are essential.[18] Without such standardization, comparisons with former or future measurements of patients and comparable studies cannot be made. Our preliminary results on fetal behavior have already been published elsewhere.[6,8,9,17]

LONGITUDINAL QUANTIFICATION OF FETAL BEHAVIOR BY 4D SONOGRAPHY

Methodology and sampling characteristics

Throughout the period April 2004–April 2005, a study was conducted at the Department of Obstetrics and Gynecology, University of Zagreb, Sveti Duh General Hospital. The longitudinal study consisted of 100 of 119 pregnant women regardless of parity with normal singleton pregnancies, who were referred for routine 2D sonography in the outpatient clinic at different gestational ages. The patients were assigned to the study if they met the following inclusion criteria: the fetus and mother were considered 'normal'; 2D sonography and clinical assessment were uneventful; and the neonates were eventually delivered at term with normal 1- and 5-minute Apgar scores. Pregnancies that were subsequently found to be complicated by congenital abnormalities, gestational diabetes, hypertensive disorders in pregnancy, preterm deliveries, and abnormal Apgar scores were excluded. Fetuses from the 2nd and 3rd trimesters whose examined parts of the body were not visualized in one region of interest were also excluded from the study.

The patients were offered 4D sonography, and signed informed consent forms for the investigation of fetal motor activity. Subjects were randomly assigned

to the investigation. All 4D examinations were performed in the morning and all patients selected for the examination during the 1st trimester were asked to come again in the 2nd and 3rd trimesters for follow-up. Pregnant women were asked not to eat within 2 hours before the beginning of the investigation.

Technology

All 4D examinations were performed by experienced operators using Voluson 730 Expert (Kretztechnik, Zipf, Austria) and Sonoline Antares (Siemens AG, Issaquah, USA) machines, with transvaginal 8 MHz transducers for examination in the 1st trimester and transabdominal 5 MHz transducers for examination during the 2nd and 3rd trimesters. After standard assessment with 2D B-mode sonography, a 4D mode was turned on and a live 3D image was built by selecting the ideal representative 2D image placed in the region of interest (ROI). The crystal array of the transducer moved mechanically over the defined ROI. The volume was automatically scanned every 2 seconds, and 4D images were displayed on the screen and recorded on videotape during the 30-minute observation period. This procedure was used for 30-minute observation of fetal movement activity and fetal facial

Table 22.1 Movements analyzed in embryos and fetuses during the 1st trimester

- General movements
- Startle
- Stretching
- Isolated arm movements
- Isolated leg movements
- Head retroflexion
- Head rotation
- Head anteflexion

Table 22.2 Movements analyzed in fetuses during the 2nd and 3rd trimesters

Facial expression	Hand and head movements
Isolated eye blinking	Head retroflexion
Mouthing	Head rotation
Yawning	Head anteflexion
Tongue expulsion	Hand-to-head direction
Grimacing	Hand-to-eye direction
Swallowing	Hand-to-mouth direction
	Hand-to-face direction
	Hand-to-ear direction

Table 22.3 Definition of some fetal movement patterns and facial expressions[4,11,18,32]

General movements	Series of movements with variable speed and amplitude; involve all parts of the body without distinctive patterning of body parts can be seen. Duration varies from a few seconds to about a minute
Startle	Quick generalized movements, starting in the limbs and spreading to the neck and trunk; only last about 1 second
Stretching	A complex motor pattern, always carried out at a slow speed and consisting of the forceful extension of the back, retroflexion of the head, and external rotation and elevation of the arms
Isolated arm or leg movements	Rapid or slow movements, and may involve extension, flexion, external and internal rotation, or abduction and adduction of an extremity, without movements in other body parts
Head retroflexion, rotation, and anteflexion	Isolated retroflexions, rotations, and anteflexions of the head not associated with general movements; usually carried out slowly, but can also be fast and jerky
Hand-to-body contact (head, mouth, eye, face, ear)	The hand slowly touches the body parts, with extension and flexion of the fingers
Grimacing	Wrinkling of the brows or face in frowning
Isolated eye blinking	A reflex that closes and opens the eyes rapidly; brief closing of the eyelids by involuntary normal periodic closing, as a protective measure, or by voluntary action
Yawning	Prolonged wide opening of the jaws, followed by quick closure, with retroflexion of the head and elevation of the arms; this movement pattern is non-repetitive
Tongue expulsion	Facial expression characterized by expulsion of the tongue
Swallowing	Indicating that the fetus is drinking amniotic fluid; swallowing consists of displacements of tongue and/or larynx
Mouthing	A facial expression characterized by mouth manipulation to investigate an object; mouthing is most common in fetus, and it may develop into a persistent, stereotyped behavior pattern

expression. Variables of maternal and fetal characteristics including gestational age, eight fetal movement patterns in the 1st trimester (Table 22.1) and 14 parameters of fetal movement and fetal facial expression patterns (Table 22.2) from the 2nd and 3rd trimesters. These were included in constructing the fetal neurologic charts.

Definitions

It is possible to identify and to understand abnormal behavior before birth only if normal behavior is entirely understood.[15,18–21] Most types of movement patterns are present between 7 and 15 weeks of gestation.[11] Once observed, the movements remain unchanged throughout the whole pregnancy. 4D sonography provided the possibility to study a full range of facial expressions, including mouthing, grimacing, and eyelid movements.[2,3,5–7,17,22] The definitions of types of analyzed movement patterns are presented in Table 22.3, following the studies by de Vries and Prechtl.[11,12,23,24]

Results

Statistical analysis of the incidence of fetal movements and facial expressions studied in the 1st trimester revealed statistically significant changes in general movements, stretching, isolated arm and leg movement, head retroflexion, head rotation, and head anteflexion ($p < 0.05$) (Figures 22.2–22.9). During the 2nd and 3rd trimesters, multiple regression and polynomial regression revealed statistically significant changes in tongue expulsion, grimacing, swallowing, head movements, and all hand-to-body contact movements ($p < 0.05$) (Figures 22.10–22.23).

At the 1st trimester, a tendency towards increased frequency of fetal movement patterns with increasing gestational age has been noticed. Only the startle movement pattern seemed to occur stagnantly during the 1st trimester (Figure 22.3). In this type of movement, there is no significant correlation with gestational age, as shown by the large dispersion of scatterpoints around the regression line ($r = 0.673$; $p = 0.506$).

At the beginning of the 2nd trimester, the fetuses tend to increase the frequency of fetal movement

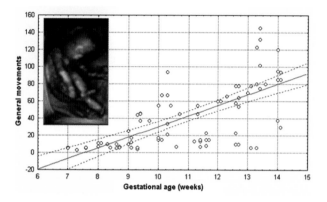

Figure 22.2 Scatterplot and multiple regression analysis of 1st-trimester frequency of general movement pattern versus gestational weeks in the formula-generating group ($y = -93.521 + 12.387x$; $r = 0.661$; $p < 0.001$)

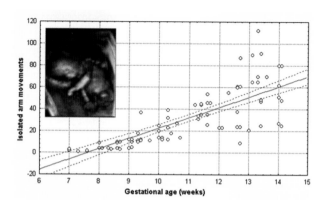

Figure 22.5 Scatterplot and multiple regression analysis of 1st-trimester frequency of isolated arm movements pattern versus gestational weeks in the formula-generating group ($y = -72.281 + 9.479x$; $r = 0.769$; $p < 0.001$)

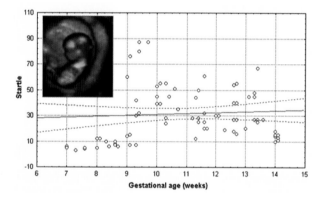

Figure 22.3 Scatterplot and multiple regression analysis of 1st-trimester frequency of startle pattern versus gestational weeks in the formula-generating group ($y = 23.863 + 0.708x$; $r = 0.673$; $p = 0.506$)

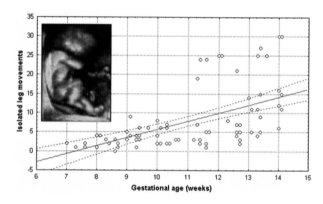

Figure 22.6 Scatterplot and multiple regression analysis of 1st-trimester frequency of isolated leg movement pattern versus gestational weeks in the formula-generating group ($y = -15.54 + 2.122x$; $r = 0.557$; $p < 0.001$)

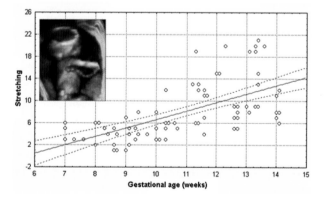

Figure 22.4 Scatterplot and multiple regression analysis of 1st trimester frequency of stretch pattern versus gestational weeks in the formula-generating group ($y = 8.743 + 1.536x$; $r = 0.600$; $p < 0.001$)

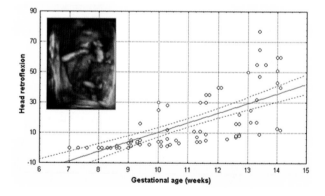

Figure 22.7 Scatterplot and multiple regression analysis of 1st-trimester frequency of head retroflexion pattern versus gestational weeks in the formula-generating group ($y = -53.363 + 6.368x$; $r = 0.664$; $p < 0.001$)

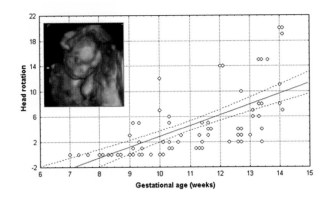

Figure 22.8 Scatterplot and multiple regression analysis of 1st-trimester frequency of head rotation pattern versus gestational weeks in the formula-generating group ($y = -14.136 + 1.699x$; $r = 0.661$; $p <0.001$)

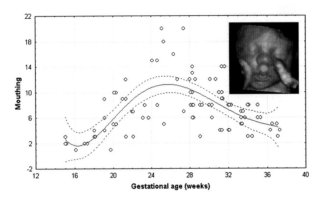

Figure 22.11 Scatterplot and polynomial regression analysis of 2nd- to 3rd-trimester frequency of mouthing pattern versus gestational weeks in the formula-generating group ($y = 722.192 - 14.949x + 11.136x^2 - 0.408x^3 + 0.007x^4$; $r = 0.117$; $p = 0.244$)

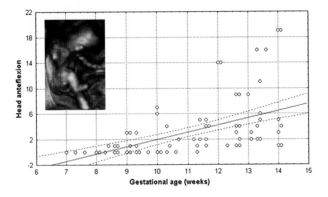

Figure 22.9 Scatterplot and multiple regression analysis of 1st-trimester frequency of head anteflexion movement pattern versus gestational weeks in the formula-generating group ($y = -9.29 + 1.125x$; $r = 0.537$; $p <0.001$)

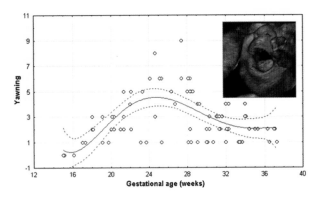

Figure 22.12 Scatterplot and polynomial regression analysis of 2nd- to 3rd-trimester frequency of yawning pattern versus gestational weeks in the formula-generating group ($y = 348.823 - 72.737x + 5.803x^2 - 0.221x^3 + 0.004x^4$; $r = 0.425$; $p = 0.674$)

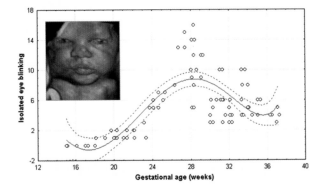

Figure 22.10 Scatterplot and polynomial regression analysis of 2nd- to 3rd-trimester frequency of isolated eye blinking pattern versus gestational weeks in the formula-generating group ($y = -34.06 + 22.032x - 3.127x^2 + 0.179x^3 - 0.004x^4$; $r = 0.478$; $p <0.001$)

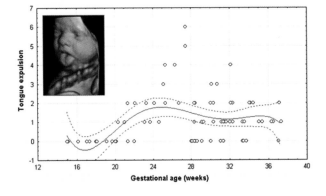

Figure 22.13 Scatterplot and polynomial regression analysis of 2nd- to 3rd-trimester frequency of tongue expulsion pattern versus gestational weeks in the formula-generating group ($y = 362.38 - 74.762x + 5.967x^2 - 0.231x^3 + 0.004x^4$; $r = 0.238$; $p = 0.017$)

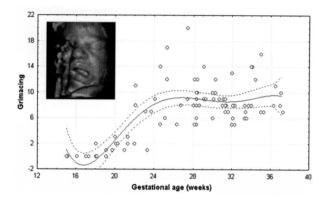

Figure 22.14 Scatterplot and polynomial regression analysis of 2nd- to 3rd- trimester frequency of grimacing pattern versus gestational weeks in the formula-generating group ($y = 1074.211 - 217.491x + 16.97x^2 - 0.64x^3 + 0.012x^4$; $r = 0.639$; $p <0.001$)

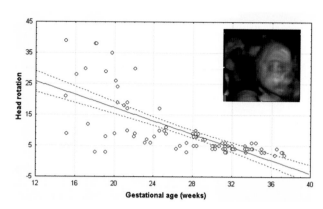

Figure 22.17 Scatterplot and multiple regression analysis of 2nd- and 3rd-trimester frequency of head rotation pattern versus gestational weeks in the formula-generating group ($y = 38.586 - 1.064x$; $r = 0.723$; $p <0.001$)

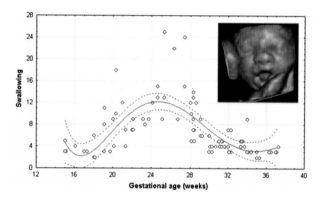

Figure 22.15 Scatterplot and polynomial regression analysis of 2nd- to 3rd-trimester frequency of swallowing pattern versus gestational weeks in the formula-generating group ($y = 1227.892 - 0.49x + 19.122x^2 - 0.71x^3 + 0.013x^4$; $r = 0.187$; $p = 0.062$)

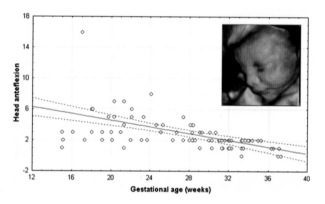

Figure 22.18 Scatterplot and multiple regression analysis of 2nd- and 3rd-trimester frequency of head anteflexion pattern versus gestational weeks in the formula-generating group ($y = 8.858 - 0.215x$; $r = 0.519$; $p <0.001$)

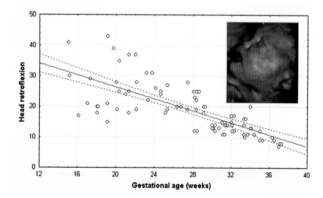

Figure 22.16 Scatterplot and multiple regression analysis of 2nd- and 3rd-trimester frequency of head retroflexion pattern versus gestational weeks in the formula-generating group ($y = 45.85 - 0.974x$; $r = 0.732$; $p <0.001$)

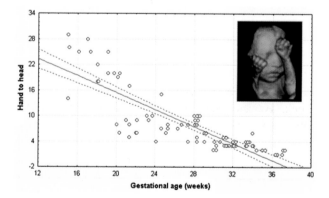

Figure 22.19 Scatterplot and multiple regression analysis of 2nd- and 3rd-trimester frequency of hand-to-head pattern versus gestational weeks in the formula-generating group ($y = 35.258 - 0.992x$; $r = 0.826$; $p <0.001$)

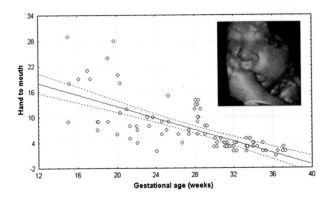

Figure 22.20 Scatterplot and multiple regression analysis of 2nd- and 3rd-trimester frequency of hand-to-mouth pattern versus gestational weeks in the formula-generating group ($y = 26.161 - 0.683x$; $r = 0.691$; $p < 0.001$)

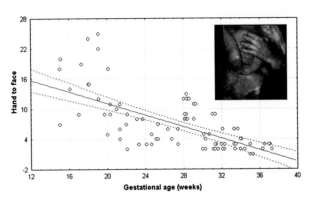

Figure 22.22 Scattergram and multiple regression analysis of 2nd- and 3rd-trimester frequency of hand-to-face pattern versus gestational weeks in the formula-generating group ($y = 22.656 - 0.578x$; $r = 0,649$; $p < 0.001$)

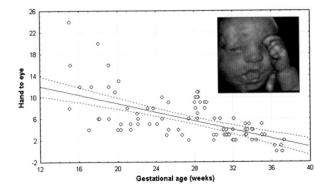

Figure 22.21 Scatterplot and multiple regression analysis of 2nd- and 3rd-trimester frequency of hand-to-eye pattern versus gestational weeks in the formula-generating group ($y = 16.826 - 0.401x$; $r = 0.593$; $p < 0.001$)

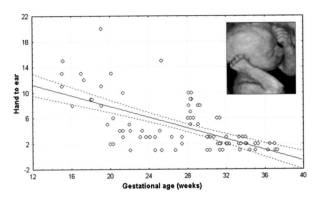

Figure 22.23 Scatterplot and multiple regression analysis of 2nd- and 3rd-trimester frequency of hand-to-ear pattern versus gestational weeks in the formula-generating group ($y = 16.302 - 0.423x$; $r = 0.636$; $p < 0.001$)

pattern. We noticed fluctuation and dispersion of the incidence of all facial expressions, as seen in the polynomial regression diagram (Figures 22.10–22.15). All types of facial expressions display a peak frequency at the end of the 2nd trimester, except isolated eye blinking, which increases at the beginning of the 24th week. At the beginning of the 3rd trimester, the fetuses display decreasing or stagnant incidence of fetal facial expression.

A statistically significant correlation was found between all head movements and hand-to-body contact patterns during the 2nd and 3rd trimesters. Figures 22.16–22.23 illustrate the relation between parameters of head movements and hand-to-body contact. The scatterplot diagrams indicate a decrease in the incidence of movements.

Discussion

The ultimate clinical application of fetal neurobehavioral assessment is to identify functional characteristics of the fetus that predict a range of subsequent developmental dysfunction. Establishing this link will require demonstration of positive and negative predictability to outcomes much beyond the immediate perinatal period.[25] Indeed, no unified neurobehavioral assessment method of the fetus currently exists. The goal of all investigations should be to gather information that reveals neural continuity from fetus to newborn.

Prenatal motility is considered to reflect the developing nervous system, but also involves functional and maturational properties of the fetal hemodynamic and muscular systems. Despite medical reports dating back over 100 years and the 25 years or more of systematic research initiated by Prechtl and colleagues, the study of prenatal behavior is still in its infancy.[20,21,23,26]

One of the most promising advances in the field of sonography is the new 4D technology. Its advance has been completed in the last few years, providing almost real-time visualization.[2,4–8,13,17,27–29] The availability of new diagnostic data has increased our knowledge about intrauterine life and substantially modified some earlier interpretations.[4]

General movements are the first complex fetal movement patterns observed by 2D sonography.[1,11] They can be recognized from 8–9 weeks of gestation onwards, and continue to be present until 16–20 weeks after birth.[15] According to Prechtl,[24] these are gross movements, involving the whole body. They wax and wane in intensity, force, and speed, and they have a gradual beginning and end.[11,18,23] The majority of extension and flexion sequences of the legs and arms are complex, and may be better assessed with 4D sonography.[1,2,5,7,17,30]

The range of first appearance of limb movements is between 8 and 12 weeks.[1,2,7,9,11,13,27] de Vries et al[11] found isolated arm and leg movements at 8 weeks of gestation. With 4D sonography, limb movements at 8 and 9 weeks were found.[9] The organization of the appearance of the movement pattern occurs with the increase in frequency.[6] It seems that fetal arms explore the surrounding environment and cross the midline, while the palmar surface is oriented towards the uterine wall. The fetal legs are also extended to the uterine wall.[2, 18,21,31] More limb joints are active and move simultaneously – for example, with extension or flexion in arm and elbow or hip and knee. Elevation of the hand and extension of the elbow joint, with a slight change in direction and rotation, can be seen simultaneously.[32]

From the 10th week onwards, the number and frequency of fetal movements increase and the repertoire of movements begins to expand. The isolated limb movements seen at 9 weeks are followed by the appearance of movements in the elbow joint at 10 weeks, changes in finger position in the 11th week, and clenching and unclenching of the fist at 12–13 weeks. Finally, at 13–14 weeks, isolated finger movements can be seen, as well as an increase in activity and strength of hand and finger movements.[16] By 14–19 weeks, fetuses are highly active, with the longest period between movements being only 5–6 minutes. In the 15th week, 15 different types of movement can be observed. Besides the general body movements and isolated limb movements, retroflexion, anteflexion, and rotation of the head can be seen.[32]

Simultaneously with the decrease in the number of general movements, an increase in facial movements, including opening or closing of the mouth and swallowing, can be observed. This pattern is considered to reflect the normal neurologic development of the fetus.[20,24,26] The application of the new technology in the examination of fetal facial movements revealed the existence of a full range of facial expressions, including grimacing, tongue expulsion, and eyelid movements similar to emotional expressions in adults.[2,3,6,7,17,22,31] This finding however, raised a number of questions, many of which are yet to be resolved. First, precise criteria for the distinction of these facial expressions in the fetus should be established. For example, in this study, a grimacing pattern appears incidentally around the 20th week of gestation. We still do not know in which period of gestation facial expressions begin to appear. In this study, we tried to determine whether there are any gestational age-related trends in their appearance. The nuclei of the facial nerve, a structure that controls these motor patterns, are developed by the end of the 1st trimester, indicating that some facial grimaces could appear rather early in gestation. The possibility of studying such subtle movements might open a new area of investigation. One potential value of the observation of facial expressions could be the possibility of detecting facial nerve paresis in utero.[3,17,22,24,31] Obviously, the story of fetal intrauterine activity is far from complete.[3,22]

Significant trends in fetal eye movement organization can also be observed during the second half of pregnancy, especially during the 3rd trimester. The earliest eye movements appear at 16–18 weeks of gestation, as sporadic movements with a limited frequency. We found in this study that an isolated eye blinking pattern appears more frequently and begins to consolidate at 24–26 weeks.

During the past few years, we have initiated research into fetal behavior in normal and pathologic pregnancies using 3D and 4D sonography. In the 1st trimester of pregnancy, 3D sonography allows precise morphologic examinations, which are important for early detection of serious fetal malformations, such as anencephalic fetus and spina bifida.[27,33,34] Using 4D sonography, quantitative assessment of fetal motility can be performed almost as precisely as by conventional 2D sonography, even in the very early period of gestation and at the onset of fetal motility. Qualitative assessment might be even more informative, because this method allows the simultaneous visualization of the whole fetal body.[1] In our previous study, fetal movements were recorded by 4D sonography in 10 term pregnancies, and neonatal spontaneous motor activity was recorded after birth.[7,17] Interestingly, we found no statistically significant differences in either quality or quantity of fetal hand-to-face movements or fetal facial movements. No movements were observed in fetal life that were not present in neonatal life, whereas the Moro reflex was present only in neonates.[6–8] This pilot study confirmed the existence of a prenatal–neonatal continuum even in subtle, fine movements such as facial mimics.

In another study, we detected the earliest embryonic movements at 7 weeks of gestation.[1] These movements, which involved the whole body, such as general movements and startles, occurred most frequently, although in 8-week-old embryos, isolated arm and leg movements could also be observed. All of the above movement patterns were also recognizable by 2D imaging in fetuses studied between 9–14 weeks of gestation.[3] Several movement patterns, such as sideway bending, hiccup, fetal breathing movements, and facial movements, could not be observed by 4D sonography, although they were clearly visible by 2D sonography. Although our previous studies showed that the full range of facial movements can be recognized by 4D sonography in the 3rd trimester of pregnancy, this investigation failed to find the same results in the 1st trimester.[1,6–8,17]

Recently, we have studied fetal behavior in all three trimesters of normal pregnancy. We noted a tendency towards decreased frequency of observed facial expressions and movement patterns with increasing gestational age.[7]

In the present longitudinal study, standard parameters of fetal movements and facial expressions in all trimesters of pregnancy are presented in Figures 22.2–22.23. In the 1st trimester, a tendency towards increased frequency of fetal movement patterns with increasing gestational age was noted, while at the beginning of the 2nd trimester, the fetuses began to display a tendency towards increased frequency of observed fetal facial expression to the end of the 2nd trimester. An oscillation and dispersion of the incidence of all facial expressions as seen in the polynomial regression diagram are shown in Figures 22.10–22.15. All types of facial expression patterns displayed a peak frequency at the end of the 2nd

trimester, except in isolated eye blinking, which began to increase at the beginning of 24 weeks of gestation because fetuses cannot open their eyelids before this period. During the 3rd trimester, the fetuses began to display a decreasing or stagnant incidence of fetal facial expression.

All types of head movements and hand-to-body contact show a tendency to decrease in frequency from the beginning of the 2nd trimester to the end of the 3rd trimester.

CONCLUSIONS

The investigation of fetal behavior and the development of 4D sonography open a new perspective in establishing normal fetal neurodevelopmental standards. According to the present results, 4D sonography could represent a significant advance in the investigation of fetal neurobehavior and understanding of the functional development of the fetal CNS. The incidence of fetal behavioral patterns correlates fairly well with gestational age, and also correlates with structural development of the CNS. The quality of fetal movements reveals the integrity of the CNS. Thus, this technique might facilitate the diagnosis of cerebral dysfunctions.

Because of its complexity, it is unlikely that a single behavioral measure will serve to detect all aspects of neural dysfunction. Furthermore, the predictive validity of specific measures for both fetal and neonatal developmental outcomes needs to be confirmed. Therefore, it is premature at present to suggest a unified fetal neurobehavioral assessment scale. However, it is our belief that recent data obtained by 4D sonography are stimulating and might result in a more effective strategy to assess development before birth. The availability of quantitative standards might be valuable for intrauterine neurologic assessment.

REFERENCES

1. Andonotopo W, Medic M, Salihagic-Kadic A, et al. The assessment of embryonic and fetal neurodevelopment in early pregnancy: comparison between 2D and 4D sonographic scanning. J Perinat Med 2005; 33: 406–14.

2. Andonotopo W, Stanojevic M, Kurjak A, Azumendi G, Carrera JM. Assessment of fetal behavior and general movements by four-dimensional sonography. Ultrasound Rev Obstet Gynecol 2004; 4: 103–14.

3. Azumendi G, Kurjak A, Carrera JM, Andonotopo W, Scazzocchio E. 3D and 4D sonography in the evaluation of normal and abnormal fetal facial expression. In: Carrera JM, Kurjak A, eds. Atlas of Clinical Application of Ultrasound in Obstetrics and Gynecology. New Delhi: Jaypee Brothers Medical Publishers, 2006: 250.

4. Carrera JM. Fetal ultrasonography: the first 40 years. Ultrasound Rev Obstet Gynecol 2004; 4: 141–7.

5. Kurjak A, Carrera JM, Andonotopo W, et al. Behavioral perinatology assessed by four dimensional sonography. In: Kurjak A, Chervenak F, eds. Textbook of Perinatal Medicine. New Delhi: Jaypee Brothers Medical Publishers, 2005: 568.

6. Kurjak A, Stanojevic M, Andonotopo W, et al. Behavioral pattern continuity from prenatal to postnatal life-a study by four-dimensional (4D) ultrasonography. J Perinat Med 2004: 32: 346–53.

7. Kurjak A, Stanojevic M, Andonotopo W, et al. Fetal behaviour assessed in all three trimesters of normal pregnancy by four-dimensional (4D) ultrasonography. Croat Med J 2005; 46: 772–80.

8. Kurjak A, Stanojevic M, Azumendi G, Carrera JM. The potential of four-dimensional (4D) ultrasonography in the assessment of fetal awareness. J Perinat Med 2005; 33: 46–53.

9. Kurjak A, Vecek N, Hafner T, et al. Prenatal diagnosis: What does four-dimensional ultrasound add? J Perinat Med 2002; 30: 57–62.

10. de Vries JIP, Visser GHA, Prechtl HFR. Fetal motility in the first half of the pregnancy. In: Prechtl HFR, ed. Continuity of Neural Functions from Prenatal to Postnatal Life. Oxford: Blackwell Scientific, 1984: 44.

11. de Vries JIP, Visser GHA, Prechtl HFR. The emergence of fetal behaviour I. Qualitative aspects. Early Hum Dev 1982; 7: 301–22.

12. de Vries JIP, Visser GHA, Prechtl HFR. The emergence of fetal behaviour II. Quantitative aspects. Early Hum Dev 1985; 12: 99–120.

13. Azumendi G, Arenas JB, Andonotopo W, Kurjak A. Three dimensional sonoembriology. In: Kurjak A, Arenas JB, eds. Textbook of Transvaginal Sonography. London: Taylor and Francis, 2005: 407.

14. Einspieler C, Prechtl HF, Ferrari F, Cioni G, Bos AF. The qualitative assessment of general movements in preterm, term and young infants – review of the methodology. Early Hum Dev 1997; 24: 47–60.

15. Hopkins B, Prechtl HF. A qualitative approach to the development of movements during early infancy. In: Prechtl HFR, ed. Continuity of Neural Functions from Perinatal to Postnatal Life. Oxford: Blackwell Scientific, 1984: 179.

16. Kurjak A, Andonotopo W, Azumendi G, Vecek N, Funduk-Kurjak B. Normal and abnormal fetal hand movements studied by 4D sonography. In: Carrera JM, Kurjak A, eds. Atlas of Clinical Application of Ultrasound in Obstetrics and Gynecology. New Delhi: Jaypee Brothers Medical Publishers, 2006: 283.

17. Kurjak A, Azumendi G, Vecek N, et al. Fetal hand movements and facial expression in normal pregnancy studied by four-dimensional sonography. J Perinat Med 2003; 31: 496–508.

18. Nijhuis JG. Neurobehavioral development of the fetal brain. In: Nijhuis JG, ed. Fetal Behaviour: Developmental and Perinatal Aspects. Oxford: Oxford University Press, 1992: 489.

19. Cioni G, Prechtl HF, Ferrari F, et al. Which better predicts later outcome in full term infants: quality of general movements or neurological examination? Early Hum Dev 1997; 50: 71–85.

20. Prechtl HFR. Ultrasound studies of human fetal behaviour. Early Hum Dev 1985; 12: 91–8.

21. Roodenburg PJ, Wladimiroff JW, van Es A, Prechtl HFR. Classification and quantitative aspects of fetal movements during the second half of normal pregnancy. Early Hum Dev 1991; 25: 19–35.

22. Azumendi G, Kurjak A. Three-dimensional and four-dimensional sonography in the study of the fetal face. Ultrasound Rev Obstet Gynecol 2003; 3: 160–4.

23. Prechtl HFR. Qualitative changes of spontaneous movements in fetus and preterm infant are a marker of neurological dysfunction. Early Hum Dev 1990; 23: 151–8.

24. Prechtl HFR. State of the art of a new functional assessment of the young nervous system. An early predictor of cerebral palsy. Early Hum Dev 1997; 50: 1–11.

25. Di Pietro JA. Neurobehavioral assessment before birth. Mental Retard Dev Disab 2005; 11: 4–13.

26. Prechtl HFR, Einspieler C. Is neurological assessment of the fetus possible? Eur J Obstet Gynecol Reprod Biol 1997; 75: 81–4.

27. Andonotopo W, Kurjak A, Azumendi G. Early normal pregnancy. In: Carrera JM, Kurjak A, eds. Atlas of Clinical Application of Ultrasound in Obstetrics and Gynecology. New Delhi: Jaypee Brothers Medical Publishers, 2006: 25.

28. Kurjak A, Carrera JM, Andonotopo W, et al. The role of 4D sonography in the neurological assessment of early human development. Ultrasound Rev Obstet Gynecol 2004; 4: 148–59.

29. Kurjak A, Carrera JM, Salihagic-Kadic A, et al. The antenatal development of fetal behavioural patterns assessed by four-dimensional sonography. J Matern Fetal Neonatal 2005; 6: 401–16.

30. Kurjak A, Vecek N, Kupesic S, Azumendi G, Solak M. Four-dimensional ultrasound: How much does it improve perinatal practice? In: Carrera JM, Chervenak FA, Kurjak A, eds. Controversies in Perinatal Medicine: Studies on the Fetus as a Patient. New York: Parthenon, 2003: 222.

31. Stanojevic M, Perlman JM, Andonotopo W, Kurjak A. From fetal to neonatal behavioral status. Ultrasound Rev Obstet Gynecol 2004; 4: 59–71.

32. Pooh RK, Ogura T. Normal and abnormal fetal hand positioning and movement in early pregnancy detected by three- and four-dimensional ultrasound. Ultrasound Rev Obset Gynecol 2004; 1: 46–51.

33. Andonotopo W, Kurjak A, Kosuta MI. Behavioral of anencephalic fetus studied by 4D sonography. J Matern Fetal Neonatal Med 2005; 17: 165–8.

34. Kurjak A, Pooh RK, Carrera JM, et al. Structural and functional early human development assessed by three-dimensional (3D) and four-dimensional (4D) sonography. Fertil Steril 2005; 84: 1285–99.

23   Fetal yawning, hearing, and learning

Aida Salihagic Kadic, Marijana Medic, and Asim Kurjak

INTRODUCTION

The application of three- and four-dimensional (3D and 4D) sonography in the investigations of embryonic and fetal activities in the natural environment has produced invaluable information on the development of fetal behavior and has therefore provided direct insight into the prenatal functional development of the central nervous system (CNS). It has been shown that all of the movement patterns of a newborn originate from the prenatal period. The onset and developmental course of the movement patterns have been studied extensively, and the interpretation of those results together with information on the structural development of the fetal brain and other organ systems has demonstrated that fetal motility reflects the maturation of the fetal CNS.[1] Furthermore, it has been shown that fetal motility is not only required for the maturation of motor functions but is also involved in the development of other organs, such as the lungs. Prenatal observation of specific reflexive behavioral patterns such as fetal yawning has given a new perspective on the purpose of this reflex. Although the characteristics of yawning in adult age have been described in detail, its role is still poorly understood. The presence of spontaneous yawning movements from the early 2nd trimester of gestation onwards indicates its evolutionary importance. Therefore, the investigation of prenatal yawning patterns could improve our understanding of the physiologic role of this reflex. On the other hand, an altered frequency of yawning has been observed in adults in relation to various brain dysfunctions, which leads to the assumption that such a relation might exist in the fetal period as well, and could be one of the indicators of brain function disturbances.

The investigation of spontaneous fetal behavior, as well as the behavior elicited by external stimulation, has expanded our understanding of the prenatal development of senses such as hearing, and has implied that prenatal exposure to sensory stimuli might contribute to the postnatal acquisition of various abilities, such as speech and language learning. Recently developed techniques of 4D sonography have enabled the recording of 3D sequences nearly in real time, which could open a new perspective on the investigation of fetal behavior (Figure 23.1). This technique brings significant improvements to the qualitative analysis of various motor patterns, while quantitative analysis can be performed with almost the same accuracy as when using standard 2D sonography.

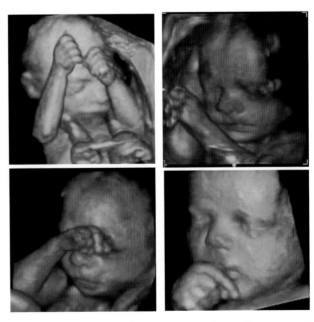

Figure 23.1 A variety of movements in the 2nd trimester of gestation seen by 3D/4D sonography

Thus, the application of 4D sonography in maternal–fetal medicine could enable even better understanding of the development of fetal motor activity and fetal senses, and even elucidation of the origins of fetal learning and memory. Recent advances in understanding the role of fetal yawning, the development of fetal hearing, and the origins of fetal learning will be presented in this chapter, based on a review of the literature and our own preliminary results.

OVERVIEW OF THE PHYSIOLOGY OF YAWNING

Yawning is a physiologic phenomenon that can be recognized in humans and many animal species. It is a phylogenetically old reflex, which can be observed in all mammals, and some components of a yawn exist even in birds and reptiles. Although this reflex has been well known since antiquity (for instance, Hippocrates interpreted it as an exhaustion of the fumes, preceding fever), its physiologic role is still poorly understood. Yawning is an easily recognizable and easily quantifiable behavioral pattern. It is represented by three distinct phases: long inspiration (4–6 seconds), brief acme (2–4 seconds) and finally, rapid expiration. The maximal duration of the whole yawn is about 10 seconds.[2] Yawning can be accompanied by stretching of the neck and arms, and sometimes the stretch can be even more generalized. Therefore, yawning is not a simple motor reflex, but has a complex spatiotemporal organization with facial, respiratory, and other components. Several anatomic structures, such as the brainstem reticular formation, the neostriatum, the hypothalamus, the hippocampus, and the neocortex, have been proposed as the participants in the control of yawning, whereas the effector structures include the inspiratory bulbar center, the motor nuclei of cranial nerves V, VII, X, and XII, as well as the phrenic nerve and nerves of the accessory respiratory muscles (for a review see reference 2).

Although yawning is present in all humans and mammals, and some of the components of this reflex can be recognized in almost all vertebrates, it appears difficult to define the purpose of such a widespread behavioral pattern. In mammals, yawning is often associated with gaping, inspiration, and stretching. In some mammals, males yawn more than females, and yawning is associated with penile erection. Dominant primate males yawn more often than other males, which could implicate the social component of

yawning, but these sexual differences have not been observed in humans. In humans, yawning can often be seen before sleeping and after waking. Other physiologic situations that can trigger yawning in humans include periods before meals (probably due to hypoglycemia) or immediately after meals, particularly if a meal is accompanied with ingestion of alcohol (drowsiness), as well as stressful situations, motion sickness, or altitude changes (for reviews, see references 2 and 3). These observations have stimulated the development of several theories about the aims of yawning, none of which has been definitely accepted. Some investigators have proposed a respiratory role, suggesting that contractions of the diaphragm and the neck during the inspiration, as well as the contractions of the limb muscles during stretching increase the venous return, whereas the concomitant bronchial dilatation stimulates the vagal terminals, thus causing the vasodilatation and increasing the cerebral blood flow and cerebral oxygenation (for a review see reference 3). However, the respiratory function of yawning was disproved in later experiments, which showed that neither breathing of pure oxygen nor inhalation of a carbon dioxide-rich mixture of gases influenced the frequency of yawning.[4] Another theory on the role of yawning is based on the observations that this reflex occurs more often at bed and waking times and in boring situations, and is accompanied with an increase in cortical electroencephalographic (EEG) activity. These observations stimulated the hypothesis that yawning is an ancestral remnant that occurs when attention is low, in order to increase the arousal.[2,5] This theory is supported by monitoring of jugular oxygen partial pressure and EEG, which showed that the appearance of yawning is preceded by slowing of posterior activity on EEG and a decreased oxygen partial pressure.[5] In another investigation, where yawning was induced by electrical and chemical stimulation of the paraventricular nucleus of the hypothalamus, a yawning response occurred only after a systematic fall of blood pressure and an EEG arousal.[6] Finally, the fact that yawning often appears in situations that people find boring, such as in listeners during boring conferences, suggests that yawning could have a social significance, being a semivoluntary act of non-verbal communication.[7]

During the past few decades, progress in the field of neuropharmacology has redirected investigators' interest to the physiologic mechanisms and roles of yawning. Namely, it has been shown that different neurotransmitters and hormones, including opioids, acetylcholine, serotonin, dopamine, nitric oxide (NO), oxytocin, adrenocorticotropic hormone (ACTH), α-melanocyte-stimulating hormone (α-MSH), and excitatory amino acids such as N-methyl-D-aspartic acid (NMDA), participate in the regulation of yawning.[5,8,9] Although the mechanisms of their action in promotion or inhibition of yawning are still quite obscure, it has become apparent that at least some of them operate on the level of the paraventricular nucleus of the hypothalamus. Briefly, it seems that oxytocinergic neurons from the paraventricular hypothalamic nucleus, which project to the extra-hypothalamic regions such as the hippocampus, pons, and/or medulla oblongata, mediate, at least in some circumstances, the expression of yawning. These neurons can be activated by dopamine, excitatory amino acids, or oxytocin itself to promote yawning, or inhibited by opioid peptides to prevent yawning. Furthermore, it seems that NO could be the intracellular messenger in these neurons. However, some other hormones, such as serotonin and ACTH–MSH peptides mediate yawning reflex through other pathways, which do not include the paraventricular nucleus, although those pathways have not been clearly identified.[5,8,9]

Apart from physiologic situations, an altered frequency of yawning can be seen in many different pathologic conditions involving the CNS. For instance, yawning occurs more frequently before, during, and after migraine attacks, basal ganglia disorders, focal brain lesions such as tumors, apalic syndrome, cerebral malformations and transtentorial herniation,[9,10] encephalitis, increased intracranial pressure, and epilepsy.

YAWNING IN THE FETAL PERIOD

The development of real-time sonography has inspired many scientific investigations, that have described in detail different motor patterns of the fetus in its natural environment. Surprisingly, fetal yawning was recognized as one of the movement patterns consistently present from the end of the 1st trimester until delivery. In their classical investigation, de Vries et al[11] studied longitudinally the development of fetal movement patterns in 11 healthy pregnant women during the 1st trimester of pregnancy. The first movements were observed during the 7th and 8th postconceptional weeks and were described as just discernible movements, and by the 9th week they

disappeared, being replaced with complex generalized and isolated limb movements. Movements of the fetal jaw and face such as jaw opening, swallowing and yawning were observed around 10–11 weeks. Fetal yawning was described as a pattern similar to the yawn observed after birth: prolonged wide opening of the jaws followed by head retroflection and rapid closure of the jaws. The earliest yawning movements were observed around 11 postconceptional weeks as an infrequent and non-repetitive movement pattern. This early onset of fetal yawning and other jaw movements coincides with the development of the lower portions of the brainstem, medulla oblongata and pons. As described in Chapter 20, major structures of medulla oblongata are fashioned by 7–8 postconceptional weeks, although its maturation continues until the 7th postconceptional month.[12] In addition to its many subnuclei, the medulla gives rise to a variety of descending spinal motor tracts and hosts the nuclei of five cranial nerves (VIII–XII). Formation of the pons begins almost simultaneously, but its maturation is more prolonged. The structures of the pons include cranial nerves V–VIII (vestibular nuclei of nerve VIII) and medial longitudinal fasciculus (MLF), pontine tegmentum, raphe nucleus and locus ceruleus, which exert widespread influences on arousal, including the sleep–wake cycle. Therefore, these structures exert tremendous influences on gross body movements, head turning, heart rate, and respiratory movements, as well as swallowing, yawning, suckling, hiccups, and facial grimacing movements.[12] Maturation of the medulla and pons could be associated with changes in the yawning pattern. Sepulveda et al[13] described repetitive sequences of yawning movements in the 27-week-old fetus in normal pregnancy, indicating that in this period of gestation, not only is yawning present but its pattern changes from non-repetitive to repetitive sequences.

Although the purpose of the yawning reflex in humans and animals is presently incompletely understood, its early appearance during fetal development and continuous presence imply its evolutionary importance. However, fetal yawning is still quite a mysterious phenomenon, and its possible relation to the pathologic conditions, particularly those affecting the fetal CNS has not been investigated so far, despite the clearly altered incidence of yawning in a wide spectrum of CNS disorders observed in adults. The increased frequency of yawning movements has been reported in fetuses suffering Rhesus immunization, fetal erythroblastosis, and severe anemia. This phenomenon was interpreted as a fetal attempt to increase venous return and thereby improve the delivery of oxygenated blood to the vital organs.[14] However, these findings should be confirmed on a larger number of high-risk fetuses.

The recent development of the advanced technique of 4D sonography opened a new perspective for research into fetal behavior and particularly facial movements. Early reports of yawning movements in the 20-week-old fetus indicated that 4D sonography might facilitate the investigation of this infrequent movement pattern.[15] In this report, fetal yawning was described as sudden opening of the jaw, accompanied by stretching of the fetal upper limbs and flexion of the head, which distinguished it from the more frequently observed swallowing pattern. However, apart from this early report, systematic investigations of fetal yawning and other facial movement patterns are still in their infancy, and the first scientific papers were published only recently. According to our results, investigation of fetal yawning movements in early pregnancy is limited by technical obstacles. In this study, the frequencies of embryonic and fetal movements recorded by 4D sonography during the 1st trimester of normal gestation were compared with movements recorded by 2D sonography in the same period. Several movements, including fetal yawning, could not be observed by 4D sonography, although they were clearly observed by 2D sonography.[16] Yawning movement appeared at the end of the 1st trimester and was one of the most infrequent movement patterns. It seems that very infrequent movements, as well as discrete or short rapid movement patterns could not be observed due to the relatively slow repetition time for data acquisition required to obtain images of satisfactory quality. Nevertheless, other studies showed that yawning movement could clearly be observed during the 2nd and 3rd trimesters[17] (Figures 23.2 and 23.3). The systematic investigations of fetal movements confirmed that all components of the fetal yawning pattern – prolonged jaw opening followed by rapid closure and accompanied by head flexion and elevation of the arms – can easily be recognized by 4D sonography in this period[18–20] (Figure 23.4). Furthermore, when fetal yawning in the 3rd trimester was compared with yawning in neonates during the 1st week of life, no differences were found in the frequencies of this reflex. All components of the yawning pattern in neonates could also be observed in the fetal period.[19,20] In our latest study, we investigated

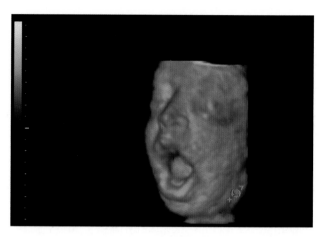

Figure 23.2 Yawning movement recorded by 3D/4D sonography in a 28-week-old fetus

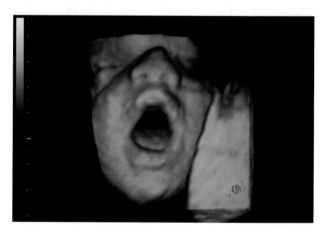

Figure 23.3 Yawning movement recorded by 3D/4D sonography in a 29-week-old fetus

longitudinally the frequency of body and facial movements in 100 fetuses from all trimesters of normal pregnancies. The frequency of yawning gradually increased between the 15th and 24th weeks, after which a short plateau was observed from the 24th to the 26th weeks, and this was followed by a slight decrease towards term.[20] This was the first study to demonstrate a clear gestational age-related trend in the frequency of yawning movements, which could be interpreted as maturation of the brainstem and possibly the acquisition of control by more cranial structures over the yawning pattern. It also defined as the normal frequency range of this as well as other movement patterns in all trimesters of gestation. Finally, these findings have provided new information about the course of neurodevelopment of this interesting but poorly understood reflex. Whether this course is altered in the case of neurodevelopmental

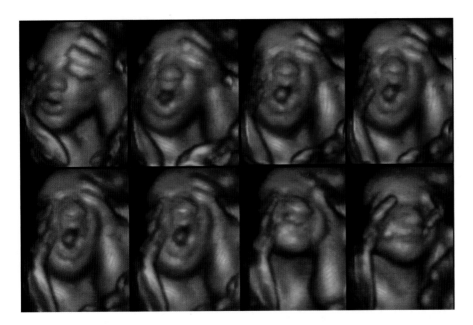

Figure 23.4 A sequence of images showing all the components of the yawning pattern recorded by 4D sonography: wide opening of the jaws, head retroflexion, flexion of the arms, and finally closing of the jaws

disturbances, and whether such alterations can give us insight into the function of the fetal nervous system in high-risk pregnancies, remain to be determined.

DEVELOPMENT OF FETAL HEARING, LEARNING, AND MEMORY

Although pregnant women have for a long time been aware that their fetuses respond with body movements to loud external sounds, the investigation of the stimuli able to produce such an effect or the characterization of fetal responses to sounds aroused only limited attention among scientists until the 1980s. Conversely, there was a prevailing opinion that the fetal environment is isolated from the noise of the outer world.[21] However, this opinion was radically changed after the development of real-time sonography, which enabled non-invasive visualization of fetal intrauterine activities. Studies performed using this method confirmed that in the 3rd trimester, the fetus is capable of registering and reacting to exogenous acoustic stimulation and that the character of fetal reactions changes as pregnancy progresses.[22] These observations have raised many questions about the characteristics of sounds that can reach the fetal ear, the exact onset of fetal hearing, and the consequences of fetal exposure to sounds such as music or speech on fetal well-being, or even about possible fetal memorization of intrauterine acoustic experiences. Numerous investigations performed on human fetuses and animal models have contributed to our under-

standing of the intrauterine acoustic environment and external sound transmission (reviewed in reference 21) Simultaneously, sonographic studies revealed that examination of fetal physiologic responses to acoustic stimulation can provide insight into fetal status, and the fetal vibroacoustic stimulation test was soon added to standard non-stress testing for the evaluation of fetal well-being. Subsequently, psychobiologic investigations led to the hypothesis that the acoustically rich environment in the uterus contributes to fetal learning.[23] Finally, it has been suggested that overexposure to noise, for instance in a woman's workplace, could place the fetus at risk for hearing loss. These suggestions imply a need to understand the principles of sound transmission to the fetus and the characteristics of fetal sound perception and responsiveness.

There are many factors that influence fetal perception of external sounds. Primarily, the components of the fetal auditory system must be developed sufficiently to enable the perception and transmission of sound waves. Furthermore, the stimulus must generate a sufficient sound pressure to penetrate the uterus, reach the fetal head, and produce the mechanical displacements of the basilar membrane of the organ of Corti that trigger the response of the hair cells and associate afferent neurons. The afferent and efferent neural pathways involved in sound perception must be sufficiently developed. Finally, the fetal response to stimulation has to be registered in order to quantify the nature of the stimulus that reaches the hearing mechanism.[21]

The perception of sound undoubtedly develops prenatally in humans as well as many other species, although the maturation of auditory organs continues during the first postnatal weeks and months and these maturational changes influence infant sound perception and discrimination. The development of the external ear canal and middle ear structures occurs during the embryonic period, although the maturation of the middle ear continues during the first postnatal months. In healthy human infants born at term, significant structural and functional changes in the color, translucency, and mobility of the tympanic membrane occur during the first 4 postnatal months. Furthermore, mesenchymal resorption in the middle ear is incomplete at birth and continues after birth, resulting in a marked decrease in tympanic membrane thickness. The decrease in tympanic membrane epithelial thickness proceeds during the first postnatal years.[24] These maturational changes in the mechanical properties of middle ear function can be documented by multiple-frequency tympanometry.[25]

Development of the inner ear structures is prolonged and proceeds in a more complex fashion. The cochlea is coiled at 9 weeks of gestation, and cochlear ducts form from the basal to the apical region during the subsequent month. The tectorial membrane is formed by 10 weeks, and 2 weeks later, perilymphatic spaces are apparent. Although the exact period of differentiation of the hair cells is unknown, the formation of their synapses with cranial nerve VIII begins around the 10th week of gestation, preceding by 2 weeks the formation of stereocilia at the apex of sensory hair cells. However, the maturation of those synapses occurs a few weeks later, around the 15th week for inner hair cells and around the 22nd week for outer cells. The 22nd week is also the period of maturation of the stereocilia, which are critical structural components in the transduction apparatus within the cochlea. It can be generally said that the maturation of the inner hair cells precedes the maturation of the outer hair cells and that the basal region of the cochlea matures approximately 1–2 weeks earlier than the apex.[26] The development of neural structures involved in the processing of acoustic stimuli, such as the cochlear nuclei within the medulla oblongata and pons, auditory colliculi of the mesencephalon, and the primary auditory cortex, is described extensively elsewhere and will be addressed only briefly here. The major structures of the brainstem are fashioned by the 7th and 8th postconceptional weeks, but their maturation is prolonged and proceeds in a caudal-to-rostral direction. As the medulla oblongata, the most caudal part of the brainstem, matures in advance of more rostral structures, reflexive movements of the head, body, and extremities, as well as breathing movements and alterations in heart rate, appear in advance of other functions. Maturation of the pons is more prolonged, which explains the delayed onset of its specific functions, such as the selective response to sounds and vibration. High levels of pontine arousal, including the perception of loud sounds, can trigger head-turning, whole-body movement, and the startle reaction in the 3rd trimester. Finally, the maturation of the midbrain does not even begin until the 2nd trimester. It consists of the dopamine-producing substantia nigra, the inferior-auditory and superior-visual colliculus, and cranial nerves III and IV, which, together with the MLF and cranial nerve VI, control eye movements. Late in gestation, the fetus becomes increasingly responsive to sound, and reflexively orients, turns the head, and reacts with lateral eye movements if sufficiently stimulated.[12] The development of the primary auditory cortex may be studied by recording of the cortical evoked potential. For instance, an early surface negative cortical auditory evoked potential can be registered in a 28-week-old premature infant. At that time, cortical axons are present in the middle third of the auditory cortex. Maturation of the auditory cortex is characterized by the appearance of surface positive evoked potentials between the 36th and 40th weeks and continues long after term.[27]

Even in the absence of external transmissions, the intrauterine milieu is not deprived of sounds. A variety of sounds, generated by maternal respiratory, cardiovascular, and intestinal movements, as well as body movements, normally reach the uterus, generating the background, or 'noise floor', above which maternal vocalizations or external sounds can reach the uterus. Placing an underwater microphone (hydrophone) into the pocket of fluid near the necks of human fetuses, Gagnon et al[28] measured sound pressure levels of 60 dB for 0.1 kHz and less than 40 dB for frequencies of 0.2 kHz and above. In pregnant ewes, internal sounds are also predominantly of low frequency (<0.1 Hz) and can reach 90 dB.[29] Therefore, the 'noise floor' in humans as well as animals is dominated by low-frequency energy less than 0.1 kHz and can reach levels as high as 90 dB. Exogenous sounds with frequency less than 0.2 kHz penetrate the uterus with very little reduction in sound pressure, whereas high frequencies of 4.0 Hz are attenuated by approximately 20 dB.[30] Over the frequency range from 0.125 to 2.0 kHz, the abdomen can be characterized as a low-pass filter, with high-frequency energy being rejected at a rate of approximately 6 dB/octave.[29]

The development of real-time 2D sonography has allowed non-invasive observations of fetal responses to the various external stimuli, and several procedures have been used to examine the development of the fetal acoustic system. Many researchers have used a device termed an 'electronic artificial larynx' applied directly to the maternal abdomen, above the fetal head, to elicit a fetal response, and this device is most commonly used in the examination of fetal reactions to stimuli as an indicator of fetal well-being. Another mode of examination is stimulation by very loud airborne sounds within the audible frequency spectrum. Examination of acoustic evoked potentials in healthy prematurely born neonates has confirmed that the cochlear function is established between 22 and 25 weeks. In other studies, fetal responses to external vibratory and acoustic stimulation were recorded around the 24th week, and consisted mainly of fetal body movements.[31,32] Applying acoustic stimulation with a wide spectrum of frequencies directly to the maternal abdomen, Shahidullah and Hepper[33] have recorded reflex movements with a short lag time in 20-week-old fetuses, and movements without a lag time in 25-week-old fetuses. This reaction can be interpreted primarily as a response to proprioceptor stimulation, as well as vibroacoustic stimulation. Nevertheless, Kisilevsky et al[34] reported an increased number of fetal movements and heart rate during stimulation with very loud airborne sound (110 dB sound pressure level) performed with a sound transmitter placed 10 cm above the maternal abdomen in 30-week-old fetuses. During the last weeks of pregnancy, the fetal response to vibroacoustic stimulation is characterized not only by alterations in the frequency of gross body movements and breathing movements, but also by an increase in fetal heart rate. For instance, 5-second vibroacoustic stimulation applied to the abdominal surface of women volunteers between 33 and 40 weeks of gestation resulted in fetal tachycardia that persisted up to 1 hour, and the onset of the response was often delayed between 10 and 20 minutes. Vibroacoustic stimulation of fetuses between 36 and 40 weeks of gestation resulted in alterations in the incidence of breathing movements.[35] Finally, a few weeks prior to term, dramatic changes in fetal behavioral states following vibroacoustic stimulation have been reported. The increasingly complex repertoire of fetal reactions to the same type of stimulus develops owing to maturation of the neural structures that participate in the perception of sounds. Another interesting feature of the auditory system of the fetus is the limited range of frequencies that it can register in comparison to the auditory system of adults. Shahidullah and Hepper[36] examined the ranges of frequencies and intensity levels required to elicit movements in human fetuses. At 27 weeks, 96% of the 450 fetuses included in the study responded to tones at 0.25 and 0.50 kHz, and between 29 and 31 weeks, they responded to tones at 1.0 and 3.0 kHz, respectively. Between 33 and 35 weeks of gestation, fetuses were responding 100% of the time to presentation of 1.0 and 3.0 kHz. As the pregnancies progressed, the fetuses responded to a progressively wider range of frequencies. There was also a significant decrease in the intensity of the stimulus required to elicit a response for all frequencies, which suggested that fetal registration of pure tones becomes progressively sensitive as pregnancy proceeds.[36] It should be borne in mind that the basal portions of the cochlea, involved in the perception of lower frequencies, mature earlier than the apical portions, responsible for the perception of higher frequencies, which could explain this developmental trend. During the last weeks of pregnancy (from the 36th week onward), the fetus can respond to external noises, even to the sound of the mother's voice, with reflexive body movements, head-turning, and heart-rate acceleration. However, these sounds have to be rather loud and high in frequency to overcome the attenuation of the uterus and amniotic fluid (for a review, see reference 12). At that age, the fetus seems to be able not only to perceive the sounds but also to discriminate between different sounds. This astonishing finding is explained by the tonotopic organization of the cochlear nuclei and by the maturation of the brainstem during the last weeks of pregnancy. Another remarkable property of the brainstem nuclei and pathways is their synaptic plasticity, which makes them easily influenced by the external auditory experience and capable of 'synaptic learning'. For example, specific midbrain neural networks and pathways are molded through the repetitive auditory stimulation, or lack thereof, and those pathways selectively respond to the stimuli that shaped them. Consequently, the fetal and neonatal brainstem becomes responsive to the sounds to which it is repeatedly exposed, while the neural pathways that fail to be stimulated eventually disappear. This might explain the reports of the selective preference of the term fetus for its mother's voice or other familiar or repetitive sounds presented up to 6 weeks before birth (for a review, see reference 12).

The intrauterine origins of learning and memory processes, indicated above, have been tested extensively in many experimental studies. Most of these studies used habituation methods, classical conditioning, or exposure learning in the assessment of fetal learning. Habituation is the decrement in response following repeated presentation of the same stimulus.[37] Despite the simplicity of the test, the decrement of responses due to habituation needs to be distinguished from sensory fatigue. In one of the classical studies that demonstrated the existence of a true fetal habituation response, fetuses at 36 weeks of gestation were stimulated with a tone played by a loudspeaker on the maternal abdomen.[38] Initially, all fetuses moved in response to sound, but after 10–15 stimulus presentations, fetuses stopped moving. When a new sound of a different frequency was presented, the fetuses moved, but after repeated presentation of this stimulus, the movements stopped. Finally, when the original sound was presented again, the fetuses initially responded to the tone but then ceased responding more rapidly and after fewer instances than when the tone was originally presented. The earliest developmental stage at which fetal habituation was demonstrated was 22 weeks of gestation.[39] This investigation used a vibroacoustic stimulus, and the onset of habituation coincided with the onset of fetal hearing, indicating that the development of audition might have been the limiting factor in the assessment of habituation and that it might have been present even earlier. Nevertheless, developmental trends in habituation have been registered, with younger fetuses requiring more presentations of the stimulus than older fetuses.[40] Fetal habituation to vibroacoustic stimuli has also been tested in high-risk pregnancies. Altered habituation was demonstrated in fetuses with Down syndrome,[38] as these fetuses required more presentations to acquire habituation than healthy fetuses of the same gestational age. Furthermore, the time required to habituate differed among fetuses with Down syndrome and was related to the neonatal outcome. A delayed habituation response to vibroacoustic stimuli was also demonstrated in fetuses from pregnancies complicated by maternal diabetes mellitus.[41] This investigation has shown that delayed habituation might indicate functional impairment of the structures involved in memorization process. Finally, in small-for-gestational-age (SGA) infants, delayed habituation 10 days prior to delivery was related to impaired individual performance on the Brazeltone Neonatal Behavior Assessment Scale performed 12

and 24 hours after delivery. Infants with normal habituation had significantly higher General Intelligence Quotients, assessed by the Griffiths Mental Development Scale at 1 year of age, than did infants with either a slow or a fast habituation pattern. This study indicated that the prenatal habituation pattern could provide insight into CNS functioning.[42]

Another method used to assess fetal learning and memory is classical conditioning, which involves the pairing of two stimuli: a conditioned stimulus (which elicits no response when presented alone) and an unconditioned stimulus (which elicits a fetal response when presented alone). Following repeated paired exposure to these two stimuli, the conditioned stimulus also elicits a response – termed a 'conditioned response'. Using a pure tone as the conditioned stimulus and a vibroacoustic stimulus as the unconditioned one, Hepper[43] was able to demonstrate a conditioned response in fetuses ranging from 32 to 39 weeks of gestation. However, the same response could be demonstrated in fetuses with anencephaly.

Exposure learning represents another method that is applicable in the assessment of fetal memory. In this case, the fetus is exposed to a stimulus, and its response after a number of exposures is registered. This response is then compared either with the response to the 'unfamiliar' sound in the same individuals or with the response of unexposed fetuses to the same stimulus. Application of this method has shown that newborn infants exhibited a preference for their mother's voice compared with an unfamiliar voice. When the mother's voice as it sounded after birth was compared with the mother's voice as it sounded in utero (different due to the sound attenuation in utero), the newborn infants showed a preference for their mother's voice as it sounded in the uterus. These studies confirmed that fetuses are able to hear and learn their mother's voice before birth.[44] It has also been shown that fetuses at 37 weeks of gestation respond differently to familiar and unfamiliar sounds, but this difference could not be observed at 30 weeks of gestation.[45]

Although these experiments have provided evidence for prenatal development of at least a short-term memory, they need to be interpreted with special caution, particularly when attributing adult-like memory qualities to the fetus. For instance, the classical conditioning response, which can be registered in healthy adults, can be elicited in anencephalic fetuses, which implies that the underlying mediation of this memory in fetuses may be very different than in adults. Furthermore, evidence for habituation as a model of learning and memory can be found in animals such as rats, and even in invertebrates. Therefore, despite the existence of scientifically reliable evidence that fetuses are able to learn and memorize stimuli, this memory should be considered rudimentary and of limited duration. The relationship between these findings and the functioning of the CNS, as well as that between memory before birth and memory evidenced after birth or later in life, remain to be investigated in the future.

REFERENCES

1. Salihagic-Kadic A, Kurjak A, Medic M, Andonotopo W, Azumendi G. New data about embryonic and fetal neurodevelopment and behavior obtained by 3D and 4D sonography. J Perinat Med 2005; 33: 478–90.

2. Daquin G, Micalleg J, Blin O. Yawning. Sleep Med Rev 2001; 5: 299–312.

3. Lehman HE. Yawning; a homeostatic reflex and its physiological significance. Bull Meninger Clinic 1979; 43: 123–36.

4. Provine RR, Tate BC, Geldmaker LL. Yawning: no effect of 3–5% CO_2, 100% O_2 and exercise. Behav Neural Biol 1987; 48: 382–93.

5. Argiolas A, Melis MR. The neuropharmacology of yawning. Eur J Pharmacol 1998; 343: 1–16.

6. Sato-suzuki I, Kita I, Oguri M, Arita H. Stereotyped yawning responses induced by electrical and chemical stimulations of the paraventricular nucleus of the rat. J Neurophysiol 1998; 80: 2765–77.

7. Askenasy JJM. Is yawning an arousal defense reflex? J Psychol 1989; 123: 609–21.

8. Bertolini A, Gessa GL. Behavioural effects of ACTH and MSH peptides. J Endocrinol Inv 1981; 4: 241–51.

9. Blin O, Azullay JP, Masson G, Aubrespy G, Serratrice G. Apomorphine induced yawning in migraine patients: evidence for central dopaminergic hypersensitivity. Clin Neuropharmacol 1991; 14: 91–5.

10. Sandyk R. Excessive yawning and progressive nuclear palsy. Int J Neurosci 1987; 34: 123–6.

11. de Vries JIP, Visser G, Prechtl HFR. Emergence of fetal behavior. Qualitative aspects. Early Hum Dev 1982; 73: 1–23.

12. Joseph R. Fetal brain and cognitive development. Dev Rev 1999; 20: 81–98.

13. Sepulveda M, Mangiamarchi M. Fetal yawning. Ultrasound Obstet Gynecol 1995; 5: 57–9.

14. Petrikovsky R, Kaplan G, Holsten N. Fetal yawning activity in high risk fetuses: a preliminary observation. Ultrasound Obstet Gynecol 1999; 13: 127–30.

15. Sherer DM, Smith SA, Abramowicz JS. Fetal yawning in utero at 20 weeks gestation. J Ultrasound Med 1991; 10: 68.

16. Andonotopo W, Medic M, Salihagic-Kadic A, et al. The assessment of fetal behavior in early pregnancy: comparison between 2D and 4D songoraphic scanning. J Perinat Med 2005; 33: 406–14.

17. Walusinsky O, Kurjak A, Azumendi G. Fetal yawning assessed by 4D sonography. Ultrasound Rev Obstet Gynecol 2005; 5: 210–17.

18. Kurjak A, Stanojević A, Andonotopo W, et al. Behavioral pattern continuity from prenatal to postnatal life – a study by 4 dimensional (4D) ultrasonography. J Perinat Med 2004; 32: 346–53.

19. Kurjak A, Stanojevic M, Andonotopo W, et al. Fetal behavior assessed in all three trimesters of normal pregnancy by four-dimensional ultrasonography. Croat Med J 2005; 46: 772–80.

20. Kurjak A, Andonotopo W, Hafner T, et al. Normal standards for fetal neurobehavioural developments – longitudinal quantification by four-dimensional sonography. J Perinat Med 2006; 34: 56–65.

21. Lecanuet JP, Schaal B. Fetal sensory competencies. Eur J Obstet Gynecol Reprod Biol 1996; 68: 1–23.

22. Hepper P, Shahidullah S. Development of fetal hearing. Arch Dis Child 1994; 71: 81–7.

23. Abrams RM, Gerhardt KJ. The acoustic environment and physiological responses of the fetus. J Perinatol 2000; 20: 30–55.

24. Ruah CB, Schachern PA, Zelterman D, Paparella MM, Yoon TH. Age related morphologic changes in the human tympanic membrane. Arch Otolaryngol Head Neck Surg 1991; 117: 627–34.

25. Holte L, Margolis RH, Cavanaugh RM Jr. Developmental changes in multifrequency tympanograms. Audiology 1991; 31: 1–24.

26. Hall JP. Development of ear and hearing. J Perinatol 2000; 20: 11–19.

27. Kostovic I, Judas M, Petanjek Z, Simic G. Ontogenesis of goal-directed behavior: anatomo-functional considerations. Int J Psychophysiol 1995; 19: 85–102.

28. Gagnon R, Benzaquen S, Hunse C. The fetal sound environment during vibroacoustic stimulation in labor: effect on fetal heart rate response. Obstet Gynecol 1992; 79: 550–5.

29. Gerhardt KJ, Abrams RM, Oliver CC. Sound environment of the fetal sheep. Am J Obstet Gynecol. 1990; 162: 282–7.

30. Querleu D, Renard X, Crepin G. Perception auditive et reactivite foetale aux stimulations sonores. J Gynecol Obstet Biol Reprod 1981; 10: 307–14.

31. Crade M, Lovett S. Fetal response to sound stimulation: preliminary report exploring use of sound stimulation in routine obstetrical ultrasound examination. J Ultrasound Med 1988; 7: 499–50.

32. Birnholz JC, Benacerraf BR. The development of human fetal hearing. Science 1983; 222: 516–18.

33. Schahidullah S, Hepper P. The developmental origins of fetal responsiveness to an acoustic stimulus. J Reprod Infant Psychol 1994; 12: 143–54.

34. Kisilevsky BS, Pang LH, Hains SMJ. Maturation of human fetal responses to airborne sound in low- and high-risk fetuses. Early Human Dev 2000; 58: 179–95.

35. Gagnon R. Stimulation of human fetuses with sound and vibration. Semin Perinatol 1989; 13: 393–402.

36. Shahidullah S, Hepper P. Frequency discrimination by the fetus. Early Hum Dev 1994; 36: 13–26.

37. Thompson RF, Spencer WA. Habituation: a model for the study of neuronal substrates of behavior. Physiol Rev 1966; 73: 16–43.

38. Hepper PG, Shahidullah S. Habituation in normal and Down syndrome fetuses. Q J Exp Physiol 1992; 44: 305–17.

39. Leader LR, Baillie P, Martin B, Vermeulen E. The assessment and significance of habituation to a repeated stimulus by the human fetus. Early Hum Dev 1982; 7: 211–19.

40. Kuhlman KA, Burns KA, Depp R, Sabbagha RE. Ultrasonic imaging of normal fetal responses to external vibratory acoustic stimulation. Am J Obstet Gynecol 1998; 158: 47–51.

41. Doherty NN, Hepper P. Habituation in fetuses of diabetic mothers. Early Hum Dev 2000; 59: 85–93.

42. Leader LR, Baille P, Martin B, Molteno C, Wynchak S. Fetal responses to vibrotactile stimulation, a possible predictor of fetal and neonatal outcome. Aust NZ J Obstet Gynaecol 1984; 24: 251–6.

43. Hepper P. Memory in utero? Dem Med Child Dev 1997; 39: 343–6.

44. Hepper P, Scott D, Shahidullah S. Newborn and fetal response to maternal voice. J Reprod Infant Psychol 1993; 11: 147–53.

45. De Casper AJ, Spence MJ. Prenatal maternal speech influences newborn's perception of speech sound. Inf Behav Dev 1986; 9: 133–50.

24 Assessment of multifetal pregnancies by 3D/4D sonography

Asim Kurjak, Guillermo Azumendi, and Pilar Prats

INTRODUCTION

The increases in both the rate and the number of multiple births in the USA and Western Europe have been well documented in the literature. Several factors seem to be responsible for the rising incidence of multiple births, including the rapid growth in the use of assisted reproductive technologies (ART) and the rise in the average age of women giving birth to their first child (older mothers have a greater likelihood of spontaneous multiple pregnancies and at the same time a greater prevalence of ART procedures).[1]

The introduction of sonography has revolutionized the antenatal diagnosis of multiple pregnancy. Thirty years ago, twins were most often overlooked, whereas triplets were diagnosed only after the delivery of the second infant. After the introduction of sonography into routine prenatal care, the confident diagnosis or exclusion of multiple pregnancies became practical reality.

Indeed, two-dimensional (2D) sonography is still the primary modality for diagnosing and evaluating multiple pregnancy. However, 2D sonography may soon be overtaken by 3D and 4D sonography. These new techniques should be accepted as complementary to 2D sonography, because additional information that assists in clinical management can sometimes be provided. Modern 4D sonography machines are capable of performing spatial imaging in near real time, providing up to 28 frames/s. 4D sonography can be used in multifetal pregnancies for detection and evaluation of intertwin contacts, because it allows simultaneous visualization of both fetuses and assessment of their motor activity. The main benefits of 4D sonography include accurate recognition of isolated motor activity of a single fetus, distinguishing between spontaneous and stimulated motor activity, and spatial visualization of the intertwin area.[2] Numerous improvements in data processing capacity during the past few years have made it possible to overcome the previous limitations of 3D/4D sonography. In other words, no fetal position precludes the acquisition of a desired section. At present, the only limitation on visualization of a desired structure is the amount of adjacent amniotic fluid.[3]

The advantages of 3D imaging in management of multiple pregnancy are described in Table 24.1.

Table 24.1 The advantages of 3D sonographic imaging

1st trimester	• Elimination of undercounting phenomenon
	• Improved prediction of spontaneous abortion
	• Improved prenatal clasification of uterine anomaly
2nd trimester	• Improved diagnosis of vanishing phenomenon
	• Early detection of fetal anomalies
	• Improved evaluation of fetal malformation
	• Improved determination of placentation

DIAGNOSIS OF MULTIPLE PREGNANCY

The diagnosis of multiple pregnancy (triplets, quadruplets, quintuplets, etc.) with 2D sonography usually requires a long examination period and an experienced ultrasonographer. If one uses transvaginal sonography (TVS), multifetal pregnancies can be diagnosed as early as the 5th to 6th weeks of gestation (Figures 24.1–24.3). An early diagnosis can be associated with

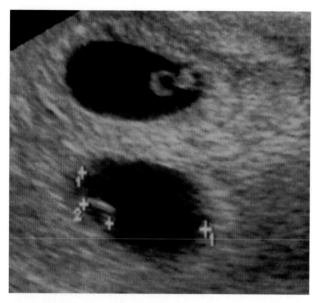

Figure 24.1 The first visible structure of dizygotic and diamniotic twins. Note the number of gestational sacs and yolk sacs

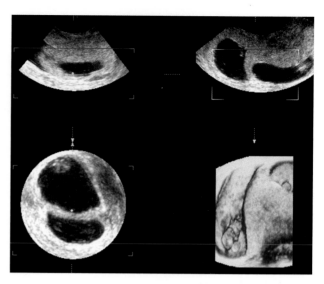

Figure 24.3 Multiplanar and surface rendering 3D sonography of a twin pregnancy at 7 weeks of gestation demonstrating the advantages of 3D sonography in the evaluation of early multiple pregnancies

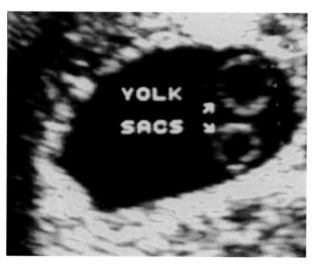

Figure 24.2 The separated yolk sacs are demonstrated in early diagnosis of monozygotic twins

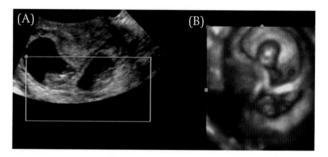

Figure 24.4 Comparison between 2D (A) and 3D (B) sonography. Both modalities provide an examiner with essential information concerning the management of twin pregnancy, including the number of fetuses and chorionic status

numerous pitfalls. One embryo usually arises from a single gestational sac. However, in monozygotic twins, two embryos arise from a single gestational sac (Figure 24.2). The number of gestational sacs always matches the number of placentas, and very often, but not always, the number of embryos. Therefore, reliable prediction of the number of embryos on the basis of the number of gestational sacs is not accurate. Even the finding of a gestational sac with a single yolk sac does not exclude monoamniotic twins. Only one (large or irregular) yolk sac can be seen in monoamniotic twin pregnancies.[4] Therefore, until the 7th week of gesta-

tion, when the embryo is recognizable sonographically, reliable counting of embryos is not possible. Only the number of embryos is important for final diagnosis of the number of multiples (Figures 24.4–24.8).

Three gestational sacs have to be recognized in the case of trichorionic–triamniotic triplets (Figures 24.6, 24.7 and 24.9). However, even when two gestational sacs are seen, a diagnosis of triplets is not yet excluded, and the possibility of dichorionic–triamniotic triplets (complex chorionicity) should be taken into consideration (Figures 24.10 and 24.11). Only counting the number of embryos is definitive in the diagnosis of triplets.

Determination of cardiac activities is another important prognostic factor. The probability of delivering twins when two chorionic sacs are seen is 57%,

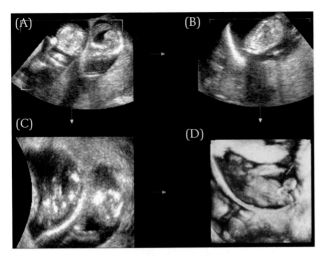

Figure 24.5 Multiplanar (A–C) and surface rendering (D) modes of a twin pregnancy

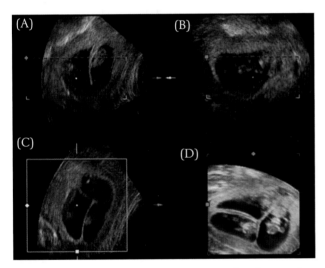

Figure 24.6 3D multiplanar view (A–C) and surface rendering (D) in the determination of the accurate number of gestational sacs in a triplet pregnancy at the 12th week of gestation

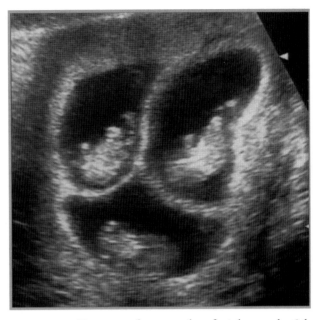

Figure 24.7 Transvaginal sonography of triplets at the 8th week of gestation: three embryos in three gestational sacs (trichorionic–triamniotic triplets)

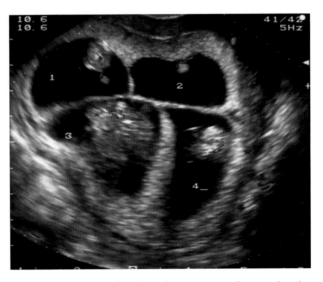

Figure 24.8 2D color Doppler imaging of a quadruplet pregnancy

but when two cardiac activities (two viable embryos) are present, it increases to 87%. Similarly, the probability of delivering triplets after visualization of three gestational sacs is 20%, but with three viable embryos, it increases to 68%.[5] The viability of each embryo can be confirmed using color Doppler imaging of the corresponding fetal circulation (Figure 24.8).

DETERMINATION OF THE NUMBER OF GESTATIONAL SACS

Sonography in early pregnancy confirms that the number of conceived multiple pregnancies exceeds the rate of multiple births. Spontaneous embryonic/fetal loss in the 1st trimester of multiple pregnancies is known as the 'vanishing twin' phenomenon[6] (Figures 24.12–24.14). Pregnancy number before the 6th week is determined by counting the number of gestational sacs. Using this method, the examiner must be aware of what has been characterized as the late-appearing twin phenomenon or 'undercounting'. The late appearance of twins is recognized on the basis of the discrepancy between two sonograms, in which comparison of an initial

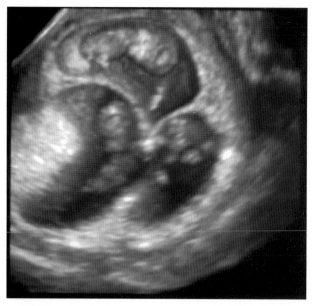

Figure 24.9 3D sonography of the same pregnancy as in Figure 24.7

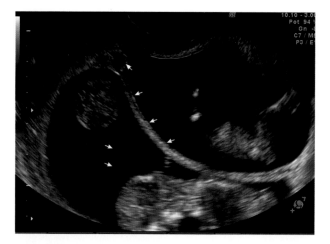

Figure 24.10 2D sonography of a dichorionic–triamniotic triplet pregnancy at 11 weeks of gestation

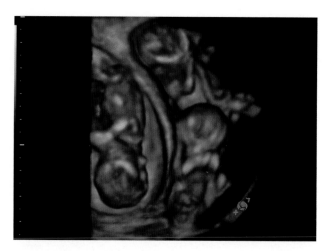

Figure 24.11 3D sonography of a dichorionic–triamniotic triplet pregnancy at 11 weeks of gestation demonstrates the advantages of 3D sonography in the evaluation of multiple pregnancy

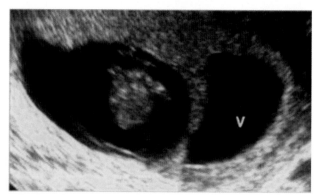

Figure 24.12 Transvaginal scan of a dichorionic twin complicated by a vanished twin (right of image)

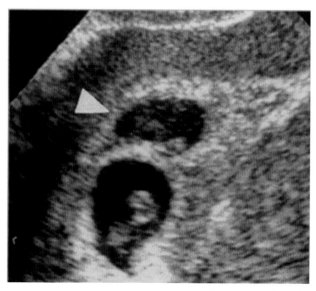

Figure 24.13 Transvaginal scan of dichorionic twin demonstrating a vanished twin in the upper part of the image

sonogram, usually obtained at 5.0–5.9 weeks, and a subsequent sonogram at 6 or more weeks demonstrates more embryos or fetuses than the previously counted gestational sacs. The outcome of successful pregnancy after three chorionic sacs have been seen is triplets 47.4%, twins 31.6%, singletons 18.4%, miscarriages 2.6%.[7] There are two types of undercounting: polyzygotic and monozygotic. A meta-analysis showed that more than 50% of pregnancies with three or more gestational sacs have spontaneous reduction before the 12th week. The surviving fetuses weigh less and are born earlier than unreduced pregnancies with the same initial number of fetuses.[8]

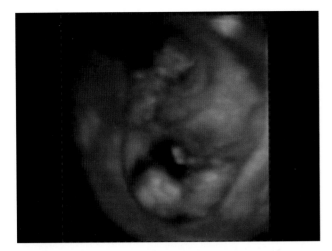

Figure 24.14 Surface rendering of a vanished triplet at 13 weeks of gestation

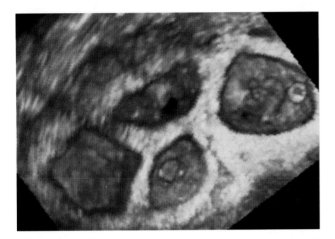

Figure 24.15 3D scan of the correct number of gestational sacs: final diagnosis of quadruplets with the 3D surface rendering mode. In contrast to 2D manual slicing, an analysis of 3D volugrams reveals the correct number of gestational sacs

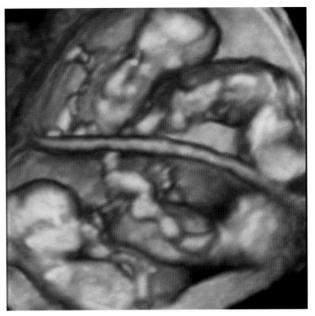

Figure 24.16 3D surface rendering showing a quadruplet pregnancy and clearly illustrating intertwin position and contacts

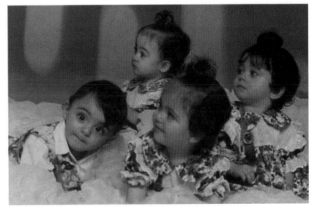

Figure 24.17 Postnatal picture of the quadruplets in Figure 24.16

Polyzygotic undercounting is a result of the limitations of 2D transvaginal sonography. The anatomy of the female reproductive tract as well as contemporary probe design limit the possible examination planes to the sagittal and transverse. Because the uterus can only be examined in these two planes, it is possible that an examiner fails to visualize the total number of gestational sacs on a single screen. In other words, one or more gestational sacs may be overlooked. This problem is enhanced in high-order multiple pregnancies in which it is impossible to visualize all gestational sacs on a single screen (Figures 24.8, 24.10, 24.11, and 24.15–24.17). Therefore, the risk of undercounting is correlated with the number of embryos. Undercounting of the number

of gestational sacs is the most common pitfall during the 1st trimester. This pitfall can be avoided either by conventional or 3D sonography.

Whenever spontaneous reduction is suspected in a high-order multiple pregnancy on conventional sonographic examination, the additional use of the surface rendering mode is recommended. With the use of this mode, distinction between spontaneous reduction and normal pregnancy in a high-order pregnancy is easy. Using 3D sonography the frontal (coronal) plane enables examination of the uterine cavity in sections that are unobtainable with conventional 2D sonography. Further, 3D sonography enables the

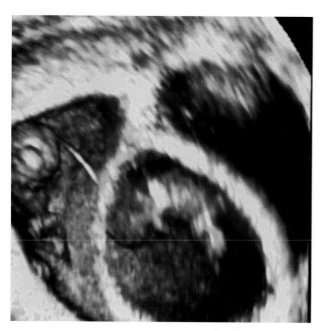

Figure 24.18 3D surface rendering demonstrating trichorionic–triamniotic triplet pregnancy

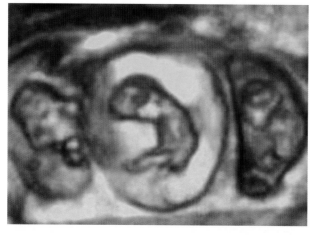

Figure 24.19 Surface features of fetuses, including yolk sacs. The spatial relationship of the fetuses to each other can be assessed easily

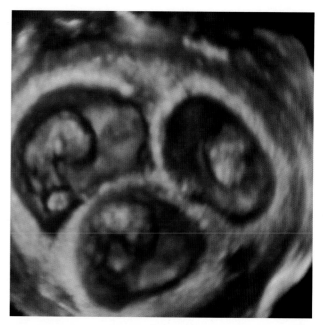

Figure 24.20 3D sonography of triplets at the 8th week of gestation: three embryos in three gestational sacs (trichorionic–triamniotic triplets)

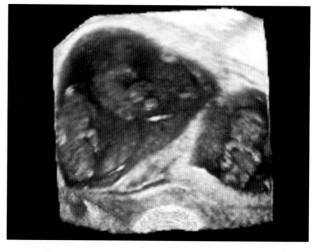

Figure 24.21 3D sonography of a triplet pregnancy at 9 weeks of gestation: three embryos in two gestational sacs (dichorionic–triamniotic triplets)

appropriate counting of gestational sacs without any risk of undercounting even for less experienced ultrasonographers (Figures 24.7–24.11, 24.15, 24.16, and 24.18–24.21). Therefore, interobserver variability in detecting the number of gestational sacs is significantly lower. Even quadruplets are recognizable without any difficulty (Figures 24.15 and 24.16). This advantage strongly suggests that 3D sonography should become the new standard in the early management of high-order multiple pregnancies. Before the introduction of 3D sonography, 11% of dichorionic twins were initially undercounted as singletons, and 16% of high-order multiple gestations were also undercounted.[9]

DETERMINATION OF CHORIONICITY AND AMNIONICITY

During the 1st and 2nd trimester chorionicity can be determined directly and indirectly (Figures

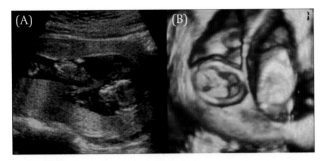

Figure 24.22 Comparison between sectional 2D imaging (A) and 3D spatial imaging (B). The advantages of 3D spatial visualization in early pregnancy include improved visualization of both fetuses and their gestational sacs

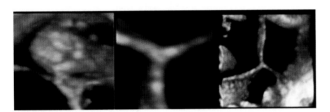

Figure 24.23 3D sonographic determination of chorionicity in the late 2nd trimester. The 'Mercedes sign' ('Y') represents the junction of the fetal membranes in the triplet pregnancy

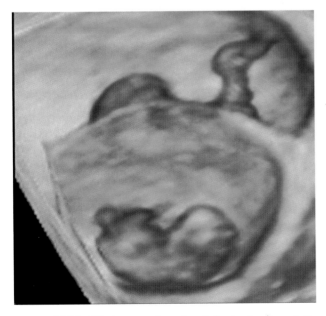

Figure 24.24 3D sonography of a dichorionic–diamniotic twin pregnancy at 8 weeks of gestation

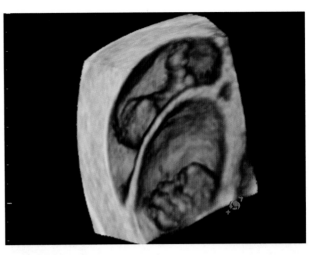

Figure 24.25 3D sonography of a dichorionic–diamniotic twin pregnancy at 8 weeks of gestation

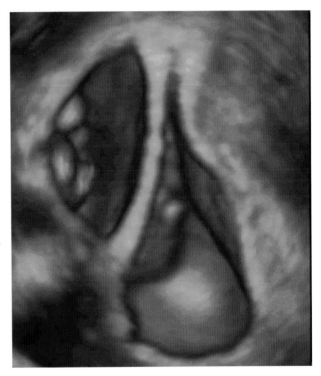

Figure 24.26 3D surface rendering illustrating a dichorionic–diamniotic pregnancy

24.6–24.11, 24.15, 24.16, and 24.18–24.35). Direct determination of chorionicity is based on counting of placentas. This method is easy to perform when the placentas are separated. However, in multichorionic pregnancies, fusion of different placentas occurs during the 2nd trimester. Distinguishing between single and fused placentas is accomplished by considering the so-called 'twin peak' sign (Figures 24.32–24.34). The 'twin peak' sign (also known as the 'lambda' sign) is a triangular projection of placental tissue beyond the chorionic surface, extending between the two chorionic layers of the intertwin

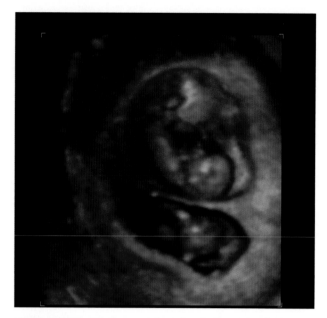

Figure 24.27 3D sonography of a dichorionic–diamniotic twin pregnancy at 12 weeks of gestation

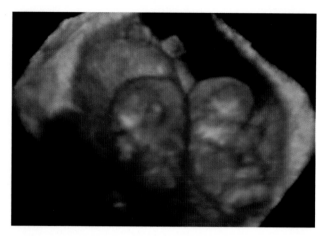

Figure 24.29 3D surface rendering demonstrating embryos in a monochorionic–monoamniotic pregnancy at 9 weeks of gestation

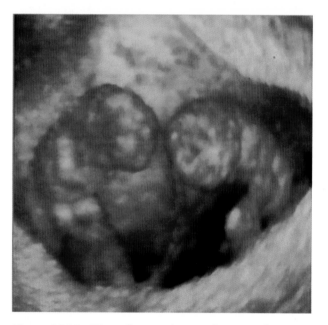

Figure 24.28 3D surface rendering of a monochorionic–monoamniotic pregnancy

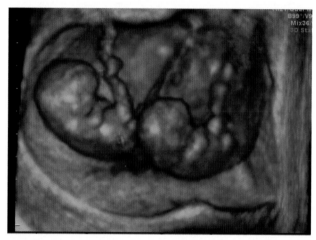

Figure 24.30 3D sonography of a dichorionic twin pregnancy at 9 weeks 3 days of gestation. The full length of two umbilical cords with their insertions and the intertwin membrane are clearly depicted

membrane. It provides reliable evidence that there are two fused placentas (dichorionic–diamniotic) rather than a single shared placenta (monochorionic–diamniotic).[10] However, with 2D sonography, membranes can be evaluated, counted, and measured only when they are at 90°. In other words, the orientation of the membranes studied should be positioned parallel to the transducer cristal array. Clearly, 3D sonography

enables one to obtain a 'perfectly' oriented picture. The rate of appropriate chorionicity determinations should be ideal (100%) in the 2nd and 3rd trimesters.

The junction of the three interfetal membranes is the 'Y' (or 'Mercedes sign') zone (Figures 24.23 and 24.35). Sepulveda and co-workers reported a complete correlation between the findings at the 'Y' zone and transvaginal ultrasonography on the 6th and 7th weeks.[11] However, in advanced pregnancy, when placentas cannot be seen, the junction between the membranes should be examined. Absence of the 'Y' zone does not exclude trichorionic triplets. In the 2nd trimester, the 'Y' zone can be absent in cases in which the interfetal membranes do not intersect. Therefore,

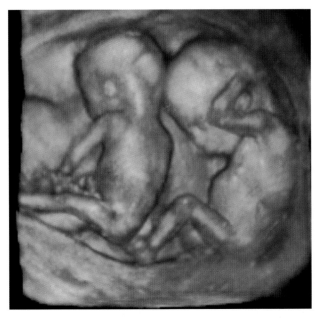

Figure 24.31 3D sonography of a monochorionic twin pregnancy at 14 weeks of gestation. The intertwin area can be assessed easily

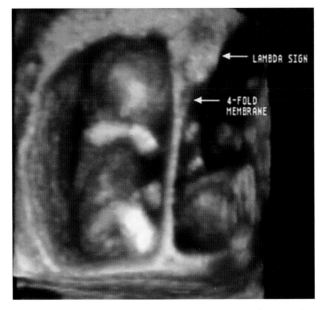

←— LAMBDA SIGN

←— 4-FOLD MEMBRANE

Figure 24.32 Spatial reconstruction of the membrane take-off site provides easier differentiation between dichorionic and monochorionic placentation. Furthermore, membrane thickness can be simultaneously evaluated. Therefore, 3D sonography is a more comprehensive tool for accurate understanding of placentation

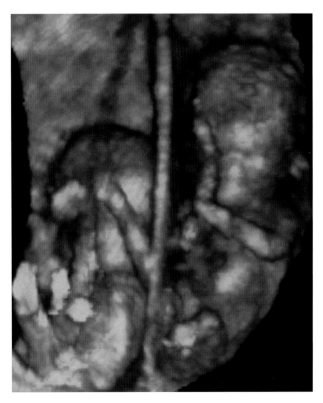

Figure 24.33 3D surface rendering illustrating fetuses not in direct contact

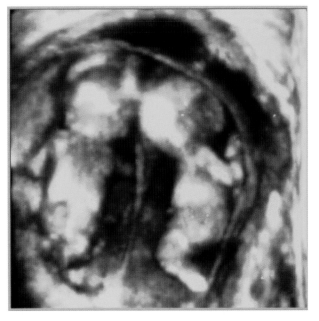

Figure 24.34 3D scan illustrating both twins seen from the back. The intertwin membrane and back surface anatomy are seen

assessment of the 'Y' zone should be combined with other parameters for determination of chorionicity.[11]

In the case of dichorionic–triamniotic triplets (complex placentation), the placenta is represented by

the 'T' sign and lambda sign, with one thin and one thick membrane (Figures 24.10 and 24.11). Using conventional sonography, it is difficult to distinguish

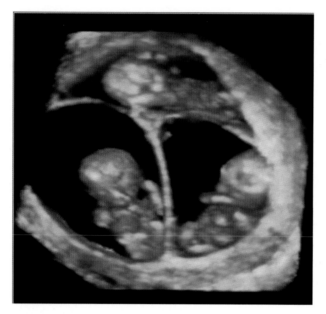

Figure 24.35 3D image of a triplet pregnancy and external frontal anatomy. The orientation of one twin with respect to the other can be simultaneously assessed

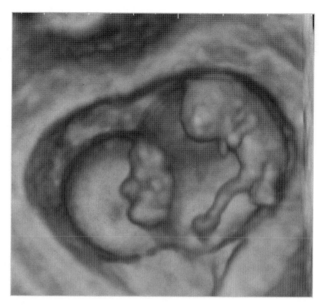

Figure 24.36 A case of discordant twins

between a single placenta and fused placentas of twins, and this is especially so in triplet pregnancy. Such complex placentation types can be examined more easily using 3D sonography, regardless of gestational age.

ULTRASOUND ASSESSMENT OF DISCORDANT GROWTH

Twin discordance, which is usually defined as a >20–30% difference in birthweight, has been associated with adverse perinatal outcome.[12] An increasing body of evidence suggests that discordant growth patterns may begin in the 1st trimester and can be detected sonographically.[13–16] A 1st trimester crown–rump length (CRL) disparity in dichorionic twin gestations is associated with an increased risk of fetal structural and chromosomal abnormalities.[12] 3D sonography improves the visualization of both twins, while the use of volumetric calculations might improve the diagnosis of discordant growth (Figures 24.36 and 24.37).

Discordant growth of multiples of over 3 mm or more than 5 days during the 1st trimester is associated with a high loss rate and/or major abnormalities.[17] Over 8 years, van Gaever et al[17] observed six twin and two triplet pregnancies with discordant growth of more than 15% between 8 and 14 weeks of gestation.

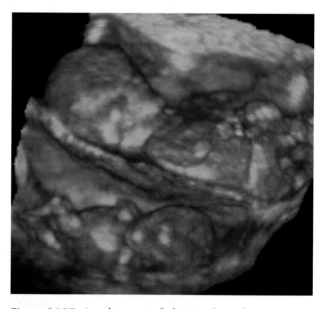

Figure 24.37 Another case of obvious discordant twins

In two dichorionic–diamniotic twin pairs, one twin had a chromosomal abnormality, and in one monochorionic–diamniotic twin pair, increased nuchal translucency and a reduced motility pattern was demonstrated – both pairs of twins died before 18 weeks in spite of a normal karyotype. In one monochorionic twin pair, twin reversed arterial perfusion (TRAP) was observed, the co-twin showed reduced motility and died at 12 weeks. In two dichorionic–diamniotic twin pairs with normal karyotype, normal nuchal translucency values, and normal behavioral patterns, growth discrepancy persisted. The outcome of one pair was normal, while in the other pair, the smaller fetus presented with VATER syndrome (vertebral anomalies, anal atresia, tracheo-esophageal fistula, radial and renal anomalies).

However, congenital malformations do not appear to be increased in cases of 1st-trimester growth-discordance twins if normal anatomy is shown at the 1st-trimester scan. Nevertheless, the rates of intrauterine growth restriction (IUGR) and growth discordance in late pregnancy are increased for this group of patients, and therefore it should be considered a high-risk subgroup among multiple pregnancies.[18]

DETECTION OF FETAL MALFORMATIONS IN MULTIPLE PREGNANCY

In a singleton pregnancy, the empiric risk for major fetal malformations is approximately 3%. In trichorionic triplets, the empiric risk for major fetal malformations within each fetus is independent of the others, so that the probability of having at least one malformed fetus is approximately 9%.[19] According to the Eurofetus study, the sensitivity of routine 2D sonography for detecting malformation is 61.4%.[20] The sensitivity is lower in multiple pregnancies as a consequence of overcrowding. 3D sonography is useful for visualizing embryos and early fetuses and for recognizing their surface morphology.[21] It also improves diagnostic capability by offering more diagnostic information in evaluating fetal malformation than fetal growth, particularly in displaying the fetal malformations of the cranium, face, spine, and extremities and body surface.[22] The ideal visualization rate of a desired structure regardless of its anatomic limitations is the major advance of 3D sonography. This advantage can be used when the findings of 2D sonography are incomplete in terms of either fetal anatomy or placentation, due to incovenient anatomic relations.

A variety of anomalies arise in multifetal pregnancies. Malformations unique for twins (MUTs) are malformations that occur exclusively in multiple pregnancies, whereas malfomations not unique for twins (MNUTs) are malformations that also occur in singletons but are more common in twins (Table 24.2).

Among MUTs, 3D sonography is useful for confirmation of suspicion of conjoined twins and fetus-in-fetu. The incidence of conjoined twins is somewhere about 1 in 100 000 births or 1 in 500–600 twin

Table 24.2 Malformations in multiple pregnancies

Unique to twinning (MUT)	Not unique to twinning (MNUT)
Conjoined twins (Figure 24.42)	Neural tube defects Hydrocephalus
Twin reversed arterial perfusion (ACARDIA)	Congenital heart disease
Fetus-in-fetu	Anorectal atresias Intersex
Twin-to-twin transfusion syndrome	Genitourinary anomalies Esophageal atresia

pregnancies, and varies between countries. Maggio et al[23] reported on the 1st-trimester sonography diagnosis of conjoined twins. Since then, several cases have confirmed the utility of proposed diagnostic criteria.[24–26] Despite great progress in the early diagnosis (in the embryonic and early fetal period), delineation of organ sharing cannot be done properly before the 2nd trimester. Moreover, the examiner must be aware that following the criteria proposed by Maggio et al[23] is sometimes problematic, because two cases of false-positive diagnosis of conjoined twins have been reported.[27,28] In the absence of clear-cut signs of fusion, additional sonographic findings summarized by Koontz et al[29] include the following:

- lack of a separating membrane
- inability to separate the fetal bodies
- detection of other anomalies in a twin gestation
- more than three vessels present in the umbilical cord
- both fetal heads persistently at the same level
- backward flexion of the cervical and upper thoracic spine
- no change in the relative position of the fetuses despite attempts at manual manipulation.

It is known that in 2D transvaginal sonography, the examination planes are limited to sagittal and transverse. Because the uterus can only be examined in these two planes, the examiner may fail to visualize the coronal section through the fetus. In other words, conjoined twins may be overlooked. This problem can be solved using both modalities of 3D sonography: multiplanar imaging and surface rendering. Using multiplanar imaging, the visualization rate for the

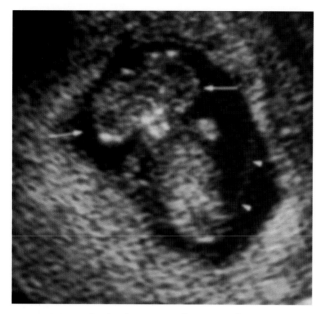

Figure 24.38 Early detection of conjoined twins by 2D sonography

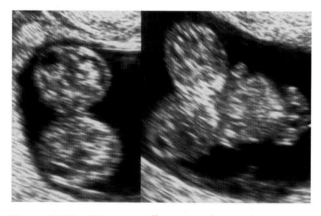

Figure 24.39 2D images illustrating thoracophagus, with double heads in a conjoined twin

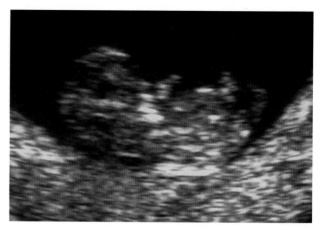

Figure 24.40 2D longitudinal sectional imaging demonstrating thoracophagus

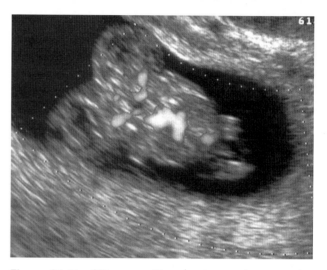

Figure 24.41 2D power Doppler image demonstrating single shared circulation in a conjoined twin

coronal section through the fetus is 100%, due to the unlimited number of sections that can be generated by data manipulation.

Maymon et al[30] reported that in a case of conjoined twins at the 10th week of gestation, the exact area could be successfully identified by transvaginal 3D sonography. Vecek et al[31] diagnosed this anomaly at 12 weeks of amenorrhea in a fetus of 27 mm maximum length, showing two separated heads with twins joined at the level of the thorax (Figures 24.38–24.41). The fetal orientation remained unchanged despite manipulation of the transvaginal probe and prolonged scanning by multiple sonographers. Early diagnosis of conjoined twins requires

detailed examination of the fetus in the sagittal, transverse, and coronal sections. Avoiding this recommendation can result in missing the diagnosis, because the appearance of conjoined twins in the sagittal section can be almost normal, as shown in Figure 24.42.

Although 2D sonography is the primary modality for diagnosing and evaluating conjoined twins, color Doppler and 3D sonography can sometimes provide additional information that assists in the clinical management of these twins. 3D sonography also provides images that are easier for parents to understand, which can help them with decision making[32] (Figure 24.42). Sepulveda et al[33] reported two cases of conjoined twins complicating a triplet pregnancy diagnosed by 2D sonography in the 1st trimester and evaluated further by 3D sonography. A review of the

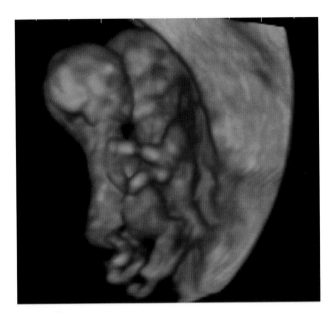

Figure 24.42 3D sonography of a twin pregnancy clearly showing a case of thoracopagus

literature over the last 30 years revealed 11 other cases diagnosed prenatally by ultrasound. On the other hand, the literature suggests that this modality does not improve on the diagnosis made by 2D sonography, and that very early prenatal diagnosis and 1st-trimester 3D imaging provide very little additional practical medical information compared with the 11–14-week sonography examinations.[34]

Development of a fetus-like mass inside a more mature fetus characterizes the fetus-in-fetu (FIF) malformation.[35] The true incidence of FIF is unknown, although it has been estimated to be 2 per million births.[36,37] Jones et al[38] in 2001 reported 3D sonographic imaging of a highly developed FIF with spontaneous movement of extremities. In contrast to the ease of the diagnosis with 3D imaging, a FIF with even an extraordinarily high degree of differentiation is very difficult to distinguish by 2D sonography. Nevertheless, an increasing number of reports use 2D sonographic examination following the minimal criteria for diagnosis proposed by Willis. These include the presence of an axial skeleton or fetus with metameric organization, skin coverage, encapsulation, and a two-vessel cord.[38] Since 3D sonography is capable of generating a 3D surface view of the structure encapsulated within a fluid-filled sac, it should be used for this purpose. With this technique, a highly fetiform shape and axialization could be recognized easily even by less experienced sonographers who could not envision FIF on the basis of 2D sonography. Distinguishing

between FIF and teratoma can sometimes be problematic. Therefore, whenever a cystic mass is recognized at specific locations within a fetus, an additional 3D examination is recommended. Prenatal sonographic differentiation between FIF and teratoma is based on the degree of differentiation of the anomaly. In highly differentiated FIF, visualization of the presence of a fetiform mass is essential. However, in a FIF with a low degree of differentiation, the diagnostic criteria are based on the presence of a rudimentary spinal architecture, which confirms the embryonic development beyond the primitive streak stage. This is in contrast to the classic embryonic concept, which postulated that teratomas do not develop beyond the primitive streak stage of 12–15 days.[39]

Among MNUTs, 3D sonography can be advantageous for confirmation of suspicion of neural tube defects. Twins may be concordant and discordant for congenital anomalies. Concordance for congenital malformations is defined as the presence of concordant anomaly in both twins, whereas discordance for congenital malformations is characterized by the presence of an anomaly in only one of a twin pair. Monozygotic twins are at higher risk for such anomalies than dizygotic twins.[40] Under these circumstances, discordance for major malformation in a twin pair does not imply dizygotic or dichorionic status.

2D sonography is the primary modality for detection of congenital anomalies. According to the Eurofetus Study, the sensitivity of routine 2D sonography for detection of malformation in a singleton pregnancy is 61.4%.[20] On the other hand, the sensitivity in multiple pregnancy has been reported as between 39–87%.[41,42] Neural tube defects include anencephaly, acrania, encephalocele, and the various forms of spina bifida. Screening for these anomalies is recommended during the 1st trimester because reports have documented successful diagnosis in the embryonic period.[43–45] The detection rates for these anomalies in singleton pregnancies is high, except for spina bifida. The morphologic anomalies of acrania and anencephalia can be confirmed even before 10 weeks of gestation. Bonilla-Musoles et al[45] reported 2D diagnosis of two cases of anencephaly at 10 weeks of gestation. Takeuchi[46] diagnosed acrania by conventional 2D sonography at 8 weeks and 5 days of amenorrhea in a fetus of 18 mm in maximum length, showing an irregular shape of the head with neither cranium nor brain vesicle development. Similar early cases are illustrated in Chapter 12. A 3D surface rendered image facilitated confirmation of this diagnosis, because it showed characteristics of the anomaly more clearly. It is generally believed that absence of the cranial vault leads to disintegration of the exposed brain during the fetal period, resulting in clinical anencephaly. Bronshtein and Ornoy[43] reported a case that detailed the progression from acrania to anencephaly. Spina bifida is associated with anencephaly in 9–30% of cases.[47] Using 3D sonography, Bonilla-Musoles[48] reported diagnosis of spina bifida at 9 weeks. Therefore, whenever anencephaly is found in the embryonic period, an additional 3D scan of the fetal spine is recommended. The multiplanar view is particularly useful in localizing spinal defects accurately in fetuses with spina bifida and in determination of the exact location of the extracranial mass and amount of extracranial tissue in fetuses with encephalocele.[44]

CORD ENTANGLEMENT

The diagnosis of cord entanglement with 2D real-time sonography (Figures 24.43 and 24.44) usually requires a long examination period. Due to the limitations of sectional imaging, examination is informative only about the quality and number of loops, and the final diagnosis is postponed. The main problem is distinguishing between adjacent and entangled cords. Cords positioned close to each other without torsion of one around the other are defined as adjacent umbilical

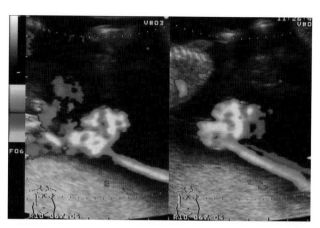

Figure 24.44 Power Doppler imaging demonstrating cord entanglement in a monochorionic–monoamniotic pregnancy

cords, whereas if such torsion is present, this is called cord entanglement.

Much more information about umbilical cords can be obtained by 3D sonography (Figure 24.45). 3D power Doppler permits imaging of curvatures of the umbilical cord, and the number of involved loops in entanglement can easily be determined. Counting the number of loops involved in the entanglement is a useful method for longitudinal evaluation of entanglement.

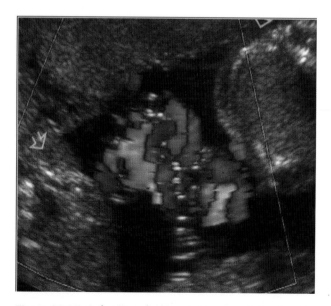

Figure 24.43 Color Doppler imaging improves visualization of cord entanglement in monochorionic–monoamniotic pregnancies

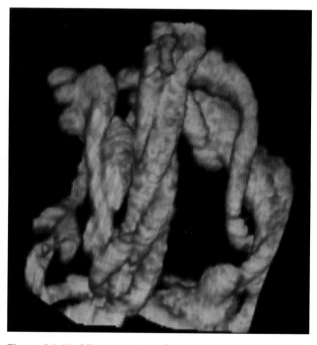

Figure 24.45 3D power Doppler reconstruction of umbilical cord with possibility of differentiating between false and true knots in multiamniotic or umbilical cord entanglement and adjacent cords in monoamniotic pregnancies

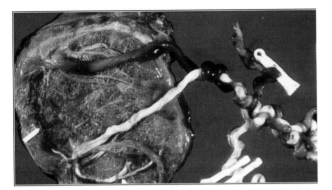

Figure 24.46 Cord entanglement demonstrated after delivery

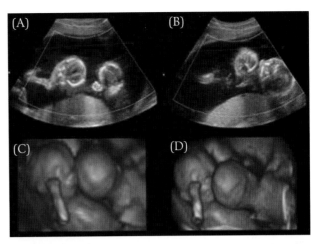

Figure 24.47 Comparison between two techniques for evaluation of fetal behavior: real-time 2D (A,B) and 4D (C,D) sonography. Hand-to-head contact together with head-to-head intertwin contact can be recognized

It is currently possible to distinguish between two types of umbilical cord knots: true and false. A focal redundancy of the vessels, which appears sonographically as a vascular protuberance that does not persist in all scanning planes, is called a false umbilical cord knot.[49] This condition should be differentiated from a true umbilical cord knot, which is a life-threatening condition (Figures 24.45 and 24.46).

ASSESSMENT OF FETAL BEHAVIOR IN MULTIPLE PREGNANCIES BY 4D SONOGRAPHY

It seems that application of 3D/4D sonography in the assessment of fetal behavior is most promising. Fetal activity such as kicking has been used as a sign of fetal viability from ancient times. It was found that fetal motor activity is present for some period before the mother feels it. Reinold[5] was one of the first to describe fetal activity using ultrasound, and he stressed the spontaneous character of early prenatal movements. The discovery by Hooker and colleagues[50] that the fetus responds to a tactile stimulus led to the hypothesis that the motor activity of a twin can be either spontaneous or induced by the co-twin. Endogenous activity is the dominant behavioral pattern in singleton pregnancies. Sometimes, the mother's movements, such as walking or running, can initiate fetal motor activity. On the other hand, in multiple pregnancies, two types of fetal activity are present: endogenous–spontaneous motor activity and motor activity that is a reaction to an exogenous stimulus.

Spontaneous motor activity precedes stimulated motor activity in terms of gestational age of onset. Activity evoked by intertwin contacts is characterized

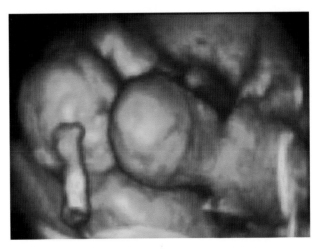

Figure 24.48 3D surface rendering demonstrating intertwin contact in a case of monochorionic–monoamniotic twin pregnancy

as stimulated activity (Figures 24.47–24.58). The effect on neurologic maturation of prenatal reactions evoked by an internal stimulus in twinning phenomenon due to intertwin contacts was the focus of interest of the systematic research initiated by Arabin et al.[51] They used real-time 2D sonography for detection and evaluation of the intertwin contacts. Due to the sectional imaging, simultaneous visualization of both fetuses and assessment of their motor activity was impossible. Therefore, it was possible to assess the motor activity of a single fetus only, and unfortunately to just a limited extent. Similarly, the intertwin area is tomographically visualized, and some intertwin contacts are overlooked. Therefore, when using this

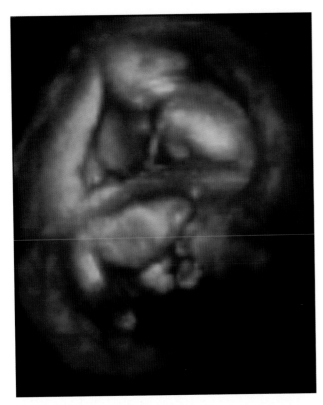

Figure 24.49 3D surface rendering illustrating reconstruction of intertwin contact activity at 13 weeks of gestation

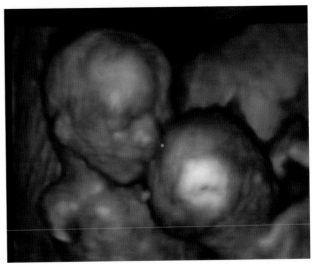

Figure 24.51 3D image demonstrating intertwin contact. Note that the second fetus seems to lean against the first (left)

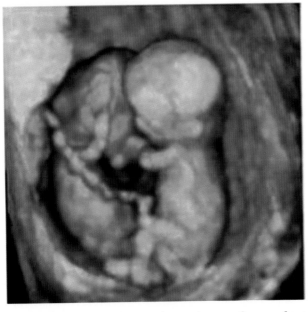

Figure 24.50 3D surface rendering showing front-to-front position of both fetuses

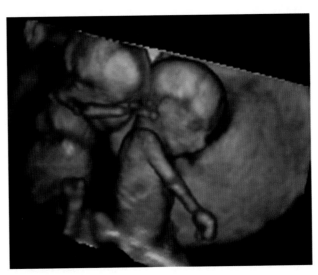

Figure 24.52 The left twin is touching the nuchal region of the right twin

method, distinguishing between spontaneous and stimulated motor activity is very difficult and sometimes impossible.

Veček et al[31] found that movement activity of each fetus in twin or multiple pregnancies can be successfully determined by 4D sonography in the 1st and early 2nd trimesters. Using this technique, it was possible for the first time to observe cases where one twin is active while the co-twin or co-triplets may or may not be active. Simultaneous visualization of the entire anatomy (head, body, and extremities) of two or more fetuses along with their movements allows characterization of the type of movement, isolated movements of each fetus, and intertwin contacts and interactions (Figures 24.59–24.71).

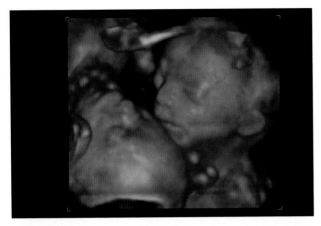

Figure 24.53 3D sonography of a twin pregnancy at 21 weeks of gestation showing head-to-head contact between the twins

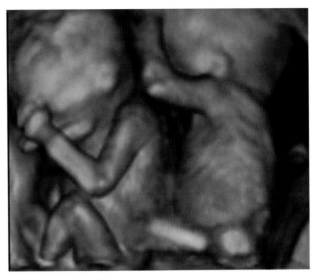

Figure 24.55 Different movements in a twin pregnancy at 21 weeks of gestation

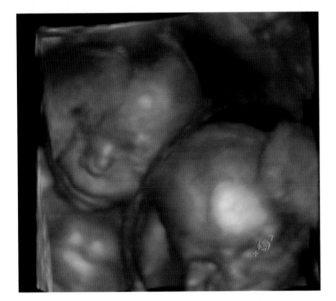

Figure 24.54 3D sonography of a triplet pregnancy at 21 weeks of gestation showing head-to-head contact between the twins. The intertwin membrane is clearly visualized

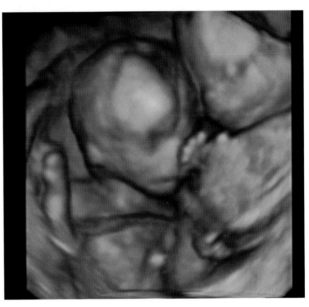

Figure 24.56 3D sonography of a twin pregnancy at 21 weeks of gestation showing head-to-head contact

Arabin et al[51] defined intertwin contacts for the first time, and differentiated between the following types of such contact and determined the gestational age of their onset: first reach and touch (first evidence of touch between twins); first reaction (first movement towards the touch of the co-twin); slow and fast arm, leg, head, or body contacts (action and reaction based on the initiating part of the body); mouth contacts; and complex interactions. Apart from the descriptive definitions, they also classified the speed of actions and reactions as slow initiations followed by slow or fast reactions, and fast initiations followed by slow or fast

reactions. Intertwin contacts may be explained by the onset of movements whereby incidental touches in utero cannot be avoided and can be defined as early reflexes. Furthermore the initiating and reacting body parts may be randomly involved. However, Piontell et al[52] stated that the existence of intrapair stimulation indicates merely the functioning of fetal tactile and propriceptive sensibility. They stressed that the existence of intrapair stimulation should not be taken to mean, as suggested by Arabin et al[51] that fetuses are

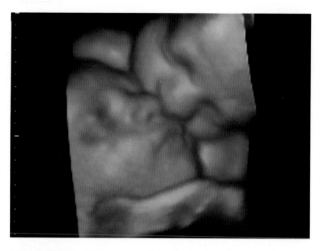

Figure 24.57 3D sonography of a twin prgnancy showing close face-to-face intertwin contact

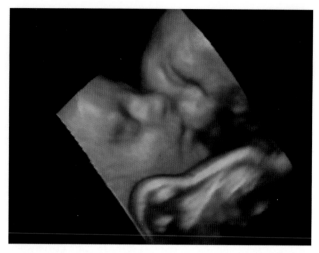

Figure 24.58 3D sonography of a twin pregnancy showing close face-to-face intertwin contact

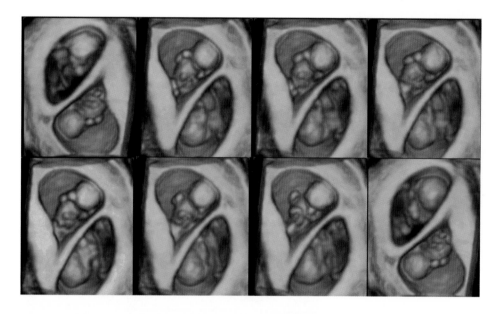

Figure 24.59 4D sonographic sequence of a dichorionic–diamniotic twin pregnancy at 10 weeks of gestation. Both twins are active, but there is no intertwin contact

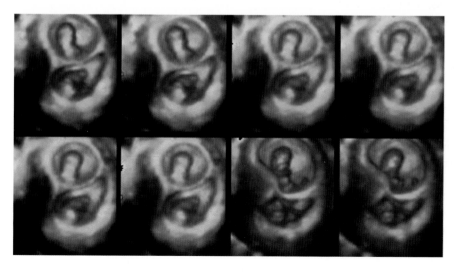

Figure 24.60 4D sequence demonstrating embryonic movements in a dichorionic–diamniotic pregnancy

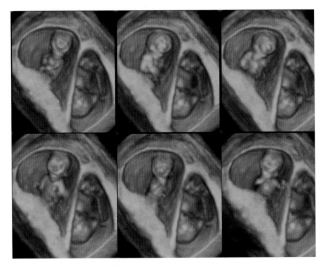

Figure 24.61 4D sequence of a dichorionic–diamniotic twin pregnancy at 10 weeks of gestation. Both twins are active, showing general body movements

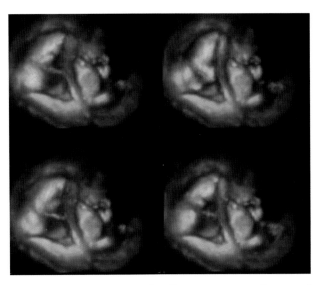

Figure 24.63 4D sonography allows separate evaluation of the fetal activity of each twin. The first twin (left) is active, whereas the second (right) is passive

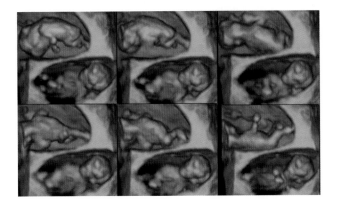

Figure 24.62 4D sequence of a dichorionic–diamniotic twin pregnancy at 12 weeks of gestation showing one fetus rotating 180° and changing its position, while the second twin shows extremity movements

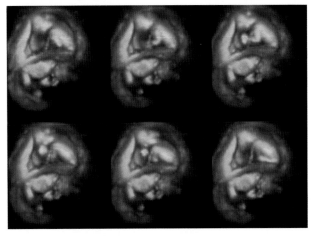

Figure 24.64 4D imaging illustrating active fetal hand movement from the first twin (A), while the second twin (B) is passive

having complex intrapair interactions, but simply that intrapair stimulation exists constantly from late 1st trimester and is an active part of the intrauterine environment. Sadovsky et al[53] proposed that movements of one twin stimulate the other to move. However, Ferrari et al[54] came to a different conclusion, namely that intertwin contacts cause increased rates of simultaneous twin activities in early pregnancy.

The distribution of the periods with or without fetal movements demonstrates the high percentage of active periods (with a mean of about 80%) in twins compared with singletons, which might be the result of intertwin stimulation.[51] The observation period was 26–36 weeks, and a 3-minute window was used. In contrast Sadovsky et al[53] found that in twin pregnancies

between 33 and 39 weeks, about 75% of the observed fetal movements were independent of the movements of the co-twin. Piontelli et al[55] found that each twin, regardless of zygosity, showed individualized behavioral styles. One twin was found to be 'dominant' in the sense of bring more active but a bit less reactive, possibly due to fewer stimuli being generated by its co-twin. Monozygotic twins, as opposed to dizygotic, showed greater similarities in activity and reactivity levels, but were never behaviorally identical and decreased in likeness with increasing age. These data suggest that so-called 'identical' twins are not behaviorally identical from early in pregnancy.[55,56]

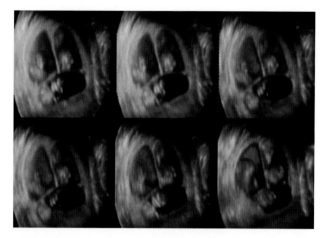

Figure 24.65 4D sequence illustrating movements of the embryos in a triplet pregnancy

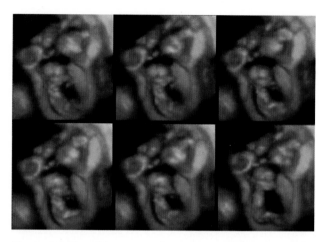

Figure 24.66 4D images demonstrating changes in the position of each embryo in a triplet pregnancy

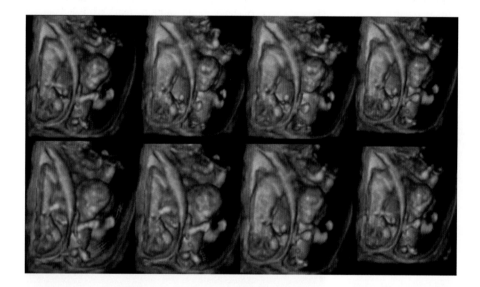

Figure 24.67 4D sonography sequence of a dichorionic–monoamniotic at 11 weeks of gestation showing gross body and extremity movements of the triplets

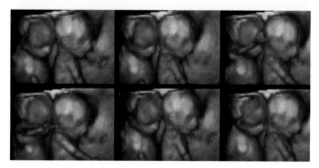

Figure 24.68 4D sequence demonstrating intertwin contact. Note the active hand movement of the first twin (left)

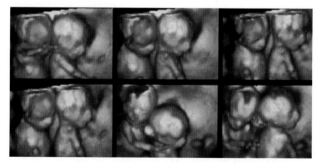

Figure 24.69 4D scan demonstrating separate evaluation of the fetal activity of each twin. The first twin (left) shows active body movements, while the second twin (right) is passive

It has been demonstrated that the membrane status has a direct impact on the onset and quantity of intertwin contacts: in monochorionic–monoamniotic twins contacts occur earlier than in monochorionic–diamniotic and dichorionic twins, which may be explained by the smaller distance between the embryos.[52] Intrapair stimulation before the 11th week of gestation can be considered a rather exceptional event, and has been

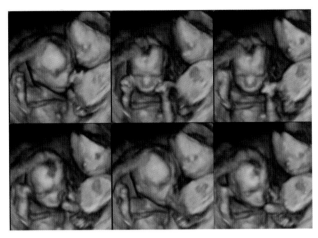

Figure 24.70 4D sonography sequence of a twin pregnancy at 21 weeks of gestation showing intertwin contact, with one fetus making a head rotation movement pattern

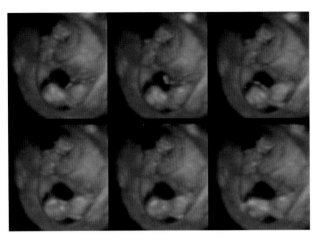

Figure 24.72 Missed triplet and isolated motor activity of only one fetus. On this 4D sequence, the activity of only one twin can be recognized. Moreover, with spatial imaging, even the type of movement can be recognized. It is isolated hand-to-fluid movement of the first triplet

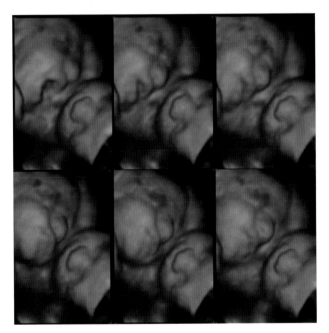

Figure 24.71 4D sequence of monochorionic twins showing a yawn of one twin

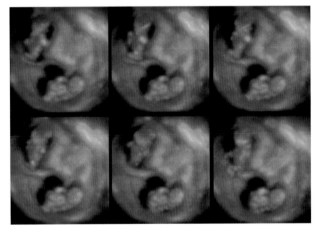

Figure 24.73 Missed triplet at 13th week of gestation by 4D sonography. In this sequence, the activity of only one twin can be recognized

noted only in monochorionic twins. From 12 weeks onward, intrapair stimulation becomes a progressively more frequent event in both monochorionic and dichorionic pregnancies. However, these results are from a 2D sonographic study, and thus movements occurring outside the plane of scan could have been missed. This is particularly relevant after 13 weeks of gestation, when simultaneous visualization of both fetal bodies is no longer possible.[51]

Furthermore, 4D sonography is useful in evaluation of altered motor development, such as in pathologic pregnancy. The delay in activity pattern is described in twins with triploidy XXX, and some activities such as yawning and stretching are not even present.[56] This is particularly important in dizygotic twinning.

MULTIPLE GESTATIONS AND CEREBRAL PALSY

Cerebral palsy (CP) is the most common physical disability in childhood, affecting about 2 per 1000 live births. The higher risk of CP in multiple births has been known for many years. The prevalence of CP is significantly higher in twins compared with singletons, although the type of CP differs, as does its etiology, between twins and singletons.[57] Multiple compared with singleton gestations have a 5–10-fold increased risk of CP.[58] Data clearly indicate that the higher the number of fetuses, the greater is the prevalence of CP. Moreover, the increase in incidence of CP with number of fetuses is exponential. When comparing twin with singleton births, the relative risk of CP is greatest and significant only for twins delivered at 37 or more weeks of gestation. Brain damage of the survivor following single-fetal demise is almost exclusively seen in monochorionic twins. in which intertwin transplacentar vascular connections are always found, and it was on this basis that the 'embolic' and 'ischemic' theories were proposed.[59]

Multiple pregnancies are related to preterm delivery, IUGR, birth defects, and intrapartal complications. Although CP can be related to all of these events, the main cause seems to be associated with preterm birth or the antenatal death of a co-twin or co-triplet[60–62] (Figures 24.12–24.14). The death of one twin can affect the neurologic development of the survivor (Figures 24.72 and 24.73). The live-born co-twin of a fetus dying in utero has a 20% overall risk of cerebral impairment. The gestational-age-specific prevalence of CP after fetal death of a co-twin is much higher than that reported for the general twin population. At particular risk are monozygotic twins, who have poorer survival rates compared with dizygotic twins. The prevalence of CP in monozygotic twins is 106 per 1000 infant survivors, while for dizygotic twins there are 29 per 1000 infant survivors.[59] Other studies showed that twins were at an approximately 4-fold increased risk of CP compared with singletons. However, at birthweight less than 2.5 kg, twins did better than singletons.[58] Approximately 70% of pregnancies with two sacs/embryos continue as twin gestations, while, in contrast, only about 50% of pregnancies with three sacs/embryos will continue as triplets, and only 38% of pregnancies with four sacs/embryos will continue as quadruplets.[63] Vanishing rates are more than twice as high in monochorionic as in dichorionic twin gestations (50% vs 21%).[64] The increasing use of sonography has drawn attention to the 'vanishing twin' phenomenon, which, in conjunction with the observation that normal-birthweight twins are at increased risk of CP compared with singletons, led to the hypothesis that CP of unknown etiology in singleton pregnancies may be attributed to the early loss of a previously unrecognized monochorionic twin.[65] Accordingly, the survivor's neurologic development is impaired throughout pregnancy, with spastic CP the resulting clinical manifestation.[65] Data are not consistently supportive of this concept, however, and indicate that the 'vanishing twin' syndrome is unlikely to account for a high proportion of cases of CP:[66] there is a lack of reported cases following multifetal pregnancy reduction, a procedure that is not unlike the 'vanishing twin' phenomenon. An attempt was made to determine whether iatrogenic fetal reduction increases the prevalence of CP, and the results revealed that the prevalence of CP among children from trichorionic triplet pregnancies reduced to twins by selective termination (13.8 per 1000) was similar to that of children from trichorionic triplet pregnancies with no loss (18 per 1000), but the pregnancies with selective termination were delivered at a later gestational age.[67] There is an urgent need for clarification of this issue and it is likely that 4D sonography will help in this.

In vitro fertilization (IVF) procedures have often been suggested as one of the main reasons for the increasing incidence of CP in multiple pregnancies. With the publication of reports of increased risks of CP after IVF in a Swedish cohort study, Finnström et al[68] found that there were no differences in type, severity of CP, or background characteristics between children born after IVF and non-IVF children. This interpretation was that etiologic factors for CP do not differ, but that the increased prevalence of CP seen after IVF is due to the high rate of multiple pregnancies and prematurity.

CONCLUSIONS

Transvaginal sonography is still a very important modality in routine prenatal care, because it allows accurate diagnosis and clinical management of multiple pregnancies during the 1st trimester. It has been found that an early diagnosis of pregnancy number and placentation type (chorionicity and amnionicity) has a positive influence on mortality and morbidity rate in multiple pregnancy.

2D sonography is still the primary modality for diagnosing and evaluating multiple pregnancies, but, due to its limitations, an additional 3D scan is recommended, because this provides more accurate and reliable diagnosis, as well as additional information important for management. 4D sonography has several advantages over real-time 2D sonography in the assessment of twin behavior. These include the capability of simultaneous visualization of both fetuses and assessment of their motor activity. The same advantage applies to the intertwin area. Therefore, 4D sonography should be considered the method of choice for accurate diagnosis of isolated motor activity of single twins.

However, before the onset of fetal movement, 3D sonography is beneficial with regard to the determination of the accurate number and size of gestational sacs, which has led to elimination of the undercounting phenomenon and improved prognosis of spontaneous pregnancy reduction. Moreover, volumetric studies in multiple pregnancies are less time-consuming. Furthermore, the 3D power Doppler technique enables confident differentiation between life-threatening cord abnormalities (e.g., cord entanglement and true umbilical cord knots) and false-positive results achieved with 2D power Doppler ultrasound.

4D sonography is undoubtly a powerful new imaging tool whose full scientific and clinical potential we are yet to discover. In the meantime, the true clinical value of this new modality should be neither under- nor overestimated.

REFERENCES

1. Alexander GR, Salihu HM. Perinatal outcomes of singleton and multiple births in the United States, 1995–98. In: Blickstein I, Keith LG, eds. Multiple Pregnancy: Epidemiology, Gestation and Perinatal Outcome. London: Taylor and Francis, 2005: 3–10.

2. Vecek N, Kurjak A, Azumendi G. Fetal behaviour in multifetal pregnancies studied by 4D sonography. Ultrasound Rev Obstet Gynecol 2004; 4: 52–8.

3. Kurjak A, Veček N. Three-dimensional sonography. In: Blickstein I, Keith LG, eds. Multiple Pregnancy: Epidemiology, Gestation and Perinatal Outcome. London: Taylor and Francis, 2005: 309–21.

4. Bromley B, Benacerraf B. Using the number of yolk sacs to determine amnionicity in early first trimester monochorionic twins. J Ultrasound Med 1995; 14: 415–19.

5. Reinold E. Clinical value of fetal spontaneous movements in early pregnancy. J Perinat Med 1973; 1: 65–72.

6. Landy HJ, Keith LG. The vanishing twin: a review. Hum Reprod 1998; 4: 177.

7. Manzur A, Goldsman MP, Stone SC, et al. Outcome of triplet pregnancies after assisted reproductive techniques: How frequent are the vanishing embryos? Fertil Steril 1995; 63: 252–7.

8. Dickey R, Taylor S, Peter YL, et al. Spoontaneous

reduction of multiple pregnancy: incidence and effect on outcome. Am J Obstet Gynecol 2002; 186: 77–83.

9. Doubilet PM, Benson CB. 'Appearing twin': undercounting of multiple gestations on early first trimeseter sonograms. J Ultrasound Med 1998; 17: 199–203.

10. Finberg HJ. The 'twin peak' sign: reliable evidence of dichorionic twinning. J Ultrasound Med 1992; 11: 571–7.

11. Sepulveda W. Chorionicity determination in twin pregnancies: double trouble. Ultrasound Obstet Gynecol 1997; 10: 79–88.

12. Kalish RB, Gupta M, Perni SC, et al. Clinical significance of first trimester crown-rump length disparity in dichorionic twin gestations. Am J Obstet Gynecol 2004; 191: 1437–40.

13. Kalish RB, Chasen ST, Gupta M, et al. First trimester prediction of growth discordance in twin gestations. Am J Obstet Gynecol 2003; 189: 706–9.

14. Smith GCS, Smith MFS, McNay MB, Fleming JEE. First trimester growth and the risk of low birth weight. N Engl J Med 1998; 339: 1817–22.

15. Isada NB, Sorokin Y, Drugan A, et al. First trimester interfetal size variation in well-dated multifetal pregnancies. Fetal Diagn Ther 1992; 7: 82–6.

16. Achiron R, Blickstein I. Persistent discordant twin growth following IVF-ET. Acta Genet Med Gemellol 1993; 42: 41–4.

17. van Gaever C, Nizard J, Arabin B. Early discordant growth in multiple pregnancy. Ultrasound Obstet Gynecol 2003; Suppl 1: 162.

18. Bartha JL, Ling Y, Kyle P, Soothill PW. Clinical consequences of first-trimester growth discordance in twins. Eur J Obstet Gynecol Reprod Biol 2005; 119: 56–9.

19. Kurjak A, Kos M, Vecek N. Pitfalls and caveates in ultrasound assessment of triplet pregnancies. In: Keith LG, Blickstein I, eds. Triplet Pregnancies and Their Consequences. Carnforth, UK: Parthenon, 2002: 85–105.

20. Grandjean H, Larroque D, Levi S. The performance of routine ultrasonographic screening of pregnancies in the Eurofetus Study. Am J Obstet Gynecol 1999; 181: 446–54.

21. Yonemoto H, Yoshida K, Kinoshita K, et al. Embryological evaluation of surface features of human embryos and early fetuses by 3-D ultrasound. J Obstet Gynaecol Res 2002; 28: 211–16.

22. Xu HX, Zhang QP, Lu MD, et al. Comparison of two-dimensional and three-dimensional sonography in evaluating fetal malformations. J Clin Ultrasound 2002; 30: 515–25.

22. Maggio M, Callan NA, Hamod KA, et al. The first-trimester ultrasonographic diagnosis of conjoined twins. Am J Obstet Gynecol 1985; 152: 833–5.

24. Lam YH, Sin SY, Lam C, et al. Prenatal sonographic diagnosis of conjoined twins in the first trimester: two case reports. Ultrasound Obstet Gynecol 1998; 11: 289–91.

25. Meizner I, Levy A, Katz M, et al. Early ultrasonic diagnosis of conjoined twins. Harefuah 1993; 124: 741–4, 796.

26. Tongsong T, Chanprapaph P, Pongsatha S. First-trimester diagnosis of conjoined twins: a report of three cases. Ultrasound Obstet Gynecol 1999; 14: 434–7.

27. Usta IM, Awwad JT. A false positive diagnosis of conjoined twins in a triplet pregnancy: pitfalls of first trimester ultrasonographic prenatal diagnosis. Prenat Diagn 2000; 20: 169–70.

28. Weiss JL, Devine PC. False positive diagnosis of conjoined twins in the first trimester. Ultrasound Obstet Gynecol 2002; 20: 516–18.

29. Koontz WL, Herbert WN, Seeds JW, Cefaloo RC. Ultrasonography in the intrapartum diagnosis of conjoined twins: a report of two cases. J Reprod Med 1983; 28: 627–30.

30. Maymon R, Halperin R, Weinraub Z, et al. Three-dimensional transvaginal sonography of conjoined twins at 10 weeks: a case report. Ultrasound Obstet Gynecol 1998; 11: 292–4.

31. Veček N, Solak M, Erceg-Ivkosic I. Four-dimensional sonography in multiple pregnancy. Gynecol Perinatol 2003; 12: 157.

32. Bonilla-Musoles F, Machado LE, Osborne NG, et al. Two-dimensional and three-dimensional sonography of conjoined twins. J Clin Ultrasound 2002; 30: 68–75.

33. Sepulveda W, Munoz H, Alcade JL. Conjoined twins in a triplet pregnancy: early prenatal diagnosis with three-dimensional ultrasound and review of literature. Ultrasound Obstet Gynecol 2003; 22: 199–204.

34. Pajkrt E, Jauniaux E. First-trimester diagnosis of conjoined twins. Prenat Diagn 2005; 25: 820–6.

35. Jeanty P, Caldwell K, Dix PM. Fetus in fetu. Fetus 1992; 65: 181–9.

36. Hoeffel CC, Nguyen KQ, Phan HT, et al. Fetus in fetu: a case report and literature review. Pediatrics 2000; 105: 1335–44.

37. Grant P, Pearn JH. Foetus-in-fetu. Med J Aust 1969; 1: 1016–19.

38. Jones DC, Reyes-Múgica M, Gallagher PG, et al. Three-dimensional sonographic imaging of a highly developed fetus in fetu with spontaneous movement of extremities. J Ultrasound Med 2001; 20: 1357–63.

39. Willis RA. The structure of teratoma. J Pathol Bacteriol 1935; 40: 1–36.

40. Hall JG, Lopez-Rangel E. Embryonic development and monozygotic twinning. Acta Genet Med Gemellol 1996; 45: 53–7.

41. Edwards MS, Ellings JM, Newman RB, et al. Predictive value of antepartum ultrasound examination for anomalies in twin gestations. Ultrasound Obstet Gynecol 1995; 6: 43–9.

42. Allen SR, Gray LJ, Frentzen BH, et al. Ultrasonographic diagnosis of congenital anomalies in twins. Am J Obstet Gynecol 1991; 165: 1056–60.

43. Bronshtein M, Ornoy A. Acrania:anencephaly resulting from secondary degeneration of a closed neural tube: two cases in the same family. J Clin Ultrasound 1991; 19: 230–4.

44. Dyson RL, Pretorius DH, Budorick NE, et al. Three-dimensional ultrasound in evaluation of fetal anomalies. Ultrasound Obstet Gynecol 2000; 16: 321–8.

45. Bonilla-Musoles FM, Raga F, Ballester MJ, et al. Early detection of embryonic malformations by transvaginal and color Doppler sonography. J Ultrasound Med 1994; 13: 347–55.

46. Takeuchi H. Two- and three-dimensional sonoembryology in the embryonic period. In: Kurjak A, Chervenak FA, Carrera JM, eds. The Embryo as a Patient. Carnforth, UK: Parthenon, 2001: 13–22.

47. Fiske CE, Filly RA. Ultrasound evaluation of the normal and abnormal fetal neural axis. Radiol Clin North Am 1982; 20: 285–9.

48. Bonilla-Musoles F. Three-dimensional visualization of the human embryo: a potential revolution in prenatal diagnosis. Ultrasound Obstet Gynecol 1996; 7: 393–7.

49. Dudiak CM, Salomon CG, Posniak HV, et al. Sonography of the umbilical cord. Radiographist 1995; 15: 1035–42.

50. Hooker D. The Prenatal Origin of Behavior. Kansas: University of Kansas Press, 1952.

51. Arabin B, Mohnhaupt A, van Eyck J. Intrauterine behavior of multiples. In: Kurjak A, ed. Textbook of Perinatal Medicine, Vol II. London: Parthenon, 1998: 1506–31.

52. Piontelli A, Bocconi L, Kustermann A, et al. Patterns of evoked behavior in twin pregnancies during the first 22 weeks of gestation. Early Hum Dev 1997; 50: 39–45.

53. Sadovsky E, Ohel G, Simon A. Ultrasonographical evaluation of the incidence of simultaneous and independent movements of twin fetuses. Gynecol Obstet Invest 1987; 23: 5–9.

54. Ferrari F, Cioni G, Prechtl HFR. Quantitative changes of general movements in preterm infants with brain lesions. Early Hum Dev 1990; 23: 193–7.

55. Piontelli A, Bocconi L, Boschetto C, et al. Differences and similarities in the intra-uterine behaviour of monozygotic and dizygotic twins. Twin Res 1999; 2: 264–73.

56. Arabin B, Bos R, Rijlaarsdam R, et al. The onset of inter-human contacts: longitudinal ultrasound observations in early twin pregnancies. Ultrasound Obstet Gynecol 1996; 8: 166–73.

57. Bonellie SR, Currie D, Chalmers J. Comparison of risk factors for cerebral palsy on twins and singletons. Dev Med Child Neurol 2005; 47: 587–91.

58. Pharoah PO. Risk of cerebral palsy in multiple pregnancies. Obstet Gynecol Clin North Am 2005; 32: 55–67.

59. Blickstein I. Cerebral palsy in multifetal pregnancies. Dev Med Child Neurol 2002; 44: 352–5.

60. Nelson KB, Grether JK. Causes of cerebral palsy. Curr Opin Pediatr 1999; 11: 487–91.

61. Pharoah PO, Adi Y. Consequences of in-utero death in a twin pregnancy. Lancet 2000; 355: 1597–602.

62. Scher AI, Patterson B, Blair E, et al. The risk of mortality or cerebral palsy in twins: a collaborative population-based study. Pediatr Res 2002; 52: 671–81.

63. Landy HJ, Keith LG. The vanishing fetus. In: Blickstein I, Keith LG, ed. Multiple Pregnancy Epidemiology: Gestation and Perinatal Outcome. London: Taylor and Francis, 2005: 108–12.

64. Benson CB, Doubilet PM, Laks MP. Outcome of twin gestation following sonographic demonstration of two heart beats in the first trimester. Ultrasound Obstet Gynecol 1993; 3: 343–45.

65. Pharoah POD, Cooke RWI. A hypothesis for the aetiology of spastic cerebral palsy – the vanishing twin. Dev Med Child Neurol 1997; 39: 292–6.

66. Newton R, Casabonne D, Johnson A, et al. A case–control study of vanishing twin as a risk factor for cerebral palsy. Twin Res 2003; 6: 83–4.

67. Dimitrou G, Pharoah POD, Nicholaides KH, Greenough A. Cerebral palsy in triplet pregnancies with and without iatrogenic reduction. Eur J Pediatr 2004; 163: 449–51.

68. Finnström O, Karl-Gösta N, Otterblaed Olausson P. Cerebral palsy in children born after IVF in Sweden 1982–1995: type of CP and maternal/obstetrical characteristics are similar to those in non-IVF children with CP. Acta Obstet Gynecol Scand 2005; 84: 1215–16.

25 General movements during prenatal and early postnatal life

Mijna Hadders-Algra

EVOLUTION IN UNDERSTANDING OF NORMAL AND DEVIANT MOTOR DEVELOPMENT

During the last century knowledge of the mechanisms governing the functions of the central nervous system (CNS) has rapidly increased. This expansion in knowledge was brought about by the development of sophisticated physiologic, neurochemical, and imaging techniques. In the field of motor control, the augmented understanding of neurophysiology resulted in a gradual shift from the concept that motor behavior is largely controlled by reflex mechanisms[1,2] towards the notion that motility is the net result of the activity of complex spinal or brainstem machineries, which are subtly modulated by segmental afferent information and ingeniously controlled by supraspinal networks.[3] For instance, nowadays it is assumed that motor control of rhythmic movements such as locomotion, respiration, sucking, and mastication is based on so-called central pattern generators (CPGs). CPGs are neural networks that are able to coordinate autonomously (i.e., without segmental sensory or supraspinal information) the activity of many muscles. Of course, in typical conditions, the CPG network does not work autonomously, but is affected by signals from other parts of the nervous system. The activity of the networks, which are usually located in the spinal cord or brainstem, is controlled from supraspinal areas via descending motor pathways.[3] The supraspinal activity itself is also organized in networks, large-scale ones, in which cortical areas are functionally connected through direct recursive interaction or through intermediary cortical or subcortical (striatal and cerebellar) structures.[4,5]

The conceptual changes in motor control have been paralleled by changes in ideas on motor development and neurologic assessment of young children. Development is no longer considered to be the result of a gradual unfolding of predetermined patterns in the CNS[6] or of increasing cortical control over so-called lower reflexes.[7] It is currently viewed as a complex process in which genetically based and environmentally driven process continuously interact.[8,9] In particular, the ideas of Edelman,[10,11] the neuronal group selection theory (NGST), proved to be helpful in gaining understanding of the mechanisms directing motor development and developmental motor disorders, such as cerebral palsy (CP).

According to NGST, normal motor development is characterized by two phases of variability.[9] The variation is not random, but is determined by criteria set by genetic information. Development starts with the phase of primary variability, during which variation in motor behavior is not geared to external conditions. Next, the phase of secondary variability takes over, during which motor performance can be adapted to specific situations. Adaptation occurs on the basis of selection guided by afferent information resulting from self-generated motor activity. The transition from primary to secondary variability occurs at function-specific ages. In terms of NGST, children with pre- or perinatally acquired lesions of the brain resulting in CP suffer from stereotyped motor behavior produced by a limited repertoire of primary cortical–subcortical networks.[12] In addition, these children have problems in selecting the most efficient neuronal activity due to deficits in the processing of sensory information.

The idea that spontaneous activity is a fundamental characteristic of neural tissue also affected the way in which young children are assessed neurologically. Traditionally, the neurologic assessment focused on muscle tone and reflexes,[7] but gradually people started to devote more attention to the observation of spontaneous behavior.[13] Heinz Prechtl was among the pioneers promoting the value of the evaluation of the quality of spontaneous motility during early human development.[14] He discovered that the quality of spontaneous movements of the fetus and young infant (i.e., the quality of general movements) may provide information on the integrity of the young nervous system.

TYPICAL DEVELOPMENT OF GENERAL MOVEMENTS DURING PRE- AND POSTNATAL LIFE

General movements (GMs) consist of series of gross movements of variable speed and amplitude, which involve all parts of the body but lack a distinctive sequencing of the participating body parts.[15] Remarkably, GMs are among the first movements that the human fetus develops, and they emerge prior to isolated limb movements.[16] GMs can already be observed before the completion of the spinal reflex arc, which is accomplished at 8 weeks' postmenstrual age (PMA).[17] This means that GMs, like other motor behaviors produced by CPG networks, can be generated in the absence of afferent information. This underscores the spontaneous or autogenic nature of the first movements[18] and refutes the long-held belief that all movements of the fetus and newborn are reflex in character.[19]

GM development from a phylogenetic perspective

Movements resembling human GMs can be observed in other species, albeit only during prenatal life. For instance, Coghill[20] described GM-like movements in the embryos of the amphibian *Amblystoma*. During the early phases of development, *Amblystoma* exhibits 'total behavior patterns' in which trunk and fore- and hindlimbs participate.

Early motor behavior has been studied especially in the embryonic chick. The basic motility type of the chick embryo is type I motility, which consists of spontaneous, seemingly uncoordinated movements.[21] During type I motility, all parts of the body can move

in any conceivable combination.[22,23] Type I motility disappears when the embryo approaches hatching age, to be absent after hatching.

In mammalian fetuses (rat,[24] rabbit,[25] and guinea pig[25]), comparable generalized motility can be recognized. In the fetal rat, generalized motility emerges 1 day after the onset of fetal motility, which starts at embryonic day 15.[24,26] A slight difference between the generalized movements of the rat fetus and those of the chick embryo has been observed. The movements of the rat are in general smoother than those of the chick.[23] After birth, rats no longer show GM-like movements. Instead, they show motility aiming at progression, i.e., weak crawling movements[27] or swimming behavior.[28] Unfortunately, no detailed reports exist on the various forms of prenatal motility in monkeys. But, like other animals, monkeys do not have GM-like movements after birth.[29] In fact, the human newborn seems to be the only newborn creature in which generalized movements persist after birth. Possibly, the human newborn can afford this type of non-goal directed motor behavior, which is especially displayed in the vulnerable supine position due to the presence of sophisticated parental care.[30]

Of course, one could query whether the prenatal general movements of the human fetus are identical to those of the chick and rat embryos. The basic description of generalized motility in various species is the same, and includes the notion that generalized movements are movements in which all parts of the body participate in a very variable way. The observation that all parts of the body participate resulted in the term 'total' or 'mass' movements (in rat[24] and human[7]), and only recently has the term 'general movements' been introduced for spontaneous movements in human preterms.[31] The very variable nature in which the various body parts are coordinated led to the descriptions 'impulsive' (various species),[25] 'seemingly uncoordinated' (chick),[23] and 'uncoordinated' (human),[31,32] and more recently to the description 'coordinated' movement pattern (human).[14] In all studies reported, generalized motility precedes the emergence of isolated limb movements. Thus, the basic features of generalized motility are shared by all hitherto studied subjects. Still, a qualitative difference seems to be present between the generalized movements of the chick and those of the human fetus and infant. The movements of the chick are described as monotonous and lacking rotatory components,[23] whereas complexity and rich variation in movement trajectory, including rotatory movements, are the hallmark of normal human GMs.[14,33] It is conceivable that the rich variety and complexity of human GMs reflect the seemingly aimless and explorative activity of the primary cortical–subcortical networks on the extensive CPG networks of the GMs in the spinal cord and brainstem. This hypothesis is supported by the finding that human GMs that lack complexity and variation (i.e., GMs that are definitely abnormal) are strong indicators of the development of CP.[33,34]

Ontogeny of GMs in the human

After their emergence during early fetal life, GMs continue to be present throughout pregnancy. The incidence of GMs first rapidly increases between 8 and 10 weeks' PMA,[35] after which it is relatively stable to decrease again after 28–32 weeks' PMA. The latter decrease has been observed in utero[36] and in preterm infants.[31] It should, however, be stressed that throughout pre- and postnatal life, the incidence of GMs is characterized by a large intra- and interindividual variation.[35–38]

GMs show age-specific characteristics (Table 25.1). Little is known about the qualitative changes of GMs during the first 2 trimesters of pregnancy. During the 3rd trimester, GMs are characterized by a large variation and complexity. The movements – described as 'preterm' GMs[39] – give the impression of a wonderfully complex ballet performance, and include many movements of the trunk. Around 36–38 weeks' PMA, a transition in GMs can be observed. The largely variable 'preterm' GMs change into the slower and more forceful 'writhing' GMs, in which the trunk participates less obviously than during the previous

GM phase.[39] The 'writhing' GMs constitute a temporary form of GMs, as they disappear around 6–8 weeks' post-term age.[40] Electromyograph (EMG) recordings of GMs[39,41] and H-reflex studies[42] indicated that the periterm period (i.e., the period from 36–38 weeks' PMA until 6–8 weeks' post-term age) is characterized by a temporary increased excitability of the motoneurons. This might explain why the motor behavior around term age was previously described as the phase of 'physiologic hypertonia'.[7] At the end of the 2nd month post term, the 'writhing' GMs are replaced by the final form of GMs, the so-called 'fidgety' GMs. The latter consist of a continuous stream of tiny, elegant movements occurring irregularly all over the body.[40] The transition from 'writhing' to 'fidgety' GMs occurs in general between 6 and 8 weeks' post-term age – thus in a relatively narrow time window. The finding that this change in GM form is more closely related to postmenstrual age than to postnatal age suggests that the transition for a major part is based on endogenous maturational processes.[40] Postnatal experience plays a minor role, as healthy preterm infants in general exhibit their 'fidgety' GMs only 1 week earlier than full-term babies do.[38] Surface EMG recordings indicated that the change from 'writhing' GMs to 'fidgety' GMs is associated with a decrease in the duration and amplitude of the phasic EMG bursts and a decrease in tonic background activity. Our group[41] suggested that the EMG changes might point to developmental changes of neuronal membranes throughout the nervous system, changes in muscle innervation (a regression of polyneural muscle innervation),[43] changes in the spinal circuitries (an increasing effect of Renshaw inhibition), and – last but not least – changes in supraspinal organization.

Table 25.1 Age-specific characteristics of normal GMs[39,40]

GM type	Period of presence (weeks PMA)	Description
Preterm GMs	From ± 28 weeks until 36–38 weeks	Extremely variable movements, including many pelvic tilts and trunk movements
'Writhing' GMs	From 36–38 weeks until 46–52 weeks	The variable movements take on a more forceful ('writhing') character. In comparison with preterm GMs, 'writhing' GMs seem to be somewhat slower and to show less participation of the pelvis and trunk
'Fidgety' GMs	From 46–52 weeks until 54–58 weeks	Basic motility consists of a continuous flow of small and elegant movements occurring irregularly all over the body – i.e., head, trunk, and limbs participate to a similar extent. The small movements can be superimposed on large and fast movements

At any GM age, the basic characteristics of normal GMs are (1) participation of all body parts and (2) movement complexity and variation

The latter idea is supported by imaging studies indicating that around the age of 3 months post term, functional activity in the cerebellum, the basal ganglia, and the parietal, temporal, and occipital cortices increases significantly.[44]

The 'fidgety' GMs disappear around 4 months post term.[40] They are gradually replaced by goal-directed movements. In terms of neural networks, the gradual change from GM activity into goal-directed behavior could mean that the widely distributed (sub)cortical networks controlling GM activity are flexibly rearranged by means of changed synaptic connectivity into multiple smaller networks.[45] In other words, the large (sub)cortical GM network is cut into various smaller networks. These smaller (sub)cortical networks form the primary neuronal repertoires for the control of specific motor behaviors, such as goal-directed motility of the arms and the legs, and postural control. Due to the dissolution of the primary neuronal network of the GMs, the development of GMs does not include a transition from a primary neuronal repertoire to a secondary repertoire. This underscores the unique position of GMs in human motor development, and supports the notion that the (sub)cortical networks involved in the control of GM activity form the neural building blocks for later motor skills.[9]

ABNORMAL GMs

Characteristics of abnormal GMs

Keywords describing the quality of GMs are variation and complexity (Figure 25.1).[14,33,39,46,47] Complexity points to the spatial variation of the movements. Complex movements are movements during which the infant actively produces frequent changes in direction of the participating body parts. The changes in movement direction are brought about by continuously varying combinations of flexion–extension, abduction–adduction, and endorotation–exorotation of the participating joints. GM variation represents the temporal variation of the movements. It means that, across time, the infant produces continuously new movement patterns. Thus, the primary parameters of GM quality evaluate two aspects of movement variation. This fits with the idea that variation is a fundamental feature of the function of the healthy young nervous system and stereotypy a hallmark of early brain dysfunction.[9,12]

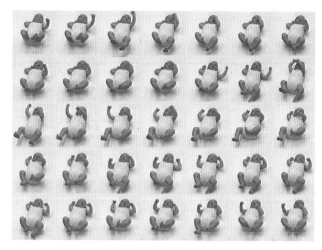

(A)

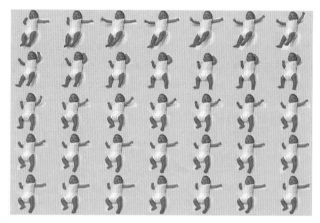

(B)

Figure 25.1 Representation of video frames with GMs of two infants at the 'fidgety' GM age. The video recording starts in the left hand upper corner and should be read like the lines in a book. The interval between the video frames is 0.24 seconds. The infant in (A) was born at term and shows normal fidgety GMs. The continuously varying positions of the limbs illustrate the rich spatial and temporal variation of normal movements. The infant in (B) was born at 28 weeks' PMA. She shows definitely abnormal GMs. The abnormal character of the movement is reflected by the lack of variation, indicated by the virtually identical frames, which induce the false impression that the infant hardly moves. (The video recordings were made in collaboration with the Department of Developmental and Experimental Clinical Psychology, Faculty of Psychological and Social Sciences; figure published with permission of the parents and the Nederlands Tijdschrift voor Geneeskunde[48])

Four classes of GM quality can be distinguished: two forms of normal GMs (normal–optimal and normal–suboptimal GMs) and two forms of abnormal GMs (mildly and definitely abnormal GMs; Table 25.2). Normal–optimal GMs are abundantly variable

Table 25.2 Classification of the quality of GMs[47]

Classification	Complexity[a]	Variation[a]	Fluency[b]
Normal–optimal GMs	+++	+++	+
Normal–suboptimal GMs	++	++	−
Mildly abnormal GMs	+	+	−
Definitely abnormal GMs	−	−	−

[a]Complexity and variation: +++, abundantly present; ++, sufficiently present; +, present, but insufficiently; −, virtually absent or absent
[b]Fluency (the least important aspect of GM assessment): +, present; −, absent

and complex. In addition, they are also fluent. Normal–optimal movements are relatively rare: only 10–20% of 3-month-old term infants show GMs of such a beautiful quality.[49,50] The majority of infants shows normal–suboptimal movements, which are sufficiently variable and complex but not fluent. Mildly abnormal GMs are insufficiently variable and complex and not fluent, and definitely abnormal GMs are virtually devoid of complexity, variation, and fluency. It is good to realize that the classification into four categories of quality is somewhat artificial. In fact, quality of movement is a continuum with at the one extreme splendidly complex, variable, and fluent movements, and at the other extreme very stereotyped movements, such as a repertoire restricted to cramped-synchronized movements.[39,51] The latter movements are characterized by a suddenly occurring en bloc movement, in which trunk and (flexed or extended) limbs stiffly move in utter synchrony. Actually, the cramped–synchronized movements are the only form of GMs that can be considered as pathologic. Their presence points to a loss of supraspinal control.[52] Thus, the presence of cramped–synchronized GMs implies that the infant shows abnormal GMs. When an infant only occasionally shows a cramped–synchronized GM within a repertoire of movements that mostly exhibit some degree of variation and complexity, GM quality can be classified as mildly abnormal. But when the infant frequently exhibits the cramped–synchronized pattern, GM quality should be considered as definitely abnormal.[53]

VALIDITY OF ABNORMAL GMs

Various pre-, peri-, and neonatal adversities, such as maternal diabetes, intrauterine growth retardation, preterm birth, perinatal asphyxia, neonatal hyperbilirubinemia, and neonatal treatment with dexamethasone, can give rise to abnormal GMs.[54]

Definitely abnormal GMs are specifically but not exclusively related to discernible lesions of the brain.[39,51,55,56] Children with Down syndrome often show mildly abnormal GMs.[57] It has also been demonstrated that movement quality is not a fixed phenomenon. It can change in various ways: movement quality can be transiently affected by illness,[58] and movement abnormalities can vanish or become more distinct with increasing age. The majority of changes in GM quality occurs in the transitional periods during which normal GMs change in form (i.e., between 36 and 38 weeks' PMA and between 6 and 8 weeks' post term).[47,59] Within the three GM phases (Table 25.1), movement quality is relatively stable (Figure 25.2).

The predictive validity of GM quality varies with the age at which the GMs are evaluated and with the type of outcome (Figure 25.2). The best prediction can be obtained by longitudinal series of GM assessments. Infants who persistently show definitely abnormal GMs, even while passing the transformational phases at

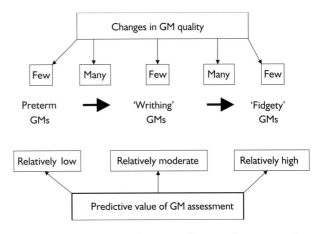

Figure 25.2 Schematic diagram indicating that GM quality is relatively stable within a specific GM phase, but changes frequently during the periods of transition (indicated by the bold arrows). Due to the frequent changes in quality, GM assessment prior to term age has relatively low predictive value

36–38 weeks' PMA and 6–8 weeks post term, have a high risk (70–85%) for the development of CP.[51,55] Infants who persistently show cramped–synchronized GMs invariably develop CP.[60] The prediction of a single GM assessment improves with increasing age. Thus, prediction is best at the age of 'fidgety' GMs (i.e., at 2–4 months post term). Studies in populations of infants at high risk for developmental disorders reported that the presence of definitely abnormal GMs at 'fidgety' age, which implies a total absence of the elegant, dancing complexity of 'fidgety' movements, predict CP with an accuracy of 85–98%.[34,47,59] Recent studies indicate that infants with definitely abnormal GMs at 'fidgety' age who do not develop CP usually show other developmental problems, such as minor neurologic dysfunction (MND), attention-deficit hyperactivity disorder (ADHD), or cognitive problems.[47,59] Mildly abnormal GMs at 'fidgety' age are related to the development of MND, in particular with respect to coordination problems and fine manipulative disability, ADHD, and aggressive behavior,[47,53,59] but the accuracy of prediction of these 'minor' problems is modest, due to the presence of relatively many false positives, resulting in a moderate specificity. The power to predict 'minor' developmental disorders improves considerably when the results of the assessment of GMs are combined with those of the infant neurologic examination.[47]

TECHNIQUE AND RELIABILITY OF GM ASSESSMENT

The assessment of the quality of GMs focuses on the amount of movement variation and complexity exhibited by the infant (Figure 25.1). These parameters can be appreciated by means of Gestalt perception of the observer.[14] Gestalt perception allows the evaluation of the repertoire of movement patterns displayed by *all* parts of the body, and does not pay special attention to particular behavior of specific body parts (e.g., fisting). GM evaluation also includes the evaluation of movement fluency (Table 25.2). But this is the least important aspect of the assessment. Regrettably, our visual system has an innate sensitivity to spot a loss of movement fluency, and this visual propensity for the detection of abnormalities in movement fluency (e.g., jerkiness, tremulousness, and stiffness) interferes to some extent with the assessment of the major components of the GMs (i.e., movement complexity and variation).

The evaluation of movement complexity and variation is demanding and requires offline assessment by means of a video recording. Assessment of the movements in 'real life' introduces errors and should be avoided.[50] Ideally, about 5–10 minutes of real-time motility is recorded with the infant in an adequate behavioral state. The absolute minimum duration of a GM video is 3 minutes with real-time behavior. Only this minimum duration allows for an evaluation of the overall variation in the infant's motor repertoire. The video has the advantage that it also offers the opportunity of movement replay at high speed, which facilitates the evaluation of movement complexity and variation. A high-speed replay produces an effect that is comparable to the effect produced by the video-frame sampling procedure of Figure 25.1.

GMs are affected by the behavioral state of the infant.[61] The optimal state for GM analysis is active wakefulness (i.e., Prechtl's state 4).[62] In this state, the splendid variation and fluency of normal GMs is expressed best. During other behavioral states, normal GMs have features reminiscent of abnormality, implying that a non-optimal state interferes with movement classification. The effects of behavioral state on normal GMs are summarized in Table 25.3. Practically, this means that GMs are preferably assessed in state 4. When a video recording only contains GMs during state 2 (or state-2-like conditions), the primary parameters of GM analysis – complexity and variation – can still be evaluated. GMs should not be assessed during crying or non-nutritive sucking, including thumb sucking.[61]

The basic principles of GM assessment can be learned in 2 days. Thereafter, it requires further practice of about 100 GM recordings to become a skilled observer.[50] Various studies reported that the intra- and inter-observer agreement of GM assessment of skilled observers is high (κ-values around 0.80, implying an excellent inter-rater and intra-rater reliability).[53,59]

Table 25.3 Effect of behavioral state on normal GMs[61]

Behavioral state[a]	Complexity and variation	Fluency
2: active sleep or REM sleep	Normal	Reduced
4: actively awake	Normal	Normal
5: crying	Reduced	Reduced
NNS[b]	Reduced	Normal

[a]Behavioral states (numbers according to Prechtl[62]) are only fully established from 36–38 weeks' PMA onwards[63]
[b]Non-nutritive sucking

CONCLUDING REMARKS

Assessment of the quality of GMs is a sensitive tool to evaluate brain function in the fetus and young infant. Currently, the application of GM assessment in the fetus is technically highly demanding: adequate assessment implies evaluation of the motor behavior of virtually all parts of the body for a period of at least 3 minutes. Most likely, future sonography machines and dedicated software programs will allow GM assessment in the fetus.

GMs have a function complementary to the traditional neurologic examination. Prediction of developmental outcome on the basis of longitudinal series of GM assessment is best. Second best is prediction on the basis of an assessment at 'fidgety' age (i.e. at 2–4 months post term). Prediction of developmental outcome on the basis of GM quality prior to term age is, however, relatively poor.

REFERENCES

1. Sherrington CS. The physiological position and dominance of the brain. In: Sherrington CS, ed. The Integrative Action of the Nervous System. London: Constable, 1906: 308–53.

2. Magnus R, De Kleijn A. Die abhängigkeit des Tonus der Extremitätenmuskeln von der Kopfstellung. Pflüger's Archiv 1912; 145: 455–548.

3. Grillner S, Deliagina T, Ekeberg Ö, et al. Neural networks that co-ordinate locomotion and body orientation in lamprey. Trends Neurosci 1995; 18: 270–9.

4. Alexander GE, Crutcher MD. Functional architecture of basal ganglia circuits: neural substrates of parallel processing. Trends Neurosci 1990; 13: 266–71.

5. Hikosaka O, Nakahara H, Rand MK, et al. Parallel neural networks for learning sequential procedures. Trends Neurosci 1999; 22: 464–71.

6. Gesell A, Amatruda CS. Developmental Diagnosis. Normal and Abnormal Child Development, 2nd edn. New York: Harper and Row, 1947.

7. Peiper A. Cerebral Function in Infancy and Childhood, 3rd edn. New York: Consultants Bureau, 1963.

8. Thelen E. Motor development. A new synthesis. Am Psychol 1995; 50: 79–95.

9. Hadders-Algra M. The Neuronal Group Selection Theory: an attractive framework to explain variation in normal motor development. Dev Med Child Neurol 2000; 42: 566–72.

10. Edelman GM. Neural Darwinism. The Theory of Neuronal Group Selection. Oxford: Oxford University Press, 1989.

11. Sporns O, Edelman GM. Solving Bernstein's problem: a proposal for the development of coordinated movement by selection. Child Dev 1993; 64: 960–81.

12. Hadders-Algra M. The Neuronal Group Selection Theory: promising principles for understanding and treating developmental motor disorders. Dev Med Child Neurol 2000; 42: 707–15.

13. Hadders-Algra M. The neuromotor examination of the preschool child and its prognostic significance. Ment Retard Dev Disabil Res Rev 2005; 11: 180–8.

14. Prechtl HFR. Qualitative changes of spontaneous movements in fetus and preterm infant are a marker of neurological dysfunction. Early Hum Dev 1990; 23: 151–8.

15. Prechtl HFR, Nolte R. Motor behaviour of preterm infants. In: Prechtl HFR, ed. Continuity of Neural Functions from Prenatal to Postnatal Life. Oxford: Blackwell Scientific, 1984: 79–92.

16. De Vries JIP, Visser GHA, Prechtl HFR. The emergence of fetal behaviour. I. Qualitative aspects. Early Hum Dev 1982; 7: 301–22.

17. Okado N, Kojima T. Ontogeny of the central nervous system: neurogenesis, fibre connection, synaptogenesis and myelination in the spinal cord. In: Prechtl HFR, ed. Continuity of Neural Functions from Prenatal to Postnatal Life. Oxford: Blackwell Scientific, 1984: 31–45.

18. Hall WG, Oppenheim RW. Developmental psychobiology: prenatal, perinatal, and early postnatal aspects of behavioral development. Annu Rev Psychol 1987; 38: 91–128.

19. Humphrey T. Postnatal repetition of human prenatal activity sequences with some suggestion of their neuroanatomical basis. In: Robinson RJ, ed. Brain and Early Behavior. New York: Academic Press, 1969: 43–71.

20. Coghill GE. Anatomy and the Problem of Behaviour. Cambridge: Cambridge University Press, 1929.

21. Hamburger V, Oppenheim R. Prehatching motility and hatching behavior in the chick. J Exp Zool 1967; 166: 171–204.

22. Hamburger V. Some aspects of the embryology of behavior. Q Rev Biol 1963; 38: 342–65.

23. Hamburger V. Anatomical and physiological basis of embryonic motility in birds and mammals. In: Gottlieb G, ed. Studies on the Development of Behavior and the Nervous System, Vol 1. Behavioral Embryology. New York: Academic Press, 1973: 52–76.

24. Angulo Y, González AW. The prenatal development of behavior in the albino rat. J Comp Neurol 1932; 55: 395–442.

25. Preyer W. Specielle Physiologie des Embryo. Leipzig: Th Griebens Verlag, 1885.

26. Narayanan CH, Fox MW, Hamburger V. Prenatal development of spontaneous and evoked activity in the rat (*Ratus norwegicus albinus*). Behaviour 1971; 40: 100–34.

27. Westerga J, Gramsbergen A. Development of locomotion in the rat: the significance of early movements. Early Hum Dev 1993; 34: 89–100.

28. Cazalets JR, Menard I, Cremieux J, Clarac F. Variability as a characteristic of immature motor systems: an electromyographic study of swimming in the newborn rat. Behav Brain Res 1990; 40: 215–25.

29. Dunbar DC, Badam GL. Development of posture and locomotion in free-ranging primates. Neurosci Biobehav Rev 1998; 22: 541–6.

30. Papoušek H, Papoušek M. Qualitative transitions in integrative processes during the first trimester of human postpartum life. In: Prechtl HFR, ed. Continuity of Neural Functions from Prenatal to Postnatal Life. Oxford: Blackwell Scientific, 1984: 220–44.

31. Prechtl HFR, Fargel JW, Weinmann HM, et al. Postures, motility and respiration of low-risk pre-term infants. Dev Med Child Neurol 1979; 21: 3–27.

32. Minkowski M. Neurobiologische Studien am menschlichen Foetus. In: Abderhalden E, ed. Handbuch der biologischen Arbeitsmethoden. Abt V: Methoden zum Studium der Funktionen der einzelne Organe im Tierischen Organismus, Teil 5B. Berlin: Urban and Schwarzenberg, 1938: 511–619.

33. Hadders-Algra M. General movements: a window for early identification of children at high risk of developmental disorders. J Pediatr 2004; 145: S12–18.

34. Prechtl HFR, Einspieler C, Cioni G, et al. An early marker of developing neurological handicap after perinatal brain lesions. Lancet 1997; 339: 1361–3.

35. De Vries JI, Visser GH, Prechtl HFR. The emergence of fetal behaviour. II. Quantitative aspects. Early Hum Dev 1985; 12: 99–120.

36. Roodenburg PJ, Wladimiroff JW, Van Es A, et al. Classification and quantitative aspects of fetal movements during the second half of normal pregnancy. Early Hum Dev 1991; 25: 19–35.

37. Cioni G, Ferrari F, Prechtl HFR. Posture and spontaneous motility in fullterm infants. Early Hum Dev 1989; 18: 247–62.

38. Cioni G, Prechtl HFR. Preterm and early postterm motor behaviour in low-risk premature infants. Early Hum Dev 1990; 23: 159–91.

39. Hadders-Algra M, Klip-Van den Nieuwendijk AWJ, Martijn A, et al. Assessment of general movements: towards a better understanding of a sensitive method to evaluate brain function in young infants. Dev Med Child Neurol 1997; 39: 88–98.

40. Hadders-Algra M, Prechtl HFR. Developmental course of general movements in early infancy. I: Descriptive analysis of change in form. Early Hum Dev 1992; 28: 201–14.

41. Hadders-Algra M, Van Eykern LA, Klip-van den Nieuwendijk AWJ, et al. Developmental course of general movements in early infancy. II. EMG correlates. Early Hum Dev 1992; 28: 231–52.

42. Hakamada S, Hayakawa F, Kuno K, et al. Development of the monosynaptic reflex pathway in the human spinal cord. Dev Brain Res 1988; 42: 239–46.

43. Gramsbergen A, Ijkema-Paassen J, Nikkels PGJ, et al. Regression of polyneural innervation in the human psoas muscle. Early Hum Dev 1997; 49: 49–61.

44. Chugani HT, Phelps ME, Maziotta JC. 18-FDG positron emission tomography in human brain. Functional development. Ann Neurol 1987; 22: 487–97.

45. Simmers J, Meyran P, Moulins M. Modulation and dynamic specification of motor rhythm-generating circuits in crustacea. J Physiol Paris 1995; 89: 195–208.

46. Einspieler C, Prechtl HFR, Bos AF, et al. Prechtl's Method on the Qualitative Assessment of General Movements in Preterm, Term and Young Infants. London: MacKeith Press, 2004.

47. Hadders-Algra M, Mavinkurve-Groothuis AMC, Groen SE, et al. Quality of general movements and the development of minor neurological dysfunction at toddler and school age. Clin Rehab 2004; 18: 287–99.

48. Hadders-Algra M. De beoordeling van spontane motoriek van jonge baby's: een doeltreffende methode voor de opsporing van hersenfunctiestoornissen. Ned Tijdschr Geneeskd 1997; 141: 816–20.

49. Bouwstra H, Dijck-Brouwer DAJ, Wildeman JAL, et al. Long-chain polyunsaturated fatty acids have a positive effect on the quality of general movements of healthy term infants. Am J Clin Nutr 2003; 78: 313–8.

50. Hornstra AH, Dijk-Stigter GR, Grooten HMJ, et al. Beoordeling van gegeneraliseerde bewegingen bij zuigelingen op het consultatiebureau: een pilot onderzoek naar (on) mogelijkheden tot implementatie. Tijdschr Jeugdgezondheidszorg 2003; 6: 108–13.

51. Ferrari F, Cioni G, Prechtl HFR. Qualitative changes of general movements in preterm infants with brain lesions. Early Hum Dev 1990; 23: 193–231.

52. Hadders-Algra M. General movements in early infancy: What do they tell us about the nervous system? Early Hum Dev 1993; 34: 29–37.

53. Groen SE, de Blécourt ACE, Postema K, et al. Quality of general movements predicts neuromotor development at the age of 9–12 years. Dev Med Child Neurol 2005; 47: 731–8.

54. Hadders-Algra, M. Evaluation of motor function in young infants by means of the assessment of general movements: a review. Pediatr Phys Ther 2001; 13: 27–36.

55. Prechtl HFR, Ferrari F, Cioni G. Predictive value of general movements in asphyxiated fullterm infants. Early Hum Dev 1993; 35: 91–120.

56. Bos AF, Martijn A, Okken A, et al. Quality of general movements in preterm infants with transient periventricular echodensities. Acta Paediatr 1998; 87: 328–35.

57. Mazonne L, Mugno D, Mazonne D. The general movements in children with Down syndrome. Early Hum Dev 2004; 79: 119–30.

58. Bos AF, Van Asperen RM, De Leeuw DM, et al. The influence of septicaemia on spontaneous motility in preterm infants. Early Hum Dev 1997; 50: 61–70.

59. Hadders-Algra M, Groothuis AMC. Quality of general movements in infancy is related to the development of neurological dysfunction, attention deficit hyperactivity disorder and aggressive behavior. Dev Med Child Neurol 1999; 41: 381–91.

60. Ferrari F, Cioni G, Einspieler C, et al. Cramped synchronized general movements in preterm infants as an early marker of cerebral palsy. Arch Pediatr Adolesc Med 2002; 156: 460–7.

61. Hadders-Algra M, Nakae Y, Van Eykern LA, et al. The effect of behavioral state on general movements in healthy full-term newborns. A polymyographic study. Early Hum Dev 1993; 35: 63–79.

62. Prechtl HFR. The behavioral state of the infant – a review. Brain Res 1974; 76: 185–212.

63. Nijhuis JG, Prechtl HFR, Martin CB, et al. Are there behavioral states in the human fetus? Early Hum Dev 1982; 6: 177–95.

26 The use of 3D and 4D sonography in the neonatal period

Milan Stanojević, Sanja Zaputovic, and Asim Kurjak

INTRODUCTION

Although sonography has recently become established as an essential method for the assessment of pregnancy, at the beginnings of its diagnostic application more than half a century ago, one-dimensional (1D) sonography failed to become an important diagnostic modality for the detection of brain tumors.[1,2] Despite this diagnostic fiasco, the investigations using sonography enabled its clinical application in obstetrics in the late 1950s, while at the same time midline encephalography became the standard diagnostic modality for the evaluation of patients with traumatic brain injuries.[1,2] The introduction of Doppler, real-time, and grayscale sonography into clinical practice in the 1970s was of substantial significance.[1,2] During the 1980s, the clinical application of Doppler sonography in blood flow studies was developed.[1,2] When performing 2D imaging, sonographers were making 3D reconstructions in their imagination, and the development of computer technology finally enabled 3D reconstruction from ultrasonic tomograms.[3,4] The normal fetal head was the first object of interest in obstetric sonography, which enabled the first prenatal diagnosis of fetal brain pathology as well.[5-9]

Novel 4D technology, introduced in the last few years, is a new tool for the observation of fetal behavior.[10-16] Although 2D sonography could examine the origin, occurrence, and developmental course of specific fetal movements, simultaneous imaging of complex movements was almost impossible using only the 2D real-time technique.[9,17] A technique was needed with the aim of enabling 3D imaging of fetal movements in a real-time mode. Human eyes are known to be able to differentiate between images up to a frequency of about 12 images/s; consequently, production of an appropriate frame rate with specially designed probes and a fast computer rendering device is required. At present, 4D sonography is not real-time, with available machines being able to reach up to about 20 images/s, depending on volume size, resolution, and the mechanics of the probe. Nevertheless, even at these relatively slow frame rates, the ability to study fetal activity and its superficial structures is better than that of 2D devices.[10-16] This means that 4D sonography integrates the advantage of spatial imaging of fetal structures with the addition of time, allowing depiction of the appearance and measurement of the duration of each movement.[10-16] This new diagnostic tool allows continuous monitoring of the quantity of fetal movements, although monitoring of their quality is still somewhat difficult.

Prenatal assessment of the fetal brain is an important component of anomaly scans in the 2nd trimester of pregnancy. The brain develops rapidly, and changes remarkably throughout the gestation. The transabdominal and transvaginal approaches enable early diagnosis of the vast majority of fetal brain disorders. As well as malformations, the fetal brain should be investigated for hemorrhage, inflammatory disorders, periventricular leukomalacia, and other rare causes of postnatal developmental disorders. From the aspect of postnatal psychomotor development, it is of substantial importance to continue the prenatal assessment of fetal brain with postnatal studies.

At the beginning of the 1980s, the opened anterior fontanel was used as an acoustic window for assessment of the brains of small premature and critically sick newborns.[5–9] This was a substantial step forward in neonatal neuroimaging diagnostics.[5–9] In comparison with radiologic X-ray imaging techniques or magnetic resonance imaging (MRI), sonography was more convenient, because of the unlimited examination frequency of critically sick newborns in isolettes, less costly, and without the need for sedation and transportation of infants.[6] The introduction of Doppler studies was an advance in the assessment of neonatal brain circulation in the late 1980s.[1,2,18] This technique enabled follow-up of the brain circulation and its dynamics.[8,19] In the 1990s, a new exciting technique of 3D and 4D brain sonography was developed, depicting the neonatal brain in the third dimension in real time.[18,20–24] Brain sonography became the most widely used technique for the evaluation of brain morphology and cerebral lesions in neonates.[18,23,24] It can confirm prenatal diagnosis and identify not only the presence of lesions but also their type and extent.[25]

Because health is understood as physical, mental, and social well-being – going much further than just the absence of acute suffering or disease – neurosonographic screening and diagnostic activities should be highly prophylactic with regard to morphologic and functional handicaps of the newborn child.

The aim of the rest of this chapter is to present the sociomedical aspects and the indications for 3D sonography in the neonatal period, with the accent on neurosonography.

THE ROLE OF SONOGRAPHIC DIAGNOSTICS IN NEONATOLOGY: SOCIOMEDICAL ASPECTS

The development of diagnostic sonography in other medical disciplines was followed by its application in neonatology, contributing to better diagnostic possibilities in a number of fields:[3,5,26–32]

- neurosonography
- echocardiography with Doppler studies
- diagnosis of developmental dysplasia of the hip
- diagnosis of kidney malformations
- ocular sonography for the detection of congenital malformations and retinopathy of prematurity
- training and education.

Sonography plays a very important role as a diagnostic tool for determination of the prognosis of

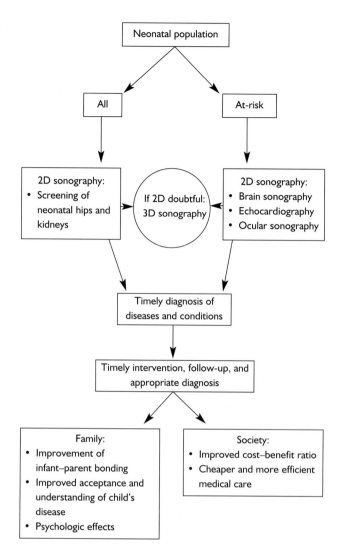

Figure 26.1 Sociomedical role of sonographic diagnostics in neonatology

diseases and conditions in newborns, and can thus possibly influence the quality of life not only of the newborns, but of the entire family as well.[3] This aspect is of crucial importance for the newborn, her or his parents and family, and the whole of society, because timely diagnosis will enable earlier and appropriate, planned and cheaper treatment, better prognosis, and better quality of life. If the quality of 2D visualization is insufficient, then 3D sonography, due to its high diagnostic potential in comparison with conventional 2D real-time techniques, deserves special attention. Sometimes, the use of 3D sonography will enable decision-making with regard to whether or not a disease is treatable, solving some diagnostic and ethical dilemmas.[20–24] Figure 26.1 illustrates sociomedical aspects of the role of sonography in neonatology.

APPLICATION OF 3D SONOGRAPHY IN FIELDS OF NEONATOLOGY OTHER THAN NEUROSONOGRAPHY

The aim of this section is to give a brief overview of the application of 3D sonography in areas of neonatology other than neurosonography. While 3D sonography has become an established modality in many specialties of adult medicine, it has not yet gained significant importance in neonatal imaging.[32] There is no doubt that 3D sonography is a valuable imaging modality for depiction of the neonatal brain, but it also appears to be useful in neonatal echocardiography, nephrology, orthopedics, ophthalmology, and other fields of pediatrics.[32] 3D sonography is used for diagnosis of neonatal spinal canal pathology, soft tissue and musculoskeletal changes, tumors, and many other conditions.[32,33] Experience with 3D sonography indicates that it is an accurate method for the assessment of volumes of many organs and pathologic changes such as the following:[32,34–41]

- renal parenchymal volume and relative renal size
- cerebral ventricular system
- cardiology
- other (tumors).

Telemedicine in pediatrics is a promising and important discipline, becoming more popular with the development of computers and telecommunication systems. It is especially well developed in pediatric cardiology, with the potential of 3D echocardiography to improve patient care.[42–44]

3D sonography is also an ideal modality for training and education, as the saved 3D volume can be retrieved from the machine without the patient's presence.[32]

A 3D sonographic reconstruction of the neonatal kidney and a 3D depiction of rhabdomyoma in the left ventricle of the heart are presented in Figures 26.2 and 26.3, respectively.

PRINCIPLES OF NEONATAL 3D NEUROSONOGRAPHY

Volume acquisition is obtained by a 3D high-resolution (5–8 MHz) sector probe, recording sets of tomograms at fixed angular increments, which are digitized and saved to the computer memory.[3,4,21,22] Specialized software enables the sonographer to generate orthogonal sets of images in any desired plane

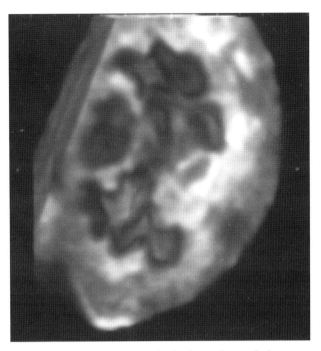

Figure 26.2 3D sonogram of a hydronephrotic kidney in a neonate

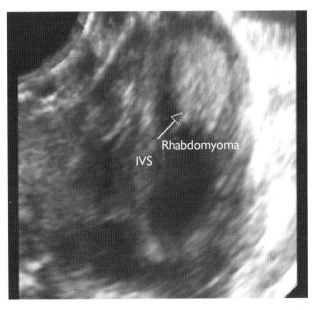

Figure 26.3 3D sonogram of a rhabdomyoma (arrow) in the left ventricle of a neonatal heart. IVS, intraventricular septum

through the 3D volume.[3,4,21,22] The acquired images are displayed in three orthogonal planes for multiplanar view analysis, with the possibility of data manipulation.[3,4,6,18–23] For better orientation during multiplanar analysis, a dot marker is always positioned in the same structure of the brain in all three orthogonal planes.

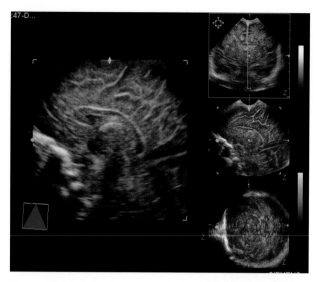

Figure 26.4 Multiplanar view (right) of the neonatal brain, with a 3D reconstruction in sagittal view (left)

After multiplanar analysis of the neonatal brain, volume rendering of the region of interest (ROI) can be performed, with direct projection of 3D data onto a 2D plane.[3,4,21,22] Different modes of volume reconstruction can be used, depending on the location of the object of interest. The surface mode is used for the depiction of the brain surface (gyri and sulci), the minimum mode is used for depiction of cystic formations, while the maximum mode is better for the depiction of calcifications.[4] There is a possibility of color and power Doppler studies of brain circulation during the examination.[18] Volumetric measurements of brain structures are sometimes important for follow-up of the brain or its structures, intracerebral cysts, and brain ventricles.[23,45,46] Figure 26.4 depicts a normal multiplanar view of the neonatal brain.

The standard sagittal and coronal planes are traditionally obtained through the anterior fontanel when 2D neurosonography is performed. Postnatal 3D neurosonography depicts the neonatal brain in coronal and sagittal planes, while the computer enables reconstruction of the axial plane.[6,18,20,23] Computer 3D reconstruction of the ROI of the neonatal brain and its depiction in a 2D plane when indicated is also possible and desirable.

INDICATIONS FOR NEONATAL 3D NEUROSONOGRAPHY

Sonography has been a very important diagnostic modality for the detection and follow-up of central nervous system (CNS) disorders of sick premature and term babies in the neonatal intensive care units for many years.[3,47–50] Although 3D neurosonography is a safe and low-risk procedure in the neonate, due to the very limited availability of equipment for 3D neurosonography (which is often connected with the necessity of newborn transportation), the benefits and risks of 3D imaging should be taken into consideration. In institutions where equipment is available and can be transported to the patient, it is the method of choice for depiction of the neonatal brain.[51–61] Indications for 3D neurosonography in the neonatal period are the same as for 2D techniques, and whenever 2D is unreliable or doubtful, 3D is indicated.[6] The main indications for 3D neurosonography in the newborn period are the following, prenatally or postnatally developed:

- intracranial hemorrhage
- hypoxic–ischemic brain damage
- inflammatory disorders of the brain and their complications
- ventriculomegaly and hydrocephaly (Doppler and volumetric studies are included)
- congenital brain defects.

In addition, this technique is used for assessment of gestational age.

Many known and unknown perinatal and social risk factors can influence the development of the neonatal brain, especially in premature infants, although abnormal prenatal neurosonography or postnatal neurologic findings in apparently well neonates can prompt neonatologists to search for ultrasound abnormalities.[25,44,48–60] A good correlation has been found between sonographic findings in the fetal and neonatal period and signs of neurologic impairment in the neonatal period and later in childhood.[5,7,25] Cranial sonography can be a good predictor of disabling and non-disabling cerebral palsy at the age of 2 years in low-birthweight infants,[48] and it can be related to impaired motor function in 5-year-old children.[7] Improved survival of very low-birthweight (VLBW) infants has contributed to the increased incidence of cerebral palsy despite the introduction of sophisticated treatment methods in intensive care units.[48,50] White matter brain lesions diagnosed sonographically have been found to be a powerful predictor of disabling cerebral palsy.[48]

NEONATAL NEUROSONOGRAPHY

The most frequently diagnosed brain lesion in neonatology is intracranial hemorrhage. On the basis of

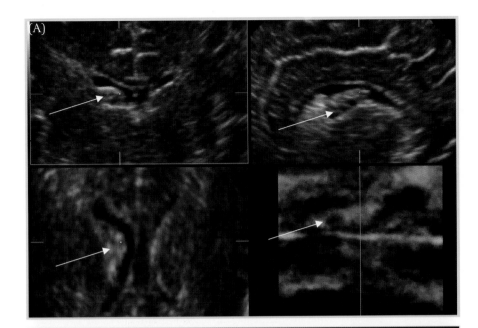

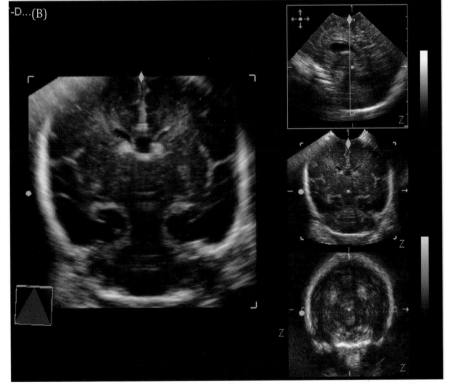

Figure 26.5 (A,B) 3D imaging of subependymal hemorrhage (white solid arrows) in a neonate (Papile grade 1)

computed tomography (CT) findings, the classical description of intraventricular hemorrhage with its grading in newborns was given by Papile et al.[9] The prevalence of intracranial hemorrhage in VLBW premature infants has tended to decrease in the last 20 years or so from as high as 60% at the beginning of the 1980s to 25% in the 1990s.[50] Intracranial hemorrhage can be detected in 3.5% of apparently normal full-term newborns.[44,62] Some new concepts in the patho-

genesis of germinal matrix hemorrhages in premature infants have enabled a better understanding of pathologic events and their prevention.[63] Most intracranial hemorrhages are postnatal in origin, although some can be detected prenatally.

Figure 26.5 shows subependymal hemorrhage in a neonate (Papile grade 1). Figure 26.6 shows intraventricular hemorrhage without dilatation of the ventricles (Papile grade 2), and Figure 26.7 shows a

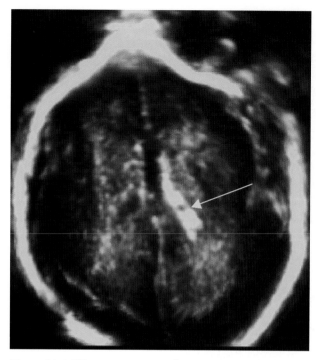

Figure 26.6 3D reconstruction of an intraventricular hemorrhage (Papile grade 2) with a small cyst inside the clot (arrow)

postnatal 3D image of a prenatally developed severe intraventricular hemorrhage with ventricular dilatation (Papile grade 3). Figure 26.8 depicts a 3D reconstruction of the most severe type of

intraparenchymal hemorrhage in a premature infant (Papile grade 4).

The prevalence of periventricular leukomalacia in VLBW infants is 9.2–14.9%,[64] while the incidence of cystic periventricular leukomalacia is 4.3–15.7% in preterm infants between 27 and 32 weeks of gestation.[50] The sonographic finding of transient hyperechogenicities of white matter – so-called 'flares' – is transient, resolving spontaneously without any subsequent developmental problems, while cystic periventricular leukomalacia is often associated with a risk of cerebral palsy of up to 50%.[50,64] Figure 26.9 shows severe cystic periventricular leukomalacia in a premature infant.

Despite improved hygiene, vaccines, and the introduction of new anti-inflammatory agents, congenital infections remain an important cause of neurologic morbidity in newborns.[65,66] Among neuroimaging diagnostic procedures, sonography has an important role to play in the detection and follow-up of neonatal TORCH infections and meningitis.[65,66] Regardless of its etiology, meningitis in VLBW infants is often caused by nosocomial agents.[65,66] The role of postnatal inflammation in the pathogenesis of the brain damage in VLBW infants still remains to be proven, while the role of prenatal inflammation in the pathogenesis of cystic PVL is beyond doubt.[50,64] Figure 26.10 depicts subdural effusion in course of nosocomial meningitis caused by multiresistant *Klebsiella pneumoniae* in a premature infant.

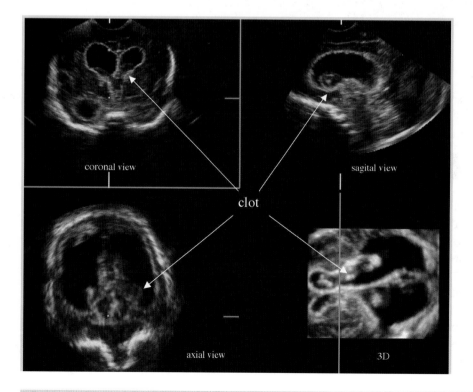

Figure 26.7 3D reconstruction of a Papile grade 3 intraventricular hemorrhage (note the markedly dilated ventricles)

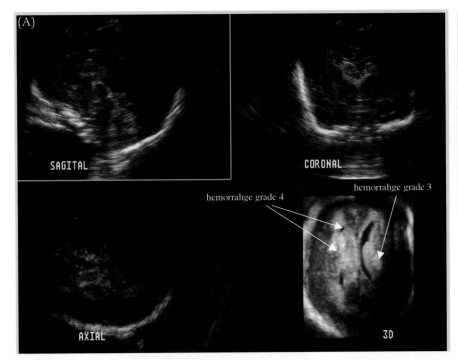

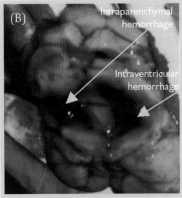

Figure 26.8 (A) 3D reconstruction of an intraventricular grade 3 and intraparenchymal grade 4 hemorrhage in a 9-day-old premature infant (27 weeks of gestation, birthweight 1.1 kg). (B) Brain specimen at autopsy

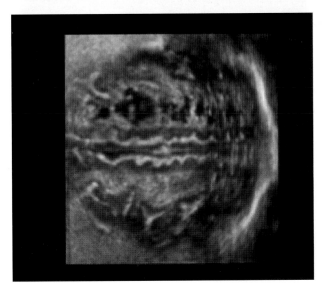

Figure 26.9 3D surface rendering of severe cystic periventricular leukomalacia (PVL) in a premature infant

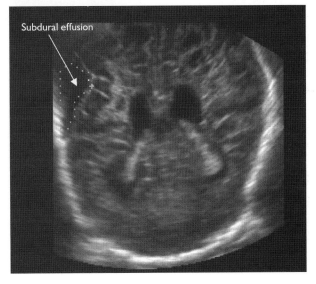

Figure 26.10 3D image of subdural effusion in the course of nosocomial meningitis caused by multiresistant *Klebsiella pneumoniae* in a premature infant

Although application of different neuroimaging modalities, among which sonography is the most frequent and suitable, has enabled prenatal and postnatal detection of hydrocephalus, its management remains a difficult challenge.[67] One major reason for this difficulty is the multifactorial nature of the conditions affecting postnatal outcome in congenital hydrocephalus.[67] A new clinicoembryologic classification of congenital hydrocephalus reflects both clinical and embryologic developmental aspects of the neuronal maturation process in the hydrocephalic infant.[67] Congenital hydrocephalus is one of the most common CNS malformations, with an incidence of 0.3–0.8 per 1000 births.[68] Neonatal ventriculomegaly, defined as an enlargement of the ventricular atrium with a width of greater than 1 cm, is often associated with numerous etiologies, ranging from underdevelopment or atrophy of intracranial structures affecting the normal

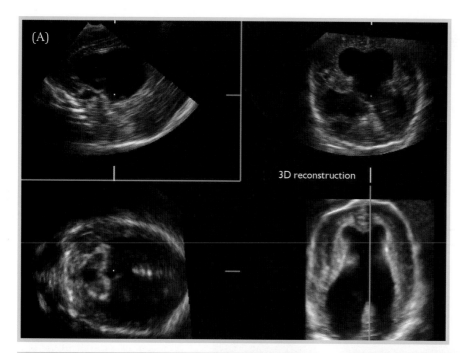

3D reconstruction

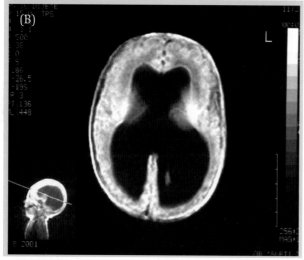

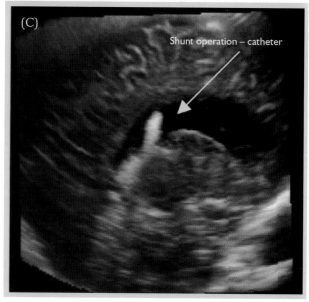

Shunt operation – catheter

Figure 26.11 3D sonographic reconstruction (A) and MRI (B) of prenatally recognized severe hydrocephalus in a term newborn. (C) Depiction of the brain by 3D sonography in the sagittal view after shunt operation

flow of cerebrospinal fluid (CSF) through the ventricular system to disorders with Mendelian inheritance.[68] In one-third of cases, ventriculomegaly is associated with additional intracranial lesions, while two-thirds have extracranial anomalies.[68] Figure 26.11 depicts 3D sonography and MRI of prenatally recognized severe hydrocephalus in a term newborn.

3D sonographic studies of fetal CNS development have improved the prenatal diagnosis of malformations and other conditions, with a sensitivity of up to 80%.[21,69–71] Nevertheless, postnatal sonography remains important for the detection of prenatally unrecognized conditions and for postnatal follow-up.

The incidence of CNS anomalies is estimated to be 0.2%.[70] Despite the possibility of a genetic diagnosis of some CNS malformations, detection of mutated genes will not be available in the near future as a screening method in clinical practice, and therefore diagnostic ultrasound remains of great importance.[72] The incidence of some common CNS anomalies such as agenesis of the corpus callosum is 2–3% of developmentally disabled individuals.[68] In 57% of cases, agenesis of the corpus callosum is associated with coexisting anomalies, while in 10% of cases it is associated with chromosomal aberrations.[68] Choroid plexus cysts have an incidence of 1–2% in the general

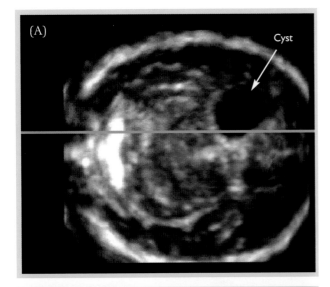

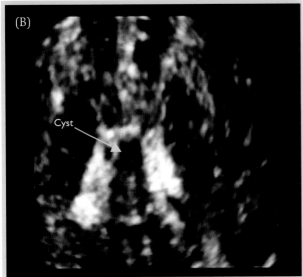

Figure 26.12 3D sonograms of large (A) and small (B) choroid plexus cysts in two newborns

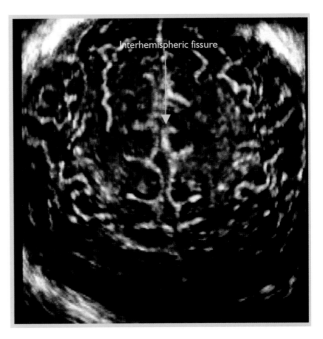

Figure 26.13 Surface mode image of normally developed gyri and sulci in a term infant

population of newborns.[68] Cysts above 5 mm in diameter have a higher rate of aneuploidy in comparison with cysts between 2 and 5 mm.[68] Figure 26.12 shows 3D sonograms of large and small choroid plexus cysts in two newborns.

There is a need for an easy and accurate clinical method to assess the gestational age in newborns. From the 24th to the 34th week of gestation, there are important identifiable changes in the cerebral surface, and the principal sulci develop and alter in complexity each week.[73,74] After 34 weeks, as the gyri increase in complexity, distinctive changes are less easy to identify.[73] Sonography is a non-invasive method of studying the important changes in the development of

the neonatal brain, with a scoring system enabling determination of gestational age.[73,74] Figure 26.13 shows the 3D surface mode of normally developed gyri and sulci in a term infant.

BENEFITS OF 3D PRENATAL AND NEONATAL NEUROSONOGRAPHY

Standard 2D neurosonography often requires 15–30 minutes to perform, exposing critically sick neonates to potentially significant stress.[18,20,23] Conventional 2D imaging of the neonatal brain is accomplished by real-time scanning with a series of representative images at selected locations of the brain anatomy, captured for electronic or film archival.[6] Neonatal neurosonography enables depiction of the brain through the anterior fontanel in coronal and sagittal planes, although acquisition of the axial plane is impossible through the anterior fontanel.[18,20,23] Interpretation of fetal and neonatal neurosonography is based on this selection, and if questions arise with regard to the diagnostic content of the examination, another session is necessary to provide additional views. 3D volume acquisition, lasting 2–5 minutes, supplies adequate diagnostic information either prenatally or postnatally, and significantly decreases the examination time.[18,20,23] The 3D method minimizes operator-dependent gaps in the information set.[18,20,23] The digital dataset is

501

saved so that it can be recalled, examined, and interpreted offline.[3,4,21,22] Furthermore, network connection enables images to be sent by telemedicine for expert consultation, without the need for patient transportation, which reduces direct and indirect medical care costs.

Although 3D images of the neonatal brain obtained by X-ray CT and MRI are quite satisfactory, sonographic imaging is in wide use, being found to be highly efficient, economical, and safe.[3] In 3D fetal and neonatal sonography, the quantity of ultrasound irradiation is decreased with shortness of examination exposure.[3] Ultrasonic equipment is much cheaper than X-ray, CT, and MRI equipment, requires little space and no special architectural accommodation, and can be operated easily.[3]

CONCLUSIONS

3D neurosonography of the neonatal brain offers significant improvements compared with conventional 2D sonography. These improvements include shorter time of data acquisition in three orthogonal planes with an unlimited number of planes, the possibility of comprehensive and thorough analysis of the obtained dataset, volume rendering, volumetric studies, and color and power Doppler studies (Figure 26.14). The possibility of sending 3D images, without the necessity to refer the patient, is a great achievement of modern technology.[3,21,22] Although 3D sonography is still not

available as the standard method for the assessment of the neonatal brain due to the relatively high cost of the equipment, it should become widely available in the near future.

REFERENCES

1. McNay MB, Fleming JEE. Forty years of obstetric ultrasound 1957–1997: from a-scope to three dimensions. Ultrasound Med Biol 1999; 25: 3–56.

2. Newman PG, Rozycki GS. The history of ultrasound. Surg Clin North Am 1998; 78: 179–95.

3. Baba K, Okai T. Basis and principles of three-dimensional ultrasound. In: Kurjak A, ed. Three-Dimensional Ultrasound in Obstetrics and Gynecology. New York: Parthenon, 1997.

4. Baba K, Satoh K, Sakamato S, Okai T, Ishii S. Development of an ultrasonic system for three-dimensional reconstruction of the fetus. J Perinat Med 1989; 17: 19–24.

5. Dubowitz LMS, Levene MI, Morante A, Palmer P, Dubowitz V. Neurologic signs in neonatal intraventricular hemorrhage: a correlation with real-time ultrasound. J Pediatr 1981; 99: 127–33.

6. Fischer AQ, Anderson JC, Shuman RM, Stinson W. Pediatric Neurosonography. Clinical, Tomographic and Neuropathologic Correlates. New York: Wiley, 1985.

7. Levene M, Dowling S, Graham M, et al. Impaired motor function (clumsiness) in 5 year old children: correlation with neonatal ultrasound scans. Arch Dis Child 1992; 67: 687–90.

8. Levene MI, Wigglesworth JS, Dubowitz V. Cerebral structure and intraventricular hemorrhage in the neonate: a real-time ultrasound study. Arch Dis Child 1981; 56: 416–24.

9. Papile LA, Burstein J, Burstein R. Incidence and evolution of subependymal and intraventricular hemorrhage: a study of infants with birth weights less than 1,500 gm. J Pediatr 1978; 92: 529–34.

10. Kumo A, Akiyama M, Yamashiro C, et al. Three-dimensional sonographic assessment of fetal behavior in the early second trimester of pregnancy. J Ultrasound Med 2001; 2: 1271–5.

11. Kurjak A, Vecek N, Hafner T, et al. Prenatal diagnosis: What does four-dimensional ultrasound add? J Perinat Med 2002; 30: 57–62.

12. Kurjak A, Vecek N, Kupesic S, Azumendi G, Solak M. Four dimensional ultrasound: How much does it improve perinatal practice? In: Carrera JM, Chervenak FA, Kurjak A, eds. Controversies in Perinatal Medicine: Studies on the Fetus as a Patient. New York: Parthenon, 2003: 222–34.

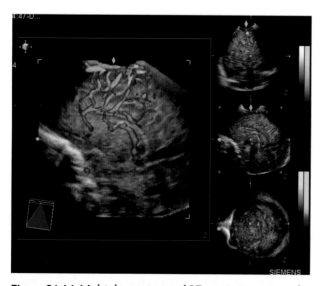

Figure 26.14 Multiplanar view and 3D reconstruction in the sagittal view of the neonatal brain, with power Doppler depiction of the brain arteries (normal anatomy)

13. Kurjak A, Azumendi G, Vecek N, et al. Fetal hand movements and facial expression in normal pregnancy studied by four–dimensional sonography. J Perinat Med 2003; 31: 496–508.

14. Azumendi G, Kurjak A. Three-dimensional and four-dimensional sonography in the study of the fetal face. Ultrasound Rev Obstet Gynecol 2003; 3: 160–9.

15. Kurjak A, Stanojevic M, Andonotopo W, Salihagic-Kadic A, Carrera JM. Behavioral pattern continuity from prenatal to postnatal life – study by four-dimensional (4D) ultrasonography. J Perinat Med 2004; 32: 346–53.

16. Kurjak A, Stanojevic M, Azumendi G, Carrera JM. The potential of four-dimensional (4D) ultrasonography in the assessment of fetal awareness. J Perinat Med 2005; 33: 46–53.

17. de Vries JIP, Visser GHA, Prechtl HFR. The emergence of fetal behaviour. I. Qualitative aspects. Early Hum Dev 1982; 7: 301–22.

18. Peng SS, Lin JH, Lee WT, et al. 3-D power Doppler cerebral angiography in neonates and young infants: comparison with 2–D Doppler angiography. Ultrasound Med Biol 1999; 25: 947–51.

19. Kurjak A, Kupesic S, Banovic I, Hafner T, Kos M. The study of morphology and circulation of early embryo by three-dimensional ultrasound and power Doppler. J Perinat Med 1999; 27: 145–57.

20. Kampmann W, Walka MM, Vogel M, Obladen M. 3-D sonographic volume measurement of cerebral ventricular system: in vitro validation. Ultrasound Med Biol 1998; 24: 1169–74.

21. Kurjak A, Hafner T, Kos M, Kupesic S, Stanojevic M. Three-dimensional sonography in prenatal diagnosis: a luxury or necessity? J Perinat Med 2000; 28: 194–209.

22. Merz E. Aktuelle technische Möglichkeiten der 3D-Sonographie in der Ginäkologie und Geburtshilfe. Ultraschall Med 1997; 18: 190–5.

23. Nagdyman N, Walka MM, Kampmann W, Stowver B, Obladen M. 3-D ultrasound quantification of neonatal cerebral ventricles in different head positions. Ultrasound Med Biol 1999; 25: 895–900.

24. Nelson TR, Pretorius DH. Three-dimensional ultrasound imaging. Ultrasound Med Biol 1998; 24: 1243–70.

25. Mercuri E, Dubowitz L, Paterson Brown S, Cowan F. Incidence of cranial ultrasound abnormalities in apparently well neonates on postnatal ward: correlation with antenatal and perinatal factors and neurological status. Arch Dis Child Fetal Neonatal Ed 1998; 79: F185–9.

26. Timor-Tritsch IE, Monteagudo A. Transvaginal fetal neurosonography: standardization of the planes and sections by anatomic landmarks. Ultrasound Obstet Gynecol 1996; 8: 42–7.

27. Monteagudo A, Reuss ML, Timor-Tritsch IE. Imaging the fetal brain in the second and third trimesters using transvaginal sonography. Obstet Gynecol 1991; 77: 27–32.

28. Monteagudo A, Timor-Tritsch IE, Moomjy M. In utero detection of ventriculomegaly during the second and third trimesters by transvaginal sonography. Ultrasound Obstet Gynecol 1994; 4: 193–8.

29. Monteagudo A, Timor-Tritsch IE. Development of fetal gyri, sulci and fissures: a transvaginal sonographic study. Ultrasound Obstet Gynecol 1997; 9: 222–8.

30. Pooh RK, Nakagawa Y, Nagamachi N, et al. Transvaginal sonography of the fetal brain: detection of abnormal morphology and circulation. Croat Med J 1998; 39: 147–57.

31. Pooh RK, Maeda K, Pooh KH, Kurjak A. Sonographic assessment of the fetal brain morphology. Prenat Neonat Med 1999; 4: 18–38.

32. Riccabona M. Pediatric three-dimensional ultrasound: basics and potential clinical value. Clin Imaging 2005; 29: 1–5.

33. Finger PT, Khoobehi A, Ponce-Contreras MR, Della Rocca D, Garcia Jr JPS. Three dimensional ultrasound of retinoblastoma: initial experience. Br J Ophthalmol 2002; 86: 1136–8.

34. Ring E, Mache CJ, Vilitis P. Future expectations – what paediatric nephrologists and urologists await from paediatric uroradiology. Eur J Radiol 2002; 43: 94–9.

35. Oswald J, Schwentner C, Lunacek A, et al. Age and lean body weight related growth curves of kidneys using real-time 3-dimensional ultrasound in pediatric urology. J Urol 2004; 172: 1991–4.

36. Riccabona M, Fritz GA, Schollnast H, et al. Hydronephrotic kidney: pediatric three-dimensional US for relative renal size assessment –initial experience. Radiology 2005; 236: 276–83.

37. Haiden N, Klebermass K, Rucklinger E, et al. 3-D ultrasonographic imaging of the cerebral ventricular system in very low birth weight infants. Ultrasound Med Biol 2005; 31: 7–14.

38. Marx GR, Sherwood MC. Three-dimensional echocardiography in congenital heart disease: a continuum of unfulfilled promises? No. A presently clinically applicable technology with an important future? Yes. Pediatr Cardiol 2002; 23: 266–85.

39. Acar P, Roux D, Dulac Y, Rouge P, Aggoun Y. Transthoracic three-dimensional echocardiography prior to closure of atrial septal defects in children. Cardiol Young 2003; 13: 58–63.

40. Franklin RC, Slavik Z. Real time three-dimensional echocardiography moves towards clinically useful neonatal cardiovascular imaging. In J Cardiol 2005; 105: 306–7.

41. Warren EK, Patronas N, Aikin AA, Albert PS, Balis FM. Comparison of one-, two-, and three-dimensional measurements of childhood brain tumors. J Natl Cancer Inst 2001; 93: 1401–5.

42. Casey FA. Telemedicine in paediatric cardiology. Arch Dis Child 1999; 80: 497–9.

43. Sable CA, Cummings SM, Schratz LM, et al. Impact of telemedicine on the practice of pediatric cardiology in community hospitals. Pediatrics 2002; 109: E3.

44. Woodson KE, Sable CA, Cross RR, Peterson GD, Martin GR. Forward and store telemedicine using Motion Picture Expert Group: a novel approach to pediatric tele-echocardiography. J Am Soc Echocardiogr 2004; 17: 1197–200.

45. Chang CH, Chang FM, Yu CH, Ko HC, Chen HY. Assessment of fetal cerebellar volume using three-dimensional ultrasound. Ultrasound Med 2000; 26: 981–8.

46. Nelson TR, Pretorius DH, Davidson TE. Initial clinical experience with an interactive volume sonography visualization system. Stud Health Technol Inform 1996; 29: 21–35.

47. Perlman JM, Risser MB, Broyles RS. Bilateral cystic perivantricular leukomalacia in the premature infant: associated risk factors. Pediatrics 1996; 97: 822–7.

48. Pinto-Martin J, Riolo S, Cnaan A, et al. Cranial ultrasound prediction of disabling and nondisabling cerebral palsy at age two in low birth weight population. Pediatrics 1995; 95: 249–54.

49. Vohr B, Ment LR. Intraventricular hemorrhage in the preterm infant. Early Hum Dev 1996; 44: 1–16.

50. Zupan V, Gonzales P, Lacaze-Masmonteil T, et al. Periventricular leukomalacia: risk factors revisited. Dev Med Child Neurol 1996; 38: 1061–7.

51. Stanojevic M, Hafner T, Kurjak A. Three-dimensional ultrasound in the assessment of the neonatal brain. In: Kurjak A, Jackson D, eds. An Atlas of Three- and Four-Dimensional Sonography in Obstetrics and Gynecology. London: Taylor and Francis, 2004: 191–200.

52. Stanojevic M. 3-D ultrasound assessment of neonatal brain. In: Carrera JM, Cabero L, Baraibar R, eds. The Perinatal Medicine of the New Millennium. Proceedings of the 5th World Congress of Perinatal Medicine, Barcelona, Spain, September 23–27, 2001. Bologna: Monduzzi Editore, 2001: 950–5.

53. Stanojevic M. Peri-intraventricular hemorrhage in premature infants diagnosed by 2D and 3D ultra-sonography. Lijec Vjesn 2004; 126(Suppl 2): 67.

54. Stanojevic M. Three-dimensional (3D) ultrasound of neonatal brain. J Perinat Med 2005; 33(Suppl 1): 41.

55. Stanojevic M, Hafner T, Kurjak A. Three-dimensional (3D) ultrasound – a useful imaging technique in the assessment of neonatal brain. J Perinat Med 2002; 30: 74–83.

56. Stanojevic M, Pooh RK, Kurjak A, Kos M. Three-dimensional ultrasound assessment of the fetal and neonatal brain. Ultrasound Rev Obstet Gynecol 2003; 3: 117–30.

57. Enriquez G, Correa F, Lucaya J, et al. Potential pitfalls in cranial sonography. Pediatr Radiol 2003; 33: 110–17.

58. de Vries LS, Gunardi H, Barth PG, et al. The spectrum of cranial ultrasound and magnetic resonance imaging abnormalities in congenital cytomegalovirus infection. Neuropediatrics 2004; 35: 113–19.

59. Haiden N, Klebermass K, Rucklinger E, et al. 3-D ultrasonographic imaging of the cerebral ventricular system in very low birth weight infants. Ultrasound Med Biol 2005; 31: 7–14.

60. Salerno CC, Pretorius DH, Hilton SW, et al. Three-dimensional ultrasonographic imaging of the neonatal brain in high-risk neonates: preliminary study. J Ultrasound Med 2000; 19: 549–55.

61. Riccabona M, Nelson TR, Weitzer C, Resch B, Pretorius DP. Potential of three-dimensional ultra-sound in neonatal and paediatric neurosonography. Eur Radiol 2003; 13: 2082–93.

62. Larcos G, Gruenwald SM, Lui K. Neonatal subependy-mal cysts detected by sonography: prevalence, sonographic findings, and clinical significance. Am J Roentgenol 1994; 162: 953–6.

63. Ghazi-Birry HS, Brown WR, Moody DM, et al. Human germinal matrix: venous origin of hemorrhage and vascular characteristics. Am J Neuroradiol 1997; 18: 219–29.

64. Dammann O, Leviton A. Duration of transient hyper-echoic images of white matter in very-low-birthweight infants: a proposed classification. Dev Med Child Neurol 1997; 39: 2–5.

65. Bale JF Jr, Murph JR. Congenital infections and nervous system. Pediatr Clin North Am 1992; 39: 669–90.

66. Frank JL. Sonography of intracranial infection in infants and children. Neuroradiology 1986; 28: 440–51.

67. Oi S, Honda Y, Hidaka M, Sato O, Matsumoto S. Intrauterine high-resolution magnetic resonance imaging in fetal hydrocephalus and prenatal estimation of postnatal outcomes with 'perspective classification'. J Neurosurg 1998; 88: 685–94.

68. Terrone DA, Perry KG Jr. Ultrasound in evaluation of the fetal central nervous system. Obst Gynecol Clin North Am 1998; 25: 479–97.

69. Monteagudo A, Timor-Tritsch IE, Mayberry P. Three-dimensional transvaginal neurosonography of the fetal brain: 'navigation' in the volume scan. Ultrasound Obstet Gynecol 2000; 16: 307–13.

70. Pilu G, Perolo A, Falco P, et al. Ultrasound of the fetal central nervous system. Curr Opin Obstet Gynecol 2000; 12: 93–103.

71. Timor-Tritsch IE, Monteagudo A, Mayberry P. Three-dimensional ultrsound evaluation of fetal brain: the three horn view. Ultrasound Obstet Gynecol 2000; 16: 302–6.

72. Tanak T, Gleeson JG. Genetics of brain development and malformation. Curr Opin Pediatr 2000; 12: 523–8.

73. Huang CC, Yeh TF. Assessment of gestational age in newborns by neurosonography. Early Hum Dev 1991; 25: 209–20.

74. Murphy NP, Rennie J, Cooke RW. Cranial ultrasound assessment of gestational age in low birthweight infants. Arch Dis Child 1989; 64: 569–72.

27 Is 3D and 4D sonography safe for the fetus?

Kazuo Maeda and Asim Kurjak

INTRODUCTION

It is well known that ultrasound may influence biologic tissues through thermal and mechanical effects, and it should be noted that teratogenicity has been reported as a consequence of the exposure of animal embryos and fetuses to high temperatures.[1] No hazardous effect is expected when the temperature rise is less than 1.5°C or the thermal index (TI)[†] is less than 1 for a long exposure, while 5 minutes' exposure of young tissue to 41°C can be hazardous.[2,3] The hazard threshold for pulsed ultrasound output power was found to be spatial peak temporal average (SPTA) 240 mW/cm^2 for cultured cells, with no suppressive effect being found below this power level in our previous studies.[4]

The non-thermal effects of ultrasound include inertial cavitation and other mechanical effects. Although cavitation in liquids can lead to free-radical formation, that does not occur in the cytoplasm because of its high viscosity, and free radicals formed in the extracellular liquid may not reach cells because of their short lifetime. However, intense mechanical effects may produce hemorrhage in the neonatal animal lung.

IS 3D SONOGRAPHY SAFE FOR THE FETUS?

Simple B-mode imaging does not produce thermal effects, because of its very low intensity (e.g., the output of B-mode machines is regulated in Japan[5,6] to be lower than SPTA 10 mW/cm^2).[2] In three-dimensional (3D) imaging, gray-level data are acquired by repeated scanning with a real-time B-mode array transducer until the whole imaging volume has been covered, the image data are stored in the computer memory for processing. Provided that the focus of the ultrasound beam is narrow and the frame interval is short, any given point of the embryo or fetus will only receive a short exposure over the whole examination. Indeed, the ultrasound exposure and possible heating of a given point caused by ultrasound should be the same as in a simple B-mode scan. Accordingly, the possible temperature rise and thermal effects in 3D sonography are almost the same as in simple B-mode sonography, and 3D techniques should be as safe as B-mode with respect to thermal effects.

Fetal 3D imaging employs pulsed ultrasound. The mechanical effect of pulsed ultrasound is the same for 3D imaging, simple B-mode imaging, and Doppler flow detection, and it is determined by its temporal peak (TP) intensity, sound pressure, and mechanical index (MI)[‡] (thermal effects are related to the time-averaged intensity). A MI of pulsed ultrasound lower than 1 is commonly recommended, particularly in the newborn lung, because pulmonary hemorrhage has been induced in animal neonates by exposure to intense pulsed ultrasound, possibly by mechanical effects on the air-containing pulmonary tissue.

[†]The thermal index (TI) is w/w_0 where w is the power of the diagnostic equipment to be tested, and w_0 is the power to raise the temperature for 1°C above 37°C in the worst case of a tissue model. A TI expresses the maximum temperature rise above 37°C in its actual use.

[‡]The mechanical index (MI) is Pr MPa/$\sqrt{f}$ MHz, where Pr is the rarefactional pressure expressed by MPa (10^6 Pascal) and f is the central ultrasound frequency expressed by MHz (10^6 Hz).

HOW SAFE IS 4D SONOGRAPHY?

Although the 4D ultrasound image is obtained by computer processing of 10–24 frames of fetal 3D pictures per second, most parts of the fetus are not expected to be exposed to ultrasound repeatedly, because the fetus is moving and thus any given point of the fetus will be continually shifting position.

With regard to thermal effects, it should be noted that both 3D and 4D imaging are based on simple B-mode scanning, for which, as mentioned above, thermal effects are not of concern.[2] Indeed, 4D sonography may be considered to be a long B-mode scan divided into short scans over periods of seconds or minutes, with any heating by ultrasound absorption being cooled by the circulation. In addition, even with repeated exposure of a given part of the fetus (e.g., due to a fetal resting state) there is no accumulated ultrasound bioeffect when exposure is intermittent. Therefore, there should be no problems due to thermal effects of ultrasound to 4D surface imaging and no need to limit sonographic examination, provided that TI <1.

As far as mechanical effects of ultrasound are concerned, 4D sonography should not be hazardous to the embryo or fetus, provided that MI <1 or the sound pressure is below 1 MPa.

COLOR AND POWER DOPPLER FLOW MAPPING

Although the World Federation of Ultrasound in Medicine and Biology (WFUMB)[2] concluded that the use of simple imaging equipment is not contraindicated on thermal grounds, the issue of ultrasound safety arose again after the introduction of Doppler flow velocity measurement, because the pulsed Doppler method requires considerably higher intensity than simple B-mode ultrasound.

The maximum intensity of commercial pulsed Doppler ultrasound for adults has generally been in the range 1–3 W/cm^2. Since this is definitely higher than in simple B-mode, potential thermal effects were of great concern with regard to the case of pulsed Doppler ultrasound in obstetrics. These effects were discussed in the context of possible teratogenicity by the WFUMB.[1,2] The International Society of Ultrasound in Obstetrics and Gynecology (ISUOG) has also discussed the safe use of Doppler ultrasound.[7]

The ultrasound intensity is less in color/power Doppler flow mapping than in pulsed Doppler due to the scanning of the ultrasound beam in color or power Doppler. The time-averaged intensity of color Doppler ultrasound has generally been lower than 720 mW/cm^2, which is less than that of pulsed Doppler, and with the limit specified by the US Food and Drug Administration.[8]

However, the American Institute for Ultrasound in Medicine (AIUM) has stated that for the current FDA regulatory limit of 720 mW/cm^2, the best available estimate of the temperature increase can exceed 2°C.[8] Therefore, it is wise to set TI <1 in color or power Doppler flow mapping for embryonic or fetal examination[9] – including 3D and 4D color/power Doppler. The examination must be limited if the TI >1: for example, if TI = 2, then the examination time should be 5 minutes or less (see below: Table 27.2 and Figure 27.1).

The initial device setting should be 'obstetric' before using the Doppler function of a new commercial 3D or 4D scanner with the purpose of examining an embryo or fetus with low ultrasound intensity. The fetal study duration can be extended if TI <1,[9] and the study duration must be documented in the patient record if the ultrasound intensity is not confirmed.

PULSED DOPPLER FETAL FLOW VELOCITY WAVEFORM

Since the intensity of pulsed Doppler ultrasound is very high, its safe use for the recording of fetal flow velocity waveform and to measure peripheral impedance to blood flow has been the subject of much discussion. The common recommendation is that the pulsed Doppler ultrasound intensity should be low and its TI <1.[9] The situation is the same in 3D and 4D techniques. However, experienced sonographers sometimes measure fetal blood flow employing more intense Doppler ultrasound (with TI >1), in order to obtain clearer and more precise fetal blood flow waves; in this case safety is ensured by using shorter exposure times than in conventional examinations (see below).

SAFE ULTRASOUND EXPOSURE TIME WITH REFERENCE TO THE AIUM STATEMENT

Although teratogenicity has been reported following exposure of animal embryos and fetuses to high temperature, the National Council on Radiation Protection (NCRP) report[1] defines hazardous and non-hazardous zones in terms of the combined factors of temperature and exposure time. No malformation is produced if the embryo or fetus is heated in the zone under the line determined by connecting the points of high temperature/short exposure and low temperature/long exposure.[1] Non-hazardous exposure can be as short as 1 minute at 43°C, but infinite at physiologic body temperature.[8] In the case of ultrasound irradiation, TI is a measure of the increase in temperature above the physiologic body temperature; therefore (for humans), the actual temperature is obtained by adding 37°C to the temperature increase derived from TI.

Guidelines on the protection of mammals against heat can be found in the revised safety statement of the AIUM,[8] which is based on the NCRP report,[1] where an inverse relation is found between hazardous temperature level and exposure time. The AIUM[9] stated that the fetus tolerates 50 hours at a 2°C rise (an actual temperature of 39°C), 16 minutes at a 4°C rise (41°C), and 1 minute at a 6°C rise (43°C). They also showed a relationship between the temperature rise T (°C) above 37°C and the non-hazardous exposure time t (min):

$$T = 6 - \frac{\log_{10} t}{0.6} \qquad (1)$$

Non-hazardous time (t) is obtained by equation (2) rearranging:

$$t = 10^{3.6 - 0.6\,T} \qquad (2)$$

The safety of ultrasound with regard to its thermal effects can be discussed in terms of the exposure time and the temperature. Heat production by Doppler ultrasound is estimated from TI, which is a measure of the temperature rise above 37°C in a standardized tissue model. The ISUOG has stated that there is no reason precluding the use of scanners that have received current FDA clearance.[7] However, the AIUM has pointed out that with the current FDA regulatory limit of 720 mW/cm², it is possible for the temperature increase to exceed 2°C.[8] Furthermore, in our studies[4] the pulsed ultrasound intensity threshold was SPTA 240 mW/cm². Thus, the FDA regulations are still controversial.

TI is a useful measure of the temperature rise induced by ultrasound exposure. Standard tissue models are exposed to ultrasound and TI is determined in the worst case; i.e., the highest temperature

rise is the basis of TI.[9] A TI of 1 represents a 1°C temperature rise; similarly, if TI = 3, the temperature rises by 3°C above 37°C (i.e., the actual temperature is 40°C). TI is further classified into soft tissue TI (TIS), bone TI (TIB), and cranial TI (TIC), according to the exposed tissue.

Ultrasound examination is completely safe with regard to thermal effects, regardless of exposure time, if TI <1 – in particular, in long fetal examinations, pregnancy screening, and research studies. If TI >1, the output power or exposure time must be reduced.[9]

The revised safety statement by the AIUM stated that the upper limit of safe exposure duration was 16 minutes at 4°C rise and 1 minute at 6°C rise above normal.[8] This statement is acceptable and useful for retrospective safety confirmation in cases where exposure time and TI were documented in the patient record. The exposure to a temperature of 41–43°C, however, is hardly acceptable, because the safety of temperatures higher than 40°C is still medically controversial. In addition, the margin of safety is too narrow to completely avoid excess heating to high temperature. We would like to propose a practically applicable safe exposure time that is preset before a Doppler examination.

PROSPECTIVE EXPOSURE TIME SETTING BEFORE DOPPLER EXAMINATION

When TI is increased to values greater than 1 in order to improve the Doppler flow wave, the exposure time must be preset before the examination to a non-hazardous value that depends on the temperature rise determined by the value of TI. The AIUM statement gives a relationship for calculating this non-hazardous

Table 27.1 Non-hazardous exposure time (t) calculated from temperature rise (T) above 37°C according to the equation given in the AIUM statement[8] (Equation (2) of text)

Temperature rise, T (°C)	Thermal index, TI	Actual temperature (°C)	Non-hazardous exposure time, t (min)
1	1	38	1000
2	2	39	251
3	3	40	63
4	4	41	16
5	5	42	4
6	6	43	1

Table 27.2 Thermal index (TI), actual tissue temperature, non-hazardous exposure time according to AIUM statement,[8] and modified non-hazardous exposure time

Thermal index, TI	Actual temperature (°C)	Non-hazardous exposure time[a] (min)	Modified non-hazardous exposure time[b] (min): Safety factor			
			3	10	50	100
6*	43*	1*	0.3*	0.1*	0.02*	0.01*
5*	42*	4*	1.3*	0.4*	0.08*	0.04*
4*	41*	16*	5*	0.2*	0.03*	0.02*
3	40	64	21	6	1	0.6
2	39	251	84	25	5	2.5

[a]According to AIUM statement[8]
[b]AIUM time divided by safety factor
*Not recommended in the safe use of diagnostic ultrasound

exposure time (Equation (2) above: see Figure 27.1): the resulting values are shown in Table 27.1. We propose, however, that this value should be modified by dividing by a 'safety factor' of 3–100 (Table 27.2). The values thus obtained are coincidentally close to those in the safety statement of the British Medical Ultrasound Society (BMUS),[10] where the exposure time is 4 minutes for TI = 2 and 1 minute for TI = 2.5.

We recommend a safety factor of 50 (although in the context of B-mode intensity, Japanese regulations specify a value of 100). Users can change the safety factor and prolong the exposure time – bearing in mind, however, that a reduced safety factor, and hence a longer time, may lead to an increased risk of thermal damage. In any case TI should not exceed 3.

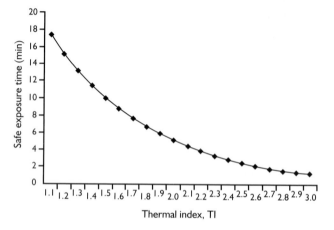

Figure 27.1 The author recommends the detailed exposure time in the TI values between 1.1 and 3.0 according to Equation (2) and Table 27.2. The safety factor was 50

OTHER THERMAL PROBLEMS

Attention should be paid to the temperature of tissue exposed to Doppler ultrasound in febrile patients, where the basic temperature is higher than 37°C. For example, if TI = 2 in a febrile patient with a body temperature of 38°C, and the temperature rise above the physiologic condition is 3°C, then this is equivalent to TI = 3 in a non-febrile normal-temperature case, and therefore only 1 minute of exposure (rather than 5 minutes) is allowed if the safety factor is 50.

Exposure duration, TI, and MI should be documented by the user in every study where the exposure time has been voluntarily increased. It is recommended that TI and MI should be documented in the 'Methods' sections of reports of Doppler ultrasound studies in human subjects. Guidelines have recently been published regarding the reports of such studies.[11]

With transvaginal scans, care should be taken concerning direct heating of the tissue due to the high surface temperature of the transducer. The transducer temperature displayed on the monitor screen should be lower than 41°C.

CONCLUSIONS

Diagnostic 3D and 4D sonography, when used for multiplanar and surface rendered imaging, do not pose any concerns with regard to thermal safety, since these techniques essentially are based on simple B-mode scanning. However, 3D and 4D color/power Doppler ultrasound requires caution in this context, and the thermal index (TI) must be less than 1 for unlimited durations of examination. The exposure time should be reduced when TI >1: for example, it should be 10 minutes or less for TI = 1.5 in a fetal study. (Longer examination is possible – but with increased risk.)

Pulsed Doppler studies require particular caution because of the high output power of the ultrasound: TI should be less than 1 when the exposure time may be prolonged (e.g., in research studies or pregnancy screening). If more precise pulsed Doppler waveforms are needed, higher values of TI are permitted, but the exposure time must be limited (and preset before the study). We recommend an upper limit of 5 minutes for TI = 2 and 1 minute for TI = 3 (for intermediate values of TI, the exposure time can be calculated from Equation (2), with an appropriate safety factor – see Table 27.2). Values of TI >3 are not presently recommended.

Care should be taken in the case of febrile patients (and their increased temperature taken into account when calculating exposure time). With transvaginal scans, the transducer temperature should be kept below 41°C.

The mechanical effects of 3D and 4D sonography are similar to those of simple B-mode and Doppler techniques. It is recommended that the mechanical index (MI) be less than 1, particularly in studies of air-containing neonatal lungs.

REFERENCES

1. National Council on Radiation Protection and Measurements. Exposure Criteria for Medical Diagnostic Ultrasound: I. Criteria Based on Thermal Mechanisms. NCRP Report 113, 1992.

2. Barnett SB, Kossoff G. WFUMB Symposium on Safety and Standardisation in Medical Ultrasound: Issues and Recommendations Regarding Thermal Mechanisms for Biological Effects of Ultrasound. Hornbick, 1991. Ultrasound Med Biol 1992; 18: v–xix, 731–814.

3. Barnett SB, Rott HD, Ter Haar GR, Ziskin MC, Maeda K. The sensitivity of biological tissue to ultrasound. Ultrasound Med Biol 1997; 23: 805–12.

4. Maeda K, Murao F, Yoshiga T, Yamauchi C, Tsuzaki T. Experimental studies on the suppression of cultured cell growth curves after irradiation with CW and pulsed ultrasound. IEEE Trans Ultrason Ferroelectr Freq Contr 1986; UFFC-33: 186–93.

5. Ide, M. Japanese policy and status of standardisation. Ultrasound Med Biol 1986; 12: 705–8.

6. Maeda K, Ide M. The limitation of the ultrasound intensity for diagnostic devices in the Japanese Industrial standards. IEEE Trans Ultrason Ferroelectr Freq Cont 1986; UFFC-33: 241–4.

7. ISUOG Bioeffects and Safety Committee. Safety Statement, 2000 (reconfirmed 2002). Ultrasound Obstet Gynecol 2002; 19: 105.

8. AIUM Official Statement Changes. Revised Statements. Clinical safety. AIUM Reporter 1998; 154(1): 6–7.

9. American Institute of Ultrasound in Medicine/National Electrical Manufacturers Association. Standard for Real Time Display of Thermal and Mechanical Acoustic Output Indices on Diagnostic Ultrasound Equipment, 1992.

10. Safety Group of the British Medical Ultrasound Society. Guidelines for the safe use of diagnostic ultrasound equipment. BMUS Bull 2000; 3: 29–33.

11. Edmonds PD, Abramowicz JS, Carson PL, Carstensen EL, Sandstrom KL. Guidelines for Journal of Ultrasound in Medicine authors and reviewers on measurement and reporting of acoustic output and exposure. J Ultrasound Med 2005; 24: 1171–9.

Index

Note: Page numbers in *italics* refer to Figures; those in **bold** refer to Tables